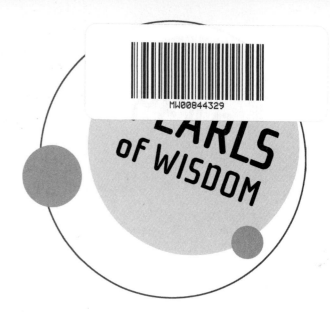

Obstetrics and Gynecology

BOARD REVIEW

Fourth Edition

Stephen G. Somkuti, MD, PhD
Associate Professor
Department of Obstetrics and Gynecology and Reproductive Sciences
Temple University School of Medicine School
Philadelphia, Pennsylvania
Director, The Toll Center for Reproductive Sciences
Division of Reproductive Endocrinology
Department of Obstetrics and Gynecology
Abington Memorial Hospital
Abington Reproductive Medicine
Abington, Pennsylvania

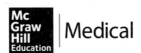 Medical

New York   Chicago   San Francisco   Athens   London   Madrid   Mexico City
Milan   New Delhi   Singapore   Sydney   Toronto

Obstetrics and Gynecology Board Review: Pearls of Wisdom, Fourth Edition

Copyright © 2014 by McGraw-Hill Education. All rights reserved. Printed in the United States of America. Except as permitted under the United States Copyright Act of 1976, no part of this publication may be reproduced or distributed in any form or by any means, or stored in a data base or retrieval system, without the prior written permission of the publisher.

1 2 3 4 5 6 7 8 9 0   QVS/QVS   18 17 16 15 14 13

ISBN 978-0-07-179928-7
MHID 0-07-179928-1

This book was set in Adobe Garamond by Aptara, Inc.
The editors were Catherine A. Johnson and Cindy Yoo.
The production supervisor was Richard Ruzycka.
Project management was provided by Abhishan Sharma.
Quad Graphics Versailles was printer and binder.

This book is printed on acid-free paper.

Library of Congress Cataloging-in-Publication Data

Obstetrics and gynecology board review / [editor] Stephen G. Somkuti. – Fourth edition.
    p. ; cm. – (Pearls of wisdom)
Includes bibliographical references and index.
    ISBN 978-0-07-179928-7 (pbk. : alk. paper) – ISBN 0-07-179928-1 (pbk. : alk. paper)
I. Somkuti, Stephen G., editor of compilation.   II. Series: Pearls of wisdom.
    [DNLM: 1. Obstetrics–methods–Examination Questions.   2. Gynecology–methods–
Examination Questions. WQ 18.2]
    RG111
    618.10076–dc23
                                                                                2013031560

McGraw-Hill Education books are available at special quantity discounts to use as premiums and sales promotions or for use in corporate training programs. To contact a representative, please visit the Contact Us pages at www.mhprofessional.com.

CONTENTS

CONTRIBUTORS

Lauren Abern, MD
Department of Obstetrics and Gynecology
Abington Memorial Hospital
Abington, Pennsylvania
Breast Disorders
Lesbian, Gay, Bisexual, and Transgender Health
Vulvar and Vaginal Carcinoma

Aroti Achari, MD
Advocare Magness & Stafford OBGYN
  Associates
Department of Obstetrics and Gynecology
Virtua Voorhees Hospital
Voorhees, New Jersey
Hysterectomy

Larry I. Barmat, MD
Assistant Professor
Department of Obstetrics and Gynecology
Temple University
Abington Reproductive Medicine
Abington Memorial Hospital
Abington, Pennsylvania
Robotic Systems and Infertility Surgery

Katherine Bohnert, DO
Department of Obstetrics and Gynecology
Einstein Hospital Medical Center
Philadelphia, Pennsylvania
First Trimester Ultrasound

Erica L. Borman, DO
Psychiatry Resident
Rowan University School of Osteopathic Medicine
Stratford, New Jersey
Amenorrhea
Hyperandrogenism

Cari Brown, MD
Resident Physician
Department of Obstetrics and Gynecology
Abington Memorial Hospital
Abington, Pennsylvania
Primary and Preventative Care
The Puerperium

Justin Chura, MD, MBA
Director, Robotic Surgery and Gynecologic
  Oncology
Cancer Treatment Centers of America
Eastern Regional Medical Center
Philadelphia, Pennsylvania
Anatomy of the Pelvis and Reproductive Tract
Uterine Sarcomas

Frank J. Craparo, MD
Associate Professor
Drexel University College of Medicine
Philadelphia, Pennsylvania
Chief, Division of Maternal Fetal Medicine
Director, Fetal Diagnostic Center
Department of Obstetrics and Gynecology
Abington Memorial Hospital
Abington, Pennsylvania
Breech
Labor and Delivery

Lindsay Curtis, MD
Abington Memorial Hospital
Abington, Pennsylvania
Ectopic Pregnancy
Postoperative Care of the Gynecologic Patient
Preoperative Evaluation and Preparation of
  Gynecologic Surgery

vi

Glen de Guzman, MD
Department of Obstetrics and Gynecology
Abington Memorial Hospital
Abington, Pennsylvania
Gastrointestinal Disorders in Pregnancy

Jennifer Deirmengian, MD
Obstetrics Faculty Teaching Group
Abington Memorial Hospital
Abington, Pennsylvania
Lactation
Rh Alloimmunization

Mitchell I. Edelson, MD
Associate Professor
Department of Obstetrics, Gynecolgy, and
    Reproductive Sciences
Temple University School of Medicine
Hanjani Institute for Gynecologic Oncology
Abington Memorial Hospital
Abington, Pennsylvania
Epithelial and Nonepithelial Ovarian Tumors
Fallopian Tube Neoplasms
Gestational Trophoblastic Disease
Gynecologic Pathology
Radiation Therapy, Chemotherapy,
    Immunotherapy, and Tumor Markers
Vulvar and Vaginal Carcinoma

Stephanie J. Estes, MD, FACOG
Associate Professor
Division of Reproductive Endocrinology and
    Infertility
Department of Obstetrics and Gynecology
Penn State Hershey Medical Center
Hershey, Pennsylvania
Disorders of Prolactin Secretion
GnRH and GnRH Analogs

Karen T. Feisullin, MD
Department of Obstetrics and Gynecology
Abington Memorial Hospital
Abington, Pennsylvania
Family Planning and Sterilization

Emily R. Goldenthal, DO
Department of Obstetrics and Gynecology
Albert Einstein Medical Center
Philadelphia, Pennsylvania
Anatomy of the Pelvis and Reproductive Tract

Remington Horesh, OMSII
Osteopathic Medical Student
Class of 2015
Lake Erie College of Medicine
Bradenton, Florida
Physiology of Normal Pregnancy

Lisa Jambusaria, MD
Resident, Department of Obstetrics and
    Gynecology
Abington Memorial Hospital
Abington, Pennsylvania
Benign Vulvar and Vaginal Lesions
Genital Tract Infections and PID
Pelvic Organ Prolapse
Urinary Incontinence and Urodynamics
Vulvodynia

Jacqueline Kohl, MD, MPH
Resident, Department of Obstetrics and
    Gynecology
Abington Memorial Hospital
Abington, Pennsylvania
Dysmenorrhea and Premenstrual Syndrome
Laparoscopy and Infertility Surgery

Kuhali Kundu, DO
Obstetrics and Gynecology Resident
Albert Einstein Medical Center
Philadelphia, Pennsylvania
Postdates Pregnancy and Fetal Demise

Richard A. Latta, MD
Maternal-Fetal Medicine
Abington Memorial Hospital
Abington, Pennsylvania
Operative Obstetrics Pearls

Vincent Lucente, MD, MBA
Clinical Professor
Department of Obstetrics and Gynecology
Temple University
Chief of Gynecology
St. Luke's University Health Network
Allentown, Pennsylvania
*Lower Urinary Tract Injuries During Gynecologic
    Surgery*
Urinary Incontinence and Urodynamics

Rahil Malik, MD
Senior Resident
Department of Obstetrics and Gynecology
Jackson Memorial Hospital
University of Miami
Miami, Florida
Adenomyosis and Endometriosis

Brielle A. Marks, BA
Student, Abington Reproductive Medicine
Holland, Pennsylvania
Robotic Systems and Infertility Surgery

Laura E. Martin, DO
Resident, Department of Obstetrics and
    Gynecology
Albert Einstein Medical Center
Philadelphia, Pennsylvania
ACOG Screening Guidelines Since 2007

Jennifer McClarren, MS, CGC
Genetic Counselor, Integrated Genetics
Philadelphia, Pennsylvania
Genetics for the Obstetrician

Alison B. McGrorty, MD
Pediatric Resident
Nemours-AI duPont Hospital for
    Children
Thomas Jefferson University Hospital
Philadelphia, Pennsylvania
Ethics, Psychosocial, and Psychiatric Pearls

Amelia McLennan, MD
Resident, Department of Obstetrics and
    Gynecology
Abington Memorial Hospital
Abington, Pennsylvania
Genetics for the Obstetrician
*Obstetrical Ultrasound and
    Fetal Abnormalities*

Marlesa R. Moore, DO
Resident Physician
Department of Obstetrics and Gynecology
Abington Memorial Hospital
Abington, Pennsylvania
Pediatric and Adolescent Gynecology

Erin M. Murphy, MD
Center for Reproductive Medicine
    and Infertility
Weill Cornell Medical College
New York, New York
Assisted Reproductive Technology
Embryology of the Genital Tract

Victoria Myers, MD
Faculty Tech Group
Abington Memorial Hospital
Abington, Pennsylvania
*Miscarriage, Recurrent Miscarriage, and
    Pregnancy Termination*

Mary C. Naglak, PhD, RD
Academic Research Specialist
Department of Medicine
Abington Memorial Hospital
Abington, Pennsylvania
Basic Epidemiology and Clinical Biostatistics

Ashwinee Natu
Medical Student, Class of 2014
Drexel University College of Medicine
Philadelphia, PA
Hypertension and Pregnancy

Neely N. Nelson, MD
Resident, Department of Obstetrics and
    Gynecology
Abington Memorial Hospital
Abington, Pennsylvania
Infertility

Jordana I. Reina-Fernandez, MD
Resident, Department of Obstetrics
    and Gynecology
Albert Einstein Medical Center
Philadelphia, Pennsylvania
*Antepartum Management and Fetal
    Surveillance*

Amanda M. Rhodes, MD
Resident, Department of Obstetrics and
    Gynecology
Abington Memorial Hospital
Abington, Pennsylvania
Labor Abnormalities

Cristina M. Saiz, MD, FACOG
Female Pelvic Medicine and Reconstructive
    Surgery Physician
The Institute for Female Pelvic Medicine and
    Reconstructive Surgery
Allentown, Pennsylvania
*Lower Urinary Tract Injuries During Gynecologic
    Surgery*

Meike Schuster, DO
Obstetrics and Gynecology Resident
Abington Memorial Hospital
Abington, Pennsylvania
Maternal Fetal Medicine Fellow
Geisinger Medical Center
Danville, Pennsylvania
Obstetric Complications

Stephen J. Smith, MD
Vice Chair and Associate Program Director
Associate Professor
Department of Obstetrics and Gynecology
Abington Memorial Hospital and
    Temple University School of Medicine
Abington, Pennsylvania
Labor Abnormalities
Postdates Pregnancy and Fetal Demise

Stephen G. Somkuti, MD, PhD
Associate Professor
Department of Obstetrics and Gynecology and
    Reproductive Sciences
Temple University School of Medicine School
Philadelphia, Pennsylvania
Director, The Toll Center for Reproductive
    Sciences
Division of Reproductive Endocrinology
Department of Obstetrics and Gynecology
Abington Memorial Hospital
Abington Reproductive Medicine
Abington, Pennsylvania
Hyperandrogenism
Pediatric and Adolescent Gynecology

Maria A. Suescum, MD
Chief Resident, Department of Obstetrics and
    Gynecology
Albert Einstein Medical Center
Philadelphia, Pennsylvania
Uterine Sarcomas

Janos L. Tanyi, MD, PhD
Assistant Professor
Division of Gynecologic Oncology
Department of Obstetrics and Gynecology
University of Pennsylvania Health System
Philadelphia, Pennsylvania
Cervical Lesions and Cancer
Endometrial Hyperplasia and Carcinoma

Kristin Van Heertum, MD
Resident, Department of Obstetrics and
    Gynecology
Abington Memorial Hospital
Abington, Pennsylvania
Amniotic Fluid
Benign Disorders of the Upper Genital Tract
Functional and Dysfunctional Uterine Bleeding
Menopause

Andrew J. Walter, MD
Attending Obstetrics and Gynecology Physician
Tampa Obstetrics, Infertility and Gynecology
Tampa, Florida
Antepartum Management and Fetal Surveillance

Chelsea Ward, MD
Obstetrics and Gynecology Resident
Abington Memorial Hospital
Abington, Pennsylvania
Hypothalamic-Pituitary-Ovarian-Uterine Axis
Multiple Gestations
The Placenta and Umbilical Cord

Karen C. Wheeler, MD
Resident Physician
Department of Obstetrics and Gynecology
Abington Memorial Hospital
Abington, Pennsylvania
Management of Medical and Surgical Conditions
    in Pregnancy

Emese Zsiros, MD, PhD
Division of Gynecologic Oncology
Department of Obstetrics and Gynecology
University of Pennsylvania
Philadelphia, Pennsylvania
Reproductive Toxicology

INTRODUCTION

Congratulations on your purchase of *Obstetrics and Gynecology Board Review: Pearls of Wisdom.* This book will help you learn some medicine. Originally designed as a study aid to improve performance on the Ob/Gyn Inservice and Written Boards examinations, this book is full of useful information. A few words are appropriate discussing intent, format, limitations, and use *Wisdom,* fourth edition.

Since *Obstetrics and Gynecology Board Review* is primarily intended as a study aid, the text is written in rapid-fire question/answer format. This way, readers receive immediate gratification. Moreover, misleading or confusing "foils" are not provided. This eliminates the risk of erroneously assimilating an incorrect piece of information that makes a big impression. Questions themselves often contain a "pearl" intended to reinforce the answer. Additional "hooks" may be attached to the answer in various forms, including mnemonics, visual imagery, repetition, and humor. Additional information not requested in the question may be included in the answer. Emphasis has been placed on distilling trivia and key facts that are easily overlooked, that are quickly forgotten, and that somehow seem to be needed on board examinations.

Many questions have answers without explanations. This enhances ease of reading and rate of learning. Explanations often occur in a later question/answer. Upon reading an answer, the reader may think, "Hmm, why is that?" or, "Are you sure?" If this happens to you, go check! Truly assimilating these disparate facts into a framework of knowledge absolutely requires further reading of the surrounding concepts. Information learned in response to seeking an answer to a particular question is retained much better than information that is passively observed. Take advantage of this!

Use this book with your preferred source texts handy and open. *Obstetrics and Gynecology Board Review* has limitations. We have found many conflicts between sources of information. We have tried to verify in several references the most accurate information. Some texts have internal discrepancies further confounding clarification. *Obstetrics and Gynecology Board Review* risks accuracy by aggressively pruning complex concepts down to the simplest kernel—the dynamic knowledge base and clinical practice of medicine is not like that! Furthermore, new research and practice occasionally deviates from that which likely represents the right answer for test purposes. This text is designed to maximize your score on a test. Refer to your most current sources of information and mentors for direction for practice.

Obstetrics and Gynecology Board Review is designed to be used, not just read. It is an *interactive* text. Use a 3 × 5 card and cover the answers; attempt all questions. A study method we recommend is oral, group study, preferably over an extended meal or pitchers. The mechanics of this method are simple and no one ever appears stupid. One person holds this book, with answers covered, and reads the question. Each person, including the reader, says "Check!" when he or she has an answer in mind. After everyone has "checked" in, someone states his/her answer. If this answer is correct, on to the next one; if not, another person says their answer or the answer can be read. Usually the person who "checks" in first receives the first shot at stating the answer. If this person is being a smarty-pants answer-hog, then others can take turns. Try it, it's almost fun!

Obstetrics and Gynecology Board Review is also designed to be reused several times to allow, dare we use the word, memorization. A hollow bullet is provided for any scheme of keeping track of questions answered correctly or incorrectly. We welcome your comments, suggestions, and criticism. Great effort has been made to verify these questions and answers. Some answers may not be the answer you would prefer. Most often this is attributable to variance between original sources. Please make us aware of any errors you find. We hope to make continuous improvements and would greatly appreciate any input with regard to format, organization, content, presentation, or about specific questions. We look forward to hearing from you!

Study hard and good luck!

S.G.S.

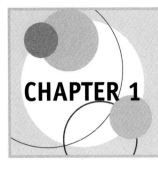

CHAPTER 1

Anatomy of the Pelvis and Reproductive Tract

Justin Chura, MD, MBA and
Emily R. Goldenthal, DO

○ **Where are Gartner ducts located?**

In the lateral walls of the vagina.

○ **Gartner duct cysts are persistent portions of what embryonic structure?**

Mesonephric duct.

○ **The portion of the gubernaculum between the ovary and the uterus becomes what structure?**

The ligament of the ovary (utero-ovarian ligament).

○ **The portion of the gubernaculum between the uterus and the labium majus becomes what structure?**

The round ligament.

○ **Failure of the development of adhesions between the uterus and what structure can result in the ovary migrating through the inguinal canal to the labium majus?**

The gubernaculum.

○ **What is the name of a pouch of peritoneum analogous to the saccus vaginalis in the male, which accompanies the gubernaculum in the inguinal canal?**

The canal of Nuck.

○ **Name the three coats of the ureter.**

Fibrous, muscular, and mucosal.

○ **The epithelium lining the ureter is of what type?**

Transitional.

○ **Name the vessels that send branches to the ureter.**

Renal, ovarian, common iliac, hypogastric, ureteric, vaginal, vesical, middle hemorrhoidal, and superior gluteal arteries.

○ **Innervation of the ureter is derived from what nerve plexuses?**

Inferior mesenteric, ovarian, and pelvic.

○ **What are the attachments between the female bladder and the pubic bone called?**

The pubovesical ligaments.

○ **Name the four coats of the bladder.**

Serosa, muscular, submucosa, and mucosa.

○ **What arteries supply the female bladder?**

Superior, middle and inferior vesical, obturator, inferior gluteal, uterine, and vaginal arteries.

○ **Name the three coats of the urethra.**

Muscular, erectile, and mucosa.

○ **What type of epithelium lines the urethra?**

Distal 1/3 = Stratified squamous epithelium that becomes transitional near the bladder (proximal 2/3).

○ **The aorta lies at what spinal level?**

L4.

○ **What are the branches of the hypogastric (internal iliac) artery?**

Posterior branch: Iliolumbar, lateral sacral, and superior gluteal.
Anterior branch: Obturator, internal pudendal, inferior gluteal, umbilical, inferior vesical, middle rectal, uterine, vaginal, and superior vesical.

○ **Arterial blood supply to the uterus is derived from what arteries?**

Uterine and ovarian arteries. The uterine artery arises from the hypogastric and the ovarian directly from the aorta.

○ **Name the visceral branches of the internal iliac artery.**

Umbilical, inferior vesical, superior vesical, middle rectal, uterine, and vaginal.

○ **What are the arcuate arteries?**

Branches of the uterine that unite with the opposite uterine artery. They supply the radial branches to the myometrium and basalis layer of endometrium. They also become the spiral arteries of the functional endometrium.

○ **What is the terminal branch of the hypogastric artery?**

Internal pudendal artery.

○ **What does the internal pudendal artery supply?**

The rectum, labia, clitoris, and perineum.

○   **Name the parietal branches of the internal iliac artery.**

Obturator, internal pudendal, iliolumbar, lateral sacral, superior gluteal, and inferior gluteal.

○   **Describe the anatomic relationship between the uterine artery and the ureter when they are at their closest position in relationship to the cervix.**

Approximately 2 cm from the cervix the uterine artery crosses above and in front of the ureter.

○   **Branches of the uterine and vaginal arteries anastomose forming median longitudinal vessels known as what arteries?**

Azygous arteries of the vagina.

○   **Name the artery from which the deep and dorsal arteries of the clitoris arise.**

Internal pudendal artery.

○   **The right ovarian vein opens into what structure?**

The inferior vena cava.

○   **The left ovarian vein flows into what structure?**

Left renal vein.

○   **Which is responsible for gluteal ischemia if hypogastric artery ligation is done incorrectly?**

Superior gluteal artery.

○   **Name the main tributaries of the external iliac vein.**

Inferior epigastric, deep circumflex, and pubic veins.

○   **The ovarian arteries arise from what structure?**

The aorta.

○   **The inferior epigastric artery is one of two main branches of what artery?**

The external iliac artery.

○   **The artery of the round ligament is a branch of what artery?**

Inferior epigastric artery.

○   **What structure crosses the obturator artery medially?**

Ureter.

○   **Where does the inferior mesenteric artery arise?**

3 cm above the aortic bifurcation.

○ **What does the inferior mesenteric artery supply?**

Parts of the transverse colon, descending colon, sigmoid, and rectum, and it becomes the superior rectal artery.

○ **The external iliac nodes receive afferent vessels from what regions?**

Lower extremity, lower anterior abdominal wall, perineum, and pelvis.

○ **Where are the common iliac nodes located?**

Medial, lateral, and posterior to the common iliac vessels extending from the external iliac nodes to the bifurcation of the aorta.

○ **The internal iliac nodes receive lymphatics from what areas?**

Drainage corresponds to the branches of the internal iliac arteries.

○ **Efferent lymphatic vessels from the cervix course to what nodes?**

Laterally to the external iliac nodes, posterolaterally to the internal iliac nodes, and posteriorly to the common iliac and lateral sacral nodes.

○ **The majority of the lymphatic vessels of the fundal corpus of the uterus drain into what nodes?**

Internal iliac nodes primarily; also aortic, lumbar, and pelvic.

○ **The upper vagina has lymphatic drainage to what nodes?**

External and internal iliac nodes.

○ **Lymphatic vessels from the middle region of the vagina terminate in what nodes?**

Internal iliac nodes.

○ **Lymphatic drainage from the vaginal orifice and vulva may terminate in what group of nodes?**

Superficial inguinal nodes.

○ **The superficial lymphatic vessels in the anal region course to what group of nodes?**

Superficial inguinal nodes.

○ **Lymphatic drainage deep in the ischiorectal fossa is to what group of nodes?**

Internal iliac nodes.

○ **Lymphatic drainage of the ovaries follows the course of the ovarian arteries to what groups of nodes?**

Lateral and preaortic lumbar nodes.

○ **Lymphatic drainage of the upper and middle portions of the fallopian tube is to what nodes?**

Lateral and preaortic lumbar nodes.

○ **Lymphatic drainage of the lower portion of the fallopian tube is to what nodes?**

Internal iliac and superficial inguinal nodes.

○ **Describe the autonomic innervations of the pelvis.**

The superior hypogastric plexus divides to form the two hypogastric nerves, which fan out to form the inferior hypogastric plexus.

○ **Name the three portions that the inferior hypogastric plexus (pelvic plexus) is divided into.**

The vesical plexus, uterovaginal plexus (Frankenhäuser's ganglion), and the middle rectal plexus.

○ **What is Frankenhäuser plexus?**

An extensive concentration of both myelinated and nonmyelinated nerve fibers located in the uterosacral ligaments and supplying primarily the uterus and the cervix.

○ **Innervation of the urinary bladder is provided by what structures?**

Fibers from the third and fourth sacral nerves and fibers from the hypogastric plexus.

○ **What is another name for the superior hypogastric plexus?**

Presacral nerve.

○ **Where is the presacral nerve located?**

It lies in the subserous fascia under the parietal peritoneum and extends from the level of the fourth lumbar to the first sacral vertebrae.

○ **Name the three supportive layers of the pelvic floor.**

Endopelvic fascia, levator ani muscles and perineal membrane/external anal sphincter.

○ **Name the external genital muscles whose primary function appears to be sexual response.**

Ischiocavernosus, bulbocavernosus, and superficial transverse perineal muscles.

○ **What constitutes the pelvic diaphragm?**

Levator ani muscles and their superior and inferior fasciae.

○ **What is the anterior midline cleft in the pelvic diaphragm called?**

Urogenital hiatus.

○ **What structures pass through the urogenital hiatus?**

Urethra, vagina, and rectum.

○ **The broad sheet of endopelvic fascia that attaches the upper vagina, cervix, and uterus to the pelvic sidewalls is known by what name?**

Cardinal and uterosacral ligaments.

○ **What three muscles constitute the levator ani muscle?**

Pubococcygeus, iliococcygeus, and puborectalis muscles.

○ **Innervation of the levator ani is from which nerves?**

Fourth sacral (sometimes, also, third or fifth sacral).

○ **Name five arteries that supply the rectum.**

(1) Superior rectal artery.

(2) Two middle rectal arteries.

(3) Two inferior rectal arteries (see the figure below).

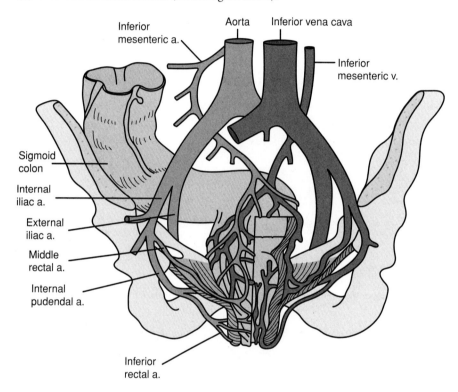

○ **Arterial blood supply to the female urethra arises from what structures?**

Inferior vesical and internal pudendal arteries.

○ **Where does the innervation of the urethra develop?**

Pudendal nerves and pelvic plexuses.

○ **What is the name of the ovarian venous plexus?**

Pampiniform plexus.

○ **The whitish folded scar on the ovary resulting from regression of a corpus luteum has what name?**

Corpus albicans.

○ **A mass of cells on one side of a mature follicle protruding into the cavity is known by what term?**
Cumulus oophorus.

○ **The surface stroma of the ovary composed of short connective tissue fibers with fusiform cells between them is known by what name?**
Tunica albuginea.

○ **What name is given to the highest of the deep inguinal lymph nodes located in the lateral part of the femoral ring?**
Cloquet node.

○ **Where is the epoophoron (parovarian) located?**
In the mesosalpinx between the ovary and the tube.

○ **The greater vestibular glands are also known by what name?**
Bartholin glands.

○ **Where are Bartholin glands located?**
4 and 8 o'clock at the vaginal introitus. They drain between the hymenal ring and the labia minora.

○ **What structure is responsible for hemorrhage associated with removal of Bartholin cyst?**
The vestibular bulb.

○ **The Bartholin glands are the female homologue of what male structure?**
Cowper bulbourethral glands.

○ **Infected Bartholin glands may cause enlargement of what lymph nodes?**
Inguinal or external iliac nodes.

○ **What is the vestibule of the vagina?**
The cleft between the labia minora and the glans of the clitoris.

○ **In the virgin the labia minora are usually joined across the midline by a fold of skin known by what term?**
Frenulum of the labia or fourchette.

○ **What is the normal weight of the non-gravid uterus?**
40 to 50 g.

○ **A retroflexed uterus is a normal variant found in what percentage of women?**
20% to 25%.

○ **Which nerve roots do the sensory fibers from the uterus enter?**
T11 and T12; referred uterine pain is often located in the lower abdomen.

○ **Which nerve roots do the sensory fibers from the cervix enter?**

S2, S3, and S4; referred pain from cervical inflammation is characterized as low back pain.

○ **What is the name of the slight constriction between the cervix and the corpus of the uterus?**

Isthmus.

○ **Name the three portions of the fallopian tube external to the uterus.**

The proximal 1/3 is the isthmus, the medial 1/3 is the ampulla, and the distal 1/3 is the infundibulum.

○ **Appendices vesiculosae of the tube are also known by what name?**

Hydatids of Morgagni.

○ **What covers the surfaces of the broad ligaments?**

Peritoneum.

○ **What structures are the boundaries of the cul-de-sac of Douglas?**

Ventrally, the supravaginal cervix and posterior fornix of the vagina; dorsally, the rectum; laterally, the uterosacral ligaments.

○ **What is the myometrium?**

The muscular wall of the uterus.

○ **What structures found in the labia majora are not found in the labia minora?**

Hair follicles.

○ **The primary tissue found in the mons pubis is what type of tissue?**

Adipose.

○ **Innervation of the uterus is primarily from where?**

Hypogastric and ovarian plexuses and the third and fourth sacral nerves.

○ **From where does the innervation of the vagina arise?**

Vaginal plexus and pudendal nerves.

○ **Name three branches of pudendal nerves and vessels.**

(1) Clitoral.

(2) Perineal.

(3) Inferior hemorrhoidal.

○ **What is the male homologue of the clitoris?**

Penis.

○ **By what cellular processes does the gravid uterus enlarge?**
Hypertrophy and hyperplasia.

○ **Skene glands are also known by what name?**
Paraurethral glands.

○ **Where are Skene glands located?**
Adjacent to the urethral opening.

○ **Skene glands are considered the homologues of what male structures?**
Prostatic glands.

○ **Which has a greater diameter, the abdominal portion or pelvic portion of the ureter?**
The abdominal (10 mm vs. 5 mm).

○ **In the female bladder, attachments directly between the bladder and the pubic bone are known by what name?**
Pubovesical ligaments.

○ **The median umbilical ligament is the remnant of what structure?**
Urachus.

○ **The anterior angle of the trigone is formed by what?**
Internal orifice of the urethra.

○ **The posterolateral angles of the trigone are formed by what?**
Orifices of the ureters.

○ **In the contracted bladder, the ureteral orifices are approximately how far apart?**
2.5 cm.

○ **Where in the female is the bulbospongiosus muscle located?**
Surrounding the lower end of the vagina.

○ **What is the blood supply to the vagina?**
It is an extensive network. The vaginal artery arises either directly from the uterine or from the internal iliac; also from the azygous arteries anastomosing from the cervical branch of the uterine.

○ **Name the four layers of the vagina.**
The mucosa: A stratified, nonkeratinized squamous epithelium.
The lamina tunica: A fibrous connective tissue.
The muscle layer: An inner circular layer and an outer longitudinal layer.
The cellular areolar connective tissue.

○ **What is the sensory innervation to the vagina?**

Pudendal nerve (S2–S4).

○ **Where is primary lymph drainage from the vagina?**

Upper 1/3: External iliac

Middle 1/3: Common/internal iliac

Lower 1/3: Common iliac, superficial inguinal, and perirectal.

○ **What is the average length of the endocervical canal?**

2.5–3 cm.

○ **What are the longitudinal folds in the mucous membrane of the endocervical canal called?**

Plicae palmatae.

○ **What is the arterial supply to the cervix?**

Cervical artery arises from the uterine artery. The cervical arteries approach the cervix at 3 and 9 o'clock.

○ **Name all the surgical cleavage spaces (7, 8, 9, 10, 11, and 12) that are filled with fatty or areolar connective tissue.**

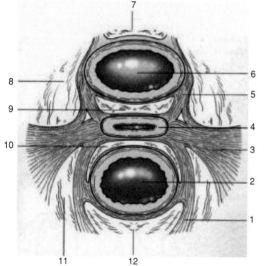

1	Uterosacral ligament
2	Rectum
3	Cardinal ligament
4	Vagina
5	Bladder pillar
6	Urinary bladder
7	
8	
9	
10	
11	
12	

Reproduced, with permission, from Smith JR. An Atlas of Gynecologic Oncology. Taylor & Francis; 2001.

7. Prevesical space

8. Paravesical space

9. Vesicovaginal space

10. Rectovaginal space

11. Pararectal space

12. Retrorectal space

○ **What is the name of the artery that supplies the round ligament?**

Sampson artery.

○ **How many oocytes are present in the human ovary at birth?**

1 to 2 million.

○ **How many oocytes eventually ovulate?**

About 300 to 400.

○ **What is the venous drainage from the ovaries?**

The pampiniform plexus to the ovarian vein.

○ **Name the spinal segments on dermatome below.**

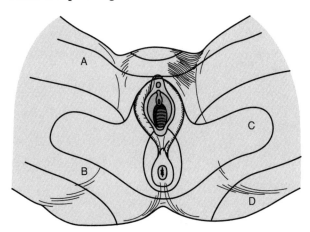

A; L2, B; S2, C; S3, D; S1.

○ **What are the three layers to the ovary?**

Cortex, central medulla, and rete ovarii.

○ **What is the tunica albuginea?**

Outer cortex of ovary.

○ **What is the ovarian fossa?**

Space between iliac vessels and ureter.

○ **When does the Müllerian tissue fuse?**

10 weeks.

○ **A woman with a bicornuate uterus has a defect that represents?**

Failure of fusion of the Müllerian system.

O **Unilateral atresia of the Müllerian system results in what type of abnormality?**
Unicornuate uterus.

O **Bilateral atresia of the Müllerian system results in what syndrome?**
Mayer–Rokitansky–Kuster–Hauser syndrome.

O **Failure of central degeneration of the fused Müllerian ducts results in what types of uterine anomalies?**
Arcuate, septum, and didelphys.

O **What are the two layers of the endometrium?**
Functionalis and basalis.

O **What is the vascular plexus around the ureter called?**
Auerbach plexus.

O **During a lymph node dissection, the external iliac vessels are displaced laterally with a vein retractor and a nerve is triggered that causes the patient's leg to move. What is the nerve?**
Obturator L2 to L4.

O **What two structures does the gubernaculum become?**
Ovarian ligament and round ligament.

O **What is the average length of the urethra in an adult female?**
3 to 4 cm.

O **A patient presents with numbness after a cesarean delivery around the area of her incision. What cutaneous nerves may have been damaged?**
Iliohypogastric and ilioinguinal nerves.

O **If a patient lost sensation to vulva or clitoris, what nerve may have been affected?**
Pudendal.

O **This nerve lies superior to the psoas muscle and is responsible for vulvar and thigh sensation.**
Genitofemoral nerve.

O **After a prolonged surgery in lithotomy position, you discover your patient has anesthesia of her anterior thigh and medial thigh and loss of patellar reflex. What do you suspect was injured?**
Femoral nerve.

O **After a prolonged surgery in lithotomy position, you discover your patient has numbness in her lower extremity and foot drop. What do you suspect was injured?**
Common peroneal nerve.

○ **During a speculum exam, you notice a lesion on the patient's cervix. It can be defined as a retention cyst of endocervical columnar cells. What do you call this lesion?**

Nabothian cyst.

○ **What structures are formed from the mesonephric duct?**

Ureter, renal pelvis, renal calyces, and collecting tubules of kidneys.

○ **What are the boundaries of the paravesical space?**

Pubic symphysis (anterior), bladder (medial), obturator internus muscle (lateral), and parametria (posterior).

○ **What are the boundaries of the pararectal space?**

Rectum (medial), parametria (anterior), sacrum (posterior), and internal iliac (lateral).

○ **How is the parametria defined during a radical hysterectomy?**

By developing the paravesical and pararectal spaces.

○ **A patient is undergoing an inguinal lymph node dissection for vulvar cancer. What are the boundaries of the inguinal triangle?**

Sartorius muscle (lateral), inguinal ligament (superior), and adductor longus (medial).

○ **What is another name for the inguinal ligament?**

Poupart's ligament.

○ **Are the inguinal lymph nodes medial or lateral to the femoral artery?**

Medial.

○ **As you start a hysterectomy and are transecting the round ligament, you encounter bleeding. What vessel is bleeding?**

Sampson's artery.

○ **You are rounding on a post-op patient who is post-op day 1 after a complicated TAH in which you used the Bookwalter self-retaining retractor for 6 hours. The patient complains of numbness of the labia and upper medial thigh without motor deficits. She also states she has paresthesias and pain that radiate down the anterior and posterior-lateral aspect of the thigh toward the knee. What nerves may have been affected?**

Genitofemoral and lateral femoral cutaneous nerves.

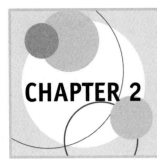

CHAPTER 2

Embryology of the Genital Tract

Erin M. Murphy, MD

○ **At what gestational age, do the primitive germ cells (oogonia) migrate to the gonadal ridge?**

Approximately 5 weeks.

○ **Do germ cells induce gonadal development?**

No. Germ cells do not induce gonadal development; however, absence of germs cell arrival to the gonadal ridge results in no gonad development and the formation of a fibrous streak (gonadal agenesis).

○ **If the indifferent gonad is destined to become a testis, at what gestational age will differentiation occur?**

6 to 9 weeks' gestation.

○ **What is the factor that determines if an indifferent gonad will become a testis?**

Testes-determining factor (TDF). TDF is a product of a gene located on the Y chromosome in the region of SRY gene.

○ **How many oogonia are present throughout a female's life?**

This is a period of rapid *mitotic* activity. A maximum of 6 to 7 million is reached at 16 to 20 weeks' gestational age. This number is reduced to approximately 1 million at birth secondary to atresia. At puberty only 300,000 remain.

○ **At what point do oogonia become oocytes?**

This begins at 11 to 12 weeks' gestational age and is completed by birth. Oogonia enter the first *meiotic* division and are arrested in prophase. These are referred to as primary oocytes.

○ **What is the mechanism of the loss of oocytes during the second half of pregnancy?**

Oocytes are lost after 20 weeks' gestation due to follicular growth and subsequent atresia, as well as degeneration of oogonia not surrounded by granulosa cells. Also, germ cells that migrate to the surface of the ovary are lost in the peritoneal cavity.

○ **After mitosis, what is required for an oocyte to become a single ovum?**

Two meiotic divisions are required with the first at ovulation and the second at fertilization.

○ **Is the rate of follicular loss constant throughout adulthood?**

No. Loss is accelerated as adults approach menopause.

○ **What happens to excess genetic material as the oocytes progress through meiotic divisions during ovulation and later fertilization?**

Excess genetic material is extruded as polar bodies.

○ **What is the chromosomal content of the primary oocyte arrested in the diplotene stage prior to ovulation?**

46 chromosomes.

○ **What is the chromosomal content of a mature oocyte after completion of meiosis II?**

23 chromosomes.

○ **Does the cycle of follicle formation, ripening, and atresia occur in the fetus?**

Yes. However, ovulation does not occur.

○ **Does the Müllerian duct development depend on fetal gonadal steroid production?**

No. The Müllerian duct development is independent of the ovary.

○ **Is the fetal hypothalamic-pituitary portal circulation functional?**

Yes. The fetal hypothalamic-pituitary portal circulation is functional by the 12th week of gestation.

○ **Do both males and females have both the Wolffian ducts and the Müllerian ducts present at any time?**

Yes. Both systems temporarily coexist until 8 weeks' gestation.

○ **Name the three stages of renal development.**

Pronephric, mesonephric, and metanephric.

○ **Are abnormalities in the development of tubes, uterus, and upper vagina associated with congenital abnormalities in any other organ system?**

Yes. These abnormalities are associated with abnormalities in the renal system, as they both require the appearance of the mesonephric ducts.

○ **What are the components of the urogenital ridge?**

Mesonephric duct and genital ridge.

○ **In the absence of any gonad, what type of development will occur?**

Internal genitalia have intrinsic tendency to feminize, as Müllerian duct development will occur.

○ **Does the development of a normal female phenotype require fetal estrogen production?**

No.

○ **What is the most common cause of an abdominal mass in a female fetus or newborn?**

Ovarian cysts.

○ **What are female infants follicle-stimulating hormone (FSH) values up to a year of life?**

FSH levels in infants are higher than normal adult levels during a menstrual cycle. FSH levels then decrease to low levels by 1 year.

○ **Before puberty, is the ovary in the female quiescent?**

No. Follicles begin to grow and frequently reach the antral stage.

○ **What are the three major anatomic parts of the ovary?**

The outer cortex, the medulla, and the hilum.

○ **Which portion of the ovary contains the oocytes?**

The inner portion of the cortex.

○ **What is the tunica albuginea?**

The outermost portion of the ovarian cortex.

○ **What three structures develop from the Müllerian ducts (paramesonephric ducts)?**

Fallopian tubes, uterus, and upper two-thirds of the vagina.

○ **What is the function of anti-Müllerian hormone (AMH)?**

AMH induces the resorption of the Müllerian ducts. It is secreted at approximately 7 weeks' gestation, when Sertoli cell differentiation occurs.

○ **Name three functions of AMH.**

AMH exerts an inhibitory effect on oocyte meiosis, helps to control the descent of the testes, and inhibits surfactant accumulation in the lungs.

○ **Is AMH completely absent in the female?**

No. AMH is not expressed prior to birth to ensure normal female differentiation. After puberty, AMH is produced and secreted by granulosa cells from small growing ovarian follicles and acts as a paracrine inhibitory factor.

○ **Which cells produce AMH?**

Sertoli cells.

○ **Which cells produce testosterone?**

Leydig cells.

○ **Do human chorionic gonadotropin (hCG) levels remain constant in the fetus throughout gestation?**

No. hCG levels are similar in the fetus to levels in maternal circulation, peaking at 10 weeks and reaching a nadir at about 20 weeks.

O **The loss of the Wolffian system in the female (including the epididymis, vas deferens, and seminal vesicle) is due to the lack of which hormone?**

Testosterone.

O **Is there any chromosome anomaly that accelerates the process of germ cell loss?**

Yes. Turner syndrome (45,X) or gonadal dysgenesis is characterized by a fibrous streak of ovarian tissue that lacks follicles.

O **Do individuals with Turner syndrome (45,X) have germ cells, which undergo mitosis and meiosis?**

Patients with Turner syndrome have germ cells, which undergo mitosis, but oogonia do not undergo meiosis.

O **Do individuals with Turner syndrome (45,X) have any follicles at birth?**

No.

O **What are the characteristic findings in someone with Turner syndrome?**

The characteristic findings include short stature, streak gonads, webbed neck, high arched palate, cubitus valgus, shield-like chest with widely spaced nipples, low hairline on the neck, short fourth metacarpal bones, renal abnormalities, and coarctation of the aorta, primary amenorrhea, lack of secondary sexual characteristics.

O **What is Swyer syndrome?**

46XY gonadal dysgenesis of the testes caused by a mutation of the SRY gene. They are found to have an XY karyotype with normal infantile female external genitalia and streak gonads.

O **Gonadal dysgenesis may also develop in individuals with a mosaic karyotype of 45X/46XX or 45X/46XY. What tumors must you be concerned about in these patients?**

Gonadoblastoma or dysgerminoma.

O **What are two conditions that cause gonadal dysgenesis but have a normal chromosome complement?**

Pure gonadal dysgenesis and gonadal agenesis (male pseudohermaphroditism).

O **What is the etiology of pure gonadal dysgenesis?**

Failure of germ cells to arrive at the gonadal ridge with subsequent failure of ovarian development.

O **In the bipotential state (6 weeks' gestation), what does the external genitalia consist of?**

Genital tubercle, a urogenital sinus, and two labioscrotal swellings.

O **External sexual differentiation is under what hormonal influence?**

Androgen secretion from the Leydig cells of the testis.

O **When do the fetal testes begin secreting androgens and when is masculinization complete?**

Testes begin secreting androgens at 8 to 9 weeks' gestation and masculinization is complete by 14 weeks' gestation.

○ **What enzyme must be present in target tissues for masculinization to occur?**

5α-reductase.

○ **What is 5α-reductase deficiency?**

46XY, autosomal-recessive deficiency resulting in decreased conversion of testosterone to the more active dihydrotestosterone (DHT), which is the necessary androgen for the target tissues at the urogenital sinus.

○ **What are the clinical manifestations of 5α-reductase deficiency?**

Decreased DHT and normal testosterone levels. Ambiguous genitalia or phenotypically female and male internal genitalia present. During puberty, increased testosterone may cause virilization with growth of a penis and descent of testes.

○ **What is the treatment of 5α-reductase deficiency?**

Individual should be raised female and undergo gonadectomy.

○ **Do male germ cells begin meiotic division prior to puberty?**

No.

○ **Which cells surround fetal spermatogonia?**

Sertoli cells.

○ **In females, androgen exposure at what gestation period may cause external ambiguity of the female phenotype?**

9 to 14 weeks' gestation.

○ **Do Leydig cell numbers remain constant throughout fetal life?**

No. Leydig cell numbers peak at 15 to 18 weeks.

○ **What is the name of the indifferent structure, which later divides into the anorectal canal and the urogenital sinus?**

The cloaca.

○ **What are the swellings on each side of the urethral fold that later develop into the scrotum in the male and labia majora in the female?**

Genital swellings.

○ **How does the phallus develop?**

Rapid elongation of the genital tubercle.

○ **Are the scrotal swellings in the male developed outside the abdominal cavity?**

No. The scrotal swellings are located initially in the inguinal region and then migrate caudally.

○ **What is the origin of the clitoris?**

The genital tubercle. In the female the genital tubercle elongates only slightly resulting in the clitoris.

○ **What is the origin of the labia minora?**

Urethral folds.

○ **What is the gubernaculum testis?**

The gubernaculum testis is the column of mesenchyme that extends from the caudal pole of the testis to the genital swelling.

○ **Is the descent of the testis under any hormonal influence?**

Yes. The descent of the testis is influenced by androgens and gonadotropins.

○ **The proliferation of the sinovaginal bulbs results in what portion of the female genital tract?**

Lower third of the vagina.

○ **What is androgen insensitivity syndrome (testicular feminization)?**

X-linked recessive, 46XY genotype, and female phenotype (male pseudohermaphroditism).

○ **What is the pathophysiology of androgen insensitivity syndrome?**

Androgen receptors are absent or defective. There is normal fetal production of testosterone and AMH. Since receptors are defective, fetal androgens are unable to cause male external genitalia formation. Production of AMH results in absence of Müllerian structures (absent fallopian tubes, uterus and upper vagina). A small vagina with a blind end pouch may be present.

○ **What are the clinical manifestations?**

Presents as primary amenorrhea. Some estrogen production results in breast development. There will be absent or sparse axillary and pubic hair. Testes will be present either in labia or inguinal canal and should be removed after puberty secondary to risk of malignancy.

○ **Should the testes in patients with testicular feminization be surgically removed?**

Yes. The testes in these patients are at increased risk of developing tumors. The recommendation is for removal following puberty between 16 and 18 years.

○ **What other condition besides androgen insensitivity syndrome gives rise to external female phenotype but absent Müllerian development?**

Müllerian agenesis (Mayer-Rokitansky-Küster-Hauser syndrome).

○ **How do you differentiate between androgen insensitivity and Müllerian agenesis?**

In Müllerian agenesis, ovaries are present; therefore secondary sexual characteristics will develop normally. A karyotype will reveal that patients with Müllerian agenesis are 46XX.

○ **What is the diagnosis characterized by development of both active ovarian and testicular tissue?**

True hermaphroditism.

○ **What percentage of true hermaphrodites are genetic females?**

70%.

○ **What develops in the male if fusion of the urethral folds is incomplete, resulting in abnormal openings along the inferior aspect of the penis?**

Hypospadias.

○ **If the caudal portions of the Müllerian ducts fail to fuse along the entire length, what uterine anomaly will result?**

Uterus didelphys.

○ **What condition is characterized by the uterus with two horns and a common vagina?**

Bicornuate uterus.

○ **What is the origin of a Gartner duct cyst?**

A Gartner duct cyst results from a Wolffian duct remnant, which may be seen in the wall of the vagina or the uterus.

○ **What is congenital adrenal hyperplasia (CAH)?**

Autosomal-recessive defect in steroid biosynthesis. Karyotype is typically 46XX. Most frequent cause of ambiguous genitalia in the newborn.

○ **Name the four enzymatic defects associated with CAH. Which is the most common?**

21-hydroxylase (most common), 11β-hydroxylase, 3β-hydroxysteroid dehydrogenase, and rarely 17α-hydroxylase.

○ **What is the pathophysiology of CAH?**

Lack of 21-hydroxylase (or others) → decreased production of cortisol → increased secretion of adrenocorticotropic hormone (ACTH) → accumulation of intermediate compounds in the pathway prior to the defect such as 17-hydroxyprogesterone → conversion to adrenal androgens (DHEA) and androstenedione that is converted peripherally to testosterone.

○ **What are the clinical manifestations?**

Ambiguous genitalia (cliteromegaly and swollen labial folds), 30% salt wasting, and 5% hypertension.

○ **How is CAH diagnosed?**

Increased plasma levels of 17-hydroxyprogesterone.

○ **How is 17α-hydroxylase deficiency different?**

Increased ACTH causes increased aldosterone production resulting in sodium retention, hypertension, and low potassium. Potentially life threatening at birth if not recognized.

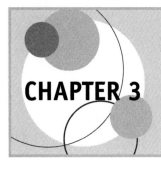

CHAPTER 3

Physiology of Normal Pregnancy

Remington Horesh, OMSII

○ **What percentage of human chorionic gonadotropin (hCG) is carbohydrate?**
30%. It has the most CHO content of all human hormones.

○ **What is the plasma half-life of intact hCG?**
24 hours.

○ **hCG is structurally related to what three other glycoprotein hormones?**
Luteinizing hormone (LH), follicle-stimulating hormone (FSH), and thyroid-stimulating hormone (TSH).

○ **How are the four hormones hCG, LH, FSH, and TSH structurally related?**
Each has an identical alpha-subunit with a unique beta subunit.

○ **What chromosome codes for the alpha-subunit of hCG?**
Chromosome 6 q12-q21 (a single gene).

○ **What chromosome codes for the beta subunit of hCG?**
Chromosome 19 (seven separate genes).

○ **What is the major source of hCG?**
Placental syncytiotrophoblast.

○ **At what gestational age, does hCG peak?**
8 to 10 weeks.

○ **What is a blood pregnancy test measuring?**
The beta subunit of the intact hCG molecule.

○ **When is hCG detectable in plasma of pregnant women?**

8 to 9 days after ovulation.

○ **Name four physiologic actions of hCG.**

(1) Maintenance of corpus luteum and continued progesterone production.

(2) Stimulation of fetal testicular testosterone secretion promoting male sexual differentiation.

(3) Stimulation of the maternal thyroid by binding to TSH receptors as its alpha-subunit is identical.

(4) Promotes relaxin secretion by the corpus luteum.

○ **During the second half of pregnancy, what effect do insulin-like growth factors (I&II) have on adrenocorticotropic hormone (ACTH)?**

IGF I&II are important in increasing adrenal responsiveness to ACTH.

○ **In early pregnancy (weeks 5–12), where is amniotic and maternal alpha-fetoprotein (AFP) produced?**

Amniotic fluid AFP is mainly from the yolk sac, while maternal circulating AFP is from fetal liver.

○ **When do AFP levels peak in fetal blood?**

At the end of the first trimester.

○ **Where can relaxin production be found other than by the corpus luteum?**

Relaxin is also produced by the placenta and myometrium.

○ **What is the most highly produced substance generated by the placenta?**

Human placental lactogen (hPL), otherwise known as human chorionic somatomammotropin (hCS) is produced in amounts as high as 1 to 4 g/day.

○ **What are the functions of hPL?**

(1) Lipolysis and an increase in the levels of circulating free fatty acids.

(2) Antiinsulin action leading to an increase in maternal levels of insulin providing mobilized sugars and amino acids.

○ **Is hPL required for successful pregnancy?**

No. Probably is a backup mechanism to ensure fetal nutrient supply.

○ **What other two hormones are homologous to hPL?**

Growth hormone (96% homology) and prolactin (67% homology).

○ **Where is hPL produced?**

Cytotrophoblast and syncytiotrophoblast.

○ **What is the biologic half-life of hPL?**

The half-life is 15 minutes.

○ **When does the corpus luteum stop producing progesterone in pregnancy?**

7 to 8 weeks of gestation.

○ **Name two consequences of excessive luteinization of the ovary.**

This may result in theca lutein cysts or a pregnancy luteoma.

○ **What is the daily rate of progesterone production in third trimester singleton pregnancy?**

250 mg/day.

○ **How is progesterone synthesized in the human placenta?**

Two-step reaction. Cholesterol is converted to pregnenolone in mitochondria by cytochrome P450 side-chain cleavage enzyme. Pregnenolone is converted to progesterone in microsomes by 3β-hydroxysteroid dehydrogenase, δ 5–4 isomerase.

○ **What is the primary source of cholesterol for placental progesterone synthesis?**

Maternal plasma low-density lipoprotein (LDL) cholesterol (90%).

○ **What is the principal estrogen found in the plasma and urine of pregnant women?**

Estriol.

○ **What are the major forms of estriol present in the amniotic fluid?**

16-glucosiduronate or 3-sulfate-16-glucosiduronate. 3-sulfate is also present in small quantities.

○ **Which hormone is decreased significantly after fetal death, umbilical cord ligation, and in anencephalic fetuses?**

Estrogen. However, measurements of estriol to predict fetuses at risk have not been shown to change perinatal morbidity or mortality.

○ **What is the average weight and volume of the nonpregnant uterus?**

Average weight is 40 to 70 g with a volume of 10 mL.

○ **What is the average weight and volume of the pregnant uterus at term?**

Average weight is 1100 to 1200 g with a volume of 5 L.

○ **What types of cellular changes occur during uterine enlargement in pregnancy?**

Hypertrophy and stretching of existing muscle. Hyperplasia is very limited. Hypertrophy results from the actions of estrogen and progesterone and occurs mostly before 12 weeks. The increase in uterine size after 12 weeks results from pressure from expanding products of conception.

○ **How many layers of muscle are in the uterus? Describe them.**

Three:

(1) An external layer that arches over the fundus to insert into the various ligaments.

(2) A middle layer of multidirectional interlacing muscle fibers between which extend blood vessels.

(3) An inner layer consisting of sphincter like fibers around the orifices of the tubes and internal os.

○ **What increased concentrations of oxytocin receptors are found in the myometrium during pregnancy at term?**
They are found to increase 300-fold as compared with prepregnancy.

○ **At what gestational age, does the uterus rise out of the pelvis?**
About 12 weeks.

○ **During a term Cesarean section you are examining the uterus before making the uterine incision. What direction of rotation are you most likely to see?**
Dextrorotation (to the right)—usually results from the presence of the rectosigmoid.

○ **In late pregnancy what is the approximate rate of blood flow to the uterus?**
450 to 650 mL/min.

○ **What are the three substances thought to take part in the regulation of uterine blood flow during pregnancy and what are their effects on the uterine flow.**
(1) Estrogen (vasodilation).
(2) Catecholamines (increased sensitivity even when controlled for blood pressure).
(3) Angiotensin II (vascular refractoriness).

○ **At term what percentage of uterine blood flow is directed toward the placenta?**
80% to 90%.

○ **What mechanism is responsible for the increased maternal-placental and fetal-placental blood flow in pregnancy?**
Maternal-placental is principally caused by vasodilation of existing vessels; and fetal-placental is principally caused by increasing numbers of placental vessels.

○ **During a strong contraction (50 mmHg) by how much is uterine blood flow reduced?**
60%.

○ **What are the normal physical changes in the cervix during pregnancy?**
Softening and cyanosis. This is known as Goodell sign.

○ **What is Chadwick sign?**
This is described as a bluish discoloration of the vagina.

○ **Microscopically, how are the cervical changes during pregnancy manifested?**
Increased vascularity and edema with hypertrophy and hyperplasia of cervical glands.

○ **What fraction of the cervical mass is composed of glands in the pregnant state?**
50%

○ **What is considered to be the main functional cell of the placenta and from what does it derive?**

The syncytiotrophoblast is the major site of hormone and protein production. It is derived from the cytotrophoblast.

○ **What is the term for the normal eversion of the endocervical glands out to the ectocervix during pregnancy?**

Ectropion.

○ **What are the changes in cervical mucous that occur in pregnancy?**

Thick tenacious mucous forms a plug blocking the cervical canal, thus preventing ascending infection (important in evaluating patients for pelvic inflammatory disease).

○ **What percentage of sodium chloride is necessary in the cervical mucous to develop a full ferning (arborization) pattern when dried on a slide?**

1%.

○ **What pattern is most likely seen on a slide of dried cervical mucous during pregnancy?**

Fragmentary crystallization or beading typical of the effect of progesterone-sodium chloride concentration that is usually <1% during pregnancy.

○ **Does the strength of the cervix decrease during pregnancy?**

Yes. Collagen is rearranged to produce a 12-fold reduction in mechanical strength.

○ **Describe the changes in vaginal secretions in pregnancy.**

Increased cervical and vaginal secretions result in thick, white odorless discharge. The pH is between 3.5 and 6.0 resulting from increased production of lactic acid from the action of *Lactobacillus acidophilus.*

○ **What is the proposed mechanism for the increased pigmentation of skin found in pregnancy? Give two examples.**

Melanocyte-stimulating hormone (MSH) is elevated from the end of the second month of pregnancy to term. Estrogen and progesterone may have melanocyte-stimulating properties. Estrogen and progesterone may also stimulate the hypertrophy of the intermediate lobe of the pituitary which is where MSH and β-endorphin are formed from the metabolism of proopiomelanocortin. Two examples are the linea nigra and the melasma gravidarum.

○ **What are the glands of Montgomery?**

Normal finding of hypertrophic sebaceous glands scattered throughout the areola of a pregnant woman's breast.

○ **What is the average weight gain in pregnancy?**

11 kg (25 lbs).

○ **What percentage of maternal weight gain is contributed by the fetus and placenta at term?**

Approximately 30%.

○   **What percentage of maternal weight gain is contributed by blood, amniotic fluid, and extravascular fluid at term?**

Approximately 30%.

○   **What percentage of maternal weight gain is contributed by maternal fat?**

30%.

○   **At term, what is the water content in liters of the fetus, placenta, and amniotic fluid?**

3.5 L.

○   **What is the total amount of extra water that a pregnant woman retains during normal pregnancy?**

6.5 L total—3.5 L for the fetus, placenta, and amniotic fluid and 3.0 L for the increased volume of blood, uterus, and breasts.

○   **Why does water retention, a normal physiologic alteration of pregnancy, and edema occur in normal pregnancy?**

Fall in plasma osmolality of 10 mOsm/kg. Prepregnancy plasma osmolality is about 290 mOsm/kg. At 4 weeks, it starts to drop and by 8 weeks it plateaus to about 280 mOsm/kg.

○   **Describe the utility of increased body protein during pregnancy.**

One half of the normal increase in body protein during pregnancy, 500 g, is contained in the fetus and placenta. The other 500 g of protein is incorporated in contractile proteins in the uterus, glands of the breast, maternal blood proteins, and hemoglobin.

○   **In a healthy pregnant woman what happens to the fasting plasma glucose level and why?**

It is decreased by 8 to 10 mg/dL in the first trimester with little change after that. This negates fetal demand as the cause; therefore, it is probably a dilutional effect.

○   **In a healthy pregnant woman how long does it take to return to fasting glucose levels after a glucose load?**

The levels peak later (55 min when pregnant vs. 30 min when not) and remain elevated longer, thereby prolonging the return to fasting level to about 2 hours (usually 1 hour in nonpregnant patients).

○   **What is the state of carbohydrate metabolism in normal pregnancy in terms of fasting glucose, postprandial glucose, insulin levels and insulin resistance?**

Mild fasting hypoglycemia, postprandial hyperglycemia, hyperinsulinemia, and increased insulin resistance.

○   **What are the changes in the pancreas seen in normal pregnancy?**

Beta cell hypertrophy, hyperplasia, and hypersecretion.

○   **In a normal pregnancy, what effect does a glucose stimulus have on glucagon levels?**

Plasma glucagon levels are suppressed.

○   **What is the general trend of serum lipid concentrations in pregnancy?**

Increase continuously throughout gestation. This includes triglycerides, cholesterol, phospholipids, and fatty acids.

○ **At what gestational age, does LDL and HDL cholesterol peak in pregnancy?**

36 weeks and 30 weeks, respectively.

○ **Are pregnant women more likely to become ketonuric after starvation compared with nonpregnant women?**

Yes. Because there are higher concentrations of lipids and lower concentrations of glucose during fasting. The lipids are preferentially metabolized to ketones. This is known as accelerated starvation.

○ **What is the effect of pregnancy on folate and B12 levels?**

Both levels decrease (there is wide variation).

○ **What is the effect of pregnancy on erythropoetin levels?**

There is a steady increase causing increased red cell mass. This is a paradoxical finding because erythropoetin is stimulated by tissue hypoxemia, an unusual finding during normal pregnancy.

○ **What is the general effect of pregnancy on electrolyte concentrations?**

Sodium, potassium, calcium, magnesium, and zinc are all mildly decreased by no greater than about 10% of nonpregnant levels.

○ **What is the effect of pregnancy on copper concentrations in serum?**

Increases from approximately 1.0 mg/L to 2.0 mg/L due to increased ceruloplasmin (copper-binding protein) levels and fetal demand. Increased estrogen levels have been shown to increase copper and ceruloplasmin.

○ **How do the bicarbonate levels change during pregnancy?**

They decrease by approximately 4 mEq/L to a level of 18 to 22 mEq/L.

○ **Why are bicarbonate levels decreased during pregnancy?**

The developing fetus must offload its bicarbonate via the mother, inducing hyperventilation with resulting respiratory alkalosis. Metabolic compensation by the kidney will restore normal pH balance by excreting bicarbonate.

○ **Which two serum protein concentrations decrease during pregnancy and why?**

(1) Total protein (70 g/L to 60 g/L—major decrease in the first trimester).

(2) Albumin (45 g/L to 35g/L—major decrease in the first trimester).

This is probably due to decreased protein synthesis in the first trimester, followed by dilutional factors during the remaining two trimesters.

○ **What is the normal total body iron content in a non-pregnant woman?**

2 g—about one half that of men.

○ **What is the total iron requirement from the beginning to the end of pregnancy?**

Approximately 1 g.

○ **What is the total iron requirement per day necessary in the latter half of pregnancy?**

6 to 7 mg/day.

○ **Describe the utilization of iron in the body during pregnancy.**

The total iron content of a healthy woman is 2 g; however, the iron stores are only about 300 mg. The fetus and placenta take 300 mg. Normal excretion accounts for 200 mg. The increase in total volume of circulating erythrocytes (450 mL) requires another 500 mg.

○ **Why is supplemental iron necessary in pregnancy?**

The iron stores and the iron absorbed from the diet are not enough to provide for the increase in red cells and as plasma volume increases, anemia will result unless exogenous iron is provided.

○ **Does the reticulocyte count normally change during pregnancy?**

Yes. It increases after 20 weeks due to moderate erythroid hyperplasia in the bone marrow, correlated with increased erythropoetin levels.

○ **Describe the changes in serum transferrin levels during pregnancy.**

Transferrin levels increase during pregnancy as do other carrier proteins. The level may increase by as much as 100% by the end of the second trimester. This is the reason that the total iron-binding capacity (TIBC) also increases 25% to 100%.

○ **Does iron supplementation decrease the TIBC to prepregnancy levels?**

No.

○ **What is thought to be the etiology of the increase in binding proteins (like transferrin and thyroid-binding globulin) during pregnancy?**

Increased levels of circulating estrogens are thought to stimulate the liver to increase binding proteins. Women taking oral contraceptives also have increased levels of binding proteins.

○ **During pregnancy, how much do the total erythrocyte volume (TEV), hemoglobin, hematocrit, and mean erythrocyte volume (MCV) change both with and without iron supplementation?**

Iron Supplementation	No Iron Supplementation
• TEV *increases* by 30%	• TEV *increases* by 15%
• Hemoglobin *decreases* by 2%	• Hemoglobin *decreases* by 10%
• Hematocrit *decreases* by 3%	• Hematocrit *decreases* by 5%
• MCV *increases* to an average of 89.7 μm^3	• MCV *does not change* from prepregnancy mean = 84.6 μm^3

○ **Does the MCV change during pregnancy?**

Without iron supplementation, the MCV does not change. With iron supplementation, the MCV increases.

○ **What hemoglobin concentration should be considered abnormal in a pregnant woman?**

Values below 11.0 g/dL are present in only 6% of normal pregnant women taking iron and are considered to be in the range for anemia in the first and third trimesters. A patient should be considered anemic in the second trimester if the hemoglobin value is <10.5 g/dL. Value less than these numbers should prompt a workup for anemia.

○ **What is the most helpful parameter to make the diagnosis of iron deficiency anemia in a pregnant woman?**

MCV, as it is one of the only hematologic parameters not changed during pregnancy in women not taking iron and is increased in women taking iron. Microcythemia is only caused by three entities—thalassemia, iron deficiency, and lead poisoning. A progressive decrease in MCV to below 82 μm^3 is usually a sign of iron deficiency as the other causes are rare and easily ruled out.

○ **Describe the normal white blood cell count in pregnancy.**

Normal range is 5,000 to 12,000/mL. During labor and the puerperium, it may increase markedly to 25,000 or more.

○ **Which type of immunity (cell mediated vs. humoral) is affected by pregnancy and how?**

Clinical evidence shows that cell-mediated immunity is weakened (Th1 responses) and humoral immunity, immunosuppression, is strengthened (Th2 responses). Th1 and Th2 cells are functionally distinct subsets of CD4+ T-lymphocytes or helper cells. The weakened cell-mediated immunity is responsible for the decreased production of IL2, gamma interferon, and tumor necrosis factor by the Th1 cells that are harmful to the maintenance of pregnancy. The strengthened humoral immunity is responsible for the increase in immunosuppressive cytokines IL4 and IL10 produced by the Th2 cells.

○ **What is the physiology of the maternal immune system in pregnancy in general terms?**

Pregnancy represents a 50% allograft from the paternal contribution. As a result there is a general suppression of immune function. Therefore, one might have increased susceptibility to infections, improvement in the humoral-mediated autoimmune diseases, and worsening of other cellular-mediated autoimmune diseases.

○ **Does the platelet count change in normal pregnancy?**

Yes. There is a moderate decrease in the number of platelets per unit volume; however, the normal range remains the same for pregnant women (150,000–450,000/mm³). The mechanism is not clear. Dilution may contribute, but there is some evidence of increased consumption in pregnancy. Thrombocytopenia is defined as platelets <100,000/mm³.

○ **Is the bleeding time affected by pregnancy?**

No. Bleeding times are not different when compared with nonpregnant women.

○ **By how much does the maternal resting heart rate increase in pregnancy?**

10 to 15 beats per minute.

○ **Describe the change in the position and size of the heart in pregnancy.**

The heart is displaced 15 degrees to the left and upward and is rotated laterally causing a larger silhouette in radiographs. The cardiac volume may increase by 10% between early and late pregnancy.

○ **Can a pericardial effusion be normal in pregnancy?**

Yes. Small effusions are considered normal in pregnancy.

○ **Stroke volume increases during pregnancy. Is this a function of an increased inotropic effect?**

No. Increased stroke volume in a singleton pregnancy is directly proportional to the increased end-diastolic volume caused by increased blood volume (Starling phenomenon). In multifetal pregnancies, however, there has been a positive inotropic effect demonstrated to further increase stroke volume.

○ **What is the prepregnancy stroke volume compared with the pregnancy stroke volume?**

Normal prepregnancy stroke volume is about 60 mL. This increases to about 70 mL in pregnancy. Remember: stroke volume = cardiac output/heart rate.

○ **What normal changes could you see on an EKG during pregnancy?**

Left axis deviation, absent Q wave in aVf, T wave flattening or inversion in lead III. All of these are caused by the positional shift of the heart. The rhythm may be irregular as atrial and ventricular extrasystoles are common.

○ **What are the normal changes in the auscultative heart examination during pregnancy?**

Exaggerated split S1 with increased loudness of both components, systolic ejection murmurs heard at the left sternal border are present in 90% of patients, soft and transient diastolic murmurs are heard in 20%, and continuous murmurs from breast vasculature are heard in 10%. The significance of murmurs in pregnancy must be carefully evaluated and clinically correlated. Harsh systolic murmurs and all diastolic murmurs should be taken seriously and worked up before being attributed to pregnancy.

○ **Why is the erythrocyte sedimentation rate (ESR) not a useful test during pregnancy?**

The ESR is elevated normally during pregnancy for unclear reasons. A plausible explanation is the increased clumping of red cells caused by increased levels of fibrinogen and globulin. The elevation is different between whole blood samples and citrated blood samples. For whole blood (red top tube) the mean is 78 mm/h with a range of 44 to 114 mm/h. For citrated blood (purple top tube) the mean is 56 mm/h with a range of 20 to 98 mm/h.

○ **Plasma volume and blood volume increase in pregnancy. By how much and at what gestational age, does the volume increase?**

	Increase (%)	Gestational Age	Plateau
Plasma volume	40–60%	12–36 weeks	34–36 weeks
Blood volume (plasma and erythrocytes)	45%	24–28 weeks (peak) starts in first trimester	34–36 weeks

○ **Which three clotting factors decrease during pregnancy?**

- Factor XI.
- Factor XIII.
- Antithrombin III (antifactor Xa).

○ **All vitamins are found in human breast milk except which one?**

Vitamin K. This is why vitamin K is administered to newborns.

Formula is also deficient in vitamin K.

○ **The increase and decrease of which factors cause the increased risk of deep vein thrombosis in pregnancy?**

Patients who are pregnant are known to have an increase in clotting factors VII, VIII, X, and XII as well as an increase in prothrombin and fibrinogen. Also, they are found to have a decrease in the anticoagulant protein S.

○ **What is the normal fibrinogen level in pregnancy?**

A normal fibrinogen (factor I) during pregnancy can reach a level of 600 mg/dL at term. This increases from a prepregnancy value of 300 mg/dL.

○ **How does pregnancy affect cardiac output?**

Cardiac output increases to its maximum in the first trimester and this increase continues to term. The increase is 1.5 L/min above the nonpregnancy average.

○ **Blood flow to most organ systems increases during pregnancy. Which vital organ system does not receive more flow during pregnancy?**

Cerebral blood flow remains unchanged.

○ **How does pregnancy affect arterial blood pressure?**

There is relatively little change in systolic blood pressure (SBP). Diastolic blood pressure (DBP) decreases from 12 to 26 weeks and increases to reach the nonpregnancy value at 36 weeks. This causes an increase in pulse pressure during the second trimester.

○ **What is the definition of mean arterial blood pressure (MAP)?**

$$MAP = \frac{SBP + 2(DBP)}{3}$$

○ **How does pregnancy affect systemic vascular resistance (SVR)?**

Both SVR and pulmonary vascular resistance are decreased. Remember: MAP = SVR × CO. MAP does not change that much in pregnancy; however, CO is very much increased. SVR must decrease by definition. By midpregnancy, the SVR is about 1000 dynes/sec/cm^5 compared with the nonpregnancy value of 1500 dynes/sec/cm^5. Be aware that SVR may increase if the patient is in the supine position due to aortic compression.

○ **Does pulmonary capillary wedge pressure (PCWP) change in late pregnancy?**

No. PCWP and central venous pressure (CVP) are not changed significantly in late pregnancy when compared with 12 weeks postpartum. Normal averages are 6 mmHg and 4 mmHg, respectively.

○ **What is the normal glomerular filtration rate (GFR) in pregnancy?**

125 cc/min. The average prepregnancy rate is 90 cc/min.

○ **At what gestational age, does the GFR reach the maximum level?**

20 weeks and then persists to term. The etiology is not well specified except that renal blood flow is increased by as much as 50% by the beginning of the second trimester. Near term there is a 15% decrement in the GFR.

○ **Does urine output change in pregnancy?**

No. Urine output changes little despite the increase in GFR indicating that the increased filtered load of water is reabsorbed efficiently.

○ **By how much does the kidney increase in size during pregnancy?**

The length increases by 1 cm.

○ **Which nutrients are lost in greater amounts in the urine of pregnant women?**

Glucose, amino acids, and water-soluble vitamins.

○ **Describe the changes in blood urea nitrogen (BUN) and creatinine during pregnancy.**

BUN and creatinine decrease in pregnancy by about 25% with the nadir at 32 weeks. This is thought to be due to an increased GFR. The normal mean creatinine for a pregnant woman is 0.68 mg/dL. The mean BUN level in pregnancy is 10 mg/dL. Renal insufficiency should be suspected with values of creatinine >0.9 mg/dL and urea >14 mg/dL.

○ **What is the best way to calculate GFR in pregnancy?**

A 24-hour urine collection for creatinine clearance is preferred as the formula because body weight is not accurate in pregnancy. In pregnancy the patient's weight does not reflect kidney size as it does in prepregnancy.

○ **What is the daily urine protein loss during normal pregnancy?**

Urinary protein loss changes little as a result of pregnancy. The normal range goes up to 300 mg/24 hrs. Losses >300 mg/24 h may be a result of urinary tract infection or preeclampsia.

○ **How is the function of the renin-angiotensin system unique in the pregnant state?**

In the nonpregnant state renin is secreted when blood flow to the kidney is compromised causing the formation of angiotensin I and its conversion to angiotensin II. Angiotensin II is a potent vasoconstrictor causing an increase in blood pressure that maintains perfusion to the kidney. Angiotensin II also stimulates the release of aldosterone that allows sodium retention and conservation of volume. Despite the hypervolemic state of pregnancy the levels of renin and angiotensin II increase during pregnancy to about five times normal. The expected vasoconstriction and increase in blood pressure does not occur rendering normal pregnancy as a state refractoriness to angiotensin II. Moreover, the negative feedback exerted by angiotensin II on renin release is not seen in the pregnant state as renin and angiotensin II levels rise simultaneously.

○ **Postpartum, how long does it take for the physiologic hydronephrosis of pregnancy to completely resolve?**

12 to 16 weeks.

○ **How does the bladder and urethra compensate for the pressure exerted by the uterus?**

Bladder pressure doubles from 8 cm H_2O to 20 cm H_2O at term and the urethra lengthens by 5mm as bladder capacity decreases. Compensation occurs by way of increasing intraurethral pressure from 70 to 93 cm H_2O.

○ **What are the normal pregnancy-induced changes known in pulmonary function tests?**

Tidal volume, inspiratory capacity, minute ventilatory volume, and minute oxygen uptake increase by as much as 40% as pregnancy advances. Respiratory rate changes little but may be slightly increased. In general, all of the residual measures are reduced-including functional residual capacity, residual volume, and expiratory reserve volume. The maximum breathing capacity, forced expiratory volume (FEV1), and peak expiratory flow rate remain unchanged.

○ **Why are the residual capacities of the lungs decreased in pregnancy?**

The resting level of the diaphragm is 4 cm higher in pregnancy.

○ **How much do oxygen requirements increase in pregnancy?**

30 to 40 mL/min.

○ **What anatomic changes occur in the pregnant lungs to facilitate maximal oxygenation?**

- Diaphragm excursion increases from 4.5 cm (prepregnancy) to 6 cm at term.
- The subcostal angle increases from 68 degrees to 100 degrees.
- The diameter of the thoracic cage increases by 2 cm.
- The pulmonary diffusing capacity or rate at which gases diffuse from the alveoli to the blood is increased.

○ **Does pCO_2 increase or decrease during pregnancy?**

There is normally a dramatic decrease in the pCO_2 from a nonpregnancy range of 35 to 40 mmHg to 28 to 30 mmHg in pregnancy. This occurs from the increased respiratory drive induced by progesterone on the respiratory center. Medroxyprogesterone has been shown to stimulate the respiratory drive in obese nonpregnant patients who hypoventilate.

○ **Describe the trend of gastric acid production in pregnancy.**

It is reduced into the second trimester (36 mg/45 min) from prepregnancy values (60 mg/45 min) but begins to increase in late pregnancy (100 mg/45 min). Keep in mind that mucous production increases with a protective effect

○ **Does peptic ulcer disease (PUD) improve or worsen during pregnancy?**

Because there is a decrease in HCl production, PUD is rarely found in pregnancy. Disease that is already present usually improves during the pregnant state.

○ **What is thought to be the cause of the decreased transit time throughout all parts of the alimentary system in pregnancy?**

Increased progesterone levels cause smooth muscle relaxation. Decreased levels of motilin cause loss of smooth muscle-stimulating effects. This is evidenced by decreased esophageal, gastric, and intestinal motility and decreased lower esophageal sphincter tone.

○ **What is epulis of pregnancy?**

A focal, highly vascular swelling of the gums that regresses spontaneously after delivery.

○ **Is gastric emptying time increased or decreased during pregnancy?**

In nonpregnant patients 60% of a meal is emptied in 90 min. This time is found almost double during pregnancy.

○ **In normal pregnancy, what two components of the liver function test change appreciably and in which directions?**

Alkaline phosphatase increases, while albumin levels decrease.

○ **If a healthy pregnant woman were to undergo a liver biopsy, what would you see histologically?**

Normal liver morphology even with electron microscopy.

○ **What is the regulator of gall bladder contraction and why is it compromised in pregnancy?**

Cholecystokinin (CCK) causes gall bladder contraction and pancreatic enzyme release. It is formed in the type I mucosal cell of the duodenum and proximal jejunum. High levels of estrogen and progesterone inhibit CCK action on smooth muscle cells in the gall bladder causing impaired contraction and high residual volume.

○ **Name two GI disorders of pregnancy that most commonly present in the third trimester.**

Acute fatty liver of pregnancy and cholestasis of pregnancy.

○ **Hyperplasia of the pituitary occurs in pregnancy. How large does the pituitary grow?**

The pituitary enlarges by 135% compared with nonpregnant controls. This does not compress the optic chiasm.

○ **Is it possible to maintain a pregnancy after a hypophysectomy?**

Yes. The pituitary gland is not necessary for the maintenance of pregnancy. Women have undergone hypophysectomy and completed pregnancy with replacement of glucocorticoids, thyroid hormone, and vasopressin.

○ **Which thyroid function tests reflect true thyroid function in pregnancy?**

TSH, free T3, and free T4 are the three tests not affected by pregnancy after the first trimester. The other parameters (total T4, total T3, and T3 uptake) are altered due to the increase in thyroid-binding globulin that occurs as a result of the high estrogen state.

○ **Name the thyroid hormones that cross the placenta.**

Thyroid-releasing hormone can cross the placenta and may stimulate the fetal pituitary to secrete TSH. There is minimal transfer, if any, of thyroxine, triiodothyroxine, or reverse triiodothyroxine from the maternal to the fetal compartment. The fetal thyroid function is independent of the maternal thyroid status except in the case of autoimmune thyroid disease when stimulatory or inhibitory IgG crosses the placenta and affects the fetal thyroid.

○ **Describe the trend of TSH in pregnancy. Does it cross the placenta.**

TSH decreases in the first trimester then normalizes throughout the rest of the pregnancy. TSH does not cross the placenta.

○ **What is the correlation between TSH and hCG levels during pregnancy?**

TSH levels are inversely correlated with hCG levels.

○ **What percentage of pregnant women will have "hyperthyroid" levels of TSH during each trimester?**

- 13% of gravidas in the first trimester.
- 4.5% in the second trimester.
- 1.2% in the third trimester.

The undetectable TSH levels occur in the absence of thyroid disease due to the effects of β-hCG.

○ **Why does rising hCG cause a decrease in the TSH level?**

Both contain a homologous alpha-subunit. The hCG may act as TSH and stimulate the pituitary to secrete thyroid hormones that in turn suppress the release of TSH.

○ **Does the basal metabolic rate increase or decrease in pregnancy and by how much?**

Increases. Oxygen consumption increases by 25% as a result of fetal metabolic activity.

○ **At what gestational age does thyroid-binding globulin plateau?**

The peak increase begins early in the first trimester with a plateau at approximately 500 nmol/L at 20 weeks until term.

○ **Describe the trend in the free T4 and free T3 levels in pregnancy.**

- Both levels decrease from 6 weeks to a nadir and plateau at 20 weeks.
- Both remain within the normal nonpregnant reference range.
- Both correspond to decreasing thyroxine-binding globulin saturation that decreases from 40% to 30%.

○ **List the six most important factors responsible for calcium metabolism in pregnancy.**

- Serum calcium levels.
- Magnesium levels.
- Phosphate levels.
- Parathyroid hormone (PTH).
- Calcitonin.
- Vitamin D.

○ **Why is pregnancy termed a "hyperparathyroid state"?**

The feto-maternal unit has the primary goal of transporting calcium across the placenta (by active transport) for fetal skeletal development. This consumes most of the maternal calcium. Calcium concentration is maintained within normal range despite the increased and expanding extracellular volume. As calcium needs are very great, PTH levels are increased by 30% to 50% to bring calcium from the maternal bone, kidney, and intestine into the serum.

○ **Describe the trend of calcitonin in pregnancy.**

Calcitonin is secreted from the parafollicular cells of the thyroid gland. Calcitonin levels have been shown to increase from 13 to 16 weeks with a peak at 25 weeks (230 pg/mL) then a return to prepregnancy levels at about 35 weeks (200 pg/mL). Not only does the level increase but the responsiveness to hyopcalcemia also increases in order to protect the maternal skeleton from calcium loss.

○ **Which form of vitamin D is increased in pregnancy and why?**

The activated form 1,25-dihydroxyvitamin D is increased in pregnancy with nonpregnant values doubling to a range of 75 to 100 pg/mL. This is a PTH-related mechanism. As PTH increases, the hydroxylation of 25-vitamin D at the 1 position is increased at the level of the kidney. In addition, vitamin D-binding protein also increases in pregnancy, which may increase 1,25 vitamin D levels.

○ **Does PTH and/or calcitonin cross the placenta?**

Neither hormone crosses the placenta.

○ **Which of the substances produced by the adrenal cortex are decreased in pregnancy?**

Dehydroepiandrosterone sulfate (DHEAS) remains unaltered or slightly decreased through extensive 16 alpha-hydroxylation. All other products (sex steroids, cortisol, and aldosterone) increase.

○ **If testosterone is increased in the maternal serum, why is the female fetus not masculinized?**

Total testosterone is doubled from nonpregnancy levels of 0.5 µg/L to 1.0 µg/L. Free testosterone levels are decreased in pregnancy by about one half. Little or no testosterone enters the fetal circulation as testosterone. There is complete conversion of testosterone to 17β-estradiol by the trophoblast. This has been documented in women who have very high testosterone levels due to androgen secreting tumors.

○ **Describe the ACTH response to pregnancy.**

ACTH levels rise in pregnancy after an initial decrease early in pregnancy. The levels rise despite a dramatically increased cortisol level (three times nonpregnancy values). This is a paradox postulated to be due to a resetting of the feedback system secondary to tissue refractoriness to cortisol.

○ **A pregnant patient complains that her contact lenses are painful to wear recently. Is this normal?**

Yes. Corneal thickness increases in pregnancy and can cause discomfort when wearing lenses fitted before pregnancy.

○ **Is vision affected by pregnancy?**

Visual acuity remains the same; however, a transient loss of accommodation has been reported during pregnancy and lactation.

○ **Which hormones, aside from hCG, increase the most in pregnancy?**

Hormone	Increase
Human placental lactogen (hPL)	5000-fold
Progesterone	1000-fold
Estradiol	400-fold
Prolactin	10-fold

○   **At what gestational age, is the breast ready for lactation?**

Lactation is possible after 16 weeks of gestation.

○   **What mechanism prevents lactation from actually occurring prior to delivery?**

The effect of prolactin is blocked by progesterone.

○   **Describe the lesions of polymorphic eruption of pregnancy.**

Also known as pruritic urticarial papules and plaques of pregnancy, these lesions consist of small erythematous papules located most commonly on the abdomen and spare the palms, soles of the feet, and periumbilical area.

○   **Other than polymorphic eruption of pregnancy, name three other dermatologic lesions that may be specific to pregnancy?**

Three other lesions are pruritic folliculitis (erythematous papules most commonly found on the back and chest), pemphigoid gestations (also known as herpes gestations characterized by pruritic bullous disease of the skin), and prurigo of pregnancy (characterized by pruritic, erythematous, nodular lesions and is frequently a diagnosis of exclusion).

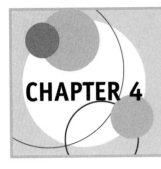

CHAPTER 4

Antepartum Management and Fetal Surveillance

Jordana I. Reina-Fernandez, MD and Andrew J. Walter, MD

○ **What is the utility of antepartum fetal surveillance?**

To assess the risk of fetal death in pregnancies complicated with preexisting maternal conditions as well as those in which complications have developed. These tests do not predict stillbirths related to acute changes in maternal-fetal status; for example, placental abruption or cord accident.

○ **What are the techniques used in antepartum fetal surveillance?**

- Fetal movement assessment.
- Nonstress test (NST).
- Contraction stress test (CST).
- Biophysical profile (BPP).
- Modified BPP.
- Umbilical artery Doppler velocimetry.

○ **At what gestational age, can antepartum testing be initiated?**

Initiating testing at 32 to 34 weeks is appropriate for most pregnancies at increased risk of stillbirth. In those pregnancies with multiple or worrisome conditions, testing may be initiated as early as 26 to 28 weeks.

○ **What are the indications of antepartum fetal monitoring?**

Maternal conditions:

- Chronic hypertension.
- Pregestational diabetes mellitus.
- Cyanotic heart disease.
- Chronic renal disease (ie, Lupus).
- Antiphospholipid syndrome.
- Hyperthyroidism.
- Hemoglobinopathies: Hemoglobin SS (sickle cell disease), Hemoglobin SC Disease.

Pregnancy-related conditions:
- Decreased fetal movement.
- Post-term pregnancy.
- Gestational hypertension or preeclampsia.
- Oligo/Polyhydramnios.
- Intrauterine growth restriction.
- Previous fetal demise.
- Multiple gestation.
- Isoimmunization.

○ **What aspects of the fetal condition might be predicted by antepartum testing?**

Perinatal death, intrauterine growth restriction, concerning fetal status, metabolic acidosis, postnatal motor and intellectual impairment, premature delivery, congenital abnormalities, and need for specific therapy.

○ **What medical factors place patients at risk of uteroplacental insufficiency?**

Post-term pregnancy, diabetes mellitus, hypertension, previous stillbirth, severe asthma, suspected intrauterine growth restriction, substance abuse (cocaine), advanced maternal age, cholestasis of pregnancy, abnormal analytes (elevated inhibin, decreased PAPP-A).

○ **When can fetal heart tones first be heard via transabdominal Doppler?**

10 to 12 weeks.

○ **When can fetal heart tones first be ascultated via nonelectronic fetoscope?**

18 to 20 weeks.

○ **By what gestational age, should all pregnant patients begin monitoring fetal activity?**

24 weeks or the currently accepted gestational age of viability.

○ **Which technique has been found to be ideal in assessing fetal movement?**

Kick counts.

○ **What maternal physiologic condition is associated with decreased fetal movement?**

Hypoglycemia.

○ **What is the count-to-ten approach in maternal assessment of fetal movement?**

The patient should count a minimum of 10 fetal movements in a 2-hour period.

○ **What are the fetal and placental factors that influence the maternal assessment of fetal activity?**

Placental location, the length of fetal movements, the amniotic fluid volume, and fetal anomalies.

○ **What placental location is associated with decreased perception of fetal movements?**

Anterior.

○ **What types of anomalies are associated with decreased activity?**

CNS anomalies and neuromuscular disorders.

○ **What maternal factors influence the evaluation of fetal movement?**

Maternal activity, **obesity**, and medications.

○ **Which position do mothers appear to appreciate fetal movements best?**

Left lateral recumbent position.

○ **Which maternal medications depress fetal movement?**

Narcotics and barbiturates.

○ **What is a CST?**

Response of fetal heart rate (FHR) to uterine contractions. Relies on the premise that fetal oxygenation will be compromised or worsened by uterine contractions.

○ **How should the CST be performed?**

The patient is placed in the semi-Fowler's position at a 30- to 45-degree angle with a slight left tilt to avoid the supine hypotensive syndrome. FHR is recorded and uterine contractions are monitored. Maternal blood pressure is determined every 5 to 10 minutes to detect maternal hypotension. Baseline FHR and uterine tone are recorded for 10 to 20 minutes. A CST then requires uterine contractions of moderate intensity, either spontaneous or stimulated, lasting approximately 40 to 60 seconds with a frequency of three in 10 minutes.

○ **How can uterine activity be stimulated?**

Nipple stimulation or intravenous oxytocin.

○ **How is oxytocin administered for the CST?**

By an infusion pump at 0.5 mU/min. The infusion rate is doubled every 20 minutes until adequate uterine contractions are produced.

○ **What is the advantage of generating uterine contractions with nipple stimulation versus intravenous oxytocin administration?**

The CST can be completed in less time (on average, 30 minutes as opposed to 90 minutes). Also, an intravenous infusion is not required.

○ **How is nipple stimulation achieved for the CST?**

One of two methods may be utilized. The patient may apply a warm moist towel to each breast for 5 minutes. If uterine activity is not adequate, the patient is asked to massage one nipple for 10 minutes. A second method involves using intermittent nipple stimulation. The patient gently strokes the nipple of one breast with the palmer surface of her fingers through her clothes for 2 minutes and then stops for 5 minutes. The cycle is repeated only as needed to achieve adequate uterine activity.

○ **How long should a patient be monitored after the CST has been completed?**

The patient should be observed until uterine activity has returned to baseline.

○ **What are the contraindications to the CST?**

Patients at high risk of premature labor such as patients with premature rupture of membranes, multiple gestation, and cervical incompetence and those patients in which uterine contractions should be avoided such as placenta previa, previous classical cesarean section, or previous uterine surgery.

○ **How is a CST interpreted?**

According to the presence or absence of late FHR decelerations.
- *Negative CST*: No late or significant variable decelerations.
- *Positive CST*: Late decelerations following 50% or more of contractions.
- *Equivocal-suspicious*: Intermittent late decelerations or significant variable decelerations.
- *Equivocal-hyperstimulatory*: FHR decelerations that occur when contraction pattern is more frequent than every 2 minutes or lasting longer than 90 seconds.
- *Unsatisfactory*: Fewer than three contractions in 3 minutes or an uninterpretable tracing.

○ **What is the incidence of perinatal death within 1 week of a negative CST?**

0.4/1000.

○ **What is the likelihood of perinatal death after a positive CST?**

7 to 15%.

○ **Is a positive CST an indication for an elective cesarean section?**

No. A trial of labor can be attempted if the cervix is favorable for induction so that FHR monitoring and uterine contractility monitoring can be carefully assessed.

○ **When should a suspicious or equivocal CST be repeated?**

Within 24 hours.

○ **How is a NST performed?**

The patient is seated in a reclining chair and tilted to the left slightly with a Doppler ultrasound transducer monitoring the FHR and a tocodynamometer detecting uterine contractions.

○ **What defines a reactive NST?**

Presence of at least two accelerations of the FHR in 20 minutes of monitoring [15 beats per minute (bpm) by 15 seconds in ≥32 weeks and 10 bpm by 10 seconds in <32 weeks].

○ **What pathway is required for a healthy fetus to exhibit accelerations above the baseline FHR?**

An intact neurologic coupling between the CNS and the fetal heart.

○ **What fetal condition can disrupt this pathway?**

Fetal hypoxia, metabolic acidosis, or CNS anomalies.

○ **What is the most common cause of absent FHR accelerations?**

Fetal sleep state.

○ **What are the other causes for absence of FHR accelerations?**

CNS depressants such as narcotics and phenobarbital and beta-blockers such as propranolol and chronic smoking.

○ **If in 20 minutes of monitoring the NST is nonreactive, what is the next step?**

The test can be extended for an additional 20 minutes.

○ **If in 40 minutes of monitoring the NST continues to be nonreactive, what is the next step?**

A CST or BPP should be performed.

○ **When is the NST most predictive?**

When it is reactive.

○ **What is the perinatal mortality rate associated with a nonreactive NST?**

30 to 40/1000.

○ **What is the false-positive rate associated with a nonreactive NST?**

75 to 90%.

○ **What percentage of NSTs are nonreactive between 24 and 28 weeks' gestation?**

As high as 50%.

○ **What percentage of NSTs remain nonreactive between 28 and 32 weeks?**

15%.

○ **How can vibroacoustic stimulation be utilized during a NST?**

Used for a nonreactive tracing in order to promote fetal accelerations. Can decrease time required to obtain reactive tracing. It has no place in practice with the presence of concerning fetal decelerations.

○ **What is the false-negative rate of a reactive NST (ie, what is the incidence of stillbirth occurring within 1 week of a reactive NST)?**

1.9 per 1000.

○ **What is a BPP?**

It is the use of real-time ultrasonography to perform an in utero physical examination and evaluate dynamic functions reflecting the integrity of the fetal CNS, within a 30-minute period.

○ **What five parameters are assessed by the fetal BPP?**

- NST.
- Fetal movement.
- Fetal breathing movements.
- Fetal tone.
- Amniotic fluid volume.

○   **How are the various BPP parameters measured?**

The presence of each parameter is given a score of 2 and the absence of each parameter is assigned 0 points.

○   **What must be present in order to receive 2 points for tone on the BPP?**

One or more episodes of active extension/flexion of fetal limbs or spine, or an episode of opening and closing of fetal hand.

○   **What must be present in order to receive 2 points for fluid on the BPP?**

A cord and limb-free pocket of amniotic fluid measuring at least 2 × 2 cm.

○   **What must be present in order to receive 2 points for movement on the BPP?**

Three or more discrete episodes of gross body movements or movements of extremities.

○   **What must be present in order to receive 2 points for breathing on the BPP?**

One or more episode of rhythmic fetal breathing movements of 30 seconds or more.

○   **What components make up a modified BPP?**

NST and amniotic fluid index (AFI). Necessary test to perform for the complaint of "decreased fetal movement" in order to establish normal fluid volume.

○   **What is the false-positive rate of a well-performed BPP?**

As low as 20%.

○   **What is the false-negative rate of a BPP?**

0.8 per 1000 tests.

○   **What is the management of BPP scores?**

- *Score 8 to 10*: Normal.
- *Score 6*: Equivocal. In a term fetus should prompt delivery, whereas in preterm fetus the BPP should be repeated in 24 hours, and administration of steroids for lung maturity should be considered if <34 weeks.
- *Score 4*: Indicates delivery should be warranted; vaginal delivery acceptable if fetal tracing allows for it.
- *Score ≤4*: Indicates expeditious delivery usually by cesarean section.

○   **In the presence of risk factors, how often should the FHR be auscultated during the active phase of the first stage of labor?**

FHR should be evaluated and recorded at least every 15 minutes after a contraction.

○   **In the presence of risk factors, how often should the FHR be auscultated during the second stage of labor?**

FHR should be evaluated and recorded at least every 5 minutes.

○   **What does an external FHR monitor measure?**

Continuous Doppler detects cardiac valve closure.

○   **What is the largest increased risk associated with continuous electronic FHR monitoring?**

Increased cesarean section rate.

FETAL HEART RATE PATTERNS AND DEFINITIONS

○   **What is the baseline FHR?**

The mean FHR rounded to increments of 5 bpm during a 10-minute window. There must be at least 2 minutes of identifiable baseline segments. Normal baseline ranges from 110 to 160 bmp. Bradycardia when baseline is <110 bpm and tachycardia when baseline is >160 bpm.

○   **What is variability?**

Fluctuations in the baseline FHR that are irregular in amplitude and frequency. Quantified as the amplitude from peak to trough.

○   **What are the different degrees of variability?**

- *Absent*: Amplitude range undetectable.
- *Minimal*: Amplitude range 1 to 5 bpm.
- *Moderate*: Amplitude range 6 to 25 bpm.
- *Marked*: Amplitude range >25 bpm.

○   **What is an acceleration?**

Visually apparent abrupt increase in FHR. Onset of acceleration to peak >30 seconds. A prolonged acceleration is ≥2 minutes but <10 minutes long.

○   **What is a deceleration? And how are they classified?**

Visually apparent decrease in FHR. Decelerations are classified into early, variable, late, and prolonged decelerations.

○   **What is an early deceleration?**

Visually apparent, symmetrical, *gradual* decrease and return of FHR baseline associated with a uterine contraction. Cause: Fetal head compression

Characteristics:
- Onset to nadir ≥30 seconds.
- Nadir of deceleration occurs at the same time as the peak of the contractions.

○   **What is a variable deceleration?**

Visually apparent *abrupt* decrease in FHR. Cause: Umbilical cord compression

Characteristic:
- Onset to nadir <30 seconds.
- Decrease in FHR is ≥15 bpm, lasting >15 seconds and >2 minutes in duration.

○ **What is a late deceleration?**

Visually apparent, usually symmetrical and *gradual* decrease and return of FHR. Cause: Uteroplacental insufficiency

Characteristics:

- Deceleration is delayed in timing with respect to the contraction; nadir of decelerations occurs after peak of contraction.
- Onset to nadir ≥30 seconds.

○ **What is a prolonged deceleration?**

Visually apparent decrease in FHR that lasts ≥2 minutes but >10 minutes.

○ **What are recurrent decelerations?**

When they occur with ≥50% of contractions in any 20-minute window.

○ **What are periodic decelerations?**

Decelerations associated with contractions.

○ **What are episodic decelerations?**

Decelerations not associated with contractions.

○ **How are uterine contractions quantified?**

- Number of contractions in a 10-minute window, averaged over 30 minutes.
  - *Normal*: ≤5 contractions in 10 minutes, averaged over 30 minutes.
  - *Tachysystole*: >5 contractions in 10 minutes, averaged over 30 minutes.

○ **What defines a FHR Category I tracing?**

Includes all the following:

- *Baseline heart rate*: 110 to 160 bpm.
- *Variability*: Moderate.
- *Accelerations*: Present or absent.
- *Early decelerations*: Present or absent.
- *Late or variable decelerations*: Absent.

○ **What defines a FHR Category II tracing?**

Includes all FHR tracings not categorized as Category I or III:

- Baseline:
  - Bradycardia not accompanied by absent variability
  - Tachycardia
- Variability:
  - Minimal
  - Absent variability not accompanied by recurrent decelerations
  - Marked variability
- Accelerations:
  - Absent

- Decelerations:
  - Recurrent variable decelerations plus minimal or moderate variability
  - Prolonged decelerations
  - Recurrent late decelerations with moderate variability

○ **What defines a FHR Category III tracing?**

- Absent variability plus any of the following:
  - Recurrent late or variable decelerations
  - Bradycardia
  Or
- Sinusoidal pattern (visually apparent, smooth, sine wavelike undulating pattern in FHR baseline that persists for >20 minutes)

○ **Fetal scalp stimulation is used to improve?**

Variability, and adequate response represents a nonacidotic fetus.

○ **What are the advantages of an internal scalp electrode monitor?**

Fetal variability is more apparent, easier to continuously follow FHR despite movement of fetus or mother, and decreased chance of inadvertently monitoring maternal pulse instead of FHR.

○ **What are the disadvantages of an internal scalp electrode monitor?**

Necessity of rupture of membranes for placement and a slightly increased risk of fetal infection or scalp hematoma. Risk of vertical transmission of infections.

○ **In what maternal conditions should application of a fetal scalp electrode be avoided?**

Hepatitis B and HIV infection.

○ **What are the potential causes of a sinusoidal FHR pattern?**

Maternal-fetal hemorrhage, Rh isoimmunization, and fetal hypoxia, often resulting from severe chronic fetal anemia, or administration of narcotic drugs to the mother.

○ **What are the potential causes of fetal tachycardia?**

Maternal fever, chorioamnionitis, fetal anemia, illicit drug use, congenital heart disease, sympathomimetic drugs (ie, terbutaline), fetal hypoxia, and acidosis.

○ **What are the potential causes of fetal bradycardia?**

Acute cord compression or prolapse, rapid descent of the fetal head in labor, uterine hyperstimulation, maternal hypotension, congenital heart block, inadvertent monitoring of maternal pulse, uterine dehiscence, severe fetal hypoxia, and placental abruption.

○ **What are the potential causes of decreased variability?**

Fetal sleep cycle, hypoxia, narcotics, CNS anomalies, and magnesium sulfate.

○   **What maneuvers should be performed for intrauterine resuscitation with late decelerations?**

Administer oxygen via face mask.

Change maternal position to lateral decubitus to minimize supine hypotension and improve uterine blood flow.

Correct hypotension if present.

Stop oxytocin infusion.

Consider terbutaline, especially in presence of uterine hyperstimulation.

Validate fetal well-being with scalp stimulation.

○   **What is the mechanism of supine hypotension?**

Uterine compression of the inferior vena cava leads to decreased return of blood to the heart (preload), decreasing maternal cardiac output, causing maternal hypotension and decreased uterine blood flow.

○   **What does this fetal heat rate monitoring tracing represent?**

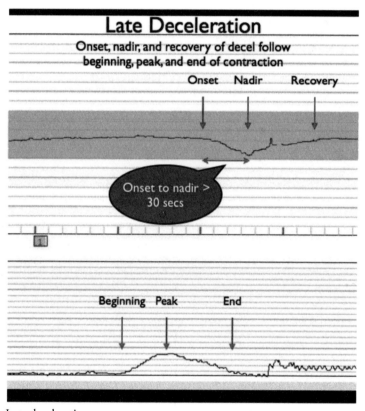

Late deceleration.

○   **What does this fetal heat rate monitoring tracing represent?**

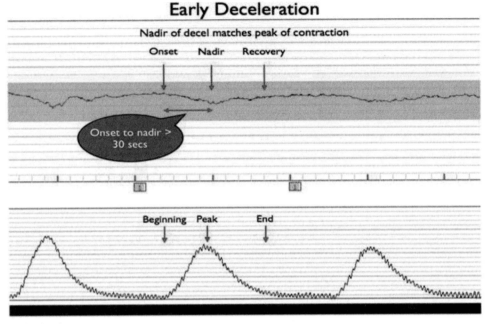

Early deceleration.

BIBLIOGRAPHY

1. American College of Obstetricians and Gynecologists. *Antepartum Fetal Surveillance.* ACOG Practice Bulletin 9, October 1999.
2. American College of Obstetricians and Gynecologists. *Intrapartum Fetal Heart Rate Monitoring: Nomenclature, Interpretation and General Management Principles.* ACOG Practice Bulletin 106, July 2009.
3. Macones G, Hankins G, Spong C, Hauth J, Moore T. The 2008 NICHD workshop report on electronic fetal monitoring: update on definitions, interpretation and research guidelines. Green Journal 2008;112(3):661–666.
4. Frederickson HL, Wilkins-Haug L, eds. *Ob/Gyn Secrets.* 2nd ed. Philadelphia, PA: Hanley & Belfus, Inc.; 1997.
5. Creasy RK. *Creasy & Resnik's Maternal-Fetal Medicine Principles and Practice.* 6th ed. Philadelphia, PA: Saunders Elsevier; 2009.

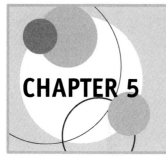

CHAPTER 5 Labor and Delivery

Frank J. Craparo, MD

○ **What is the definition of labor?**

Labor is defined with the initiation of regular and rhythmic contractions that result in serial dilatation and effacement of the cervix.

○ **How many stages of labor exist?**

Labor is traditionally divided into three stages and some consider there to be a fourth stage.

○ **What is the definition of the first stage of labor?**

The first stage of labor is defined as the onset of regular contractions that result in cervical change. This stage ends when the cervix is fully dilated.

○ **What is the definition of the second stage of labor?**

The second stage of labor is defined from the time of full dilatation of the cervix until delivery of the infant.

○ **What is the definition of the third stage of labor?**

The third stage of labor begins with delivery of the infant and ends with the delivery of the placenta.

○ **Is there a fourth stage of labor?**

Some consider the 1 to 2 hours time period after delivery of the placenta to be the fourth stage. This is not part of the traditional description of labor.

○ **What is a common complication of this "fourth stage"?**

This is a time when postpartum hemorrhage is most likely to occur.

○ **What is the latent phase of labor?**

The latent phase of labor is the initiation of contractions with slow cervical change that continues until accelerated cervical change occurs.

○   **Is there a time difference in the latent phase for nulliparous versus multiparous patients?**

In the nulliparous patient, the average latent phase is 6.4 hours. In the multiparous patient, the average is 4.8 hours.

○   **What is the definition of the active phase of labor?**

The active phase of labor is defined as when the expected phase of maximal slope has been accomplished. The majority of patients (90%) are in this phase when they are approximately 5 cm dilated.

○   **What is the average cervical change during the active phase for a nulliparous patient?**

The expected cervical dilatation in the nulliparous patient is ≥1.2 cm/h.

○   **What is the average cervical change for a multiparous patient?**

The expected cervical change in a multiparous patient in the active phase of labor is 1.5 cm/hour.

○   **What is the average length of time pushing for a multiparous patient?**

The multiparous patient usually pushes for no >1 hour. However, this may be extended to 2 hours if there is regional anesthesia.

○   **What is the average length of time pushing for a nulliparous patient?**

The average time may last up to 2 hours in the nulliparous patient or extended to 3 hours if the patient has had regional anesthesia.

○   **What is the definition of precipitous labor?**

Traditionally, this is defined as labor resulting in delivery in <3 hours. In a nulliparous patient, labor is also considered precipitous if the cervical dilatation is >5 cm/h.

○   **What is "failure to progress"?**

"Failure to progress" is defined as labor not resulting in cervical dilatation or descent of the fetus.

○   **What is cephalopelvic disproportion?**

Cephalopelvic disproportion is the difference in the dimensions of the fetal head and the maternal pelvis resulting in obstruction of labor.

○   **What is protracted labor?**

Protracted labor can be the result of protracted dilatation or protracted descent. Protracted dilatation is progress <1.2 cm/h in a nulliparous patient and <1.5 cm/h in a multiparous patient. Protracted descent is defined as descent <1 cm/h in a nulliparous patient or <2 cm in the multiparous patient.

○   **What is the Bishop score?**

The Bishop score is a description of the cervix to help evaluate "ripeness."

○   **How is the Bishop score defined?**

There are five parts to the Bishop score including dilatation, effacement, station, consistency, and the position of the cervix in the pelvis.

○ **What is considered a favorable Bishop score?**

≥9.

○ **What is considered an unfavorable Bishop score?**

Four or less is considered unfavorable.

○ **How are dilatation and effacement defined?**

Dilatation is defined in centimeters. Effacement is defined in percentages and refers to the thinning of the cervix.

○ **How frequently is the fetus vertex at term?**

95% of all patients at term present as vertex.

○ **What do the cardinal mechanisms of labor refer to?**

They refer to the changes in the position of the fetal head as it passes though the birth canal.

○ **Why does the fetal head need to change position at this time?**

These changes are needed secondary to the asymmetric shape of the fetal head and maternal bony pelvis.

○ **How are these changes accomplished?**

The changes occur as the result of the propulsive forces of uterine activity during labor.

○ **How many changes occur during the cardinal movements?**

Seven.

○ **Name the cardinal movements of labor.**

Engagement, descent, flexion, internal rotation, extension, external rotation, and expulsion.

○ **How is engagement defined?**

Engagement occurs when the descent of the biparietal diameter (BPD) is below the level of the pelvic inlet.

○ **What is the average distance between the pelvic inlet and the ischial spines?**

The average distance is 5 cm.

○ **When does the greatest rate of descent occur?**

It most often occurs during the deceleration phase of the first stage of labor and during the second stage of labor.

○ **How does flexion usually occur?**

Flexion usually occurs as a passive motion.

○ **Approximately what percentage of pregnant patients have factors that can be identified prenatally that place the patient at increased risk?**

Approximately 20% of patients have identifiable risk factors.

○ **Of the patients identified with risk factors, how many of these will result in a poor outcome?**

Twenty percent of patients identified with risk factors may account for >50% of poor outcomes.

○ **What percentage of patients are identified with risk factors when they present in labor?**

An additional 5% to 10% will be identified at this time.

○ **How many of these will result in poor outcomes?**

These patients account for approximately 20% to 25% of poor outcomes.

○ **What percentage of patients with a poor outcome have no identifiable risk factors?**

20%.

○ **What are the goals of assisted spontaneous deliveries?**

Assisted spontaneous deliveries should result in decreased maternal trauma and decreased fetal injury.

○ **What are the "proposed advantages" of routine episiotomy?**

The "proposed advantages" include easier repair of a surgical incision, reduction in the second stage of labor, and reduction in trauma to the pelvic floor musculature.

○ **What are the "proposed disadvantages" to episiotomy?**

The "proposed disadvantages" include increased blood loss, increased maternal pain and unnecessary surgical incision.

○ **What are the four types of the pelvic shapes?**

Gynecoid, anthropoid, android, and platypelloid.

○ **What are Leopold maneuvers?**

Palpation of the uterus to determine fetal lie and position.

○ **What is the definition of prolonged latent phase?**

The latent phase is defined as prolonged if this period lasts >20 hours in a nulliparous patient or >14 hours in a multiparous patient.

○ **What is the most common treatment of prolonged latent phase of labor?**

Maternal rest.

○ **What percentage of patients will proceed to active labor following maternal rest?**

Approximately 85% will proceed to active labor and approximately 10% will stop having contractions.

○ **How is dysfunctional labor defined?**

Dysfunctional labor is defined when the active phase of dilatation is in the <5th percentile.

○ **What is the <5th percentile for nulliparous patients?**

<.2 cm/h.

○ **What is the <5th percentile for multiparous patients?**

<1.5 cm/h.

○ **What is the definition of the secondary arrest of labor?**

It is defined as lack of cervical change for 2 hours following normal dilatation.

○ **What are the most common units used to describe uterine activity?**

Montevideo units, a uterine activity unit.

○ **How are these units defined?**

Montevideo units refer to the strength of contractions in mm of mercury multiplied by the frequency per 10 minutes. The uterine activity unit is defined as 1 mmHg/min.

○ **When is oxytocin indicated?**

When uterine activity is <50 mgHg every 3 minutes or <200 Montevideo units.

○ **What is the duration (half-life) of intravenous oxytocin?**

The half-life is 3 to 4 minutes.

○ **Name a maternal systemic effect of oxytocin.**

Antidiuresis.

○ **An anthropoid pelvis is often associated with what presentation?**

Occipitoposterior.

○ **An android pelvis is often associated with?**

Deep transverse arrests.

○ **A transverse presentation is frequently seen with which pelvis type.**

Platypelloid.

○ **What percentage of women have a gynecoid pelvis?**

Approximately 50% making this the most common pelvis type.

○ **The critical distance of the anterior-posterior diameter of the pelvis is?**

10 cm.

○ **The uterus receives what percentage of cardiac output at term?**

Approximately 10%.

○ **What is the average blood flow to the uterus at term?**

Approximately 600 mL/min.

○ **Name the principal prostaglandins produced by the amnion and the decidua.**

The principal prostaglandin of the amnion is PGE2. The principal prostaglandin produced by the decidua is PGF2alpha.

○ **When the fetal vertex enters the pelvis, and what is the most common position?**

Left occiput transverse.

○ **In what percentage of pregnancies are there a nuchal cord?**

10% to 25%.

○ **After delivery, signs of placental separation may include?**

A gush of blood, lengthening of the umbilical cord, and anterior-cephalad movement of the uterine fundus.

○ **What are the classifications that describe the changes that occur with placental separation?**

Latent phase, contraction phase, detachment phase, and expulsion phase.

○ **What is the definition of the latent phase of placental separation?**

The latent phase is defined as from the time of delivery until the initiation of contractions leading to separation.

○ **Describe the contraction phase of normal placental separation.**

Contraction at the placental site myometrium.

○ **What occurs during the detachment phase?**

As the result of contraction of the myometrial insertion site, the placenta is sheared off the uterus.

○ **How is the expulsion phase defined?**

The phase is defined as when the placenta is extruded from the uterus into the vagina.

○ **What is the average length of the third stage of labor?**

<10 minutes, 90% within <15 minutes, and 97% within 30 minutes.

○ **What complication is associated with increase in duration of the third stage of labor?**

Postpartum hemorrhage.

○ **Name the two approaches for the management of the third stage of labor.**

Expectant and active.

○ **Expectant management is defined as?**

Spontaneous delivery of the placenta without the use of pharmacologic agents or physical traction of the cord.

○ **Components of the active management of the third stage of labor include?**

Early clamping of the umbilical cord, placing traction of the cord, manual massage of the uterus, and the use of pharmacologic agents.

○ **Name two of the more commonly used pharmacologic agents used in the active management of the third stage.**

Oxytocin and ergot alkaloids.

○ **Oxytocin may be administered by what routes?**

Intravenous and intramuscular.

○ **Ergot alkaloid agents should not be used in women with these?**

Hypertension, a history of migraines, a history of Raynaud phenomenon.

○ **What is the definition of retained placenta?**

Retained placenta is one that has not been expelled with 30 to 60 minutes after delivery of the infant.

○ **What is the incidence of retained placenta?**

0.5% to 1.0%.

CHAPTER 6

Operative Obstetrics Pearls

Richard A. Latta, MD

○ **What type of needle tip should be used to close the fascia of a Pfannenstiel skin incision?**

Taper needles. Cutting needles or reverse cutting needles increase the risk of pull through. Blunt needles are used for friable tissues.

○ **What tissues are disrupted in a first-degree laceration?**

This is defined as superficial laceration of the vaginal mucosa or perinatal body not requiring suturing.

○ **What tissues are involved in a second-degree laceration or episiotomy?**

This involves the vaginal mucosa and perineal skin and deeper subcutaneous tissue and requires suturing.

○ **Define a fourth-degree laceration.**

This involves extension of an episiotomy or laceration into the rectal mucosa.

○ **True or False: Episiotomy increases the risk of disruption of the rectal sphincter.**

True.

○ **Myonecrosis of the deep fascia is most often associated with infection by which organism?**

Clostridium perfringens.

○   **What type of locking devices is shown with the forceps in the figure?**

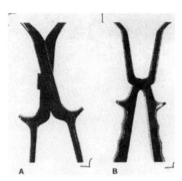

    A. Kielland forceps with a sliding lock

    B. Simpson forceps with a fixed English lock

○   **Modern forceps were developed by this family in England (that maintained forceps as their family secret until the late 18th Century).**

The Chamberlen family.

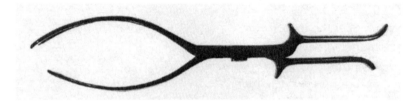

○   **What type of forceps is shown above?**

Kielland forceps.

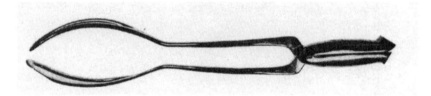

○   **The forceps demonstrated above is utilized for delivery in what situation?**

Breech.

○   **What is the name of the forceps from the last question?**

Piper forceps.

○   **How would you describe a delivery from a +2 station with a 35-degree rotation?**

Low forceps, nonrotational delivery.

○ **How would you describe a forceps delivery with a sagittal suture in the anteroposterior diameter with the fetal scalp visible at the introitus?**

Outlet forceps.

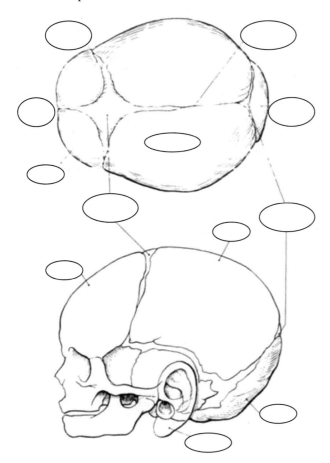

○   **Label the structures on the associated figure.**

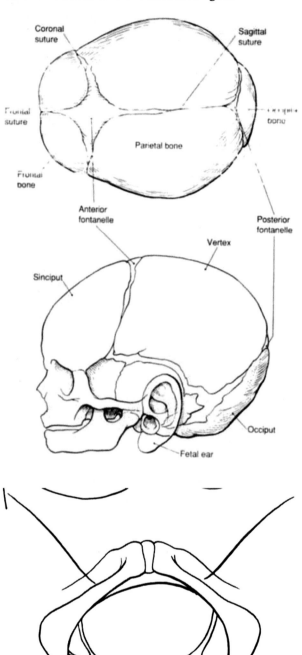

○ **Describe the presentation of the fetus in figure above.**

Left occiput transverse with anterior asynclitism.

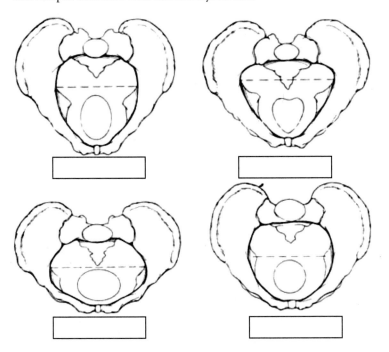

○ **Label the pelvis types noted above.**

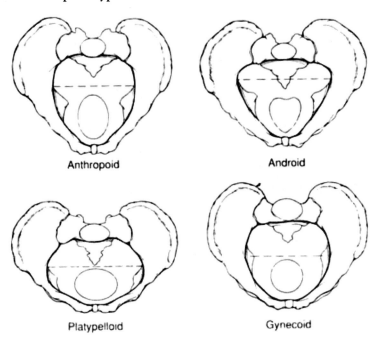

Anthropoid

Android

Platypelloid

Gynecoid

○ **What are the common contraindications to cervical cerclage?**

Active bleeding, premature labor, ruptured membranes, chorioamnionitis, hydramnios, or confident diagnosis of a lethal fetal anomaly.

○ **What are the common intrapartum complications associated with cervical cerclage placement?**

Cervical lacerations occurring in 3 to 13% of patients, and cervical stenosis secondary to scarring in approximately 5% of patients.

○ **What type of cervical cerclage is currently the most common?**

McDonald.

○ **What cervical cerclage involves the dissection of the anterior cervicovaginal mucosa just distal to the bladder refection?**

Shirodkar.

○ **Define cervical incompetence.**

A repetitive, acute, painless, second trimester evacuation of the uterus without associated bleeding or contractions.

○ **How does the stroma of the cervix differ from the uterine corpus?**

There is a relative lack of smooth muscle compared with the amount of collagenous and elastic tissue.

○ **Specify at least one indication for cervical cone biopsy during pregnancy.**

Suspected microinvasion on colposcopy or colposcopy directed biopsy, or persistent cytologic evidence of invasive disease not explained by colposcopy or cervical biopsy or adenocarcinoma in situ.

○ **What is the current maternal mortality associated with legal abortion in the United States?**

<1 in 100,000.

○ **Osmotic dilators used for dilating the cervix prior to abortion include laminaria tents. What are laminaria tents derived from?**

Dried seaweed of the Japonicum species.

○ **What four complications almost equally contribute to the mortality related to legal abortion?**

Embolism, infection, hemorrhage, and anesthesia.

○ **What is the reported incidence of uterine perforation at abortion?**

0.2 per 100. However, the real incidence may be higher because of asymptomatic and unsuspected perforations.

○ **What are the two most common causes of post abortal hemorrhage?**

Uterine hypotonus and retained products of conception.

○ **What is the treatment of post abortal bleeding if uterine atony is suspected to be the cause?**

General uterine massage and parenteral uterotonics (oxytocin, methylergonovine, and 15-methylprostaglandin F2 alpha).

○ **What combination of medications is approved for the use of "medical abortion" in the United States?**

A combination of mifepristone (RU-486) and misoprostol.

○ **True or False: The FDA-approved combination of mifepristone and misoprotol has an efficacy of approximately 92% in women with pregnancies up to 49 days of gestation.**

True.

○ **The majority of midtrimester abortions are performed in the United States by what technique?**

Dilation and evacuation.

○ **What is the safest method for termination of pregnancy in terms of mortality and morbidity between 13 and 16 weeks' gestation?**

Dilation and evacuation.

○ **Of the procedures curettage, D&E, instillation procedures, and hysterotomy, what procedure is associated with the highest case fatality rate?**

Hysterotomy.

○ **At what gestational age, should elective repeat cesarean delivery be performed?**

American college of obstetrics and gynecology(ACOG) recommends elective delivery at or beyond 39 weeks with the following criteria met: (1) normal menstrual cycles; (2) no recent oral contraceptive use; (3) one of the following: fetal heart tones auscultated by 10 menstrual weeks, positive pregnancy test by 4 menstrual weeks, and ultrasound confirming menstrual dates prior to 20 weeks' gestation.

○ **What is the most frequent indication for primary cesarean delivery in the United States?**

Labor dystocia.

○ **What are the three common uterine incisions utilized to perform a cesarean delivery?**

Low transverse, low vertical, and classical.

○ **What is the most common abdominal operation performed in the United States?**

Cesarean delivery.

○ **List the ACOG practice bulletin indications for operative vaginal (there are four indications).**

- Prolonged second stage for a nulliparous woman: Lack of continuing progress for 3 hours with regional anesthesia, or 2 hours without regional anesthesia.
- Prolonged second state for a multiparous woman: Lack of continuing progress for 2 hours with regional anesthesia, or 1 hour without regional anesthesia.
- Suspicion of immediate or potential fetal compromise.
- Shortening of the second stage for maternal benefit.

○ **True or False: In 1988, ACOG redefined the classification of station and types of forceps deliveries. The revised classification uses the level of the leading bony point of the fetal head in centimeters at or below the level of the maternal ischial spines to define station (0–5 cm), instead of the previously used method of describing the birth canal in terms of thirds (0–3+).**

True

○ **The definition of midforceps is?**

Station is above +2 cm but head is engaged.

○ **True or False: According to the ACOG practice bulletin, vacuum extractors are designed to limit the amount of traction on the fetal skull because detachment can occur. Nevertheless, traction achieved with vacuum extraction is substantial (up to 50 lb) and can result in significant fetal injury if misused.**

True.

○ **The two FDA recommendations for the use of the vacuum device that rocking movements or torque should not be applied to the device; only steady traction in the line of the birth canal should be used and clinicians caring for the neonate should be alerted that a vacuum device has been used so that they can adequately monitor the neonate for the signs and symptoms of device-related injuries.**

True.

○ **According to the ACOG practice bulletin, the lowest rate of neonatal intracranial hemorrhage is associated with: Vacuum delivery alone, cesarean delivery with labor, cesarean delivery without labor, or forceps delivery alone.**

Cesarean delivery without labor.

○ **True or False: Ophthalmologic screening should be performed in all vacuum and forceps deliveries.**

False.

○ **According to the ACOG practice bulletin, the lowest rate of neonatal death is associated with: Vacuum delivery alone, cesarean delivery with labor, cesarean delivery without labor, or forceps delivery alone.**

Vacuum delivery alone.

○ **True or False: The vacuum extractor is associated with an increased incidence of complications including neonatal cephalohematoma, facial nerve palsy, retinal hemorrhages, and jaundice when compared with forceps delivery.**

False. Neonatal cephalohematoma, retinal hemorrhages, and jaundice are greater with the vacuum extractor but facial nerve palsy is increased with forceps delivery.

○ **True or False: Assuming that there is adequate operator experience, both forceps and vacuum extractors are acceptable and safe instruments for operative vaginal delivery.**

True.

○ **The definition of nonrotational low forceps requires (two-part answer)?**

Leading point of fetal skull is at station ≥+2 cm and rotation is 45 degree or less.

○ **The single greatest risk factor for third- or fourth-degree lacerations is?**

The performance of a median episiotomy.

○ **True or False: Episiotomy has been identified as an independent risk factor for dyspareunia or delayed return to sexual activity when compared with equally severe perineal trauma in women who did not have an episiotomy.**

False.

○ **True or False: Restricted use of episiotomy is preferable to routine use of episiotomy.**

True.

○ **True or False: Mediolateral episiotomy is associated with higher rates of injury to the anal sphincter and rectum than is median episiotomy.**

False.

○ **True or False: Currently the major known benefit of routine episiotomy helps to prevent pelvic floor damage leading to incontinence.**

False.

○ **True or False: To avoid anal sphincter or rectal injury, mediolateral episiotomy is superior to median episiotomy.**

True.

○ **True or False: According to the ACOG practice bulletin, the fetal benefits of episiotomy include cranial protection, especially for premature infants, reduced perinatal asphyxia, less fetal distress, and better Apgar scores.**

False. *None* of the above are benefits of episiotomy.

○ **True or False: Operative vaginal delivery is contraindicated if the fetus is known to have osteogenesis imperfecta.**

True.

○ **True or False: Operative vaginal delivery is contraindicated if the fetus is known to occiput posterior.**

False.

○ **True or False: Operative vaginal delivery is contraindicated if the fetus is known to have alloimmune thrombocytopenia.**

True.

○ **True or False: Operative vaginal delivery is contraindicated if the fetus is known to have von Willebrand disease.**

True.

○ **True or False: Comparing fetuses delivered by cesarean delivery during labor versus fetuses delivered by cesarean delivery after attempted vacuum or forceps the relative risk of intracranial hemorrhage is approximately three times greater.**

True.

○ **True or False: The American and Gynecologist practice bulletin would consider patients with two previous low transverse cesareans and no prior vaginal deliveries to be a candidate for vaginal birth after cesarean delivery College of Obstetricians.**

True.

○ **The rate of uterine rupture for a classical uterine incision is approximately?**

4% to 9%.

○ **The rate of uterine rupture for a T-shaped uterine incision is approximately?**

4% to 9%.

○ **The rate of uterine rupture for a low vertical uterine incision is approximately?**

1% to 7%. There is limited available data; health-care providers and patients may choose to proceed with TOLAC in the presence of a documented prior low vertical uterine incision.

○ **The rate of uterine rupture for a low transverse uterine incision is approximately?**

0.5% to 0.9%.

○ **True or False: Patients with pregnancies complicated by known HIV infection should be counseled that vertical transmission to the fetus is ~2%with zidovudine and scheduled cesarean delivery.**

True.

○ **True or False: Patients with pregnancies complicated by known HIV infection should be counseled that vertical transmission to the fetus is approximately 2% among women with viral loads <1000 copies/mL, even without systematic use of scheduled cesarean delivery.**

True.

○ **Placenta accreta has increased __ fold in the last 10 years.**

10-fold.

○ **Risk factors for placenta accreta include?**

(1) Prior cesarean delivery.

(2) Placenta previa.

(3) Prior myomectomy.

(4) Asherman syndrome.

(5) Submucous leiomyomata.

(6) Maternal age >35.

○ **What is the term used for the tendency of suture material to return to its original shape after deformation, for example, tying?**

Memory.

○ **What is the term used for a suture's tendency to return to original form after stretching?**

Elasticity.

○ **What are the three surgical needle types that are currently available?**

Swaged, controlled release ("pop-off"), and open.

○ **Of the forceps (pickups) dressing, tissue, or Russian, which may be utilized to grab the needle?**

None. Although occasional use of the forceps to grab a needle is of little consequence, none of these should be used for grasping the needle.

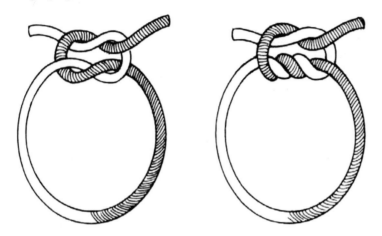

○ **Name the types of knots pictured.**

A is a square knot and B is a surgeon's square knot (2 = 1).

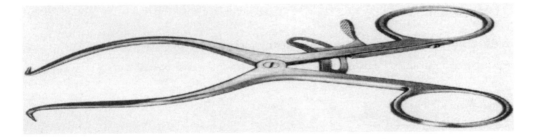

○ **What is the name of this self-retaining perineal retractor that may be utilized to provide retraction for repair of vaginal tears?**

Gelpi.

○ **What is the National Research Council's classification of surgical wounds for a cesarean delivery in labor?**

Contaminated.

○ **What is the name of the maneuver utilized to control the fetal breech head where the obstetrician applies the index finger and middle finger of one hand over the maxilla, with two fingers of the other hand hooked over the fetal neck and grasping the fetal shoulders?**

Mauriceau-Smellie-Viet maneuver.

○ **The Pinard maneuver is sometimes utilized in the case of a frank breech. Describe the maneuver.**

The obstetrician's fingers are kept parallel to the femur. Pressure is placed in the popliteal fossa, resulting in flexion of the fetal knee.

○ **Entrapment of the fetal head is potentially life threatening to a breech delivery. Describe a surgical correction of this problem.**

Duhrssen incision. The technique involves two or three incisions in the cervix at the 2, 6, and 10 o'clock positions.

○ **Of frank breech, complete breech, or footling breech, which presentation has the highest frequency of umbilical cord prolapse?**

Footling breech; 15% to 18%.

○ **True or False: Congenital anomalies are two to three times greater with a fetus in the breech presentation compared with the cephalic presentation.**

True.

○ **In approximately what percentage of twin deliveries are both twins cephalic/cephalic?**

40%.

○ **What is the approximate incidence of shoulder dystocia?**

0.6% to 1.4% of vertex deliveries, although there is a wide variation in the definition and methods of reporting.

○ **List at least three interpartum risk factors for shoulder dystocia.**

(1) First-stage labor abnormalities, including protraction disorders or arrest disorders.

(2) Prolonged second stage of labor.

(3) Oxytocin augmentation of labor.

(4) Midforceps and midvacuum delivery.

○ **What is the approximate incidence of shoulder dystocia in a patient with diabetes mellitus and a fetus >4500 g birth weight?**

50%.

○ **Name at least three antepartum risk factors for shoulder dystocia.**

(1) Fetal macrosomia.

(2) Maternal obesity.

(3) Diabetes mellitus.

(4) Post term pregnancy.

(5) Male gender.

(6) Advanced maternal age.

(7) Excessive weight gain.

(8) Prior shoulder dystocia.

(9) Platypoid pelvis or contracted pelvis.

(10) Prior macrosomic infant.

○ **What is the first necessity in the management of shoulder dystocia?**

Additional help is summoned, including anesthesia and pediatrics.

○ **What is the name of the maneuver in which the legs are sharply flexed upon the abdomen in an attempt to relieve shoulder dystocia?**

McRoberts maneuver.

○ **What is a common iatrogenic risk factor for the development of puerperal hematomas?**

Episiotomy, predominantly left medial lateral.

○ **True or False: A history of shoulder dystocia is associated with an increased recurrence rate but the studies vary widely in risk, ranging from 1% to 16.7%.**

True.

○ **True or False: Fundal pressure may further worsen impaction of the shoulder during a shoulder dystocia and also may result in uterine rupture.**

True.

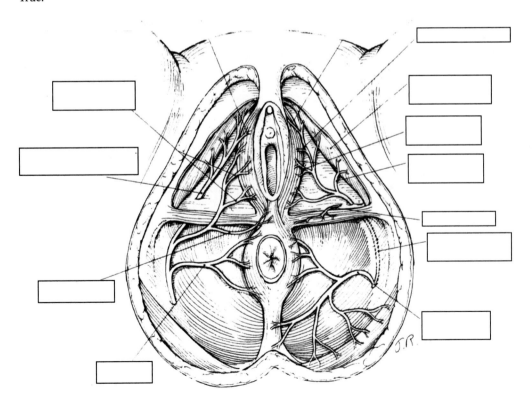

○   **Label the structures of the pelvis.**

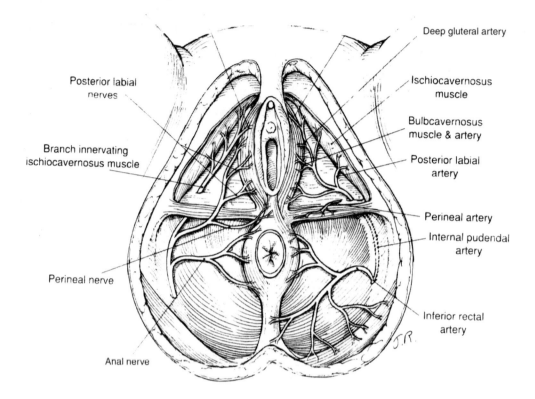

○   **What are the blood vessels most commonly injured during vulvar hematomas?**

Branches of the pudendal artery: Inferior rectal, transverse perinatal, and posterior labial arteries.

○   **In patients with placenta previa in the current pregnancy, the risk of accreta is approximately __% for those undergoing their third cesarean deliveries**

40%.

○   **What is the most frequent cause of serious postpartum hemorrhage?**

Uterine atony.

○   **In the management of postpartum uterine atony, fundal compression has not stopped the bleeding. At what dose, would you request oxytocin to be begun?**

Oxytocin, up to 40 units per liter, with rapid infusion.

○   **Several surgical techniques are available to control bleeding during a cesarean delivery including (4):**

(1) Hypogastric artery ligation.

(2) Bilateral uterine artery ligation (O'Leary sutures).

(3) B-Lynch technique.

(4) Hysterectomy.

○ **What are the common contraindications and relative contraindications to routine newborn circumcision?**

Low birth weight, <2500 g, bleeding abnormalities, family history of bleeding disorder not ruled out in the infant, infection, unstable infant, hypospadias and other genitourinary abnormalities, abnormal body temperature, and abnormal feeding.

○ **True or False: Recommendation of American Academy of Pediatrics is that the existing evidence is insufficient to recommend routine neonatal circumcision.**

True.

○ **What is the name of this device used for circumcision?**

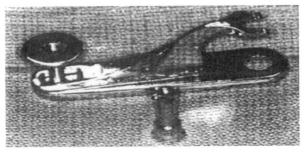

Gomco.

○ **What is the name of this device used for circumcision?**

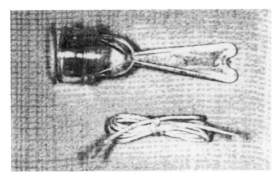

Plastibell.

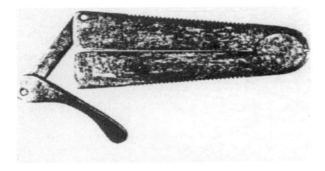

○ **What is the name of this device used for circumcision?**

Mogan.

CHAPTER 7 Multiple Gestations

Chelsea Ward, MD

○ **What percentage of all pregnancies are twins and higher order multiple gestations?**

3.3% of all live births in the United States, about 3% worldwide.

○ **How has the incidence of multiple gestations changed?**

At least 65% increase in twins and 500% increase in triplets and higher order births since 1980.

○ **What is the risk of multiple gestation with infertility treatments?**

Up to 25% assisted reproductive technology (ART) pregnancies result in multiples.

○ **What is the incidence of multiple pregnancies with the use of clomiphene citrate?**

8% with <1% triplets or higher order gestations.

○ **What is the incidence of multiple pregnancies with the use of gonadotropin therapy?**

25% with approximately 1% to 2% triplets or higher order gestations.

○ **What percentage of multiple infants births from ART represent triplets or higher order gestations?**

4% to 5% of all live births.

○ **What are the different etiologies of multiple fetuses?**

Fertilization of two separate ova (dizygotic, 70%) or from a single fertilized ovum that subsequently divides (monozygotic, 30%).

○ **What is superfecundation?**

Fertilization of two ova within a short period of time but not at the same coitus, nor necessarily the sperm from the same male.

○ **What is the difference between chimera and mosaicism?**

Chimera: Individual whose cells originated from more than on fertilized ovum

Mosaicism: Two or more cell lines from different chromosomal composition arise from the same zygote as a consequence of nondisjunction

○ **How does the timing of division of the fertilized ovum affect monozygotic twins?**

≤3 days after fertilization: Diamniotic, dichorionic

4 to 8 days: Diamniotic, monochorionic

8 to 13 days: Monoamniotic, monochorionic

13 days: Conjoined twins

○ **How does examination of the placenta aid in the determination of zygosity of like-sex twins?**

Evaluation of the amnion(s) and chorion(s).

○ **Other than opposite sex, what is the most predictive way to diagnose mono versus dichorionic gestations via ultrasound?**

Membrane character and thickness.

Dichorionic: The dividing membrane is >2 mm with 3 to 4 layers identified and a "twin peak" sign seen on ultrasound, where the chorion attaches to the amnion

Monochorionic: The dividing membrane is <2 mm and "hair-like" with only two layers and a "T" sign is noted where the chorion and amnion attach

○ **What type of monozygotic twinning is most common?**

Monochorionic–diamniotic.

○ **Which type of twinning has the highest morbidity?**

Monoamniotic–monochorionic.

○ **Which type of twin placenta is at highest risk of vascular communications?**

Monochorionic.

○ **What is the perinatal mortality rate of dichorionic-monoamniotic twins?**

25%.

○ **What is the mortality rate of mono-mono twins?**

50% to 60%.

○ **What is the recommended method of delivery for mono-mono twins?**

Cesarean delivery.

○ **What is the biggest mortality risk to mono-mono twins?**

Cord entanglement.

○ **After what gestational age does cord entanglement mortality become significantly reduced?**

32 weeks.

○ **What physiologic effects can occur in twins affected with twin-to-twin transfusion syndrome?**

Donor twin: Underperfused, anemic, growth restricted, microcardiac, hypotensive, and develops oligohydramnios.
Recipient twin: Overperfused, polycythemic, hypertensive, and develops polyhydramnios.

○ **What are the stages of twin-to-twin transfusion syndrome?**

Stage 1: Donor twin bladder still visible, fetal Doppler values normal
Stage 2: Donor twin bladder no longer visible, fetal Doppler values normal
Stage 3: Donor twin bladder no longer visible, fetal Doppler values critically abnormal
Stage 4: Presence of hydrops
Stage 5: Intrauterine death of one or both fetuses

○ **What is the prognosis of twin-to-twin transfusion syndrome?**

The earlier in gestation it develops the worse the prognosis. If diagnosed before approximately 28 weeks mortality is 60% to 80%.

○ **What antenatal factors predict a poor outcome in pregnancies with twin-to-twin transfusion syndrome?**

Early gestation at time of diagnosis, severe polyhydramnios requiring multiple therapeutic amniocenteses, hydrops or absent or reversed end-diastolic flow.

○ **What is an arteriovenous shunt?**

The most important anastomosis in twin-to-twin transfusion syndrome: A cotyledon is fed by the artery of one twin and drained by the vein of the other twin.

○ **How does the incidence of twinning affected by age?**

Increases with maternal age.

○ **The incidence of twins peak at what age?**

35 to 40 years of age.

○ **What maternal changes are more frequently observed with multiple gestations?**

(1) Anemia often develops secondary to a greater demand of iron from the fetuses
(2) Respiratory tidal volume is increased, but women pregnant with twins often feel "breathless," possibly secondary to a higher progesterone level
(3) Marked uterine distension and increased pressure on adjacent viscera.
(4) Theca-lutein cysts forms more frequently during multiple gestations as a result of higher levels of chorionic gonadotropin
(5) Urinary tract infection is at least twice as common

○   **Has bed rest been shown to reduce the risk of preterm delivery in twins?**
No.

○   **Should maternal dietary intake change in multifetal pregnancies?**
Maternal dietary intake should increase by approximately 300 kcal above that for singleton gestations.

○   **What is the recommended weight gain for women carrying twins?**
35 to 45 pound total weight gain at term.

○   **What complications of multiple gestations affect pregnancy outcome?**
   (1) Increased incidence of spontaneous abortion
   (2) Increased incidence of malformations
   (3) Intrauterine growth restriction
   (4) Increased incidence of preterm birth
   (5) Placenta previa is more frequently encountered because of large size of placenta or placentas
   (6) Gestational hypertension. The risk is increased three to four times more in multiple gestations than in single pregnancies
   (7) Gestational diabetes
   (8) Acute fatty liver
   (9) Pruritic urticarial papules and plaques of pregnancy (PUPPS)
   (10) Pulmonary embolus
   (11) Uterine atony
   (12) Abruption
   (13) Malpresentation

○   **What is the recommended gestational age to deliver twins?**
By 39 weeks.

○   **What is the most common cause of neonatal morbidity and mortality in twins?**
Preterm delivery.

○   **What percentage of twins are born preterm (before 37 weeks' gestation)?**
Almost 50% of twin gestations are born preterm.

○   **What is the mean duration of gestation in twins and triplets and quadruplets?**
Twins: 35 weeks, triplets: 32 weeks, and quadruplets: 29 weeks.

○   **What is the incidence of very premature delivery (before 32 weeks) in singletons, twins, and triplets?**
Singletons: 1.6%, twins: 12%, triplets: 36%.

○ **How much greater is the risk of cerebral palsy in twins and triplets compared with singletons?**

Increased by 4 times in twins and 17 times in triplets.

○ **How much greater is the perinatal death rate for twins compared with singletons?**

Three times greater for twins compared with singletons.

○ **How much greater is the perinatal death rate for monozygotic twins compared with dizygotic twins?**

2.5 times greater for monozygotic twins compared with dizygotic twins.

○ **If one twin dies, what complications can occur to the surviving twin?**

Recent evidence suggests that death or morbidity in the surviving twin is due to acute hypotension and partial exsanguination into the dying twin. The surviving twin can develop renal cortical necrosis, multicystic encephalomalacia, or disseminated intravascular coagulation.

○ **What percentage of twins are affected by intrauterine growth restriction?**

14 to 25%.

○ **What criteria are used to diagnose intrauterine growth restriction in twins?**

Estimated fetal weight below the 10% for a singleton gestation or when there is discordance of >20% between the twins.

○ **What antenatal monitoring should be done once intrauterine growth restriction has been diagnosed?**

Serial ultrasounds with umbilical artery Doppler velocimetry, twice-weekly nonstress tests with supplemental biophysical profiles. Early delivery should be considered if absent or reversed end-diastolic flow is discovered.

○ **What is the frequency of spontaneous reduction, or "vanishing twin"?**

Ultrasound findings show 36% of twins, 53% of triplets, and 65% of quadruplets.

○ **What is the most common clinical presentation for a vanishing twin?**

First-trimester bleeding.

○ **What is the pregnancy loss rate in multifetal reduction?**

Pregnancy loss rates range from 5% to 25% depending on the starting number of gestations.

○ **What gestational age is multifetal reduction performed?**

Multifetal reduction is performed around 10 to 12 weeks' gestational age.

○ **What percentage of twin-to-twin contamination occurs when chorionic villus sampling (CVS) is performed on a twin gestation?**

Approximately 5% of cases.

○ **What is the positive predictive value of routine cervical exams or sonographic cervical measurements in predicting preterm delivery?**

75%.

○ **Does fetal fibronectin have a predictive value in multiple gestations?**

Most studies show a high negative predictive value and fairly high positive predictive value.

○ **Do twins develop pulmonary maturity at the same rate as singletons?**

Twins appear to develop pulmonary maturity 3 to 4 weeks earlier than singletons.

○ **What are the two most common presentations of twins at the time of delivery?**

The most common presentation of twins at the time of delivery is vertex-vertex (approximately 40%) followed by vertex-breech (approximately 25%).

○ **How should vertex-vertex twins be delivered?**

Vaginal delivery is recommended.

○ **How should vertex-nonvertex twins be delivered?**

The delivery of vertex-nonvertex twins is controversial. Some data suggests that the Apgar scores are lower and perinatal complications are increased by vaginally delivering the second nonvertex twin.

○ **What are the vaginal delivery options for the vertex-breech delivery?**

Delivery options for second twin in a vertex-breech delivery include external cephalic version of the second breech twin or internal podalic version and breech extraction.

○ **How should a nonvertex-presenting twin be delivered?**

In general, cesarean delivery is the method of choice when the first twin is nonvertex.

○ **What is the minimum estimated fetal weight of a nonvertex second twin that you would consider attempting a vaginal delivery?**

>1500 g.

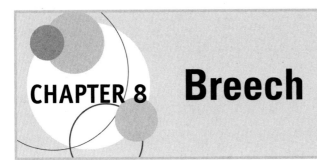

CHAPTER 8 Breech

Frank J. Craparo, MD

○ **How many types of breech presentations are there?**
Three

○ **Name the three types of breech presentations.**
Complete, incomplete, and frank.

○ **Complete breech presentation is defined as?**
Both hips and knees are flexed.

○ **Frank breech presentation is defined as?**
Both hips are flexed, knees are extended, and feet are adjacent to the fetal head.

○ **Incomplete breech presentation is defined as?**
One or both hips are NOT completely flexed.

○ **At term, the most common type of breech presentation is?**
Frank, 50% to 70%.

○ **The least common breech presentation at term is?**
Complete, 5% to 10%

○ **Label the type of breech presentations in the diagrams.**

(Figures reproduced, with permission from Cunningham FG et al. *Williams Obstetrics*, 22nd ed. New York: McGraw-Hill, 2005, pp. 566–567.)

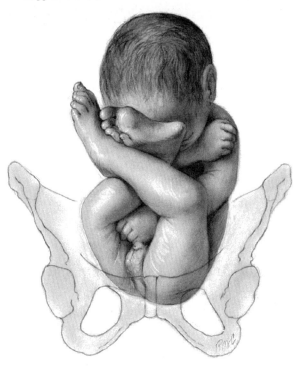

Frank breech

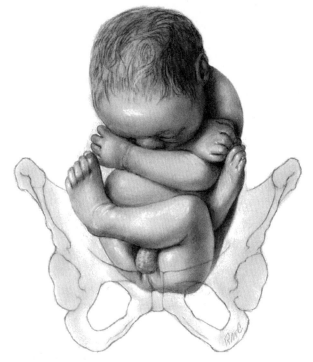

Complete breech

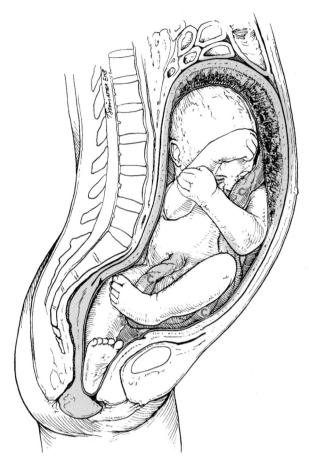

Footling breech

○ **Fetal risks associated with breech presentations include?**

Cord compression and dystocia

○ **A breech presentation is noted during a routine anatomy ultrasound performed at 18 weeks' gestation. What is the risk that the fetus will be breech at term?**

3% to 4%.

○ **Ultrasound performed at 36 weeks' gestation demonstrates a breech presentation. The chance of spontaneous version to cephalic is?**

25%.

○ **Name four risk factors or breech presentation.**

Preterm, abnormal uterine contour or volume, altered fetal shape, and impaired fetal mobility.

○ **Examples of altered intrauterine contour or volume include?**

- Uterine abnormalities.
- Fibroids.

Placental abnormalities

- Multiparty.
- Abnormal fluid levels, both oligo and polyhydramnios.

○ **Factors associated with altered fetal mobility include?**

Multiple gestation, neurologic impairment, short umbilical cord, and fetal asphyxia.

○ **Uterine/fetal abnormalities are associated with what % of breech presentations?**

<15%.

○ **What percentage of infants with breech presentation will have congenital anomalies?**

6% to 18% (whereas vertex presentation is 2–3%).

○ **If a patient's first pregnancy was a term breech, is there an increased risk in future pregnancies?**

Yes. 9% in next pregnancy, >20% if two breech presentations, >30% if three consecutive breech presentations.

○ **True or False: Perinatal mortality and morbidity is higher in breech presentation compared to cephalic presentation.**

True.

○ **Optimal conditions for a planned vaginal breech delivery include?**

- No prior C/S.
- No contraindications to vaginal delivery, i.e., placenta previa.
- Estimated fetal weight >2000 to 2500 g, but < 4000 g.
- Gestational age >36 weeks.
- Fetal head is not hyperextend.
- Frank or complete breech.
- Spontaneous labor.

○ **True or False: Incomplete breech presentation is not a contraindication to attempt vaginal delivery.**

False.

○ **Describe the three ways to deliver a breech vaginally.**

Spontaneous—infant is delivered without traction or manipulation.

Assisted breech extraction—infant is delivered spontaneously to the umbilicus with the rest of the body being extracted.

Total breech extraction—entire body of the infant is extracted.

○ **What is the best indicator of pelvic adequacy for a breech delivery?**

Satisfactory progression of labor.

○ **What is the only indication of total breech extraction?**

Total breech extraction should be used only for a noncephalic second twin.

○ **Total breech extraction is associated with an injury rate in what percent for a singleton breech?**

The injury rate is 25%.

○ **What is the mortality rate associated with total breech extraction of a singleton breech?**

The mortality rate is approximately 10%.

○ **Describe the steps for a frank breech delivery.**
- Episiotomy is generally performed.
- Spontaneous delivery of posterior hip, delivery of anterior hip, and delivery of legs.
- Fetal bony pelvis is grasped with both hands using a towel (with fingers resting on superior iliac crest and thumbs on the sacrum).
- Apply gentle downward traction until scapulas are visible.
- Once one axilla is visible, the anterior shoulder and arm should be delivered.
- Rotate trunk to deliver other shoulder and arm.
- The fetal head is then delivered by maintaining flexion with suprapubic pressure provided by an assistant with simultaneous pressure on the maxilla by the operator.

○ **Staffing for an assisted vaginal breech delivery should include?**

An obstetrician with an assistant, an anesthesiologist, and a pediatrician.

○ **The maneuver where the index and middle finder are placed over the maxilla to flex the head is termed?**

Mauriceau-Smellie-Veit maneuver.

○ **If the Mauriceau maneuver cannot be easily accomplished, what type of forceps can be applied?**

Piper forceps.

○ **This complication of the fetal head can occur during a vaginal breech delivery?**

Head entrapment (88/1000), head circumference is greater than abdominal or thoracic circumference at about 36 weeks.

○ **If head entrapment is encountered, these two maneuvers can be performed to facilitate delivery?**

(1) Duhrssen incisions.
(2) Abdominal rescue.

○ **Describe why and how to perform Duhrssen incisions.**

If attempts to slip the cervix over the entrapped head are unsuccessful, cervical incisions are made at 2, 6, and 10 o'clock.

○ **What are the two most common complications of Duhrssen incisions?**

Maternal hemorrhage and extension into the lower uterine segment.

○ **Hyperextended heads are noted in what percentage of breech fetuses that are present in labors?**

3% to 5%.

○ **When there is hyperextension of the head, what is the risk of spinal cord injury?**

21%.

○ **Describe the Prague maneuver?**

The Prague maneuver is performed by using two fingers of one hand to grasp the shoulders of the back-down fetus, the other hand is then used to draws the feet up out of the abdomen.

○ **When is the indication of Prague performed?**

It is used when the fetal trunk fails to rotate anteriorly.

○ **What is the Pinard maneuver?**

The Pinard maneuver is used with frank breech presentations to deliver a foot into the vagina or through the uterine incision during cesarean delivery.

○ **What is the reason to delay performing artificial rupture of membranes (AROM) during vaginal breech deliveries?**

Intact membranes may decrease the risk of cord prolapse and may also assist in the dilation of the cervix.

○ **Name the types of breech presentation with the lowest rate and with the highest risk for cord prolapsed.**

(1) Lowest incidence: Frank breech (0.5%).

(2) Highest incidence: Footling breech (10%).

○ **A nuchal arm is defined as?**

When either one or both fetal arms are around the fetal neck.

○ **Describe three maneuvers to facilitate delivery when a nuchal arm is present.**

(1) Two fingers are placed over the humerus and are then used to sweep the arm over the chest; the humerus should be splinted with the operator's fingers in an effort to reduce the risk of fracture.

(2) The fetus may be rotated 180 degrees, so that elbow is drawn toward the face, allowing delivery of the arm.

(3) The arm can be forcibly extracted by hooking a finger over the arm; however, this is associated with an increase risk of fracture of humerus/clavicle.

○ **Name tree common maternal complications associated with vaginal breech delivery.**

Infection (secondary to intrauterine maneuvers).

Cervical laceration.

Perineal tears and/or extension of episiotomy.

○ **What are some common fetal complications associated with a vaginal breech delivery?**

Fracture of either the humerus or clavicle.

Skull fractures.

Paralysis of the arm.

Testicular injury.

Increased risk of sudden infant death syndrome.

○ **Name a condition when a vaginal breech delivery of a singleton should be considered.**

A patient presents in active labor, with advanced cervical dilation and delivery appears.

○ **True or False: Planned cesarean section is the recommended mode of delivery for a persistent breech presentation.**

True.

○ **In the United States, the percentage of breech presentations who are delivered by u cesarean section?**

90%.

○ **Required conditions to consider for external cephalic version (ECV)? (New)**

- Breech presentation.
- Reassuring fetal heart tracing.
- No contraindications for vaginal delivery.
- ≥36 weeks' gestation.

○ **What is the most favorable factor associated with successful ECV?**

Parity.

○ **Factors associated with an unsuccessful version include?**

- Diminished amniotic fluid.
- Obesity.
- Anterior placenta.
- Cervical dilation.
- Descent of breech into the pelvis.
- Positioning of the fetal spine.

○ **Name three absolute contraindications for ECV.**

- Contraindications to vaginal delivery, ie, previa.
- Multiple gestations with a breech presenting fetus.
- Nonreassuring fetal status.

○ **Relative contraindications for ECV include?**

- Abnormal fluid, both poly and oligohydramnios.
- Fetal growth restriction.
- Fetal anomaly.

○ **Common reasons to discontinue ECV include?**
- Maternal discomfort.
- Persistent abnormal fetal heart rate.
- Multiple failed attempts.

○ **Is D-immune globulin indicated for a D-negative unsensitized woman after attempted version?**
Yes.

○ **Is regional anesthesia required for attempted ECV?**
There is insufficient evidence to require the use of regional anesthesia during ECV.

○ **What test is performed after ECV, whether or not it was successful?**
Non stress test (NST).

○ **What are possible complications associated with attempted ECV?**
- Placental abruption.
- Uterine rupture.
- Fetal distress.
- Fetomaternal hemorrhage.

○ **What is the quoted overall success rate of ECV?**
58%.

○ **What is the average cesarean delivery rate among those undergoing an attempted version?**
37%.

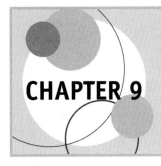

CHAPTER 9

Postdates Pregnancy and Fetal Demise

Kuhali Kundu, DO and
Stephen J. Smith, MD

○ **Define post-term pregnancy.**

A pregnancy that has extended to or surpassed 42 weeks of gestation or 294 days from the first day of the last menstrual period.

○ **Name the most common cause of post-term pregnancy.**

Error in dating the pregnancy accurately.

○ **What is Naegele Rule?**

A method used to calculate the estimated date of confinement. Using the date of the first day of the last menstrual period as the starting point, subtract 3 months and then add 7 days.

○ **During which trimester is pregnancy dating most accurate?**

First trimester.

○ **What is the margin of error for an ultrasound evaluation of pregnancy dating based on gestational age?**

The margin of error can be:
- ± 7 days up to 20 weeks of gestation.
- ± 14 days between 20–30 weeks of gestation.
- ± 21 days beyond 30 weeks.

○ **What is the incidence of post-term pregnancy?**

Approximately 5 to 10%.

○   **List the risk factors for post-term pregnancy.**

Primiparity.

Prior post-term delivery with increasing risk with each subsequent post-term delivery.

Fetal anencephaly.

X-Linked placental sulfatase deficiency.

Fetal male gender.

Prepregnancy BMI ≥25.

Adrenal hypoplasia.

Recurrence across generations.

○   **List the fetal risks associated with post-term pregnancy.**

Increased perinatal mortality (approx twice the risk compared to term).

Uteroplacental insufficiency leading to oligohydramnios and intrauterine growth restriction.

Meconium aspiration.

Intrauterine infection.

Macrosomia.

Postmaturity syndrome.

Increased risk of death within 1 year of life.

Increased neonatal intensive care unit admissions.

Neonatal seizures.

○   **What is the cause of postmaturity syndrome?**

Skin changes are due to loss of the protective effects of vernix caseosa.

Placental senescence and placental apoptosis.

Decreased fetal oxygenation as evident by increased cord blood erythropoietin levels in post-term pregnancy

Oligohydramnios.

Fetal growth restriction.

○   **What is the incidence of postmaturity syndrome in post-term pregnancy?**

Approximately 10% between 41 and 43 weeks.

Increases to 33% at 44 weeks.

○   **Describe the appearance of the infant with dysmaturity syndrome.**

Dry and wrinkled, parchment-like skin with desquamation.

Wasted, malnourished appearance with long, thin arms.

Meconium staining in some cases.

Long nails.

Sparse or absent lanugo.

Increased alertness with "wide-eyed" look.

○ **What intrapartum and neonatal complications are observed in the infant with postmature syndrome?**

Intrapartum: Umbilical cord compression from oligohydramnios.

Meconium aspiration.

Nonreassuring fetal heart tracing.

Neonatal: Hypoglycemia.

Seizures.

Respiratory insufficiency.

○ **What fetal heart rate tracing patterns are concerning for oligohydramnios leading to intrapartum fetal distress in post-term pregnancies?**

Prolonged decelerations.

Variable decelerations.

Saltatory baseline (oscillations exceeding 20 bpm).

○ **List the maternal complications associated with post-term pregnancy.**

Labor dystocia.

Perineal injury.

Cesarean delivery.

These complications are due to the higher risk of macrosomia.

○ **What maternal complications are seen with higher frequency following cesarean section versus vaginal delivery?**

Endometritis.

Hemorrhage.

Thromboembolism.

○ **What form of antenatal surveillance may be used to assess the post-term fetus?**

Options include: Nonstress test.

Biophysical profile.

Modified biophysical profile.

Contraction stress test.

No single method has been shown to be superior, but an assessment of amniotic fluid volume should be incorporated into the surveillance scheme.

○ **What are the components of the biophysical profile?**

Nonstress test with ultrasound assessment of gross fetal body movements, fetal tone, fetal breathing, and amniotic fluid volume.

○ **What is the modified biophysical profile?**

Nonstress test plus amniotic fluid volume estimation.

○ **What are the criteria for oligohydramnios requiring delivery in the post-term pregnancy?**

Amniotic fluid index <5 cm

OR

Largest vertical pocket of amniotic fluid <2 × 2 cm

○ **What is the most reasonable management plan for the patient with a favorable cervix at 42 weeks' gestation?**

Induction and delivery.

○ **In the patient with an unfavorable cervix, what are the potential benefits to labor induction at 41 to 42 weeks' gestation versus continued expectant management?**

Lower perinatal mortality rate.

Reduced risk of meconium-stained fluid.

Higher patient satisfaction.

○ **The intrapartum fetal heart rate tracing of a patient at 42 weeks' gestation is shown below. What intrapartum complication does this tracing suggest?**

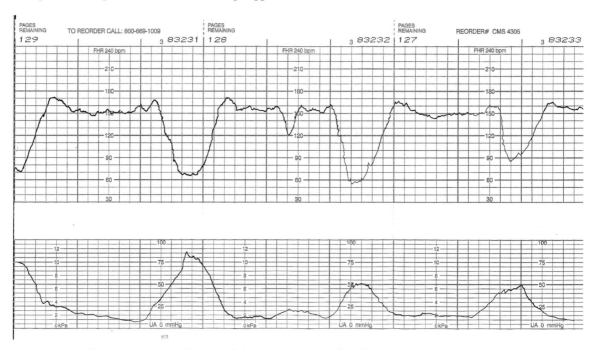

Recurrent variable decelerations indicative of oligohydramnios and umbilical cord compression.

○ **The nonstress test shown below was performed on a patient at 41 weeks' gestation. The amniotic fluid index was 10 cm. Her cervix is uninducible. What are the options for management?**

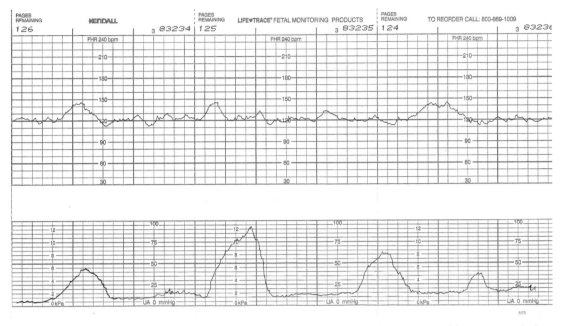

This is a reactive nonstress test in a patient with normal amniotic fluid volume. Reasonable options include continued expectant management or induction of labor.

○ **What risk factors are associated with stillbirth?**

Non-Hispanic black race

Nulliparity

Advanced maternal age

Obesity

Maternal medical disorders such as hypertension, diabetes, lupus, renal disease

Smoking

Multiple gestation

Preeclampsia

○ **What are causes for stillbirth?**

Fetal growth restriction

Placental abruption

Chromosomal/genetic abnormalities

Infection such as CMV, listeria, parvovirus, syphilis, malaria

Cord events

○   **What are the most important tests in the evaluation of stillbirth?**

Autopsy

Pathology evaluation of the placenta

Karyotype evaluation

○   **True or False: Since 1990, the rate of stillbirth in the United States has decreased?**

True

○   **Antepartum fetal surveillance is performed routinely in the patient with a history of stillbirth in a prior pregnancy. What is the primary risk of this strategy?**

The 1–2% risk of iatrogenic prematurity due to false-positive test results.

○   **In the low risk patient with a prior unexplained stillbirth, what is the risk for recurrent stillbirth?**

Less than 1%.

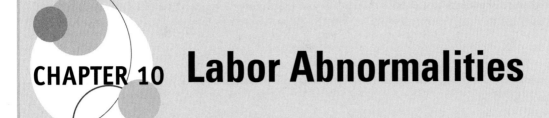

CHAPTER 10 Labor Abnormalities

Stephen J. Smith, MD and
Amanda M. Rhodes, MD

○ **What is the definition of labor?**

The presence of uterine contractions of sufficient intensity, frequency, and duration to cause effacement and dilation of the cervix.

○ **What is the definition of labor dystocia?**

Abnormal labor resulting from abnormalities in "power, passenger, or passage."

○ **In the United States, the most common indication of primary cesarean delivery is?**

Arrest of first or second stage of labor.

○ **Many repeat cesarean deliveries are performed after primary cesarean delivery for labor arrest in the first or second stage. Taking this fact into account, what percentage of all cesarean deliveries performed in the United States are attributable to the diagnosis of dystocia?**

25–55%.

○ **What is one of the most important steps in active management of patients that has been found to increase the rate of successful vaginal delivery and decrease the cesarean delivery rate?**

Delaying admission until active labor is established.

○ **According to the data by Friedman, latent phase is considered prolonged if?**

It exceeds 20 hours in nulliparas or 14 hours in multiparas.

○ **According to the contemporary data by Zhang, the active phase begins when the cervix is?**

6 cm. dilated.

○ **Management of choice for prolonged latent phase is?**

Therapeutic rest induced with morphine.

○   **What percentage of patients treated with therapeutic rest for prolonged latent phase will progress to active phase?**

85%.

○   **List the risk factors for protraction and arrest disorders in the first stage of labor.**

Advanced maternal age.

Diabetes.

Hypertension.

Oligohydramnios.

Previous perinatal death.

Premature rupture of the membranes.

Chorioamnionitis.

Macrosomia.

Epidural anesthesia.

Pelvic contractures.

Nonreassuring fetal heart rate pattern.

○   **List the risk factors for arrest in the second stage of labor.**

Occiput posterior presentation.

Prolonged first stage of labor.

Epidural analgesia.

Nulliparity.

Short maternal stature.

Increased maternal body mass index.

Macrosomia.

High station at complete cervical dilation.

○   **Is amniotomy beneficial for the patient with prolonged latent phase?**

Amniotomy can shorten the latent phase of labor if used with active management of labor protocols. One meta-analysis found that it shortened the first stage by up to 39 minutes.

○   **Describe the effect of amniotomy (performed during the active phase) on labor duration, maternal fever, cesarean delivery, and nonreassuring fetal heart rate patterns.**

Labor duration: Reduction by 1 to 2 hours.

Maternal fever: Increased incidence.

Cesarean delivery: No effect.

Nonreassuring fetal heart rate patterns: No effect.

○   **According to Friedman's original data, the lower limit (5th percentile) for rate of cervical dilation in the active phase is?**

1.2 cm per hour in nulliparas and 1.5 cm per hour in multiparas. The most recent research by Zhang suggests that these limits may no longer be valid and that labor may be longer than these numbers indicate.

○ **Complete the table, indicating the criteria for second-stage arrest in nulliparas and multiparas.**

	No Regional Anesthesia	**Regional Anesthesia**
Nullipara	_____ hours	_____ hours
Multipara	_____ hours	_____ hours

	No Regional Anesthesia	**Regional Anesthesia**
Nullipara	__3__ hours	__4__ hours
Multipara	__2__ hour	__3__ hours

○ **The most commonly used unit of uterine activity is?**

The Montevideo unit.

○ **A Montevideo unit is defined as?**

Peak of contractions in millimeters of mercury minus baseline uterine pressure multiplied by the frequency of contractions per 10-minute period.

○ **Can Montevideo units be calculated based on the contractions depicted from the traditional external tocodynamometry?**

No. The external monitoring can determine length and frequency of contractions, but not their strength. An intrauterine pressure catheter must be used to calculate Montevideo units, and can be placed after rupture of membranes has occurred.

○ **Traditionally, what two criteria must be met to diagnose an arrest disorder in the first stage of labor?**

(1) At least 6 cm dilated.

(2) Uterine contraction pattern exceeding 200 Montevideo units for at least 4 hours without cervical change calculated using an intrauterine pressure catheter.

○ **True or False: In making the diagnosis of active phase arrest, 4 hours of sustained uterine contractions without cervical change may be more appropriate than the traditional "2-hour rule."**

True.

○ **Are the cut-off time as listed above for second-stage arrest absolute?**

No. If the fetal heart tracings are reassuring, there have been no excess findings of neonatal morbidity associated with a prolonged second stage. If there is steady progress, there is no need to conform to these cut-offs.

○ **With that in mind, after how many hours in the second stage has it been shown that the chance of vaginal delivery significantly decreases while maternal morbidity increases?**

4 hours. The incidence of vaginal delivery with a second stage <2 hours is 99%, 2 to 4 hours is 91%, and >4 hours is only 66%.

○ **Treatment of active phase arrest includes?**

Amniotomy and/or oxytocin augmentation.

○ **Minimally effective uterine activity is defined as?**

Three contractions per 10 minutes of at least 25 mm of mercury above baseline or a contraction pattern exceeding 200 Montevideo units per 10-minute window without cervical change.

○ **Tachysystole is defined as?**

More than 5 contractions in 10 minutes, averaged over a 30-minute window.

○ **What is oxytocin?**

A peptide hormone made in the hypothalamus and released from the posterior pituitary in a pulsatile manner.

○ **What is the mechanism of action of oxytocin?**

On binding to its receptor, phospholipase C is activated. This increases intracellular calcium by stimulating the release of intracellular calcium and by initiating influx of extracellular calcium.

○ **Mean plasma half-life of oxytocin is?**

3 to 4 minutes, but shorter when high doses are infused.

○ **The interval to reach a steady-state concentration of oxytocin in plasma is approximately?**

24 minutes.

○ **True or False: X-ray pelvimetry is generally considered of little value in the treatment of active phase arrest.**

True.

○ **Maximal dose of oxytocin is generally considered to be?**

30 to 40 mU/min.

○ **In patients with documented disorders of labor, what percentage responds to oxytocin infusion resulting in a vaginal delivery?**

80%.

○   **Calculate the Montevideo units for the 10-minute window in this illustration (round to the nearest 50). Assume an internal pressure transducer is being used.**

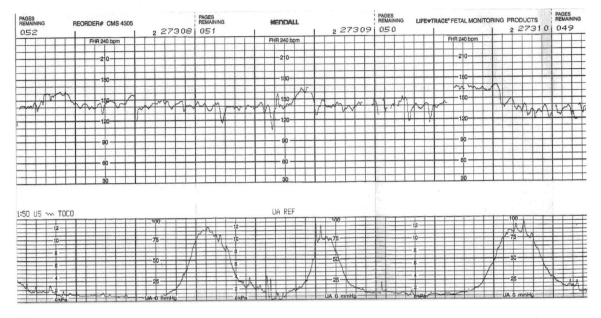

250.

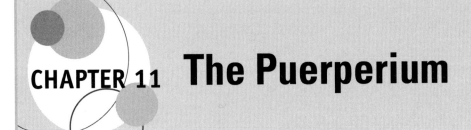

CHAPTER 11 The Puerperium

Cari Brown, MD

○ **Define the puerperium.**

The period that extends from delivery of the placenta to 6 weeks postpartum.

○ **How many weeks does it take for the uterus to regain its nonpregnant size?**

The uterus regains its nonpregnant size about 4 weeks after delivery.

○ **What is the process called by which the uterus shrinks to its nonpregnant size?**

Involution.

○ **What is the term used to describe the arrest of the normal process of uterine involution?**

Subinvolution. Subinvolution is recognized on exam by the presence of a uterus that is larger and softer than normal for the particular postpartum time. It is usually associated with irregular or excessive uterine bleeding.

○ **What are the two most common causes of subinvolution?**

Retained placental fragments and uterine infection.

○ **What is the typical size of the placenta, and what is the typical size of the implantation site following delivery of the placenta?**

The typical placenta has a diameter of 18 cm, and the placental implantation site is 9 cm in diameter after delivery of the placenta.

○ **What is the definition of puerperal fever?**

Temperature ≥100.4°F on any two of the first 10 postpartum days, exclusive of the first 24 hours.

○ **What are the risk factors for postpartum uterine infection?**

Mode of delivery, prolonged rupture of membranes, multiple cervical exams, prolonged labor, internal fetal monitoring, intra-amniotic infection, lower socioeconomic class, vaginal colonization with Group B streptococcus, *Chlamydia*, *Mycoplasma*, *Ureaplasma*, and *Gardnerella*.

○ **True or False: Postpartum uterine infection is usually caused by a single organism.**
False.

○ **What organism most commonly causes late onset postpartum metritis?**
Chlamydia.

○ **What are the clinical signs of postpartum uterine infection?**
Fever, fundal tenderness, tachycardia, foul-smelling lochia, and elevated white blood count of 15,000 to 30,000.

○ **What is the incidence of bacteremia associated with post cesarean uterine infection?**
10% to 20%.

○ **List the organisms most commonly causing postpartum uterine infection.**
Aerobes:
   Enterococcus.
   Staphylococcus aureus.
   Group A, B, D streptococci.
   Gram-negative bacteria—*Escherichia coli, Klebsiella, Proteus.*
Anaerobes:
   Peptococcus species.
   Peptostreptococcus species.
   Bacteroides species.
   Clostridium species.
   Fusobacterium species.
Other:
   Mycoplasma.
   Gonorrhea.
   Chlamydia trachomatis.

○ **What are the risk factors for post cesarean section wound infection?**
Obesity, diabetes, corticosteroid therapy, immunosuppression, anemia, wound hematoma, and uterine infection.

○ **What is the treatment of wound infection?**
Antibiotics and surgical drainage.

○ **What is necrotizing fasciitis?**
A rare complication of wound infection involving the deep soft tissues, including muscle and fascia.

○ **What are the risk factors for necrotizing fasciitis?**
Diabetes, obesity, intravenous drug use, age >50, hypertension, malnutrition, malignancy, cirrhosis, and peripheral vascular disease.

○ **True or False: Wound infection resulting in necrotizing fasciitis is usually monobacterial.**

False. Usually polymicrobial, caused by the anaerobes and aerobes listed in Question 8. If monobacterial, usually a result of Group A beta-hemolytic streptococcus.

○ **Name five common extrapelvic causes of puerperal fever.**

Atelectasis, pneumonia, pyelonephritis, breast engorgement, and thrombophlebitis.

○ **In a woman with post cesarean wound infection, what is the most common presenting symptom, and how many days after cesarean section does the symptom usually occur?**

Fever on postoperative, day 4.

○ **List complications of postpartum uterine infection that result in persistent fever.**

Wound infection, peritonitis, pelvic abscess, parametrial phlegmon, pelvic hematoma, septic pelvic thrombophlebitis, and antibiotic-resistant bacteria.

○ **How long after delivery does ovarian abscess complicating postpartum uterine infection usually present?**

1 to 2 weeks.

○ **True or False: Ovarian abscess complicating postpartum uterine infection is usually bilateral.**

False.

○ **What is the parametrial phlegmon?**

An area of induration in the broad ligament resulting from parametrial cellulitis and postpartum metritis.

○ **What is the approximate incidence of wound infection following cesarean section?**

3% to 15%

○ **True or False: Enigmatic fever is associated with postpartum septic thrombophlebitis.**

True.

○ **What is the one constant clinical characteristic of enigmatic fever?**

Hectic fever spikes following initial response to antimicrobial treatment of postpartum pelvic infection.

○ **What are the clinical features of ovarian vein thrombosis?**

Lower abdominal or flank pain on postpartum day 2 to 3, possible fever, and possible palpable tender adnexal mass.

○ **What is the incidence of episiotomy infection or breakdown after vaginal delivery?**

<1%.

○ **What is the primary cause of episiotomy breakdown?**

Infection.

○   **What are the three most common symptoms of episiotomy infection?**

Pain, purulent discharge, and fever.

○   **How is episiotomy infection treated?**

Open and drain wound and broad-spectrum antibiotics.

○   **True or False: Vulvar hematomas most commonly result from injury to the branches of a descending uterine artery.**

False. Pudendal artery.

○   **What is the most common presenting symptom of vulvar hematoma?**

Pain.

○   **True or False: Surgical drainage is the best treatment of a 3 cm nonexpanding hematoma in a patient experiencing a mild degree of pain.**

False. Expectant management is appropriate.

○   **What is the definition of primary postpartum hemorrhage?**

Postpartum hemorrhage occurring within 24 hours of delivery.

○   **What is the most common cause of primary postpartum hemorrhage?**

80% of cases are due to uterine atony.

○   **What other etiologies should be considered in primary postpartum hemorrhage not responsive to uterine massage, expelling of clots, and medical management?**

Retained placenta, placenta accreta, coagulation deficits, uterine inversion, and lower genital tract laceration.

○   **What are common risk factors for primary postpartum hemorrhage?**

Prolonged labor, augmented labor, rapid labor, history of postpartum hemorrhage, preeclampsia, operative delivery, chorioamnionitis, and uterine distention (ie, twin gestation, macrosomic infant, and polyhydramnios).

○   **What are options for medical management of postpartum hemorrhage?**

Oxytocin, Methergine, Hemabate, Dinoprostone, or Cytotec.

○   **In the event of failure of medical management, what steps can be taken for a patient experiencing postpartum hemorrhage?**

Examination in operating room for lacerations or uterine inversion, dilation and evacuation of retained placenta, placement of an O'Leary stitch (uterine artery ligation), B-lynch suture, or a Bakri balloon can also be used to achieve hemostasis. Analysis for coagulopathy should additionally be considered.

○   **What is the definition of secondary postpartum hemorrhage?**

Postpartum hemorrhage occurring >24 hours and <6 to 12 weeks after delivery.

○ **What are the three main causes of secondary postpartum hemorrhage?**

Abnormal involution of the placenta site, retained placenta, and uterine infection.

○ **True or False: For late postpartum hemorrhage, uterine curettage is the initial treatment of choice.**

False. Curettage is reserved for failed medical management.

○ **True or False: Breastfeeding is contraindicated in women with HIV infection due to the risk of transmission.**

True. The frequency of breast milk transmission is estimated to be 15% to 20%; thus, breastfeeding is contraindicated in situations where formula is available and can be reconstituted with water safe for the infant's consumption.

○ **True or False: Breastfeeding is contraindicated in hepatitis B.**

False. Breastfeeding is not contraindicated if hepatitis B immune globulin and vaccine are given to the infants of seropositive mothers.

○ **True or False: Breastfeeding is contraindicated in the mother with active herpes simplex virus.**

False. Breastfeeding is appropriate if there are no breast lesions and the mother is meticulous about hand washing before handling the infant and breastfeeding.

○ **True or False: Weight loss compromises a woman's ability to supply her infant with sufficient nutrition while breastfeeding.**

False. Breastfeeding is not compromised by moderate amounts of weight loss.

○ **How many days or weeks postpartum is mastitis most commonly seen?**

4 to 5 weeks.

○ **True or False: Mastitis is usually bilateral.**

False.

○ **What are the clinical signs and symptoms of mastitis?**

Marked breast engorgement, fever, chills, and hard reddened painful area of the affected breast.

○ **What is the approximate incidence of abscess complicating mastitis?**

10%.

○ **What is the most common organism causing mastitis?**

Staphylococcus aureus.

○ **True or False: A woman with mastitis should discontinue breastfeeding due to the possibility of infecting the infant.**

False. The causal organisms typically originate from the infant's nasopharynx, and discontinuation of breastfeeding increases maternal risk of abscess formation.

○   **True or False: About 50% of childbearing women experience postpartum blues.**

True.

○   **List some factors that most likely contribute to the development of postpartum blues.**

Hormonal changes of the puerperium
The discomforts of the puerperium
A new mother's anxieties over her capabilities for caring for her infant
Fatigue from loss of sleep
Fears that she has become less attractive
The emotional letdown following the anticipation and excitement of delivery

○   **List some common symptoms of postpartum blues.**

Transient feelings of feeling overwhelmed, anxious, depressed, irritable, and having trouble sleeping despite tiredness.

○   **What is the most common time frame for a woman to experience postpartum blues?**

3 to 4 days postpartum.

○   **Postpartum depression is estimated to occur in what percentage of women?**

10 to 15%.

○   **Postpartum depression may be associated with what types of symptoms?**

Feelings of being overwhelmed, anxious, depressed, decreased interest/pleasure in life, guilt, appetite change, difficulty sleeping, decreased libido, suicidal or infanticidal thoughts, and agitation.

○   **What is the time frame for occurrence of postpartum depression?**

Onset can occur anytime up to 6 months postpartum, with symptoms persisting for >2 weeks.

○   **What are risk factors for postpartum depression?**

History of previous major depressive disorder, history of postpartum depression, family history of mood disorder, marital discord, stressful life events occurring in the previous year, and lack of social support network.

○   **True or False: Adolescent women have an increased risk of postpartum depression.**

True.

○   **True or False: Thyroid dysfunction should be considered in the differential of postpartum depression.**

True. As with the initial evaluation of any depressive disorder, hypothyroidism should be considered as part of the differential.

○   **What are risk factors for postpartum psychosis?**

Personal or family history of bipolar disorder, schizophrenia, or schizoaffective disorder.

○   **Postpartum psychosis is estimated to occur in what percentage of women?**

0.2%.

○ **What is the typical timing of postpartum psychosis?**

Onset within 2 to 4 weeks postpartum, with symptoms persisting for several days to months.

○ **What symptoms are associated with postpartum psychosis?**

Anxiety, suicidal/infanticidal thoughts, agitation, decreased need for sleep, confusion, disorientation, hallucination, hyperactivity, hypersexuality, unusual thoughts, and behaviors.

○ **True or False: Women given the diagnosis of postpartum psychosis should be referred to a psychiatrist for outpatient management.**

False. Postpartum psychosis is a psychiatric emergency requiring inpatient management.

○ **How long should antibiotics be given for mastitis?**

Antibiotics should be given for 10 to 14 days for mastitis.

○ **What is the first-line antibiotic for treatment of mastitis?**

Dicloxacillin.

○ **What is the predominant immunoglobulin found in breast milk?**

Secretory immunoglobulin A.

○ **True or False: Bromocriptine is indicated for lactation inhibition.**

False. Bromocriptine is not recommended for that indication as it has been shown to have significant side effects like stroke, myocardial infections, seizures, and psychiatric disorders.

○ **What is the treatment of breast engorgement?**

Ice packs, well fitting brassiere, and oral analgesics for 12 to 24 hours.

○ **What is the most common neuropathy associated with deliveries?**

Lateral femoral cutaneous.

○ **True or False: Elective cesarean section delivery should be considered after pubic symphysis separation in prior delivery.**

True. Recurrence is >50% in subsequent pregnancy.

○ **True or False: In the event of pubic symphyseal separation, orthopedic intervention is generally necessary.**

False. Supportive measures should be initiated for care of pubic symphyseal separation, including a binder positioned around the woman's hips, and NSAIDs for pain relief until symptoms improve.

○ **What is the most important criterion for the diagnosis of postpartum metritis?**

Fever.

○ **What is the preferred treatment of pelvic infection following cesarean section?**

Clindamycin 900 mg + gentamicin 1.5 mg/kg IV q 8 h.

○   **True or False: Antepartum treatment of asymptomatic women with vaginal infection has been shown to prevent postpartum endometritis.**

False.

○   **What is the layer that is separated in a wound dehiscence?**

Fascia.

○   **What is the treatment of wound dehiscence?**

Secondary closure of incision in OR.

○   **How can you diagnose septic pelvic thrombophlebitis?**

CT or MRI of the pelvis.

CHAPTER 12 Obstetric Complications

Meike Schuster, DO

○ **Beta-sympathomimetics may cause which electrolyte abnormalities?**

Hypokalemia and hypocalcemia.

○ **Antidote for magnesium sulfate toxicity?**

1 g calcium gluconate IV push.

○ **Name the contraindication to terbutaline.**

Maternal cardiac disease (structural, ischemic, dysrhythmia), hypertensive disease, antepartum hemorrhage, uncontrolled diabetes mellitus, and uncontrolled maternal hyperthyroidism.

○ **What is the incidence of preterm birth in the United States?**

11.8%.

○ **What endogenous substances have been linked to preterm labor?**

Bacterial endotoxins (lipopolysaccharides), platelet activating factor, interleukins 1 and 6, and tumor necrosis factor.

○ **What substance is released when the amnion begins to separate from the decidua?**

Fetal fibronectin.

○ **What is the significance of testing cervical secretions for fetal fibronectin?**

Negative predictive value 95% of not delivering within 14 days when test negative
Positive predictive value 40% of delivery when test positive in symptomatic women

○ **Low-lying placenta with a marginal insertion, soft abdomen, a minimal amount of bleeding, and acutely distressed fetus suggests?**

Vasa previa.

○ **What is perinatal mortality associated with an undiagnosed vasa previa?**
60%.

○ **What percentage of vasa previa is detected by antepartum ultrasound?**
<10%.

○ **What is the signature of hepatic lesion of preeclampsia?**
Periportal necrosis.

○ **When do convulsions occur during eclampsia?**
50% before the onset of labor, and the other 50% equally divided between intrapartum and postpartum.

○ **What are the benefits of antepartum corticosteroids in premature babies?**
• Increased lung compliance, increased surfactant production, and less respiratory distress syndrome.
• Less intraventricular hemorrhage.
• Less necrotizing enterocolitis.
• Less neonatal mortality.

○ **What are the NIH recommendations for steroid use in preterm premature rupture of membranes?**
Recommended for <30 to 32 weeks in the absence of chorioamnionitis.

○ **Of all intrauterine growth restriction (IUGR) babies, how many show symmetric growth lag?**
20%.

○ **Of all IUGR babies, how many are affected by a chromosomal abnormality, congenital malformation, or genetic syndrome?**
10%.

○ **What metabolic problems are commonly found in IUGR neonates?**
Hypocalcemia, hypoglycemia, hyponatremia, hypothermia, and polycythemia.

○ **At what gestational age, does maternal immunoglobulin G (IgG) begin to crossover the placenta and provide protection for the fetus?**
16 weeks. By 26 weeks fetal and maternal IgG serum levels are similar.

○ **How is *Toxoplasma gondii* infection diagnosed in the fetus?**
Cord blood fetal anti-Toxoplasma IgM, or amniotic fluid polymerase chain reaction.

○ **What percentage of adults in the US has antibodies (and thus immunity) to Toxoplasma?**
40% to 50%, and the prevalence is highest in lower socioeconomic populations.

○   **What percentage of childbearing age women show immunity to varicella zoster (chicken pox)?**

95%.

○   **What life-threatening complications can affect a patient with adult onset varicella infection?**

Encephalitis and pneumonia.

○   **What is the role of varicella zoster immunoglobulin (VZIG) and varicella vaccine in pregnancy?**

VZIG is administered within 96 hours of significant exposure, and is 60% to 80% effective in preventing infection. Varicella vaccine is an attenuated live virus, and should NOT be given during pregnancy. Acyclovir can also be effective in preventing varicella when given prophylactically (800 mg po 5 × day for 5 to 7 days).

○   **What is the fetal effect of maternal parvovirus B-19 infection in pregnancy?**

Most fetuses are unaffected. An increased risk of miscarriage is seen with early exposure, and rarely, a syndrome of nonimmune hydrops can be seen. Parvo B-19 is thought to cause anemia by reducing supply rather than increasing destruction of erythrocytes. Treatment is intrauterine blood transfusion.

○   **What is missing on microscopic examination of the placenta when placenta accreta, increta, and percreta?**

Nitabuch layer, a line of separation between myometrium and invading trophoblasts.

○   **Name risk factors for placental abruption.**

Smoking, trauma, cocaine, hypertension, preterm premature rupture of membranes, retroplacental fibroids, multiple gestation, inherited thrombophilia, and possibly advanced age/parity, trauma, dysfibrinogenemia, hydramnios, and intrauterine infections.

○   **The occurrence rate of placental abruption is?**

1%.

○   **What is the recurrence rate of placental abruption?**

15- to 20-fold higher.

○   **How accurate is U/S at detecting placental abruption?**

50%.

○   **What complications can be anticipated in the use of a cell-saver autotransfusion for uterine or adnexal surgery in the pregnant patient?**

Potential amniotic fluid contamination (minimal after processing) and Rh incompatibility between maternal and fetal blood.

○ **Virtually all postpartum patients with septic shock have a source of infection requiring surgical drainage. What microorganisms are associated with each clinical picture?**

Endomyometritis: *Prevotella* (was *Bacteroides*) biviens and/or Gardnerella (60%), aerobic gram-negative bacilli (*Escherichia coli*, *Klebsiella pneumoniae*, *Proteus*), and Group B *Streptococcus*.

Late onset endomyometritis: *Chlamydia* and *Mycoplasma*.

Pelvic abscess: *Prevotella* and *Bacteroides*.

Necrotizing fasciitis.

Group A *Streptococcus* + *Staphylococcus*.

Mixed aerobe + anaerobes including *Clostridia*.

Group B *Streptococcus* + anaerobes.

○ **Postpartum patient presenting with mild fever, hip tenderness, and paravaginal tenderness. Delivery record shows an uncomplicated vaginal delivery with a pudendal block for anesthesia. What's going on?**

Retroperitoneal mixed aerobe and anaerobic abscess following needle track along trochanter and/or psoas muscle. Start antibiotics and confirm with CT.

○ **What is the average gestational age for delivery/multiple gestations beyond 24 weeks?**

Twins: 36 to 37 weeks.

Triplets: 33 to 34 weeks.

Quadruplets: 30 to 31 weeks.

Three or more fetuses reduced to twins: 35 to 36 weeks.

○ **At what gestational age, it is generally not recommended to use a vacuum to assist delivery?**

34 weeks or less.

○ **What is the risk of using a vacuum below this age limit?**

Intraventricular hemorrhage.

○ **What is the incidence of placenta previa?**

03 to 0.5%.

○ **What is the risk of placenta accreta in women who have a placenta previa?**

After first C/S: 3%.

After second C/S: 11%.

After third C/S: 40%.

After fourth C/S: 61%.

○ **What is the maternal mortality rate associated with placenta accreta?**

7%.

○ **What is the difference between placenta accreta, increta, and percreta?**

Accreta: Placental villi are attached to the myometrium with absent Nitabuch layer.

Increta: Invasion of placental villi into the myometrium.

Percreta: Invasion penetrates thru the full thickness of the myometrium.

○ **How sensitive is U/S for placenta accrete?**

79% (95% positive predictive value).

○ **What are the pathognomonic findings of placenta accreta on U/S?**

Irregular shaped placental lacunae within the placenta, "Swiss cheese" or moth-eaten" appearance.

○ **What is the technique for replacement of the uterus in an inverted uterus when replacement is refractory to manual replacement?**

Huntington technique: Perform a laparotomy with a tenaculum placed on the uterus to sequentially replace the fundus. If the cervical band is too tight, use the Haultain technique. This is incising the ring posteriorly (to avoid the bladder) and correct the inversion.

○ **Most fetal survivors of a perimortem C/S are delivered within what time frame?**

5 minutes of cardiac arrest.

○ **What are the two leading causes of anesthesia-related maternal morbidity and mortality?**

Failed intubation and pulmonary aspiration.

○ **What is the recurrence risk of shoulder dystocia?**

1% to 16.7%

○ **What is the advantage of placing heroin-addicted pregnant women on methadone during pregnancy?**

(1) It avoids the risks of STDs such as HIV and hepatitis from IV drug use.

(2) It decreases the risk of intrauterine demise from cyclical withdrawal.

○ **What is the incidence of conjoined twins? When does the embryonic division occur in conjoined twins?**

1/50,000 births days 13 to 15 after fertilization.

○ **Who should be tested for antiphospholipid antibody syndrome?**

(1) History or current diagnosis of vascular thrombosis.

(2) Pregnancy complications

    (a) 1 or more unexplained fetal death >10 weeks.

    (b) 1 or more premature birth secondary to preeclampsia before 34 weeks.

    (c) 3 or more consecutive spontaneous abortions before 10 weeks.

○ **What are the three tests to screen for to diagnose antiphospholipid antibody syndrome?**

Lupus anticoagulant, anticardiolipin antibodies, and anti-beta 2 glycoprotein I antibodies.

○ **How long do you anticoagulate someone with antiphospholipid syndrome (APAS)?**
Duration of their pregnancy and the 6 weeks postpartum.

○ **What type of birth control is contraindicated in someone with APAS?**
Any estrogen containing birth control

○ **Who should be tested for inherited thrombophilias?**
(1) Personal history of venous thromboembolism associated with a nonrecurrent risk factor (fractures, surgery, prolonged immobilization).
(2) First-degree relative with a history of high-risk thrombophilia or venous thromboembolism before age 50.

○ **What tests should you order to screen on a patient for inherited thrombophilias?**
(1) Factor V Leiden mutation.
(2) Prothrombin gene mutation.
(3) Protein C deficiency.
(4) Protein S deficiency.
(5) Antithrombin III deficiency.

○ **Which thrombophilia should not be screened for in pregnancy?**
Protein S deficiency.

○ **What is the neonatal complication of protein C deficiency?**
Neonatal purpura fulminans (requiring lifelong anticoagulation).

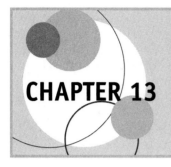

CHAPTER 13

Hypertension and Pregnancy

Ashwinee Natu

○ **What is the incidence of hypertensive disease in pregnancy?**

12% to 22%.

○ **What is gestational hypertension?**

A systolic blood pressure level of 140 mmHg or higher or a diastolic blood pressure level of 90 mmHg or higher that occurs after 20 weeks of gestation in a woman with previously normal blood pressure, and blood pressure returns to normal within 12 weeks postpartum.

○ **How should gestational hypertension be definitively diagnosed?**

The elevated blood pressure should be documented on two separate occasions at least 6 hours apart, but no >7 days apart.

○ **What is preeclampsia?**

Hypertension (as defined before) with proteinuria (urinary excretion of 300 mg protein or higher in a 24-hour urine specimen or persistent 1+ or more on dipstick in random urine samples).

○ **What is eclampsia?**

Presence of new onset grand mal seizures (that cannot be attributed to other causes) in a woman with preeclampsia.

○ **What is superimposed preeclampsia?**

New onset proteinuria in a woman with hypertension before 20 weeks of gestation, a sudden increase in proteinuria if already present in early gestation, a sudden increase in hypertension, or the development of HELLP syndrome.

○ **What is HELLP syndrome?**

Hemolysis, elevated liver enzymes, and thrombocytopenia that may occur independently or in up to 20% of cases of severe preeclampsia.

○ **What are the criteria for diagnosis of severe preeclampsia?**

One or more of the following:

- Systolic blood pressure of 160 mmHg or higher or diastolic 110 mmHg or higher on two occasions at least 6 hours apart while the patient is on bed rest.
- Proteinuria of 5000 mg or higher in a 24-hour urine specimen or 3+ or greater on two random urine samples collected at least 4 hours apart.
- Oliguria of <500 mL in 24 hours; cerebral or visual disturbances.
- Pulmonary edema or cyanosis.
- Epigastric or right upper quadrant pain.
- Impaired liver function.
- Thrombocytopenia.
- Fetal growth restriction.

○ **What is the diastolic blood pressure?**

The pressure when the sound disappears (Korotkoff phase V).

○ **What is an appropriate size cuff?**

Length 1.5 times upper arm circumference or a cuff with a bladder that encircles 80% or more of the arm.

○ **How should the blood pressure be measured?**

In an upright position (or left lateral recumbent position with the patient's arm at the level of the heart) after 10 minutes or longer rest period.

○ **What external factors may cause a falsely elevated blood pressure measurement?**

Elevation limited to the clinical setting (white-coat syndrome) and use of tobacco or caffeine <30 minutes prior to the measurement.

○ **What is the incidence of preeclampsia?**

5% to 8%.

○ **What are some risk factors for preeclampsia?**

First pregnancy, multifetal gestations, preeclampsia in a previous pregnancy, chronic hypertension, pregestational diabetes, vascular and connective tissue disease, nephropathy, antiphospholipid antibody syndrome, obesity, age 35 years or older, and African American race.

○ **What is the pathophysiology of preeclampsia?**

Vascular endothelial damage with vasospasm, transudation of plasma, and ischemic and thrombotic sequelae.

○ **Name a few suggested etiologies for the development of preeclampsia.**

Abnormal (incomplete) trophoblastic invasion of uterine vessels, immunological intolerance of fetoplacental tissue, maladaption to inflammatory or cardiovascular changes of pregnancy, and dietary deficiencies and genetic influence.

○ **What term is used to describe the arterial changes noted in preeclampsia?**

Atherosis.

○ **How does the prostacyclin: thromboxane angiotensin 2 ratio change in preeclampsia?**

It decreases; thus, there is increased sensitivity to infused angiotensin 2, which results in vasoconstriction.

○ **What is the effect of gestational hypertension on blood volume during pregnancy?**

In average size women, there is an expected increase in the blood volume at the end of normal pregnancy from 3500 to 5000 mL. With gestational hypertension, a normal blood volume is expected.

○ **What is the effect of preeclampsia on blood volume during pregnancy?**

Different degrees of hemoconcentration are expected with preeclampsia depending on the severity.

○ **What is the effect of eclampsia on blood volume during pregnancy?**

Absence of much or all of the anticipated volume excess is expected with eclampsia.

○ **What renal changes are associated with preeclampsia during pregnancy?**

As a result of vasospasm, the normal expected increase in glomerular filtration rate and renal blood flow and the expected decrease in serum creatinine may not occur in women with preeclampsia, especially if the disease is severe.

○ **Why does oliguria occur in preeclampsia?**

Oliguria is secondary to the hemoconcentration and decreased renal blood flow. Rarely, persistent oliguria may reflect acute tubular necrosis, which may lead to acute renal failure.

○ **What is the characteristic hepatic lesion associated with gestational hypertension?**

Periportal hemorrhage in the liver periphery.

○ **What clinical manifestations can be associated with preeclampsia?**
- Vascular hypertension
- Hemoconcentration
- Intense vasospasm
- Hematologic thrombocytopenia
- Hemolysis
- Hepatic elevated aspartate aminotransferase (AST) and alanine transaminase (ALT)
- Hyperbilirubinemia
- Hepatic hemorrhage
- Neurologic temporary blindness
- Headache
- Blurred vision
- Scotomata
- Hyper-reflexia
- Eclampsia
- Renal oliguria
- ATN
- Absence of decrease in serum creatinine
- Fetal intrauterine growth restriction (IUGR)
- Oligohydramnios
- Placental abruption
- Nonreassuring fetal status

○ **Name a few imitators of severe preeclampsia/HELLP syndrome.**

Acute fatty liver of pregnancy, thrombotic thrombocytopenic purpura, hemolytic-uremic syndrome, and acute exacerbation of systemic lupus erythematosus.

○ **What may a high fever associated with preeclampsia indicate?**

A central nervous system hemorrhage.

○ **What is the recommended screening test for preeclampsia?**

No screening test is currently recommended. Tests of interest have been studied and include uric acid level, fibronectin level, plasminogen activator inhibitor-1 levels and ratio, and homocysteine level.

○ **Can preeclampsia be prevented?**

No. Treatment is currently recommended to prevent preeclampsia, but a study regarding treatment with vitamin C and vitamin E showed promising findings that should be confirmed in a larger study.

○ **Is there a role for medications in the prevention of preeclampsia?**

The Cochrane review reports a 15% reduction in the risk of preeclampsia associated with the use of antiplatelet agents. Low-dose aspirin has not been shown to prevent preeclampsia in women at low risk and therefore is not recommended.

○ **Name a few experimental treatments that may prevent preeclampsia.**

Calcium supplementation, fish oil, low-dose aspirin, and antioxidants.

○ **What is the definitive treatment of preeclampsia?**

Delivery of the fetus is the cornerstone of treatment but maternal and fetal risks must be optimized prior to making this decision.

○ **Does the severity of preeclampsia guide management?**

For mild disease with a preterm fetus continued observation may be appropriate. It may include weekly nonstress test (NST) and/or biophysical profile (BPP) (or twice weekly for suspected IUGR or oligohydramnios), and ultrasound for growth scan and amniotic fluid assessment every 3 weeks. Maternal evaluation should include platelet count, liver enzymes, and renal function and 24-hour urine collection for protein weekly. If continued observation is chosen for a severe disease (remote from term), it may include daily evaluation of fetal and maternal status including laboratory evaluation, depending on the severity and the progression.

○ **When should antihypertensive treatment be given during expectant management of preeclampsia?**

When systolic blood pressure is above 150 to 160 mmHg or diastolic blood pressure above 100 to 110 mmHg, since at these levels there is a higher risk of maternal complications such as cerebral hemorrhage.

○ **Is there a role for antihypertensive medications in mild preeclampsia?**

The only proven effect of treatment of mild preeclampsia is a reduced incidence of severe preeclampsia.

○ **What is the initial treatment of severe preeclampsia prior to 34 weeks?**

Hospitalization to evaluate maternal and fetal status: Blood pressure monitoring, strict documentation of intake and output, 24-hour urine collection and laboratory studies such as complete blood count (CBC), basic metabolic panel, liver function tests and possibly lactate dehydrogenase (LDH), uric acid, albumin, and coagulation studies. The fetal status is evaluated by NST, amniotic fluid index (AFI), fetal growth, and possible umbilical artery Doppler velocimetry. Corticosteroids should be administered and magnesium should be given for seizure prophylaxis.

○ **How should preeclampsia with onset before 23 to 25 weeks be managed?**

Pregnancy should be delivered with no role of expectant management.

○ **Who is a candidate for expectant management?**

Asymptomatic women with laboratory abnormalities that resolve within 24 to 48 hours, severe preeclampsia due to severe proteinuria alone, severe preeclampsia based solely on fetal growth restrictions, and severe preeclampsia based solely on blood pressure criteria.

○ **What are contraindications to expectant management (in which the pregnancy is not even prolonged enough to receive the second dose of steroids)?**

Women with eclampsia, pulmonary edema, disseminated intravascular coagulation (DIC), renal insufficiency, abruptio placentae, abnormal fetal testing, HELLP syndrome, or persistent symptoms of severe preeclampsia. For women with severe preeclampsia before the limit of viability, expectant management has been associated with frequent maternal morbidity with minimal or no benefits to the newborn.

○ **Who can be managed on an outpatient basis for preeclampsia?**

Ambulatory management is possible for those women with mild gestational hypertension or preeclampsia remote from term who are also compliant with their management plan.

○ **What is the medical management of preeclampsia during labor and delivery?**

Magnesium sulfate is the treatment of choice for severe preeclampsia and is aimed at preventing seizures or eclampsia and controlling hypertension. Antihypertensive treatment is recommended for diastolic blood pressure of 105 to 110 mmHg or higher or systolic blood pressure over 160 mmHg.

○ **Why is the use of magnesium sulfate in mild disease controversial?**

The risk of seizures in this group is considered low, and is balanced against the toxicity of magnesium. However, a report from Parkland in 2006 demonstrated an increase in the incidence of eclampsia following their decision not to treat mild gestational hypertension with magnesium.

○ **What is the mechanism of action of magnesium sulfate in seizure prophylaxis?**

The exact mechanism of action is unclear but is thought to affect cardiovascular and neurological functions by altering calcium metabolism. Magnesium sulfate may also act as a vasodilator, which relieves vasoconstriction, protects the blood-brain barrier, decreases cerebral edema formation, and acts as a cerebral anticonvulsant.

○ **Name the two most common antihypertensive medications used for acute therapy.**

Labetalol (20 mg IV followed by 40, 80, and 80 as needed with 10 minutes interval) or hydralazine (5–10 mg IV every 15–20 minutes).

○   **What is the optimal mode of delivery for mild preeclampsia?**

Vaginal delivery.

○   **What is the optimal mode of delivery for severe preeclampsia?**

Mode of delivery should be individualized with some recommending a scheduled cesarean delivery for pregnancies at <30 weeks with a low Bishop score.

○   **What is the preferred method of anesthesia?**

For preeclampsia and eclampsia the preferred method is regional anesthesia. This is contraindicated in the presence of coagulopathy or severe thrombocytopenia (platelet count <50,000/mm^3).

○   **When does the blood pressure usually normalize?**

Within the first week postpartum for gestational hypertension and within 2 weeks for preeclampsia

○   **Describe the classic eclamptic seizure.**

Generalized tonic-clonic. Usually begins with facial twitching, followed after a few seconds by a phase of generalized muscular contraction for 15 to 20 seconds. During the clonic phase, which may last about a minute, all the muscles contract and relax alternately, usually starting at the jaws and the eyelids. The movements then gradually subside, becoming smaller and less frequent until the woman eventually lies motionless.

○   **How should eclampsia be managed?**

The first steps will include supportive care, maintaining an open airway and maternal oxygenation (supply oxygen at 8 to 10 L/min). Magnesium sulfate (IV or IM) should be used to control convulsions and prevent recurrence. Antihypertensive medications should be used for diastolic blood pressure of 105 to 110 mmHg or higher. Delivery should be done in a timely fashion.

○   **What is the regimen of magnesium IV?**

Loading dose of 4 to 6 g over 15 to 20 minutes, followed by maintenance of 2 g/h. The magnesium level is measured every 4 to 6 h to adjust the level to 4.8 to 8.4 mg/dL.

○   **When should magnesium sulfate be discontinued?**

Usually 24 hours after delivery or after the onset of convulsions. A randomized controlled trial published in 2006 (Ehrenberg & Mercer, 2006) concluded that for mild preeclampsia discontinuation of magnesium 12 hours after delivery was associated with infrequent disease progression and a clinical course similar to that with 24-hour therapy.

○   **How is magnesium cleared?**

Renal excretion.

○   **What is the main side effect of magnesium?**

Flushing.

○   **At what level, do the patellar reflexes disappear?**

9.6 to 12 mg/dL.

○ **How should magnesium toxicity be treated?**

Calcium gluconate 1 g IV over 5 to 10 minutes.

○ **Can magnesium be used in association with calcium channel blockers, such as nifedipine?**

The simultaneous use of these drugs may, on very rare occasions, result in profound neuromuscular blockade, including cardiac depression and muscle weakness (reversal can be achieved with 10% solution calcium gluconate).

○ **How does magnesium affect the fetal heart rate pattern?**

It may decrease the variability.

○ **How should you treat a recurrent eclamptic seizure in spite of magnesium treatment (approximately 10% of cases)?**

An additional 2 g dose of magnesium should be given IV and may be repeated once in some women. If seizure activity is still present, then traditional anticonvulsant therapy should be initiated

○ **When should sodium amobarbital be used?**

250 mg intravenously over 3 to 5 minutes may be used to treat recurrent convulsions in spite of adequate magnesium therapy.

○ **What percentage of eclamptic seizures develop before overt proteinuria is identified?**

10% to 14%.

○ **Can eclampsia occur without hypertension?**

In 16% of the eclamptic cases, hypertension is absent. (It is severe in 20–54% and mild in 30–60%.)

○ **When does eclampsia develop?**

>90% develop at or beyond 28 weeks. 38% to 53% develop antepartum, 18% to 36% intrapartum, and 11% to 44% postpartum.

○ **Which condition may be associated with eclampsia prior to 20 weeks?**

Molar pregnancy.

○ **Name some common symptoms that may precede eclampsia.**

Persistent occipital or frontal headaches, blurred vision, photophobia, epigastric pain, and right upper quadrant pain.

○ **When is cerebral imaging indicated?**

For patients with focal neurological deficits or prolonged coma, and for patients with atypical features of eclampsia, such as onset before 20 weeks, late postpartum eclampsia or eclampsia refractory to adequate therapy with magnesium sulfate.

○ **What conditions are in the differential diagnosis of eclampsia?**

Hypertensive encephalopathy, seizure disorder, brain tumors, hypoglycemia, thrombophilia, thrombotic thrombocytopenic purpura, vasculitis, encephalitis, meningitis, and ruptured cerebral aneurysm.

○ **What percentage of eclamptic seizures occur in late postpartum eclampsia (beyond 48 hours postpartum but <4 weeks)?**

25% (attributed to improved prenatal care).

○ **Is fetal bradycardia following a seizure an indication for a stat cesarean?**

No. Fetal bradycardia is common after a seizure due to maternal hypoxemia and lactic acidemia. This usually resolves after 3 to 5 minutes of intrauterine resuscitation. If persistent over 10 minutes, then an imminent delivery must be considered, as it may indicate other complications such as placental abruption.

○ **What patterns of fetal heart rate may be noted during and after a seizure?**

Bradycardia, transient late decelerations, and decreased beat-to-beat variability.

○ **Name the maternal complications that may follow a seizure.**

Pulmonary edema, aspiration pneumonitis, cerebral hemorrhage resulting in hemiplegia or sudden death, blindness, psychosis, placental abruption, DIC, acute renal failure, and cardiopulmonary arrest.

○ **What is the rate of preeclampsia in a subsequent pregnancy after eclampsia in the index pregnancy?**

25%.

○ **What is the rate of recurrent eclampsia?**

2%.

○ **What are the diagnostic criteria of HELLP syndrome?**

Criterion	Laboratory Findings	Associated Clinical Findings (Nondiagnostic)
Hemolysis—microangiopathic hemolytic anemia	Abnormal peripheral smear—schistocytes and burr cells Elevated indirect bilirubin in the serum Low serum haptoglobin levels Elevated LDH (isoforms 1 and 2) Significant drop in hemoglobin level	Malaise
Elevated liver function tests	Elevated AST and ALT (usually more than two times the upper limit of normal) Abnormal bilirubin levels	Right upper quadrant or epigastric pain Nausea Vomiting
Low platelet count	<100,000/mm^3	Mucosal bleeding Hematuria Petechial hemorrhages Ecchymosis

○ **Is HELLP syndrome always associated with hypertension?**

No.

○ **Hypertension may be absent in 12% to 18%. It may be only mild in 15% to 50%. Is HELLP syndrome always associated with proteinuria?**

No. It may be absent in up to 14%.

○ **What is the differential diagnosis for a patient with HELLP syndrome?**

Acute fatty liver of pregnancy, thrombotic thrombocytopenic purpura, hemolytic-uremic syndrome, immune thrombocytopenic purpura, systemic lupus erythematosis, antiphospholipid syndrome, cholecystitis, viral hepatitis, pancreatitis, upper respiratory infection, disseminated herpes simplex, hemorrhagic or septic shock.

○ **What maternal morbidities are associated with HELLP syndrome?**

Pulmonary edema, acute renal failure, DIC, placental abruption, liver hemorrhage or failure, adult respiratory distress syndrome, sepsis, stroke, and death (1%).

○ **What is the reported perinatal mortality rate associated with HELLP?**

7.4% to 20.4% mainly due to severe prematurity.

○ **What is the rate of prematurity in HELLP syndrome?**

70%.

○ **How is a suspected case of HELLP syndrome managed?**

Immediate hospitalization and observation. Diagnostic measures include blood tests such as CBC, a peripheral smear, coagulation studies, AST, ALT, creatinine, glucose, bilirubin, and LDH. Therapeutic measures are those for severe preeclampsia including magnesium for seizure prophylaxis and antihypertensives to keep blood pressure below 160/105 mmHg.

○ **What is the definitive treatment of HELLP syndrome?**

The cornerstone of treatment is delivery, especially beyond 34 weeks (and prior to 24 weeks) gestation.

○ **What is the role of expectant management in HELLP syndrome?**

Some may advocate expectant management in selected stable patients prior to 34 weeks (ie, in the absence of multiorgan dysfunction, DIC, liver infarction or hemorrhage, renal failure, placental abruption, or nonreassuring fetal condition). This management might include delivery in 24 to 48 hours, thus allowing completion of steroid course or may include prolonging the pregnancy even further, until other indications for delivery occur. Expectant management for >48 hours was found to be associated with significant rate of fetal death, and no improvement in overall perinatal outcome, compared with those who were delivered within 48 hours.

○ **What is the role of steroids in the treatment of HELLP syndrome?**

As with severe preeclampsia, steroids prior to 34 weeks improve perinatal outcome, and may also be associated with transient improvement of the thrombocytopenia.

○ **How should steroids be administered for HELLP syndrome?**

There are two possible regimens: 12 mg of betamethasone IM every 24 hours for two doses or 6 mg of dexamethasone IM every 12 hours for a total of 4 doses.

Other regimens of steroids including high dose treatment after 34 weeks or postpartum are experimental. There is insufficient evidence to determine whether adjunctive steroid use in HELLP syndrome decreases maternal and perinatal mortality.

○ **Which methods for pain control are contraindicated in HELLP syndrome?**

Pudendal block in contraindicated due to the risk of bleeding and hematoma formation. Epidural anesthesia is contraindicated, especially when thrombocytopenia is <75,000/mm^3.

○ **What are the indications for platelet transfusion?**

A level <20,000/mm^3 or the presence of significant bleeding. Some recommend transfusion of six units of platelets prior to surgery if the level is <40,000/mm^3.

○ **What is the recommended postpartum treatment?**

Supportive therapy with continuation of magnesium sulfate prophylaxis for 24 to 48 hours and the use of antihypertensives to keep blood pressure below 155/105 mmHg.

○ **What is the rate of preeclampsia in subsequent pregnancies?**

Approximately 20%.

○ **What is the rate of recurrent HELLP syndrome?**

2% to 19%.

○ **How is chronic hypertension defined?**

Hypertension (systolic pressure of 140 mmHg or above, diastolic pressure of 90 mmHg or above) present before the 20th week of gestation (not attributable to gestational trophoblastic disease) or hypertension present before pregnancy with the use of antihypertensive medications, or hypertension that persists longer than 12 weeks postdelivery.

○ **What are the criteria for diagnosing mild and severe chronic hypertension?**

- Mild: Systolic blood pressure 140 to 159 mmHg or diastolic blood pressure 90 to 109 mmHg.
- Severe: Systolic blood pressure 160 mmHg or greater or diastolic blood pressure 110 mmHg or greater.

○ **How is chronic hypertension classified according to the Joint National Committee (2003)?**

Prehypertension (systolic 120–139 or diastolic 80–90), stage 1 hypertension (140–159 or 90–99) and stage 2 hypertension (160 or above or 100 or above).

○ **What are some benefits associated with antihypertensive treatment in nonpregnant women?**

Decreased mortality and stroke and major cardiac events.

○ **Describe some lifestyle modifications recommended for managing hypertension.**

Weight reduction, physical activity, dietary sodium reduction, smoking cessation, and moderation of alcohol consumption.

○ **What is the most common cause of chronic hypertension in pregnant women?**

Essential or familial hypertension (>90%).

○ **Which pregnancy complications are associated with chronic hypertension?**

Premature birth, IUGR, small for gestational age, fetal demise, placental abruption (1–2% and up to 8.4% with severe chronic hypertension), cesarean delivery, superimposed preeclampsia, and perinatal mortality.

○ **What are the effects of preeclampsia on the fetus?**

As a result of impaired uteroplacental blood flow or placental infarction, effects on the fetus may include IUGR, oligohydramnios, placental abruption, and nonreassuring fetal status demonstrated on antepartum surveillance.

○ **Is a history of prior preeclampsia a risk factor for superimposed preeclampsia?**

In women with chronic hypertension, a history of preeclampsia does not increase the rate of superimposed preeclampsia, but is associated with an increased rate of delivery at <37 weeks.

○ **Name a few risk factors for the development of superimposed preeclampsia.**

Severe hypertension in early pregnancy, hypertension for at least 4 years, and abnormal uterine artery Doppler velocimetry (increased impedance at 16–20 weeks).

○ **When does the physiologic decrease in blood pressure reach its lowest level?**

At 16 to 18 weeks of gestation.

○ **Which clinical tests are useful in the initial evaluation of a pregnant woman with chronic hypertension?**

Recommendations include electrocardiography, echocardiography, ophthalmologic examination, and renal ultrasonography. Baseline laboratory evaluations include serum creatinine, blood urea nitrogen, and 24-hour urine evaluation of total protein and creatinine clearance. Uric acid of at least 5.5 mg/dL could indicate an increased likelihood of having superimposed preeclampsia. Some would also recommend checking urinalysis, urine culture, glucose, and electrolytes in an attempt to rule out etiologies such as renal disease or chronic pyelonephritis or to identify comorbidities, such as diabetes.

○ **What are the guidelines for treatment of mild chronic hypertension during pregnancy?**

Women with mild hypertension generally do not require antihypertensive medications. It is reasonable to either stop or reduce medication in women who are already taking antihypertensive therapy, but therapy could be increased or reinstituted for women with blood pressures exceeding 150–160 mmHg systolic or 100–110 mmHg diastolic.

○ **What are the guidelines for treatment of severe chronic hypertension during pregnancy?**

In women with severe hypertension (systolic of 180 mmHg or more or diastolic of 110 mmHg or more), antihypertensive therapy should be initiated or continued for maternal indications. End-organ dysfunction diastolic blood pressure of 90 mmHg or higher may be considered an indication for treatment.

○ **Which antihypertensive medications are contraindicated during pregnancy?**

Angiotensin converting enzyme (ACE) inhibitors, angiotensin II receptor blockers, the beta-blocker atenolol, nitroprusside, and diuretics in the presence of uteroplacental insufficiency.

○ **What are the teratogenic effects associated with ACE inhibitors?**

Underdeveloped calvarial bone, renal failure, oligohydramnios, anuria, renal agenesis, pulmonary hypoplasia, IUGR, fetal death, neonatal renal failure, and neonatal death.

○ **Why is atenolol not recommended in pregnancy?**

Atenolol may be associated with growth restriction.

○ **Why is nitroprusside contraindicated during pregnancy?**

Nitroprusside in the later stages of pregnancy may cause fetal cyanide poisoning.

○ **Which medications should not be used postpartum if the patient is breastfeeding?**

ACE inhibitors and angiotensin receptor antagonists should be avoided in the first few weeks. Diuretics should be avoided as they can reduce the milk volume.

○ **Name a few acceptable medications for treatment of chronic hypertension during pregnancy.**

Methyldopa, Labetalol, and nifedipine.

○ **What are the limitations of using antihypertensive agents for the treatment of chronic hypertension during pregnancy?**

Chronic hypertension with or without treatment during pregnancy is an independent and significant risk factor for adverse perinatal outcomes such as IUGR, small for gestational age, and preterm delivery.

○ **What is the recommended fetal surveillance for pregnancies complicated by chronic hypertension?**

It should be individualized. Some investigators recommend baseline ultrasound at 18 to 20 weeks, then repeat at 28 to 32 weeks, and then monthly for fetal growth. NST or BPP is recommended in case of IUGR or superimposed preeclampsia.

BIBLIOGRAPHY

1. Chronic hypertension in pregnancy. Practice Bulletin No. 125. American College of Obstetricians and Gynecologists. *Obstet Gynecol.* 2012;119:396-407.
2. Diagnosis and management of preeclampsia and eclampsia. ACOG Practice Bulletin No. 33. American College of Obstetricians and Gynecologists. *Obstet Gynecol.* 2002;99:159-167.
3. Orbach H, Matok I, Gorodischer R, et al. Hypertension and antihypertensive drugs in pregnancy and perinatal outcomes. *Obstet Gynecol.* 2012;S0002–9378(12)02066-2.
4. Sibai BM. Evaluation and management of severe preeclampsia before 34 weeks' gestation. *Obstet Gynecol.* 2011;205(3):191-198.
5. Sibai BM, Koch MA, Freire S, et al. The impact of prior preeclampsia on the risk of superimposed preeclampsia and other adverse pregnancy outcomes in patients with chronic hypertension. *Obstet Gynecol.* 2011;204(4):345.
6. Cunningham FG, Leveno KJ, Bloom SL, et al., eds. Hypertensive Disorders in Pregnancy. *Williams Obstetrics.* 22nd ed. New York, NY: McGraw-Hill; 2005:761-808.

7. Cunningham FG, Leveno KJ, Bloom SL, et al., eds. Chronic Hypertension. *Williams Obstetrics.* 23rd ed. New York, NY: McGraw-Hill; 2010.

8. Compendium of selected publications. 2007 Cochrane Database of Systematic Reviews, 2007 Up to date.

9. Alexander JM, McIntire DD. Selective magnesium sulfate prophylaxis for the prevention of eclampsia in women with gestational hypertension. *Obstet Gynecol.* 2006;108(4):826-832.

10. Sibai BM. Imitators of severe preeclampsia. *Obstet Gynecol.* 2007;109(4):956-966.

11. Ehrenberg HM, Mercer BM. Abbreviated postpartum magnesium sulfate therapy for women with mild preeclampsia. *Obstet Gynecol.* 2006;108(4):833-838.

12. Sibai BM. Diagnosis, prevention and management of eclampsia. *Obstet Gynecol.* 2005;105(2):402-410.

13. Sibai BM. Diagnosis, controversies and management of the syndrome of hemolysis, elevated liver enzymes and low platelet count. *Obstet Gynecol.* 2004;103(5):981-991.

Management of Medical and Surgical Conditions in Pregnancy

CHAPTER 14

Karen C. Wheeler, MD

CARDIOVASCULAR CONDITIONS

○ **What is the leading cause of death in women ages 25 to 44?**

Cardiovascular disease.

○ **Cardiac output increases by how much in pregnancy?**

50%.

○ **What is the most common heart murmur in pregnancy?**

Systolic flow murmur.

○ **What changes occur in the EKG in pregnancy?**

15 degree left axis deviation and mild ST changes in the inferior leads due to elevation of the diaphragm, and increased frequency of premature atrial and ventricular contractions.

○ **What are predictors of cardiac complications in pregnancy?**

(1) Prior heart failure, transient ischemic attack (TIA), arrhythmia, or stroke

(2) Baseline NYHA class III or IV disease or cyanosis

(3) Left-sided obstruction (mitral valve area <2 cm^2, aortic valve area <1.5 cm^2, or peak left ventricular outflow tract (LVOT) gradient above 30 mmHg)

(4) Ejection fraction <40%

○ **Is delivery by cesarean indicated for patients with class I or II heart disease?**

No. Vaginal delivery and induction of labor are considered safe in class I and II heart disease.

○ **Is delivery by cesarean indicated for patients with class III or IV heart disease?**

No. Cesarean delivery should be performed only for obstetric indications.

○ **Are porcine or mechanical valves preferred in pregnancy?**

Porcine valves are safer because they do not require anticoagulation.

○ **What is the maternal mortality rate for women with mechanical valves?**

3% to 4%, largely due to thromboembolic events and hemorrhage.

○ **What are the risks and benefits of using warfarin for anticoagulation in pregnancy?**

Warfarin is teratogenic, causing fetal malformations 6% of the time. Warfarin also may cause stillbirth (7%) and miscarriage (32%). However, it is the most effective method of anticoagulation for women with mechanical heart valves.

○ **What anticoagulation regimen is recommended for women with mechanical valves in pregnancy?**

Twice daily low molecular weight heparin (LMWH), twice daily unfractionated heparin (UFH), or if high risk of thromboembolism, LMWH/UFH until >13 weeks' gestation, then warfarin until close to delivery when heparin is resumed.

○ **What complication of mitral stenosis occurs in pregnancy?**

Heart failure due to volume overload from increased preload and cardiac output in pregnancy.

○ **Why must tachycardia be avoided in patients with mitral stenosis?**

Tachycardia shortens ventricular filling time, which is critical to maintain adequate stroke volume in patients with mitral stenosis. Thus, tachycardia can lead to pulmonary edema and should be treated with beta blockade.

○ **Does mitral regurgitation typically improve or worsen during pregnancy, and why?**

Mitral regurgitation tends to improve in pregnancy because decreased systemic vascular resistance leads to less regurgitation.

○ **What is the safest form of analgesia in labor for women with severe aortic stenosis?**

Narcotic analgesia is safer than epidural analgesia because of possible hypotension associated with epidural analgesia. Women with aortic stenosis require end-diastolic ventricular filling pressures to be maintained in order to maintain systemic perfusion.

○ **What is the most common heart condition seen in pregnancy?**

Congenital heart disease.

○ **What is the most concerning complication of a patent foramen ovale in pregnancy?**

Paradoxical embolism—passage of a venous clot through the patent foramen ovale into the systemic circulation

○ **What is the maternal mortality rate for women with Eisenmenger syndrome?**

30% to 50%, therefore pregnancy is not recommended.

○ **For women with unrepaired ventricular septal defects (VSDs), what is recommended?**

Antibiotic prophylaxis for bacterial endocarditis.

○ **While pregnancy may be attempted after surgical repair of congenital cyanotic heart defects, what are some of the risks?**

Preterm delivery, miscarriage, worsening of maternal heart disease (heart failure, arrhythmias), and maternal death.

○ **What are the causes of pulmonary hypertension in reproductive aged women?**

Idiopathic, collagen vascular disease, left-sided heart disease, and interstitial lung disease.

○ **Is pregnancy recommended for women with pulmonary hypertension?**

Only if mild and not idiopathic, or primary pulmonary hypertension.

○ **Are there any special considerations with mitral valve prolapse in pregnancy?**

If there is valvular damage or regurgitation, consider prophylaxis for bacterial endocarditis.

○ **What are the diagnostic criteria for peripartum cardiomyopathy?**

(1) Development of cardiac failure in the last month of pregnancy or within 5 months after delivery

(2) Absence of an identifiable cause for the cardiac failure

(3) Absence of recognizable heart disease prior to the last month of pregnancy

(4) Left ventricular systolic dysfunction demonstrated by classic echocardiographic criteria such as depressed shortening fraction or ejection fraction

○ **What conditions are commonly associated with peripartum cardiomyopathy?**

Chronic hypertension, preeclampsia, obesity, and myocarditis.

○ **What are presenting symptoms of peripartum cardiomyopathy?**

Dyspnea, orthopnea, cough, palpitations, and chest pain.

○ **How is peripartum cardiomyopathy managed?**

Diuresis, afterload reduction, prevention of thromboembolism, and supportive care to maintain oxygenation.

○ **What is the most important prognostic factor for women with peripartum cardiomyopathy?**

Return of left ventricular ejection fraction to >50% within 6 months.

○ **What types of dental procedures require antibiotic prophylaxis for certain women?**

Procedures that involve manipulation of the gingiva, oral mucosa, or periapical tooth region.

○ **Women with what types of cardiac conditions require antibiotic prophylaxis for invasive dental procedures?**

Prosthetic heart valves or prior history of infective endocarditis, prosthetic material used for repair of congenital heart defects for 6 months after repair or if residual defect adjacent to the prosthetic material, and unrepaired cyanotic congenital heart defects.

○ **Is antibiotic prophylaxis indicated during delivery for women with prosthetic heart valves?**

Only if active infection or suspected bacteremia.

○ **Is chemical or electrical cardioversion safer for supraventricular tachycardia in pregnancy?**

Adenosine for termination of supraventricular tachycardia is considered safe in pregnancy. Electrical cardioversion must be approached with caution; it has been reported to lead to sustained uterine contractions and prolonged fetal heart rate deceleration.

○ **What lifestyle modifications are recommended for patients with chronic hypertension?**

Weight reduction, restriction of dietary sodium and fat, physical activity, limitation of alcohol consumption, and smoking cessation.

○ **What workup is recommended for pregnant women with chronic hypertension?**

Ophthalmologic evaluation and echocardiogram in any patient with prolonged hypertension or prior complications, 24-hour urine protein, and serum creatinine.

○ **What is the maternal mortality rate for women with chronic hypertension?**

230 per 100,000 live births.

○ **What are the risk factors for the development of superimposed preeclampsia in patients with chronic hypertension?**

Prolonged hypertension (>4 years) and history of superimposed preeclampsia in previous pregnancy.

○ **Chronic hypertension increases the risk of which pregnancy outcomes?**

Intrauterine growth restriction, preterm delivery, infant NICU admission, and perinatal mortality.

○ **At what blood pressure, should medication be started for chronic hypertension?**

Systolic 150 to 160 mmHg or diastolic 100 to 110 mmHg.

○ **What medications are recommended for management of chronic hypertension in pregnancy?**

Labetalol, methyldopa, and nifedipine are used most often. Diuretics are not recommended due to the theoretical risk of decreased volume expansion in pregnancy. Angiotensin-converting enzyme inhibitors are teratogenic and are contraindicated in pregnancy.

○ **What is the rate of superimposed preeclampsia in patients with chronic hypertension?**

Approximately 25%.

○ **How is the diagnosis of superimposed preeclampsia made?**

New onset neurologic symptoms, proteinuria, oliguria, elevated transaminases, or low platelets are suggestive of superimposed preeclampsia. Increasing blood pressures in the third trimester are not necessarily due to superimposed preeclampsia, and antihypertensive medications may be initiated or increased in the absence of other signs or symptoms of preeclampsia.

○ **When should delivery be planned for women with chronic hypertension?**

If the hypertension is well controlled, it is safe to await labor at term.

PULMONARY CONDITIONS

○ **What is the prevalence of asthma in pregnancy?**

4% to 8%.

○ **How often do symptoms occur in mild intermittent asthma?**

Twice per week or less. Nocturnal symptoms may occur twice per month or less.

○ **What severity of asthma correlates with daily symptoms?**

Moderate persistent asthma.

○ **What is the forced expiratory volume after 1 second (FEV1) in severe persistent asthma?**

<60% of predicated, and variability >30%.

○ **What is the effect of pregnancy on asthma?**

Approximately one-third of pregnant women's asthma improve, 1/3 remain unchanged, and 1/3 worsen.

○ **How should pregnant women with asthma be monitored?**

Women with moderate or severe asthma should measure their peak expiratory flow rate (PEFR) or FEV1 twice daily.

○ **What is the typical PEFR in pregnancy?**

380 to 550 L/min. Women who are at >80% of their predicted PEFR require no additional treatment.

○ **How can asthma affect maternal and perinatal outcomes?**

Women with severe asthma or who require use of oral corticosteroids have an increased risk of preterm delivery. Asthma also increases the risk of preeclampsia, cesarean delivery, gestational diabetes, and small for gestational age infants.

○ **What is the stepwise care therapeutic approach?**

The goal is to use the least pharmacologic intervention that is required to control a patient's asthma symptoms.

○ **When is a burst of oral corticosteroids indicated?**

Exacerbations not responding to initial beta 2 agonists regardless of asthma severity.

○ **Describe a short course of oral corticosteroids.**

Oral prednisone 40 to 60 mg per day for 1 week, followed by a 7 to 14-day taper.

○ **What is the preferred treatment of mild intermittent asthma?**

Inhaled beta agonists as needed.

○ **What is the preferred treatment of pregnant women with persistent asthma?**

Inhaled corticosteroids.

○   **Which inhaled corticosteroid is preferred?**

Budesonide (class B), because there is more data for its safety in pregnancy.

○   **What is the definition of status asthmaticus?**

Severe asthma not responding to 30 to 60 minutes of intensive therapy. Intensive care admission and intubation when necessary to maintain oxygenation are important next steps.

○   **Which malformation has been associated with oral corticosteroid use during the first trimester?**

Isolated cleft lip with or without cleft palate.

○   **When are stress dose steroids required?**

When a woman has had >20 mg/day of prednisone for 3 weeks or more.

○   **What is the most effective treatment of allergic rhinitis?**

Intranasal corticosteroids.

○   **What fetal monitoring should be considered for patients with moderate-to-severe asthma?**

Serial ultrasounds for fetal growth.

○   **What medication used for postpartum hemorrhage must be avoided in patients with asthma?**

Hemabate, or prostaglandin F2, because it may cause significant bronchospasm.

○   **What is a complication of viral upper respiratory infection that may have severe consequences in pregnancy?**

Pneumonia.

○   **What are typical symptoms of pneumonia?**

Cough, sputum production, dyspnea, and pleuritic chest pain.

○   **What diagnostic test should be ordered when a pregnant woman is suspected to have pneumonia?**

Chest X-ray.

○   **What are the most common bacteria that cause pneumonia?**

Streptococcus pneumonia. Other causes include Mycoplasma and Chlamydophila.

○   **What are criteria for severe pneumonia for which ICU admission is suggested?**

Relative risk (RR) ≥30/min, PaO_2/FiO_2 ratio ≤250, multilobular infiltrates, confusion or disorientation, uremia, leukopenia (WBC <4000/μL), hypothermia, and hypotension.

○   **What is the treatment of severe pneumonia?**

A respiratory fluoroquinolone (levofloxacin, moxifloxacin, or gemifloxacin) or a beta lactam plus a macrolide (amoxicillin clavulanate, Augmentin, or ceftriaxone plus azithromycin, clarithromycin, or erythromycin). Uncomplicated pneumonia may be treated with macrolide monotherapy.

○ **For whom is the pneumococcal vaccine recommended?**

Immunocompromised women, those with HIV, smoking history, diabetes, asplenia, or cardiac, pulmonary, or renal disease.

○ **What is the treatment of influenza in pregnancy?**

Supportive treatment as well as oseltamivir 75 mg bid for 5 days.

○ **For whom is influenza vaccination recommended?**

All pregnant women should receive influenza vaccination.

○ **Which women should receive testing for tuberculosis?**

Healthcare workers, history of contact with infected persons, foreign-born, HIV-infected, working or living in homeless shelters, alcoholics, illicit drug use, detainees, and prisoners.

○ **What is the next step for women with a positive purified protein derivative (PPD)?**

Chest X-ray to determine if there is evidence of active disease.

○ **When should pregnant women be treated for a positive PPD?**

In general treatment should be delayed for 3 to 6 months postpartum. In cases of a known recent conversion or HIV-positive women should be treated right away because they are at higher risk of developing active TB. They should be given isoniazid 300 mg daily for 1 year.

○ **What is the treatment of active tuberculosis in pregnancy?**

Three-drug regimen with isoniazid, rifampin, and ethambutol for 9 months

GASTROINTESTINAL

○ **What is the definition of hyperemesis gravidarum?**

Vomiting sufficiently severe to cause weight loss, dehydration, metabolic alkalosis, and hypokalemia.

○ **What is the recurrence rate of hyperemesis requiring hospitalization?**

Up to 20% of women have a recurrence of hyperemesis in a subsequent pregnancy.

○ **What is the treatment of hyperemesis?**

Inpatient management with intravenous (IV) hydration if vomiting persists, antiemetics such as promethazine, prochlorperazine, ondansetron, or metoclopramide. Short courses of steroids may decrease readmission rates.

○ **What is the management of women with peptic ulcers in pregnancy?**

Antacids, H2-receptor blockers, or proton pump inhibitors. If *Helicobacter pylori* infection is identified, it should be treated with an antibiotic regimen that does not include tetracycline.

○ **What is the management of ulcerative colitis in pregnancy?**

5-Aminosalicyclic acid or mesalamine both may be used for active colitis.

○ **What medications for Chron's disease may be used in pregnancy?**

Azathioprine, 6-mercaptopurine, and cyclosporine are safe in pregnancy. Methotrexate should not be used.

○ **What is the effect of pregnancy on inflammatory bowel disease?**

Pregnancy has not been shown to have any effect on Chron's disease or ulcerative colitis.

○ **What is the rate of appendicitis in pregnancy?**

1/1000 to 1500 pregnancies.

○ **Is the risk of appendiceal rupture affected by pregnancy?**

There is a higher risk of appendiceal rupture in pregnancy, 8%, 12%, and 20% in the first, second, and third trimesters, respectively.

○ **How is appendicitis diagnosed in pregnancy?**

Clinically, persistent abdominal pain and tenderness are suggestive. Ultrasound should be undertaken, and if nondiagnostic, CT or MRI imaging should be obtained. Surgical exploration is necessary if the diagnosis is likely.

○ **What is the risk of fetal loss after appendectomy?**

Approximately 23%; however, surgical intervention should not be delayed because appendicitis can quickly progress to peritonitis.

RENAL/UROLOGIC SYSTEMS

○ **What is the most common bacterial infection during pregnancy?**

Urinary tract infection.

○ **What is the prevalence of asymptomatic bacteriuria in pregnancy?**

5% to 8%.

○ **When does asymptomatic bacteriuria usually present?**

At the first prenatal visit.

○ **What are the possible consequences of untreated asymptomatic bacteriuria?**

Low birth weight, prematurity, and pyelonephritis.

○ **What antibiotic regimen is recommended for suppression in women with persistent or frequent urinary tract infections?**

Nitrofurantoin 100 mg at bedtime for the remainder of the pregnancy.

○ **What is the probable cause of an infection in a woman with frequency, urgency, dysuria, and pyuria, but with a negative urine culture and mucopurulent cervicitis?**

Chlamydia trachomatis.

○ **On which side is pyelonephritis more common?**

Pyelonephritis is unilateral and right sided in more than half of cases.

○ **What are the most common organisms causing pyelonephritis?**

Escherichia coli is isolated in 70% to 80% of infections, *Klebsiella pneumoniae* in 3% to 5%, *Enterobacter* or *Proteus* in 3% to 5% and gram-positive organisms including group B *Streptococcus* (GBS) in up to 10%.

○ **How often is bacteremia present in women with acute pyelonephritis?**

15% to 20%.

○ **What are the complications of pyelonephritis?**

20% of patient develop renal dysfunction, 1/3 develop acute anemia due to hemolysis, and 1% to 2% develop respiratory insufficiency that may lead to acute respiratory distress syndrome (ARDS).

○ **What is the initial treatment of acute pyelonephritis in pregnancy?**

Hospital admission, blood and urine cultures, IV hydration to ensure adequate urine output, empiric IV antibiotics with ampicillin and gentamicin or cefazolin or ceftriaxone.

○ **After a woman with pyelonephritis is afebrile, what are the next steps in management?**

She should be changed to oral antibiotics. Discharge can be considered when she has been afebrile for 24 hours. Antibiotics should be continued for 7 to 10 days and a repeat urine culture should be obtained 1 to 2 weeks after treatment is completed.

○ **What should be done if a woman does not improve clinically within 48 to 72 hours after initiation of treatment of pyelonephritis?**

Urinary tract imaging to rule out an obstruction.

○ **Which stones are most common during pregnancy?**

Calcium phosphate.

○ **What are indications for kidney stone removal?**

Obstruction, infection, intractable pain, and heavy bleeding.

○ **Which stones are associated with *Proteus* or *Klebsiella*?**

Struvite stones.

○ **How does acute glomerulonephritis affect pregnancy?**

There is an increased rate of fetal loss and perinatal mortality, prematurity and growth restriction, hypertension, and worsening of proteinuria.

○ **What are the two most important factors in predicting pregnancy outcome in women with chronic renal disease?**

Degree of hypertension and renal insufficiency.

○   **Which pregnancy complications are associated with chronic renal disease?**

Hypertension, anemia, preeclampsia, preterm delivery, and fetal growth restriction.

○   **When should dialysis be initiated?**

When serum creatinine levels are 5 to 7 mg/dL.

○   **Women who have received kidney transplants should achieve what goals before attempting pregnancy?**

Good general health for 2 years after transplant, serum Cr <2.0 with none to minimal proteinuria, and absent or easily controlled hypertension.

○   **What is the most common cause of acute renal failure in pregnancy?**

Severe preeclampsia/eclampsia.

INFECTIONS

○   **How do you define vertical transmission of an infection?**

Passage of infection from mother to fetus through the placenta, during labor and delivery, or postpartum via breastfeeding.

○   **When does fetal immunity develop?**

Between 9 and 15 weeks' gestation.

○   **What is the incubation period of herpes?**

2 to 12 days.

○   **What are the three stages of herpes simplex virus (HSV) infection?**

Primary: Infection in a patient without preexisting antibodies to HSV 1 or 2
Recurrent: Reactivation with homologous antibodies present
Nonprimary first episode: Infection with one type of HSV in the presence of antibodies to the other type

○   **What is the incidence of new HSV infection among susceptible pregnant women?**
Approximately 2%.

○   **What is the reason for most neonatal HSV infections?**
Delivery through an infected birth canal, most often in asymptomatic mothers.

○   **What is the classification of neonatal HSV infection?**

(1) Localized disease of the skin, eye, and mouth—the most common (45%). Not associated with neonatal mortality

(2) CNS disease with or without skin, eye, and mouth disease (30%). 4% mortality

(3) Disseminated disease (25%). 30% mortality

○ **What is the maternal fetal vertical transmission rate?**

Primary: 30% to 60%, nonprimary first episode: 33%, recurrent 0% to 3%.

○ **What is the risk of transmission for women with a history of recurrent disease and no visible lesions at delivery?**
2:10,000.

○ **In what situations should cesarean delivery be considered for prevention of neonatal HSV?**

Cesarean delivery should be performed for women with active genital lesions or symptoms such as vulvar pain or burning at delivery, which may indicate an impending outbreak.

○ **Is cesarean delivery recommended for women with recurrent HSV lesions on the back, thigh, or buttock?**

No. These lesions may be covered with an occlusive dressing.

○ **What is the most common congenital infection in the United States?**

Cytomegalovirus (CMV).

○ **How can vertical transmission of CMV occur?**

Transplacental infection, exposure to contaminated genital tract secretions at parturition or breastfeeding.

○ **When is the risk of transmission of CMV the highest?**

Primary maternal infection has a risk of transmission of 30% to 40%, while a recurrent infection has a risk of 0.15% to 2%. The overall risk of infection is greatest in the third trimester (but is more severe when infection occurs in the first trimester).

○ **What are symptoms of congenital CMV syndrome?**

Growth restriction, microcephaly, intracranial calcifications, chorioretinitis, sensorineural defects, hepatosplenomegaly, jaundice, hemolytic anemia, thrombocytopenia purpura, and mental retardation.

○ **What is the sensitivity of CMV immunoglobulin M (IgM) serologic assays?**
50% to 90%.

○ **What are possible consequences of fetal acquisition of parvovirus B19 infection?**

Spontaneous abortion, hydrops fetalis, and stillbirth.

○ **When does hydrops develop due to parvovirus B19?**

Within 10 weeks of maternal infection.

○ **What fetal monitoring should be done for women diagnosed with parvovirus B19?**

Serial ultrasounds should be performed every 2 weeks. MCA Doppler should be used to diagnose fetal anemia.

○ **What are the characteristics of congenital varicella syndrome?**

Skin scarring, limb hypoplasia, chorioretinitis, and microcephaly.

○ **During what weeks of pregnancy is the risk of congenital varicella syndrome the highest?**

Between 13 and 20 weeks when 2% of fetuses of women with primary varicella develop the syndrome.

○ **What is the most dangerous time for varicella zoster virus (VZV) infection in regard to neonatal death?**

When the maternal infection develops between 5 days prior to delivery and 48 hours postpartum (these infants should receive VZIG).

○ **What is the treatment of maternal varicella?**

Oral acyclovir. A chest X-ray should be performed to look for varicella pneumonia, and if present women should be hospitalized and given IV acyclovir.

○ **How should a susceptible woman exposed to varicella be managed?**

VZIG should be given as soon as possible, ideally within 96 hours of exposure.

○ **Is screening for maternal toxoplasmosis recommended?**

Only in women with HIV.

○ **What is the rate of vertical transmission of toxoplasmosis?**

10% to 15% in the first trimester, 25% in the second trimester, and 60% in the third trimester. The earlier the fetus is infected the more severe the disease.

○ **What is the treatment of maternal toxoplasmosis infection?**

Spiramycin. If fetal infection is established, pyrimethamine, sulfadiazine, and folic acid are added.

○ **What antibiotic should be given during labor to a woman who is GBS positive and developed a rash when given penicillin as a child?**

Cefazolin 2 g initially then 1 g every 8 hours until delivery.

○ **If GBS status is unknown, what risk factors should be used to determine which women should receive prophylaxis?**

Previous infant with invasive GBS disease, GBS bacteriuria during current pregnancy, delivery at <37 weeks' gestation, amniotic membrane rupture ≥18 hours, and intrapartum temperature ≥100.4°F.

○ **What foods should pregnant women avoid to prevent listeriosis?**

Raw vegetables, coleslaw, apple cider, melons, milk, fresh Mexican-style cheese, smoked fish, and processed foods, such as pâté, hummus, wieners, and sliced deli meats.

○ **What are characteristics of maternal and fetal listeriosis?**

Maternal listeriosis may present similarly to meningitis, pyelonephritis, or influenza. Fetal infection is characterized by disseminated granulomatous lesions with microabscesses.

○ **What is the most common route of fetal acquisition of syphilis?**

Transplacental. Infection may also be caused by contact with lesions at delivery.

○ **What are the stages of syphilis?**

Primary: Painless chancre

Secondary: Disseminated disease with macular rash and condylomata lata, fever, myalgias, and malaise

Latent: Untreated primary or secondary syphilis that has no clinical manifestations but may be diagnosed by serologic testing

Tertiary: Characterized by gummas, neurosyphilis, or cardiovascular syphilis

○ **What is the treatment of syphilis and what reaction may occur when treatment is given to pregnant women?**

Penicillin G is the only proven effective treatment of syphilis. Women with anaphylaxis to penicillin should be desensitized. Women treated for syphilis in pregnancy may develop a Jarisch-Herxheimer reaction involving uterine contractions and late fetal heart rate decelerations. These resolve within 24 hours.

○ **To which HIV-infected pregnant woman should antiretroviral treatment be offered?**

All HIV-infected women regardless of T cell count or viral load.

○ **How should HIV RNA levels be monitored?**

Four weeks after initiation of a change in treatment, monthly until undetectable, then every 3 months including a value near term.

○ **What is the regimen of zidovudine antepartum?**

100 mg orally five times daily, 200 mg three times daily, or 300 mg twice daily.

○ **When should IV zidovudine be started prior to elective cesarean delivery?**

3 hours prior to surgery.

○ **What is the maternal treatment if the HIV RNA level is >1000 copies/mL?**

Combination antiretroviral therapy.

○ **What is the recommended mode of delivery?**

Scheduled cesarean delivery as early as 38 weeks is recommended for HIV-infected women with over 1000 copies/mL of HIV RNA. Cesarean delivery is unlikely to offer additional benefit when the HIV RNA levels are below 1000 copies/mL.

○ **Who should be screened for gonorrhea and what is the treatment of a positive result?**

All women should be screened for *Gonorrhea* and *Chlamydia* at the first prenatal visit. Treatment of gonorrhea in pregnancy is ceftriaxone 250 mg IM and 1 g of azithromycin orally due to increasing prevalence of ceftriaxone resistant gonorrhea. A test of cure should be conducted 1 week after treatment.

○ **When should women with bacterial vaginosis be treated?**

Symptomatic women should be treated with metronidazole, 500 mg bid for 7 days. Vaginal metronidazole or clindamycin may also be used. Treatment does not decrease the rate of preterm birth.

○   **When should women with trichomoniasis be treated and what is the risk of treatment?**

Treatment should be given to symptomatic women. 2 g of metronidazole in a single dose is the most effective regimen. Treatment may increase the risk of preterm birth; however, the exact risk remains unknown.

ENDOCRINE

Diabetes

○   **When should the 50 g 1-hour oral glucose challenge test be administered?**

24 to 28 weeks gestation.

○   **What is the cutoff value that gives 90% sensitivity for gestational diabetes?**

130 mg/dL. 140 mg/dL cutoff is 80% sensitive.

○   **What is the diagnostic test for gestational diabetes?**

Women who screen positive in the glucose challenge test should receive the 100 g, 3-hour oral glucose tolerance test, which should be performed in a fasting state.

○   **What are the Carpenter-Coustan criteria for the diagnosis of gestational diabetes mellitus?**

Fasting: 95 mg/dL, 1 hour: 180 mg/dL, 2 hours: 155 mg/dL, 3 hours: 140 mg/dL. Two or more abnormal values give a diagnosis of gestational diabetes.

○   **What is the rate of recurrence of gestational diabetes in a subsequent pregnancy?**

33% to 50%.

○   **What is the effect of primary dietary therapy for gestational diabetes on fetal growth and neonatal outcomes?**

There is no significant effect on birth weight >4000 g or cesarean delivery.

○   **When should medical intervention be considered for gestational diabetes mellitus?**

When fasting blood sugars are >95 mg/dL or 2-hour postprandial values are >120 mg/dL.

○   **What is the prevalence of pregestational diabetes in the United States?**

1% of all pregnancies.

○   **Is insulin resistance increased or decreased during pregnancy?**

Insulin sensitivity is enhanced late in the first trimester by higher levels of estrogen, but later in pregnancy insulin resistance increased and is greatest in the third trimester.

○   **Which hormones contribute to the increase in insulin resistance?**

Placental hormones including human placental lactogen (hPL), progesterone, prolactin, placental growth hormone, and cortisol. TNF alpha and leptin also contribute.

○ **What does hemoglobin A1c reflect?**

It reflects the glycemic control over the past 2 to 3 months. A HbA$_{1c}$ level of 8% indicates a mean glucose level of 180 mg/dL, with each 1% higher or lower equal to a change of 30 mg/dL.

○ **When should regular insulin be given?**

30 minutes prior to eating.

○ **How does pregnancy affect diabetic retinopathy?**

It may cause acute progression of retinopathy.

○ **What are the laboratory findings associated with diabetic ketoacidosis?**

Low arterial pH (<7.3), a low serum bicarbonate level (<15 mEq/L), an elevated anion gap, and positive serum ketones.

○ **What does the treatment of diabetic ketoacidosis include?**

Laboratory assessment, IV insulin, IV hydration, repletion of glucose, potassium, and bicarbonate as needed.

○ **What is the loading dose of insulin?**

0.2 to 0.4 units/kg, followed by maintenance of 2 to 10 units per hour.

○ **Does glyburide cross the placenta?**

No.

○ **What are the pharmacokinetics of glyburide?**

Onset is 4 hours and duration is 10 hours.

○ **When should antenatal testing be initiated?**

At 32 to 34 weeks, or earlier in complicated pregnancies. Testing should include twice weekly nonstress tests. Doppler velocimetry of the umbilical artery may be useful in cases with vascular complications and poor fetal growth.

○ **When should cesarean delivery be considered in a gestational diabetic patient?**

When EFW is >4500 g.

THYROID DISEASE

○ **Which of the thyroid function tests increase during pregnancy?**

Thyroid-binding globulin (TBG), total thyroxine (TT4), and total triiodothyroxine (TT3).

○ **When does the fetal thyroid begin concentrating iodine?**

Between 10 and 12 weeks; however, maternal thyroxine (T4) remains important throughout pregnancy. Maternal thyroxine accounts for 30% of thyroxine in the fetal serum at term.

○ **Which thyroid hormone is the least likely to cross the placenta?**

Thyroid-stimulating hormone (TSH).

○ **What is the most common etiology of hyperthyroidism in pregnancy?**

Graves disease.

○ **Name general signs and symptoms of hyperthyroidism.**

Tremors, nervousness, tachycardia, frequent stools, sweating, heat intolerance, weight loss, goiter, insomnia, palpitations, and hypertension.

○ **What are symptoms and signs specific to Graves disease?**

Ophthalmopathy (including lid lag and lid retraction) and dermopathy (including localized or pretibial myxedema).

○ **What complications may result from inadequately treated thyrotoxicosis?**

Preterm delivery, severe preeclampsia, heart failure, low birth weight infant, and fetal loss.

○ **What effect may maternal Graves disease have in the neonate?**

The neonate may have either immune-mediated hypothyroidism or hyperthyroidism due to inhibitory immunoglobulin (TBII) or thyroid-stimulating immunoglobulins, (TSI) respectively, which cross the placenta.

○ **What medications can be used to manage hyperthyroidism and what are their mechanisms of action?**

Methimazole and propylthiouracil (PTU) both inhibit thyroperoxidase, which is necessary for addition of iodine to tyrosine to form T3 and T4.

○ **What is the side effect of major concern for women taking the thioamines PTU or methimazole?**

Agranulocytosis, which occurs in 0.1% to 0.4% of patients taking thioamines, usually presents with fever and sore throat. Thrombocytopenia, hepatitis, vasculitis, rash, fever, nausea, and loss of sense of smell or taste are other possible side effects.

○ **What is the recommended treatment of hyperthyroidism in pregnancy and why?**

PTU should be used in the first trimester because methimazole has been associated with choanal and esophageal atresia. After the first trimester PTU should be converted to an equivalent dose of methimazole because PTU can cause hepatotoxicity.

○ **What is the treatment of hyperthyroidism in contraindicated in pregnancy?**

Iodine 131 because it may also cause fetal thyroid gland destruction. Women should avoid pregnancy for 6 months after receiving radioactive iodine ablation.

○ **What is the clinical presentation of thyroid storm?**

Fever; tachycardia out of proportion to fever; altered mental status—restlessness, nervousness, confusion, seizures; vomiting; diarrhea; cardiac arrhythmia. Thyroid storm complicated 1% of pregnancies with hyperthyroidism.

○ **How is thyroid storm treated?**

(1) PTU 600 to 800 mg orally STAT, then 150 to 200 mg orally every 4 to 6 hours. Alternatively, methimazole rectal suppositories may be used if oral administration is not possible

(2) 1 to 2 hours after PTU administration 2 to 5 drops of saturated solution of potassium iodide every 8 hours, sodium iodide 0.5 to 1.0 g IV q8 h, Lugol solution, 8 drops q6h, or lithium carbonate, 300 mg po q6h.

(3) Dexamethasone, 2 mg IV or IM q6h × 4 doses

(4) Propranolol 20 to 80 mg orally q4 to 6 h or 1 to 2 mg IV q5 min for a total of 6 mg, then 1 to 10 mg IV q4h. Alternatively reserpine, guanethidine, or diltiazem may be used if the patient has a history of severe bronchospasm.

(5) Phenobarbital 30 to 60 mg orally q6 to 8 h for extreme restlessness

○ **Name some signs and symptoms of hypothyroidism.**

Fatigue, constipation, cold intolerance, muscle cramps, hair loss, dry skin, prolonged relaxation phase of deep tendon reflexes, carpal tunnel syndrome, weight gain in spite of decreased appetite, intellectual slowness, voice changes, and insomnia. Untreated hypothyroidism may progress to myxedema coma.

○ **What neonatal condition is associated with iodine deficient hypothyroidism?**

Congenital cretinism.

○ **What is the most common etiology of hypothyroidism in developed countries?**

Hashimoto disease.

○ **What antibodies are associated with Hashimoto disease?**

Thyroid antimicrosomal and antithyroglobulin antibodies.

○ **What laboratory values should be measured in pregnant women suspected to have thyroid disease?**

TSH and free T4, or free thyroxine index (FTI).

○ **How often should the dose of levothyroxine be adjusted?**

It takes 4 weeks for the effects of levothyroxine to be reflected in the TSH level, so doses should not be adjusted more frequently than every 4 weeks.

○ **Is treatment of subclinical hypothyroidism of any benefit?**

Studies have shown no benefit in IQ scores of children born to women with subclinical hypothyroidism that were treated versus untreated. There is no recommendation to treat subclinical hypothyroidism in pregnancy.

○ **How should thyroid cancer be managed in pregnancy?**

Surgery can often be delayed until after delivery due to the indolent course of most thyroid cancers and the risk of preterm delivery due to surgery.

○ **What is the incidence of postpartum thyroiditis, and what is the treatment?**

Postpartum thyroiditis occurs in 5% of pregnancies. The first phase occurs 2 to 6 months postpartum and is characterized by a hyperthyroid phase due to rebounding immune function and increased levels of thyroid-stimulating antibodies. Intervention is not usually required other than possibly a short course of beta blockers for symptomatic management. The second phase involved hypothyroidism and occurs between 3 and 12 months postpartum, and resolves by 12 months postpartum. Levothyroxine treatment may be necessary but can be discontinued 1 year after delivery.

RHEUMATOLOGY

Systemic Lupus Erythematosus

○ **How is systemic lupus erythematosus (SLE) diagnosed?**

Four of the following eleven criteria must be fulfilled, in which case a diagnosis of SLE can be made with a sensitivity of 95% and specificity of 75%.

- Malar rash
- Discoid rash
- Photosensitivity
- Oral ulcers
- Arthritis (joint pain and swelling of two or more joints)
- Serositis (pleuritis or pericarditis)
- Kidney disorder (persistent proteinuria or cellular casts in the urine)
- Neurologic disorder (seizures or psychosis)
- Hematologic disorder (anemia, leukopenia, lymphopenia, or thrombocytopenia)
- Immunologic disorder (positive anti-dsDNA, anti-Sm, or antiphospholipid antibodies)
- Abnormal antinuclear antibodies

○ **How does pregnancy affect lupus?**

A third of women experience improvement in their disease, however a third have worsening disease and a third stay the same.

○ **When is the prognosis for mother and child best?**

When the disease has been quiescent for 6 months prior to conception, there is no active renal involvement, superimposed preeclampsia does not develop, and there is no evidence of antiphospholipid antibody activity.

○ **How is worsening lupus differentiated from preeclampsia?**

Decreased complement levels or increased anti-DNA antibody titers are useful in identifying a lupus flare. Elevated serum levels of liver enzymes and uric acid, as well as decreased urinary excretion of calcium, are more suggestive of preeclampsia.

○ **What is the incidence of preeclampsia in women with SLE?**

Chronic hypertension complicates 30% of pregnancies of women with SLE. Superimposed preeclampsia develops in 13% to 35%, and is higher in women with lupus nephritis or antiphospholipid antibodies.

○ **What is the recommended laboratory workup in the first prenatal visit for a woman with SLE?**

In addition to routine blood work there should also be a measurement of disease activity (C3, C4, CH50, anti-ds DNA antibodies), risk of neonatal lupus (anti-SSA and anti-La antibody (SSB)), risk of fetal loss (lupus anticoagulant, anticardiolipin antibodies), and risk of renal function (24-hour urine protein).

○ **Which factors increase the risk of fetal loss?**

Hypertension, active lupus, lupus nephritis, hypocomplementemia, elevated levels of anti-DNA antibodies, antiphospholipid antibodies, or thrombocytopenia. Fetal loss usually occurs after 10 weeks' gestation.

○ **What is the most serious complication of neonatal lupus, and which maternal antibody is it associated with?**

Congenital heart block in the neonate is associated with maternal anti-Ro or SSA antibodies that cross the placenta. The recurrence risk of congenital heart block is 15%.

○ **What fetal monitoring should be done for pregnant women with lupus?**

Ultrasounds to evaluate fetal growth, weekly monitoring of the fetal heart rhythm after 16 weeks to monitor for heart block, and biweekly nonstress tests beginning at 28 weeks.

○ **What medications to treat SLE are safe during pregnancy?**

NSAIDs prior to 24 weeks and antimalarial drugs, which can be useful for skin manifestations of lupus. Corticosteroids and azathioprine may also be used in pregnancy.

○ **What congenital malformation is associated with glucocorticoid use in pregnancy?**

Cleft palate.

○ **What medications used for SLE should be avoided in pregnancy?**

Cyclophosphamide is teratogenic and should be avoided, although in severe cases may be used after 12 weeks. Methotrexate and mycophenolate mofetil should also be avoided.

ANTIPHOSPHOLIPID ANTIBODY SYNDROME

○ **What are the two antiphospholipid antibodies?**

Lupus anticoagulant and anticardiolipin antibodies.

○ **What is antiphospholipid antibody syndrome?**

Antiphospholipid antibodies may be found in asymptomatic patients with or without lupus; however, when they are present and associated with recurrent thrombosis, thromobocytopenia, or second trimester fetal loss, the diagnosis of antiphospholipid antibody syndrome is made. Anticardiolipin antibodies or lupus anticoagulant must be identified on two occasions, at least 6 weeks apart.

○ **What percentage of women with normal, unaffected, pregnancies are positive for antiphospholipid antibodies?**

5%.

○ **What is the risk of pregnancy-related thrombosis in women with antiphospholipid antibody syndrome?**

5% to 12% during pregnancy or the puerperium.

○ **What percentage of women with antiphospholipid antibody syndrome will develop preeclampsia?**

Approximately one-third of women.

○ **What is the treatment of antiphospholipid antibody syndrome in pregnancy?**

Low-dose aspirin daily concurrently with low-dose heparin twice daily during pregnancy and continued until 6 to 8 weeks postpartum. This treatment regimen may reduce pregnancy loss by 54%.

○ **What antepartum testing is recommended for women with antiphospholipid antibody syndrome?**

Serial ultrasounds for growth and biweekly nonstress tests starting at 32 weeks.

OTHER RHEUMATOLOGIC CONDITIONS

○ **How does pregnancy affect rheumatoid arthritis?**

90% of women with rheumatoid arthritis have symptomatic improvement in pregnancy. However, postpartum exacerbation is common.

○ **What medications may be used for rheumatoid arthritis in pregnancy?**

NSAIDs may be used prior to 24 weeks' gestation, but not after due to concern for premature closure of the ductus arteriosus. Aspirin may be used and low-dose corticosteroids. Disease-modifying drugs are usually avoided during pregnancy due to their teratogenicity; however, azathioprine is considered safe during pregnancy.

○ **What effect does pregnancy have on scleroderma-associated dysphagia and reflux esophagitis?**

Dysphagia and reflux are worsened by pregnancy; however, all other manifestations of the disease are stable in pregnancy.

○ **Can vaginal delivery be attempted in women with systemic sclerosis?**

Yes, unless soft tissue thickening of the vulva produces dystocia.

○ **What is the preferred method of anesthesia for cesarean delivery for women with scleroderma?**

Epidural or spinal anesthesia, given the limited ability to open the mouth wide for endotracheal intubation.

○ **Which rheumatologic disorder is associated with increased frequency of dissecting and ruptured aneurysms during pregnancy?**

Marfan syndrome.

○ **What pregnancy complications are associated with Ehlers-Danlos syndrome?**

Preterm premature rupture of membranes, prematurity, and antepartum and postpartum hemorrhage.

HEMATOLOGIC

○ **What cutoff is used for anemia in pregnancy and why is it lower than in nonpregnant women?**

11g/dL in the first and third trimesters and 10.5 in the second trimester, which is lower than nonpregnant values due to expansion of the blood volume to a greater degree than the red blood cell mass in pregnancy.

○ **How much iron is required in pregnancy?**

1000 mg per day; 300 mg for the fetus and placenta, 500 mg for maternal hemoglobin, and 200 mg lost through the GI tract.

○ **What ethnic groups are at higher risk of hemoglobinopathies?**

African, Southeast Asian, and Mediterranean.

○ **What is hemoglobin S and hemoglobin C?**

Hemoglobin S is a tetramer of 2 normal alpha chains and two beta chains with a single mutation of valine for glutamic acid at codon 6. Hemoglobin C has a substitution of lysine for glutamic acid at the same position.

○ **What is the inheritance pattern of sickle cell disease?**

Autosomal recessive.

○ **What is the prevalence of sickle cell trait in people of African origin?**

1:12 African Americans have sickle cell trait. 1:40 are heterozygous for hemoglobin C.

○ **What obstetric complications occur in pregnant women with sickle cell disease?**

Renal failure, gestational hypertension, and fetal growth restriction.

○ **What is the recommended dose of folic acid supplementation for patients with sickle cell disease?**

4 mg per day.

○ **What is acute chest syndrome?**

Pleuritic chest pain, fever, cough, hypoxia, and pulmonary infiltrate in a patient with sickle cell disease that may be caused by infection, infarction, atelectasis, or fat embolism.

○ **What fetal monitoring is recommended for women with sickle cell disease?**

Serial ultrasounds for growth as well as antenatal testing.

○ **What are thalassemias?**

Impaired production of normal hemoglobin chains.

○ **How many alpha globin genes are there?**

Four.

○ **How is alpha thalassemia diagnosed?**

By genetic testing only, it cannot be diagnosed on hemoglobin electrophoresis. The diagnosis should be considered in women with microcytic anemia who are not iron deficient and do not have beta thalassemia.

○ **What is hemoglobin Bart?**

A tetramer of four gamma chains that is moderately insoluble and accumulates in red cells. It has a high oxygen affinity and sequesters oxygen, leaving little to be delivered to tissues.

○ **What are the two forms of alpha thalassemia minor, and which is potentially worse for inheritance?**

Alpha thalassemia minor is deletion of two out of the four alpha globin genes. These can be on the same (cis) or opposite (trans) chromosomes. If both parents have the cis-form, there is a 50% risk of alpha thalassemia major.

○ **What are the different types of alpha thalassemia?**

Alpha thalassemia trait: Deletion of one alpha globin gene, which is usually asymptomatic

Alpha thalassemia minor: Deletion of two alpha globin genes, either on the same or opposite chromosomes. This causes mild to moderate microcytic anemia.

Hemoglobin H disease: Deletion of three of four alpha globin genes, leading to a mixture of hemoglobin Bart ($\gamma 4$), hemoglobin H ($\beta 4$), and hemoglobin A. Patients have moderate to severe hemolytic anemia

Alpha thalassemia major: Deletion of all four alpha globin chains, which are incompatible with extrauterine life.

○ **What is beta thalassemia?**

Impaired production of beta globin chains, causing precipitation of alpha globin in red blood cells.

○ **What are characteristics of beta thalassemia major (Cooley anemia)?**

The infant born with beta thalassemia major is healthy at birth but as hemoglobin F levels fall it develops anemia and failure to thrive.

○ **Elevated hemoglobin F (>2%) and A2 (>3.5%) are associated with which condition?**

Beta thalassemia minor.

○ **How is von Willebrand disease inherited?**

Most variants are inherited in an autosomal dominant fashion.

○ **What is Virchow triad?**

Conditions that lead to an increased risk of venous thrombosis are (1) stasis, (2) vessel trauma, and (3) hypercoagulability.

○ **Which clotting factors rise in pregnancy?**

Factors I, VII, VIII, X, von Willebrand factor, and plasminogen activator inhibitors 1 and 2, which are all procoagulants.

○ **Which clotting factors diminish during pregnancy?**

Protein S, an anticoagulant.

○ **What is the most common inherited thrombophilia?**

Heterozygous factor V Leiden mutation.

○ **Who should be screened for thrombophilia?**

Women with a personal or family history of venous thromboembolic disease. Women with unexplained fetal loss at >20 weeks, severe preeclampsia or HELLP prior to 34 weeks, or with severe growth restriction had previously been screened for thrombophilia; however, this is no longer recommended because there is a lack of data showing that anticoagulation reduced recurrence.

○ **Screening for inherited thrombophilias should include which conditions?**

Factor V Leiden, prothrombin G20210A mutation, as well as antithrombin III, protein C and protein S deficiencies, as well as antiphospholipid antibodies.

○ **Which thrombophilia carries the highest risk of pregnancy-related thromboembolism?**

Antithrombin III deficiency, with a risk of up to 40% in women with a history of previous venous thromboembolism (VTE).

○ **What prophylaxis should be given to women with inherited thrombophilias in pregnancy?**

Treatment should be individualized depending on the severity of the thrombophilia and the patient's personal history of VTE. In general, a patient with a low-risk thrombophilia with no history of prior VTE can be observed without prophylactic heparin. Patients with a high-risk thrombophilia with history of 0 to 1 VTE events can be treated with prophylactic dose of LMWH. In cases of two or more episodes of VTE, therapeutic doses should be given.

○ **How should women with a history of VTE with no inherited thrombophilia be treated in pregnancy?**

Prophylactic dose of LMWH.

○ **How long after delivery can LMWH be restarted?**

4 to 6 hours after vaginal delivery or 6 to 12 hours after cesarean delivery.

○ **When should anticoagulant therapy be stopped prior to induction of labor?**

24 hours prior.

○ **What is the reversal method for anticoagulant therapy?**

Protamine sulfate is given for UFH and fresh frozen plasma for LMWH.

○ **In what case should continuation of Coumadin therapy in pregnancy be considered?**

In women with mechanical heart valves due to the greatly increased risk of thrombosis. Most other women on long-term anticoagulation can be safely switched to LMWH or UFH in pregnancy.

○ **Can women on Coumadin breastfeed?**

Coumadin, LMWH, and UFH are all compatible with breastfeeding.

○ **The risk of thromboembolism increases by how much in pregnancy?**

Four to fivefold.

○ **What percentage of maternal deaths in developed countries are caused by thromboembolic disease?**

9%.

○ **What is the recommended duration of anticoagulant therapy after VTE in pregnancy?**

At least 6 months after the first episode. Postpartum treatment should last from 6 weeks to 3 months.

○ **What thromboprophylaxis is recommended for women undergoing cesarean delivery?**

Pneumatic compression devices.

DERMATOLOGY

○ **What are some changes that occur in the skin during pregnancy?**

Hyperpigmentation of the skin, striae gravidarum, and increased hair growth.

○ **What is the most common pruritic pregnancy-specific dermatosis?**

Pruritic urticarial papules and plaques of pregnancy (PUPPP). It is also called polymorphic eruption of pregnancy (PEP).

○ **Where do the lesions of PUPPP usually develop first?**

On the abdomen, usually around striae. The lesions may then spread to the buttocks, thighs, and extremities.

○ **How is PUPPP treated?**

Oral antihistamines, skin emollients, and topical corticosteroids. 10% may require systemic steroids.

○ **What are risk factors for developing PUPPP?**

Caucasian race, nulliparity, multifetal gestation, and is more common with a male fetus.

○ **What is herpes gestationis?**

It is a rare, noninfectious, autoimmune blistering skin condition that occurs in 1:10,000 to 50,000 pregnancies. It occurs more commonly in women with HLA-DR3 and HLA-DR4 antigens and is characterized by IgG antibodies against the epidermal basement membrane.

○ **How is herpes gestationis treated?**

Topical corticosteroids and oral antihistamines are first line, but most women require systemic steroids and occasionally cyclosporine or intravenous immunoglobulin (IVIG).

○ **What is the effect of pregnancy on psoriasis?**

Psoriasis improves in 40% of women, is unchanged in 40% and worsens in 20%.

○ **What medications for psoriasis are safe in pregnancy?**

Topical corticosteroids, calcipotriene, anthraline, or tacrolimus, ultraviolet B (UVB) phototherapy, and oral cyclosporine. Methotrexate and mycophenolate mofetil should not be used in pregnancy.

○ **How is acne treated in pregnancy?**

Oral retinoic acid derivatives are strictly contraindicated in pregnancy because they are highly teratogenic. Topical tretinoin cream is poorly absorbed and is considered to pose little teratogenic risk. Topical benzoyl peroxide is safe in pregnancy.

NEUROLOGIC

○ **How does pregnancy affect migraine headaches?**

50% to 70% of women report improvement in migraine headaches during pregnancy, although occasionally migraine headaches may arise for the first time during pregnancy.

○ **How are migraine headaches treated in pregnancy?**

Minor headaches can be treated with acetaminophen, more severe headaches with IV hydration and antiemetics. Triptans may be used safely in pregnancy. Women with frequent headaches may be treated with amitriptyline, propranolol, or labetalol for prophylaxis.

○ **Does epilepsy improve or worsen during pregnancy?**

Epilepsy improves or is stable in 80% of women; however, levels of antiepileptics must be monitored closely in pregnancy. Because of the increased plasma volume in pregnancy, medication doses often must be adjusted.

○ **Which antepileptic medications are associated with congenital anomalies and what can be done to decrease the risk?**

Phenytoin, carbamazepine, lamotrigine, and phenobarbital increase the rate of congenital anomalies two- to threefold. Valproate can increase the risk of anomalies four- to eightfold and is associated with decreased cognitive function. Monotherapy should be used whenever possible to decrease fetal medication exposure.

○ **The risk of stroke is increased by how much in pregnancy?**

There is almost a 100-fold increased risk of stroke in pregnancy. 10% develop antepartum, 40% intrapartum, and 50% postpartum.

○ **What is the most common risk factor for stroke in pregnancy?**

Some form of hypertensive condition—chronic, gestational, or preeclampsia.

○ **How is multiple sclerosis treated in pregnancy?**

Acute attacks may be treated with IV and oral steroids IVIG, exchange transfusion, or immunomodulating agents may be used. IVIG may be given routinely postpartum to decrease the relapse rate.

○ **How is Bell palsy treated in pregnancy?**

Corticosteroids.

○ **Is Bell palsy associated with any adverse pregnancy outcomes?**

It is associated with a fivefold increased risk of gestational hypertension.

○ **What is autonomic dysreflexia and which patients are at risk?**

It is a large, disordered sympathetic stimulation that occurs with stimuli from structures beneath a spinal cord lesion that is above T5-6. Women with these lesions should be given an epidural at the start of labor to avoid development of autonomic dysreflexia.

○ **Selective serotonin reuptake inhibitors are associated with what congenital anomaly?**

Fetal cardiac defects.

○ **How is postpartum psychosis treated?**

Hospitalization, pharmacologic therapy, and long-term psychiatric follow-up.

INTENSIVE CARE/TRAUMA

○ **What are the major causes of pulmonary edema in pregnancy?**

Gestational hypertension and preeclampsia, sepsis, acute hemorrhage, and tocolysis, especially with beta agonists such as terbutaline.

○ **What is the most common cause of respiratory failure in pregnancy?**
ARDS

○ **Name the most frequent causes of sepsis in pregnancy.**

Pyelonephritis, chorioamnionitis, and puerperal pelvic infection.

○ **What are the goals of ventilation of a pregnant woman?**

Maintain the partial pressure of oxygen in arterial blood (PaO_2) at or above 60 mmHg and the oxygen saturation >90% at <50% oxygen content of inspired air, along with positive end-expiratory pressures <15 mmHg.

○ **What percentage of pregnant women experience physical trauma?**
10% to 20%.

○ **When is screening for intimate partner violence recommended during pregnancy?**
All women should be screened at the initial prenatal visit, each trimester, and again postpartum.

○ **What is the most common cause of serious life threatening or fatal blunt trauma during pregnancy?**
Motor vehicle accidents.

○ **How frequent is traumatic placental abruption?**
Some degree of abruption complicates 1% to 6% of "minor" injuries and up to 50% of major injuries.

○ **What are signs and symptoms of traumatic placental abruption?**
Uterine tenderness and uterine contractions (greater than one every 10 minutes is concerning). Vaginal bleeding may be present or absent

○ **How common is uterine rupture due to blunt trauma?**
<1%.

○ **What is the most common cause of fetal maternal hemorrhage associated with blunt trauma?**
Placental tear or "fracture" caused by stretching of the placenta.

○ **How long after a trauma should a pregnant woman be monitored, and what conditions should be met for discharge?**

Monitoring can be discontinued after 4 hours if coagulation studies are normal and uterine contractions are less than one every 10 minutes. If contractions are more frequent than every 10 minutes, there is a 20% risk of placental abruption.

○ **Name indications for prolonged monitoring posttrauma.**

Frequent uterine contractions, nonreassuring fetal heart tracing, vaginal bleeding, uterine tenderness, serious maternal injury, and ruptured membranes.

○ **What is the incidence of maternal visceral injury with penetrating trauma?**

15% to 40%.

○ **When performing cardiopulmonary resuscitation (CPR) on a pregnant woman what is one important difference than a nonpregnant patient?**

It is critical to place the patient in a left lateral position to avoid compression of the vena cava and restrict cardiac output.

○ **How long after the beginning of CPR should a cesarean delivery be performed?**

Within 4 to 5 minutes if the fetus is viable.

○ **What volume of fetal blood does one vial of Rh-immune globulin neutralize?**

15 mL of fetal packed red blood cells, or 30 mL of fetal whole blood.

○ **How soon after trauma should Rh-immune globulin be administered?**

Within the first 72 hours.

○ **Should a seat belt be worn during pregnancy?**

Yes. The lap belt portion should be placed under the pregnant woman's abdomen, over both anterior superior iliac spines and the pubic symphysis. The shoulder harness should be positioned between the breasts.

CHAPTER 15
Gastrointestinal Disorders in Pregnancy

Glen de Guzman, MD

○ **What are the excess energy requirements during pregnancy (kcal/day)?**

Pregnancy increases energy requirements by 340 kcal/day and 452 kcal/day[1] in the second and third trimester, respectively. Lactation increases energy requirements by 500 kcal/day.

○ **What dietary micronutrients are needed in much greater amounts during pregnancy?**

Nutrient	Recommended Daily Intake	Add This in Pregnancy/Lactation
Riboflavin	0.6 mg/1000 kcal	0.3–0.5 mg
Niacin	6.6 mg niacin equivalents/1000 kcal	2–5 niacin equivalents
Pyridoxine	1.6–2.0 mg	1 mg
Folic acid	3g/kg	400 g
Vitamin B12	2 g	0.2–0.6 g
Ascorbic acid	60 mg	10 mg (pregnancy), 35 mg (lactation)
Iron	15 mg	15 mg
Zinc	0.6 mg/1000 kcal	0.3–0.5 mg

○ **What are the benefits of multiple-micronutrient supplementation during pregnancy?**

Multiple-micronutrient supplementation is associated with a significant decrease in the number of low birth weight (LBW) and small-for-gestational-age babies, as well as of maternal anemia, when compared with supplementation with two or less micronutrients. There was, however, no additional benefits obtained when compared with the WHO-recommended iron-folate supplementation.

○ **What are the most common gastrointestinal (GI) symptoms associated with pregnancy?**

Gingivitis 40% to 100%, reflux 30% to 50%, constipation 11%, hemorrhoids 30% to 40%, nausea and vomiting 70% to 85%. The following GI symptoms are also significantly more common among pregnant women: xerostomia, heartburn, eructation, improved appetite, early satiety, epigastric pain, nocturnal pain, and black stools.

○ **What GI motility disturbances may occur during pregnancy?**

  (1) Abnormal esophageal motility with increased nonpropulsive motor activity and decreased contraction wave amplitude and velocity.

  (2) Decreased lower esophageal sphincter pressure.

  (3) Decreased LES sensitivity to pharmacologic and physiologic stimulation.

  (4) Decreased secretion of acid and pepsin by the stomach.

  (5) Prolonged transit through the stomach and small bowel.

  (6) Prolonged intervals between interdigestive small bowel myoelectric complexes.

  (7) Increased villus height, gut hypertrophy, and increased activity of brush border enzymes in the small intestine.

  (8) Slower colonic transit.

  (9) Enhanced colonic absorption of sodium and water.

 (10) Slower gallbladder emptying.

○ **What is the differential diagnosis of nausea and vomiting in pregnancy?**

  (1) GI causes: Gastroenteritis, gastroparesis, achalasia, biliary tract disease, hepatitis, small bowel obstruction, peptic ulcer disease, pancreatitis, and appendicitis.

  (2) Genitourinary causes: Pyelonephritis, uremia, ovarian torsion, nephrolithiasis, kidney stones, and degenerating fibroids.

  (3) Metabolic disease: DKA, porphyria, Addison disease/crisis, and hyperthyroidism.

  (4) Neurologic disorders: Pseudotumor cerebri, vestibular lesions, migraines, and CNS tumor.

  (5) Pregnancy-related conditions: Acute fatty liver of pregnancy and preeclampsia.

  (6) Miscellaneous: Drug toxicity/intolerance and psychological.

○ **Which hormones influence nausea and vomiting in pregnancy?**

Peak levels of human chorionic gonadotropin (hCG) correlate temporally with the peak symptoms of nausea and vomiting. The extent of its emetogenic stimulus may be increased in conditions where there is an increased placental mass, such as in multiple gestation or molar pregnancy. Estrogen and progesterone levels are also correlated with the frequency of nausea and vomiting. These hormones relax smooth muscle and slow GI transit time. Estrogens[2] in oral contraceptive pills (OCPs) show a dose-response relationship for nausea and vomiting, and women thus sensitized have an increased likelihood of exhibiting nausea and vomiting in pregnancy. Cigarette smokers are less likely to have nausea and vomiting in pregnancy, which may be due to the associated lower levels of both hCG and estradiol, compared with nonsmokers.

○ **What features are associated with a higher risk of nausea and vomiting of early pregnancy?**

Primigravid status, multiple gestations, younger age, nonsmokers, obesity, <12 years of education, previous nausea with OCP use, history of acid reflux, and corpus luteum primarily on the right ovary.

○ **What physical findings suggest that nausea and vomiting in a pregnant woman may be due to an independent disease process?**

Abdominal pain or tenderness that is worse than the mild epigastric discomfort that occurs after retching, fever, headache, goiter, or an abnormal neurologic examination. A caveat: severe nausea and vomiting may rarely cause a neurologic abnormality, such as thiamine-deficiency encephalopathy or central pontine myelinolysis.

○ **What are the adverse effects of severe nausea and vomiting on the mother and her fetus?**

Significant morbidity to the mother might include Wernicke encephalopathy, splenic avulsion, esophageal rupture, pneumothorax, and acute tubular necrosis. A higher incidence of LBW is associated with hyperemesis gravidarum, but not with mild to moderate vomiting. Both maternal and fetal deaths are very rare.

○ **What features distinguish hyperemesis gravidarum from the more common nausea and vomiting that occurs during early pregnancy?**

The following criteria are often used to diagnose hyperemesis gravidarum: persistent vomiting not related to other causes, acute starvation with large ketonuria, loss of at least 5% the prepregnancy weight, and electrolyte abnormalities. Hyperemesis is also associated with abnormal liver function tests. Serum bilirubin can be increased up to five times the upper normal limit. Transaminases and alkaline phosphatase (ALP) can show mild to moderate increases. Serum amylase may be increased; however, the origin of this is mainly the salivary glands.

○ **What are the risk factors for hyperemesis gravidarum?[3]**

Risk factors include increased placental mass including advanced molar gestation and multiple gestation, family history, history of hyperemesis gravidarum, female fetus, history of motion sickness, or migraines.

○ **What are the fetal complications of hyperemesis gravidarum?**

Infants born of women who had been admitted for hyperemesis gravidarum are more likely to be LBW, small for gestational age, born prematurely, and have a 5-minute APGAR <7. These effects are largely attributable to poor maternal weight gain, defined as <7 kg.

○ **What are some common treatments of hyperemesis gravidarum?[3]**

Nonpharmacologic therapies: Avoidance of sensory stimuli, frequent and small meals, avoiding spicy or fatty foods, eliminating pills with iron, eating bland or dry foods, high-protein snacks, crackers in the morning before arising. Acustimulation has conflicting results.

Pharmacologic therapies: Pyridoxine (vitamin B6) or in combination of doxylamine, and ginger capsules effectively reduces nausea and vomiting and should be considered first-line pharmacotherapy. Other commonly used medications include ginger capsules, promethazine, dimenhydrinate, metoclopramide, and ondansetron. Oral methylprednisolone was found to reduce hospital readmission rates; caution should be taken especially during first trimester secondary to its teratogenic effects.

○ **True or False: *Helicobacter pylori* infection is responsible for symptomatic dyspepsia in pregnancy.**

False. In a study of 416 pregnant patients, although 42% were found to be seropositive for *H. pylori*, they were no more likely to experience dyspepsia than seronegative controls.

○ **Describe the factors that lead to the decreased risk of peptic ulcer disease in pregnant women.**

(1) Avoidance of NSAIDs and smoking during pregnancy.

(2) Protective effect of estrogen on gastric and duodenal mucosa.

(3) Immunological tolerance to *H. pylori*, thus decreasing the inflammatory response.

○ **What antisecretory medications are safe for use during pregnancy?**

H_2 receptor antagonists are pregnancy category B. Proton pump inhibitors have documented safety and are category B, except for omeprazole that is category C. Regarding other drugs, metoclopramide and sucralfate are both category B.

○   **What effect does inflammatory bowel disease have on fertility?**

Women with ulcerative colitis have a similar fertility rate compared with the general population. An exception is women who have undergone proctocolectomy with ileoanal anastomosis with J-pouch. This group has a longer time to pregnancy, probably stemming from surgery-related pelvic adhesions. Women with Crohn disease may have a lower fertility compared with the general population. Fertility is highest in those in remission, or following surgical resection of active disease.

○   **What is the risk of relapse of ulcerative colitis in a patient with inactive disease during pregnancy and the puerperium?**

The same as it is in the nonpregnant state. The most likely time for relapse of inflammatory bowel disease during pregnancy is the first trimester. The postpartum period is not necessarily a high-risk time for relapse; the degree of postpartum disease activity correlates with activity at term.

○   **What are the risks to the pregnancy when Crohn disease is active at the time of conception?**

Increased rates of spontaneous abortion, premature delivery, LBW, and neonatal vitamin K deficiency. A case report published in 2001 linked a fetal subdural hematoma diagnosed at 22 weeks to maternal vitamin K deficiency secondary to Crohn disease.

○   **True or False: An ileostomy precludes a vaginal delivery.**

False. The rate of cesarean delivery is not affected by the diagnosis of inflammatory bowel disease, and the decision should generally be based on obstetric indications. One exception is women with active or inactive perirectal, perianal, or rectovaginal fistulas, who may have poor wound healing at the episiotomy site.

○   **What medications for inflammatory bowel disease are safe in pregnancy?**

Category B: Balsalazide, loperamide, mesalamine, metronidazole, Remicade, and sulfasalazine.

Category C: Corticosteroids (budesonide, prednisone, prednisolone), ciprofloxacin, cyclosporine, diphenoxylate, and olsalazine.

Category D: Azathioprine and 6-mercaptopurine.

Category X: Methotrexate.

○   **What are the normal changes in liver function tests that occur in pregnancy?**

Albumin may decrease by 1 g/dL, while bilirubin and the transaminases may be normal or decreased. These changes are due to hemodilution caused by the increased plasma volume between the 6th and 32nd weeks of gestation. ALP is increased due to both increased bone turnover and the leakage of placental ALP into the maternal circulation. Fibrinogen, transferrin, ceruloplasmin, and cholesterol are all increased.

○   **True or False: Spider angiomata and palmar erythema are signs of liver disease in pregnancy.**

False. These are normal findings in up to 60% of pregnant women, and disappear rapidly after delivery. Their etiology is thought to be related to the hyperestrogenemia of pregnancy.

○   **True or False: Hepatomegaly is normal during pregnancy.**

False. Pregnancy has little effect on liver size and architecture; therefore, a finding of hepatomegaly should prompt a search for an underlying pathology.

○ **What is the differential diagnosis of hepatomegaly in pregnancy?**

(1) Infiltrative disease: Acute fatty liver of pregnancy

(2) Inflammatory condition: Hepatitis

(3) Passive congestion: Right-sided heart failure or Budd-Chiari syndrome

(4) Malignancy (rare)

○ **What is the differential diagnosis of jaundice in pregnancy?**

(1) Viral hepatitis: Serum transaminases increased mild to moderate range, positive serology, and prominent inflammatory infiltrate on liver biopsy with cellular disarray.

(2) Acute fatty liver of pregnancy: Serum transaminases minimally increased and prominent microvesicular fat deposition on liver biopsy.

(3) Toxic injury: History of exposure to tetracycline, isoniazid, erythromycin, or methyldopa.

(4) Cholestasis of pregnancy: Pruritus and bile salt elevation.

(5) Severe preeclampsia: Hypertension, proteinuria, thrombocytopenia, elevated creatinine, uric acid, and transaminases.

(6) Mononucleosis: Flu-like symptoms, elevated transaminases, and positive heterophile antibody.

(7) CMV hepatitis: Elevated transaminases, positive viral culture or PCR, CMV antibodies.

(8) Autoimmune hepatitis: Elevated transaminases, antibodies, and liver-kidney microsomal antibodies.

○ **What is the rate of maternal-fetal transmission of hepatitis B?**

Several factors modify the perinatal transmission rate of hepatitis B. In the absence of immunoprophylaxis, 10% to 20% of women who are seropositive for hepatitis B surface antigen (HbsAg) alone will transmit the virus to their fetus; this rate increases to 90% in women who are seropositive for both HBsAg and hepatitis B e antigen (HbeAg). The age of gestation when the illness occurs also affects transmission rates for acute hepatitis B: it is 10% during the first trimester and increased to 80% to 90% during the third trimester. Intrapartum transmission of the infant via exposure to contaminated blood and genital secretions accounts for 85% to 95% of cases of perinatal transmission; and the rest comes about from hematogenous dissemination, breastfeeding, and close physical contact between the mother and her neonate.

○ **True or False: Immunoprophylaxis of hepatitis B is necessary for the infants of HbeAg-negative and HBsAg-positive mothers.**

True. While on average the risk of transmission is lower in this group, it is still significant. Therefore, infants of HBsAg-positive mothers, regardless of HbeAg status, should receive both hepatitis B immune globulin and hepatitis B vaccine within 12 hours after birth, followed by two injections of hepatitis B vaccine during the first 6 months of life.

○ **True or False: Cesarean delivery should be performed in all pregnant women with chronic hepatitis B.**

False. Appropriate immunoprophylaxis of the infant after delivery is sufficient.

○ **True or False: Breastfeeding is contraindicated in women with hepatitis.[4]**

False. Breastfeeding is allowed in women with hepatitis A infection given appropriate hygienic precautions, in women chronically infected with hepatitis B and the infant has received both passive and active prophylaxis, or in women with hepatitis C infection.

○ **What is the rate of maternal-fetal transmission of hepatitis C?[4]**

The rate of perinatal transmission of hepatitis C is proportional to the maternal viral titers. The overall risk of vertical transmission rates is 2% to 8%. In women who were hepatitis C RNA negative, vertical transmission was rare. Breastfeeding has not been associated with an increased risk of neonatal hepatitis C infection.

○ **Does cesarean delivery decrease the risk of perinatal transmission of hepatitis C?[4]**

The route of delivery has not been shown to influence the risk of vertical hepatitis C transmission, and cesarean delivery should be performed in women with hepatitis C only for obstetric indications.

○ **What is the role of interferon alpha therapy for hepatitis during pregnancy?**

Interferon alpha has been shown to produce clinical improvement in 28% to 46% of patients with hepatitis C, and has also been shown to alter the natural history of hepatitis B and D infection. However, it has abortifacient properties and should be avoided in pregnancy.

○ **What are typical features of fulminant hepatic failure due to herpes simplex occurring during the third trimester of pregnancy?**

Herpes simplex hepatitis can result in fulminant hepatic failure with a 40% mortality rate, with half of the reported adult cases occurring during pregnancy. The clinical and biochemical features are usually indistinguishable from other causes of acute liver failure; however, jaundice is characteristically absent. Typical skin lesions are evident in less than half of patients, and diagnosis may ultimately rest on liver biopsy, cultures, and serology.

○ **True or False: Treatment of Wilson disease should be discontinued during pregnancy.**

False. Discontinuing penicillamine treatment of Wilson disease increases the risk of maternal hepatic and neurologic failure and hemolysis, and has been associated with fatal relapses. The drug itself is usually well tolerated by both the mother and her fetus. Trientine seems to be safe as well, although fewer data are available. Zinc therapy is also effective in preventing relapse in pregnancy.

○ **True or False: A history of Budd-Chiari syndrome precludes a subsequent normal pregnancy.[5]**

False. Successful pregnancy has been described in women with Budd-Chiari syndrome; however, there are substantial risks of fetal loss and preterm birth.

○ **List the cholestatic disorders of pregnancy.**

Hyperemesis gravidarum, intrahepatic cholestasis of pregnancy, acute fatty liver of pregnancy, preeclampsia, and HELLP (hemolysis, elevated liver tests, low platelets) syndrome.

○ **True or False: Pregnancy is contraindicated in patients with chronic cholestatic liver diseases.**

False. Cholestasis may worsen but can be managed and usually returns to baseline after delivery in primary biliary cirrhosis, Dubin-Johnson syndrome, and the familial intrahepatic cholestatic syndromes such as Alagille syndrome.

○ **True or False: Liver transplant is a contraindication to pregnancy.**

False. Pregnancy planned at least 2 years after liver transplant with stable allograft function can have excellent maternal and neonatal outcomes, although the risks are significant. Transplant recipients considering pregnancy should be counseled that pregnancy complications include preterm delivery (19–20%), fetal growth restriction (10%), congenital malformations (4–16%) spontaneous abortions (11%), graft rejection (10%), HELLP syndrome (8%), hypertension (up to 20%), preeclampsia (4–20%), cesarean delivery (45%), and maternal deaths (up to 3%). These numbers are higher than in the general population but lower than the corresponding outcomes quoted before 1998.

○ **Which malformations are associated with immunosuppressive therapy after liver transplantation?**

The occurrence of meningocele, urogenital defects, cleft palate, hypospadias, multicystic dysplastic kidneys, and membranous ventricular septal defect has been associated with immunosuppression after a liver transplant. No consistent pattern has, however, been identified in these patients.

○ **What is the most common cause of upper GI hemorrhage during pregnancy?**

Mallory-Weiss tear, followed by erosive esophagitis.

○ **What is the most common cause of lower GI bleeding during pregnancy?**

Hemorrhoids.

○ **What are the abdominal causes of acute volume loss (with or without abdominal pain) during pregnancy?**

(1) Ruptured ectopic pregnancy.

(2) Placental abruption.

(3) Ruptured liver.

(4) Ruptured splenic artery aneurysm.

○ **What causes of pancreatitis may be exacerbated during pregnancy?**

The incidence of gallstones is increased during pregnancy although pancreatitis is rare (occurring in 0.03% of pregnancies.[6] Pregnancy may worsen underlying hypertriglyceridemia and precipitate pancreatitis. Hyperparathyroidism may first become manifest during pregnancy and cause pancreatitis.

○ **At what stage of pregnancy, is pancreatitis most likely to occur?**

During the third trimester and the postpartum period.

○ **What presentations of gallstone disease are common during pregnancy? Which are rare?**

Biliary colic and acute cholecystitis are common; jaundice and acute pancreatitis are rare.

○ **When is cholecystectomy safe during pregnancy?**

Laparoscopic cholecystectomy is the most common laparoscopic procedure in pregnancy. Several studies have shown no increased risk of preterm delivery or adverse outcome after first trimester laparoscopic cholecystectomy. The laparoscopic approach is also feasible in the third trimester. Nonoperative management of symptomatic cholelithiasis is associated with higher recurrence of symptoms necessitating hospitalization, increased risk of gallstone pancreatitis (associated with a 10–20% rate of fetal loss), increased risk of miscarriage, preterm labor and preterm delivery compared with those undergoing laparoscopic cholecystectomy. Furthermore, such nonsurgical approaches like bile acid therapy, lithotripsy, and dissolution with methyl terbutyl ether are not recommended during pregnancy due to the lack of safety data.

○ **What is the most frequent cause of an acute abdomen in pregnancy?**

Acute appendicitis, which approximates 1 in 1500 deliveries, can occur at any time, with a slight predominance during the second trimester. Maternal mortality is rare, but the rate of fetal loss is 10% to 20%, due to preterm labor or IUFD. Preterm labor usually occurs within 5 days of surgery, and could either be due to the disease or the inflammatory response to surgery. The differential diagnosis includes pyelonephritis, cholecystitis, renal or ureteral calculi, adnexal torsion, degenerating myoma, extrauterine pregnancy, and placental abruption.

○ **What is the most common symptom of appendicitis in pregnancy?**

Right lower quadrant pain is the most common presentation in all three trimesters. The dictum that appendicitis presents as right upper quadrant pain during the third trimester has not been validated by studies.

○ **Why is acute appendicitis more hazardous to the mother during pregnancy than in the nonpregnant state?**

Local perforation may be contained by the uterine wall on one side and result in premature delivery with free perforation and generalized peritonitis after the uterus empties and pulls away from the appendiceal abscess.

○ **Why should a normal appendix found at laparotomy during pregnancy not be removed?**

Removal of a normal appendix has been associated with a tripling of the risk of fetal loss.

○ **What is the cause of acute granulomatous peritonitis in pregnancy or the puerperium?**

Rupture of fetal contents into the peritoneum or meconium spillage during cesarean delivery.

○ **Name the maternal and fetal risks experienced by obese women during pregnancy.[7]**

In pregnancy, obese women are at higher risk of gestational diabetes, preeclampsia, cesarean delivery, and infectious morbidity. Fetal risks include congenital anomalies, growth abnormalities particularly fetal macrosomia, miscarriage, stillbirth, and neonatal death.

○ **What is the benefit of exercise for obese pregnant women?**

Exercise is beneficial for the primary prevention of gestational diabetes, especially in women with a BMI >33. It is also useful in maintaining euglycemia in gestational diabetes patients who fail diet control alone. The following relative contraindications to aerobic exercise should be kept in mind: extreme morbid obesity, poorly controlled type 1 diabetes, history of extremely sedentary lifestyle, and orthopedic limitations

○ **What effects does bariatric surgery have on future fertility?[7]**

Subsequent weight loss after bariatric surgery leads to higher fertility rates secondary to improvements of conditions such as polycystic ovarian syndrome, anovulation, and irregular menses. Studies have shown higher number of unintended pregnancies occurring after the procedure relating to decreased absorption of OCPs from anatomical and physiological alterations. It is advisable to wait 12 to 24 months after surgery before conceiving so that the fetus is not exposed to rapid maternal weight loss; as well as to supplement with vitamin B12, folate, iron, and calcium.

○ **What are risks and benefits of various abdominal imaging modalities in pregnancy?[8]**

Nonionizing radiation that includes ultrasonography and magnetic resonance imaging is considered safe. However, the sensitivity of an ultrasound is highly dependent on patient anatomy and operator proficiency. Gadolinium contrast should be avoided during the first trimester. Ionizing radiation such as plain X-rays, fluoroscopy, angiography, computed tomography, and nuclear medicine may lead to adverse fetal outcomes. However, concern about possible effects should not prevent medically indicated diagnostic procedures; when necessary, techniques such as positional alterations, use of protective shields, and limiting exposure time.

○ **What are the some effects of ionizing radiation on the fetus?[9]**

Based on case reports and past experience, especially from Japanese atomic bomb survivors, potential deleterious consequences of ionizing radiation include pregnancy loss (miscarriage, stillbirth), malformation, disturbances of growth or development, and mutagenic and carcinogenic effects?

○ **A middle-aged woman presents with a 3-day history of generalized cramping abdominal pain later becoming colicky in character, and accompanied by intractable nausea and vomiting. On examination, she has right lower quadrant tenderness, a 10-week-size midline uterus, and right adnexal fullness. Diagnostic laparoscopy revealed findings in the right pelvis. What is the diagnosis?**

Torsion of the appendix. It is a rare case mimicking the more common torsion of the ovary; diagnostic laparoscopy would have been performed nonetheless to yield the final diagnosis.

○ **A woman presents with malaise, headache, nausea, poor appetite, and abdominal pain during the third trimester, and later develops hepatic failure with jaundice and encephalopathy. How would you describe the pattern of fat deposition in the liver biopsy?**

Tissue from liver biopsy shows both microvesicular and macrovesicular fat deposition on Oil red O stain, characteristic of acute fatty liver of pregnancy.

REFERENCES

1. Institute of Medicine. *Dietary Reference Intakes: The Essential Guide to Nutrient Requirements.* Washington, DC: National Academies Press; 2006.
2. Lagiou P, Tamimi R, Mucci LA, Trichopoulos D, Adami HO, Hsieh CC. Nausea and vomiting in pregnancy in relation to prolactin, estrogens, and progesterone: a prospective study. *Obstet Gynecol.* 2003;101(4):639.
3. American College of Obstetricians and Gynecologists. Nausea and vomiting of pregnancy. ACOG Practice Bulletin No. 52. *Obstet Gynecol.* 2004;103:803–815.
4. American College of Obstetricians and Gynecologists. Viral hepatitis in pregnancy. ACOG Practice Bulletin No. 86. *Obstet Gynecol.* 2007;110:941–955.
5. Rautou PE, Angermayr B, Garcia-Pagan JC, et al. Pregnancy in women with known and treated Budd-Chiari syndrome: maternal and fetal outcomes. *J Hepatol.* 2009;51(1):47.
6. Chamarthi B, Greene MF, Dluhy RG. A problem in gestation. *The New England Journal of Medicine.* Sept 2011;365:843-848.
7. American College of Obstetricians and Gynecologists. Bariatric surgery and pregnancy. ACOG Practice Bulletin No. 105. *Obstet Gynecol.* 2009;113:1405–1413.
8. Gabbe SG, Niebyl JR, Simpson JL. Obstetric: normal and problem pregnancies. Chapter 43: Hepatic and Gastrointestinal Disease. Philadelphia, PA: Churchill Livingstone, Elsevier; 2007.
9. Yamazaki JN, Schull WJ. Perinatal loss and neurological abnormalities among children of the atomic bomb. Nagasaki and Hiroshima revisited, 1949 to 1989. *JAMA.* 1990;264(5):605.

CHAPTER 16 | First Trimester Ultrasound

Katherine Bohnert, DO

○ **What techniques may be applied to perform a first trimester ultrasound?**

- Transabdominal.
- Transvaginal.
- Transperineal.

○ **What are the advantages of using transvaginal ultrasound (TVUS) versus transabdominal ultrasound?**

The probe is closer to the pelvic organs, allowing a higher frequency (5–10 MHz), which improves resolution and a full bladder is not required. Transabdominal ultrasound uses a lower frequency (3–5 MHz).

○ **What are the disadvantages of using TVUS versus transabdominal ultrasound?**

- At higher resolution, a shorter distance from the probe is seen.
- TVUS is more invasive.

○ **What is the discriminatory zone?**
The hCG serum level above which a gestational sac should be visualized if an IUP is present.

- The threshold level is the lowest value for which certain observation CAN be detected by ultrasound.
- The discriminatory level is the lowest value for which a certain observation should ALWAYS be detected.

○ **What is the first ultrasound landmark of pregnancy?**

Gestational sac.

○ **Using TVUS, what size is the threshold for detecting a gestational sac?**

2 to 3 mm.

○ **Does the presence of an intrauterine fluid-filled area confirm an intrauterine pregnancy (IUP)?**

No. It could be a decidual reaction or "pseudogestational sac."

○ **How can one calculate the gestational age from the mean sac diameter (MSD) from 5 to 11 weeks' gestation?**

- MSD (in mm) + 30 = gestational age in days.
- Example: using a gestational sac size of 6 mm, the calculated gestational age would be 36 days.

○ **What is the discriminatory size of the gestational sac (MSD) at which one would expect to see the yolk sac?**
- MSD = 8 mm via TVUS (5.5 weeks).
- MSD = 20 mm via transabdominal ultrasound (7 weeks).

○ **What are several reasons for an irregular appearing gestational sac?**
Uterine contractions, enlarged bladder, fibroids, implantation bleed, and failed pregnancy.

○ **What structure is the arrow pointing to in the ultrasound image?**

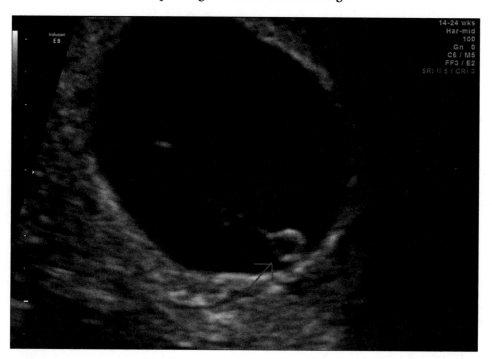

Yolk sac.

○ **What are the three known functions of the yolk sac?**
(1) Provides nutrients for the embryo.
(2) Initial site of hematopoiesis.
(3) Contributes to developing gut and reproductive systems.

○ **Which is superior in confirming an IUP: a yolk sac within the gestational sac or the double decidual sac sign (DDSS)?**
The yolk sac within the gestational sac.

○ **After identification of a gestational sac, what is the next visible landmark for pregnancy dating?**
The yolk sac.

○ **What is the embryonic disk?**

The thickened region along the outermost margin of the yolk sac that becomes visible at 1 to 2 mm in length. It correlates with a gestational age of 5 to 6 weeks.

○ **At what human chorionic gonadotropin (hCG) level will you typically see an intrauterine gestational sac?**

1000 to 2000 mIU/mL.

○ **The embryonic phase of development is between _____ and _____ weeks' gestation?**

6 and 10.

○ **The chorionic cavity normally obliterates between _____ and _____ weeks' gestation?**

12 and 16.

○ **What is the discriminatory size of the gestational sac (MSD) at which one would expect to see the embryo?**

- MSD = 20 mm via TVUS.
- MSD = 25 mm via transabdominal ultrasound.

○ **How can one calculate the gestational age from the crown-rump length (CRL) from 6 to 9.5 weeks' gestation?**

CRL (in mm) + 42 = gestational age in days.

○ **What is the approximate growth rate of the embryo (CRL) and the gestational sac diameter between 6 and 10 gestational weeks?**

1 mm/day.

○ **Which is a more accurate indicator of gestational age: CRL or mean gestational sac diameter?**

CRL.

○ **How accurate is the first trimester CRL measurement in predicting gestational age?**

Within 3–5 days.

○ **When should ultrasound-established dates take preference over menstrual dating?**

When the discrepancy is >7 days in the first trimester.

○ **Is it true or false that cardiac pulsations may be seen when performing TVUS before the embryo itself is identified?**

True.

○ **Cardiac activity should normally be seen when the embryonic pole has achieved what size? This corresponds to what gestational age and what MSD?**

4 to 5 mm, 6.0 to 6.5 weeks, and 13 to 18 mm.

○ **How does the fetal heart rate change in the first trimester?**

It increases from 100 to 115 beats per minute (bpm) before 6 weeks to 145 to 160 bpm at 8 weeks' gestation after which it plateaus at 135 to 145 bpm. The variability also increases during this time.

○ **The term-missed abortion has been replaced by what term(s)?**

Embryonic or fetal demise.

○ **What is the percentage chance for miscarriage after cardiac activity seen in an 8 weeks' gestation?**

2% to 3%.

○ **What are some common synonyms for an intrauterine blood collection in the first trimester?**

Subchorionic hemorrhage or hematoma, implantation hemorrhage, and perigestational hemorrhage.

○ **In the presence of an intrauterine hematoma, the risk of a spontaneous abortion is associated with?**

(1) Increasing size of the hematoma

(2) Advanced maternal age

(3) Earlier gestational age

(4) Structural uterine anomalies

(5) History of miscarriage

○ **True/False: An abnormal appearing yolk sac is associated with early pregnancy failure?**

True.

○ **Recurrent miscarriage is defined as?**

Three or more consecutive first trimester spontaneous losses.

○ **What is the arrow in this first trimester ultrasound pointing to?**

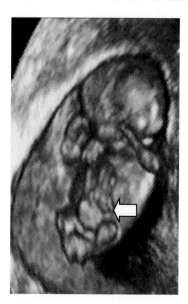

Physiologic herniation of the midgut.

○ **Is this a normal or abnormal finding?**

Normal.

○ **What abnormality could it be mistaken for?**

Abdominal wall defects, such as omphalocele and gastroschisis (which should not be diagnosed until the second trimester).

○ **The midgut typically returns to the abdomen at what week gestation?**

11 to 12 weeks.

○ **When can the midgut be seen?**

Seen from 8 to 11 weeks with herniation of the fetal bowel into the base of the umbilical cord and 90-degree counter-clockwise rotation of the bowel around the base of the superior mesenteric artery.

○ **What is the arrow in this first trimester ultrasound pointing to?**

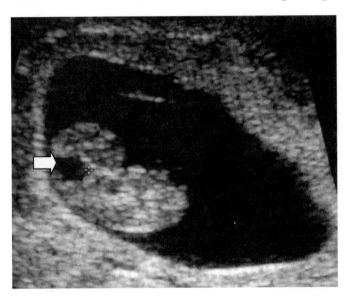

The developing rhombencephalon.

○ **Is this a normal or abnormal finding?**

Normal.

○ **What abnormality could it be mistaken for?**

Dandy-Walker malformation or hydrocephalus (which should not be diagnosed until the second trimester).

○ **When can it be seen?**

Seen from 7 to 9 weeks, it will eventually contribute to the fourth ventricle, brain stem, and cerebellum.

○ **What sign are the large arrows pointing to in this first trimester ultrasound?**

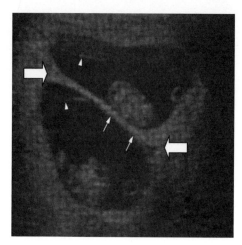

Lambda sign or twin peaks sign.

○ **What does this sign tell us about the chorionicity and amnionicity of this twin gestation?**
It is dichorionic (and diamniotic).

○ **How would you describe the amnionicity and chorionicity of this first trimester pregnancy?**

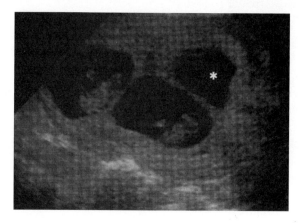

Trichorionic and triamniotic.

◯   **How would you describe the amnionicity and chorionicity of this first trimester pregnancy?**

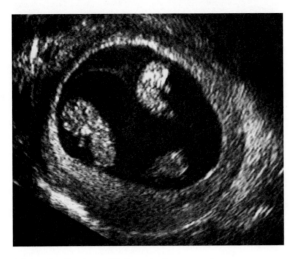

Monochorionic and triamniotic.

◯   **How are the number of yolk sacs and amnionicity related?**
The number of yolk sacs equals the number of amniotic sacs.

◯   **What is the chance of delivering twins if two gestational sacs are seen on early US studies?**
57%.

◯   **What does this percentage increase to if two embryonic poles with cardiac activity are visualized?**
87%.

◯   **When is the best time to determine amnionicity and chorionicity in a multiple gestation?**
8 to 10 weeks (the earlier the better).

◯   **What structure are the arrows pointing to in the ultrasound images?**

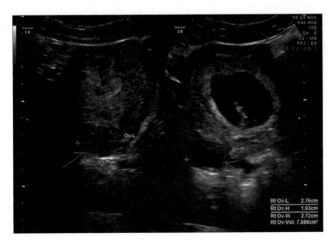

Corpus luteum cysts.

○ **What is the most common adnexal mass visualized during a first trimester ultrasound?**

The corpus luteum.

○ **The resistance index (RI) and pulsatility index (PI) of the uterine artery decline from 6 to 12 weeks' gestation due to?**

Establishment of the intervillous circulation.

○ **Name some fetal anomalies that can be detected with reliability in the first trimester.**

Large encephalocele, holoprosencephaly, ectopia cardis, and conjoined twins.

○ **Name a few major malformations that should NOT be diagnosed in the first trimester.**

Renal agenesis, anencephaly, Dandy-Walker malformation, hydrocephalus, and omphalocele.

○ **Nuchal translucency (NT) is performed between which gestational weeks?**

10 to 14 weeks.

○ **What variables are used to calculate the Down syndrome risk when performing NT?**

The NT measurement, the CRL, the gestational age, and the age of the mother.

○ **What value for NT is generally considered abnormal?**

3 mm or greater.

○ **What percentage of fetuses with an abnormal NT will have aneuploidy?**

About 75%.

○ **Which congenital abnormality is associated with an abnormal NT, but normal karyotype?**

Congenital heart disease (in 27%).

○ **Fetuses with abnormal NT and normal karyotype and anatomy may be at increased risk of what?**

Preterm delivery and growth restriction.

○ **What are the advantages of first trimester aneuploidy screening?**

The potential for earlier diagnosis, which can be confirmed by CVS, allowing for earlier, less traumatic termination with more privacy.

○ **What is the difference between NT and nuchal skin fold (NSF) measurements?**

NT is a first trimester measurement, while NSF is a second trimester measurement.

○ **How does the NT change with gestational age?**

It increases from 10 to 14 weeks' gestation.

○ **What are the requirements for a good NT image?**

- CRL between 45 and 84 mm.
- Fetus in midsagittal plane in neutral position.
- Distinguish between fetal skin and amnion.
- Magnified so fetus occupies 75% of the screen.
- Place calipers on inner margins of skin to soft tissue.

○ **What structure is the arrow pointing to in the ultrasound image?**

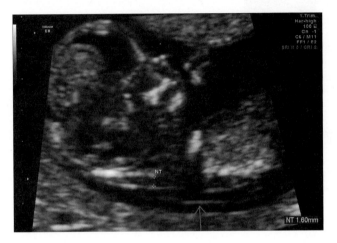

Amnion.

○ **Is TVUS required for NT measurement?**

No. Often abdominal ultrasound is successful in 80% of cases.

○ **How does neck flexion and extension affect the NT?**

Neck flexion decreases the NT by about 0.4 mm, while hyperextension increases the NT by about 0.6 mm.

○ **What first trimester biochemical analytes, along with NT, constitute an effective screening strategy for aneuploidy?**

PAPP-A (pregnancy-associated plasma protein A) and hCG (free or totalhCG).

○ **In pregnancies affected with Down syndrome, the hCG will be ____, and the PAPP-A will be _____. NT will be increased.**

Increased, decreased.

○ **In pregnancies affected with Trisomy 18, the hCG will be ____, and the PAPP-A will be ____. NT will be increased.**

Decreased, decreased.

○   **What NT is greater than the 99th percentile throughout the measured gestational ages?**
3.5 mm.

○   **While performing NT, what structure shown below may be a useful marker for detection of aneuploidy?**

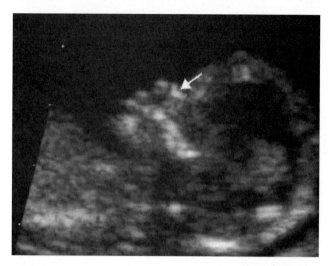

Nasal bone.

○   **What technique should be utilized for nasal bone (NB) measurements?**
• Fetus magnified so that only the head and upper thorax are in the screen.
• Precise midsagittal view of the fetal profile.
• Fetal spine down with slight neck flexion.
• Transducer parallel to the direction of the fetal nose (45–135 degrees).
• Three distinct lines should be seen.

○   **What is the ductus venosus?**
A trumpet-shaped vein connecting the umbilical sinus to the hepatic veins and the IVC, directing high velocity oxygenated blood returning from the placenta to the left atrium via the foramen ovale.

○   **What is the normal Doppler waveform pattern in the ductus venosus?**
Biphasic pulsatile continuously forward flow.

○   **What heart abnormalities may be apparent in the first trimester, but may be resolved by the third trimester?**
Muscular ventricular septal defect.

CHAPTER 17

Obstetrical Ultrasound and Fetal Abnormalities

Amelia McLennan, MD

○ **How is ultrasound produced?**

It is the vibrations of crystals in response to electrical current generate sound waves. This is known as the piezoelectric effect.

○ **True or False: The frequencies of the transvaginal transducers are typically higher than the transabdominal.**

True. The transabdominal probes are typically 3 to 7 MHz and the transvaginal probes 5 to 9 MHz. With higher frequencies, there is greater resolution but decreased penetration.

○ **Is ultrasound safe?**

With the widespread use, no biological effects have been confirmed on the fetus with the frequencies used in obstetrical ultrasound. The level of ultrasound intensity that is defined as safe is <100 mW/cm^2. It has been shown to cause thermal effects and mechanical changes via cavitation in animal studies.

○ **What serum analytes are used in conjunction with ultrasound to screen for aneuploidy?**

In the first trimester serum pregnancy-associated plasma protein A (PAPP-A) and free beta human chorionic gonadotropin (hCG) levels and in the second trimester unconjugated estriol, beta hCG and inhibin A are also measured. In Down syndrome, the serum beta hCG (free and total) and inhibin A levels are increased and the levels of PAPP-A, uE3, and AFP are decreased.

○ **Increased nuchal translucency is associated with which fetal abnormalities?**

Trisomy 13, 18, and 21.

○ **What is the most accurate measurement to estimate gestational age in first trimester?**

Crown-rump length is better than the gestational sac and yolk sac measurements.

○ **What is the most accurate measurement to estimate gestational age in the second trimester?**

Head circumference.

○ **At what crown-rump length should embryonic cardiac activity be observed?**

5 mm or greater.

○ **If only one ultrasound can be done, what is the optimal gestational age at which it should be done?**

18 to 20 weeks.

○ **What parameters are commonly used to assess gestational age in the second and third trimester?**

Biparietal diameter, head circumference, abdominal circumference, and femur length.

○ **How is the biparietal diameter measured?**

From the outer edge of the proximal skull to the inner edge of the distal skull at the level of the thalami and cavum septi pellucidi. The cerebellar hemispheres should not be visible. The head circumference is also measured at this level.

○ **At what level is the abdominal circumference measured?**

The image should be at the level of the junction of the umbilical vein and portal sinus with the fetal stomach visible.

○ **Why does femur appear to be bowed in normal fetus?**

It is the inability to see the full thickness of the femoral diaphysis that gives the impression that the femur farther away from the transducer is bowed. The femoral length should only include the diaphysis and metaphysis.

○ **After what gestational age can femur length be accurately measured?**

14 weeks.

○ **What is asymmetric intrauterine growth restriction (IUGR)?**

Estimated fetal weight less than the 10th percentile with decreased ratio of abdominal circumference to head circumference.

○ **What is the margin of error of estimated fetal weight by ultrasonography in the second and third trimesters?**

15% to 20%.

○ **Which Doppler study is used to follow fetuses with IUGR?**

Umbilical artery velocimetry. It has also been shown that the increase in flow resistance in the umbilical artery is correlated with decreased flow resistance in the middle cerebral artery (MCA) and this has been attributed to the brain sparing response of the IUGR fetus.

○ **Which imaging modality measures fetal anemia?**

MCA Doppler. With anemia there is increased fetal cardiac output, which is attributed to decreased blood viscosity and decreased peripheral vascular resistance. These allow for delivery of larger volume of less oxygenated blood. Hence, the blood flow velocity in the MCA is increased.

○ **What Doppler measurement must be followed when indomethacin is given for preterm labor?**

Ductus arteriosus. Indomethacin has been shown to cause premature constriction of the ductus arteriosus. This is seen by increase in peak systolic velocity (PSV) and decrease in pulsatility index (PI). The effect is considered reversible and abnormal Doppler should lead to discontinuation of the indomethacin.

○ **Other imaging modalities that can be used to evaluate placenta accreta are?**

Color Doppler and MRI.

○ **Macrosomia due to maternal diabetes is associated with?**

Increased abdominal circumference to head circumference ratio.

○ **What ultrasound-estimated fetal weight is the cut-off for suspected macrosomia?**

4500 in association with maternal diabetes or 5000 g without diabetes.

○ **How can amniotic fluid volume be evaluated?**

Single vertical pocket with normal being between 2 and 8 cm and the amniotic fluid index with is the sum of the largest vertical pockets in four quadrants.

○ **What abnormalities cannot be ruled out on four-chamber view of the heart?**

Small atrial septal defects (ASDs) and ventricular septal defects (VSDs) and abnormalities of the great vessels. Hence, the right and left ventricular outflow tracts should also be visualized. The chamber closest to the spine is the left atrium. The mitral valve appears to be at a higher level than the tricuspid valve. Important information regarding the size, position, and the axis of the heart can be obtained from this single view.

○ **What follow-up study should be performed on a fetus with increased nuchal translucency?**

Fetal echocardiogram as there is an increased risk of cardiac defects even in fetuses with normal karyotype.

○ **Multicystic mass posterolateral to the fetal neck?**

Cystic hygroma. Risk of aneuploidy is 60% to 75%, the most common being Turner syndrome.

○ **What is Potter sequence?**

Severe oligohydramnios or anhydramnios leading to multiple anomalies including hypoplastic lungs, limb deformities, and abnormal facies. Most commonly associated with bilateral renal agenesis or second trimester ruptured membranes.

○ **Single umbilical artery is associated with?**

15% to 20% incidence of cardiovascular abnormalities. It is seen in over 50% of fetuses with trisomy 18. Found in 1/200 newborns. Color flow Doppler of the umbilical arteries at the level of the fetal bladder is used to confirm a three-vessel cord.

○ **Cervical length of > ___ mm has good negative predictive value of preterm labor.**

25.

○ **Should all women be routinely offered cervical length screening?**

While there is evidence that shortened cervix on ultrasound is a predictor of preterm birth in women at high risk, current data does not support routine cervical length screening in low-risk populations.

○ **Ultrasound at 7 weeks demonstrates a midgut herniation. This finding is most likely?**

Normal.

○   **At which gestational age should the fetal abdomen be intact?**

12 weeks.

○   **Which anterior abdominal wall defect is associated with aneuploidy?**

With an omphalocele, there is a 30% to 40% risk of aneuploidy. It is a midline defect resulting in the herniation into the base of the cord, which is unlike gastroschisis where the herniation is lateral to the cord insertion and not associated with aneuploidy.

○   **What is an Arnold-Chiari malformation and what is it associated with?**

Displacement of the cerebellum, fourth ventricle, and the medulla. It is associated with open neural tube defects.

○   **Characteristic ultrasound findings associated with Arnold-Chiari malformation?**

Lemon sign and banana sign.

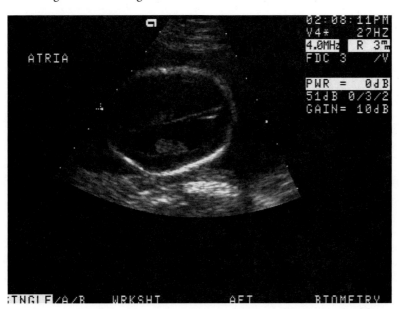

○ **What substances are elevated in the amniotic fluid of a fetus with open neural tube defect?**

AFP and acetyl cholinesterase.

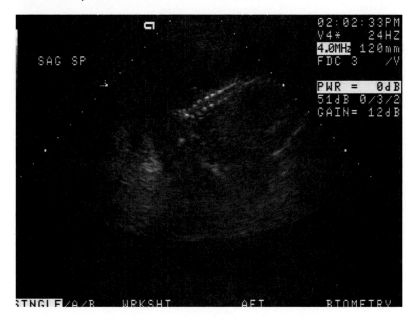

○ **Three-dimensional/four-dimensional ultrasound is useful in the assessment of?**

Fetal facial abnormalities. Cleft lip and palate when found as an isolated anomaly follow a multifactorial inheritance. They have been associated with folate deficiency.

○ **This ultrasound demonstrates?**

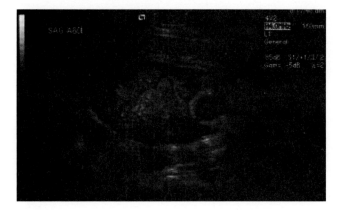

Fetal hydrops.

○ **This ultrasound in association with fetal isoimmunization indicates?**

Severe fetal anemia leading to cardiac failure.

○   **What are some of the causes of nonimmune hydrops?**

Chromosomal abnormalities, twin-to-twin transfusion syndrome, cystic hygroma, cardiac anomalies, congenital cystic adenomatoid malformation, congenital infection and hemoglobinopathies.

○   **Echogenic bowel is associated with?**

Cystic fibrosis, abnormal karyotype, congenital infections, and fetal ingestion of bloody amniotic fluid.

○   **What type of defect is anencephaly?**

It is an open neural tube defect and results from the failed fusion of the rostral neuropore. The recurrence risk 2% to 3% and patient should receive 4 mg of folic acid supplementation prior to next pregnancy.

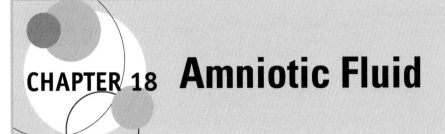

CHAPTER 18 Amniotic Fluid

Kristin Van Heertum, MD

○ **What are the five major functions of amniotic fluid?**

(1) Helps to protect the fetus from trauma.

(2) Cushions the umbilical cord from compression between the fetus and uterus.

(3) Antibacterial properties that provide some protection from infection.

(4) Serves as a reservoir of fluid and nutrients for the fetus.

(5) Provides the necessary fluid, space, and growth factors to permit normal development of the fetal lungs and musculoskeletal and gastrointestinal (GI) systems.

○ **What is the major source of amniotic fluid production in the first trimester?**

An ultrafiltrate of maternal plasma—passes through the fetal membranes by osmosis and hydrostatic forces.

○ **What is the major source of amniotic fluid production in the second half of pregnancy?**

Fetal urination.

○ **What other sources contribute to amniotic fluid production in the second half of pregnancy?**

Secretions from the fetal respiratory tract, including the lungs and oral-nasal cavity and intramembranous flow.

○ **What is the major pathway of clearance of amniotic fluid in the last half of pregnancy?**

Fetal swallowing.

○ **Significant amounts of water and solutes are not transferred across the fetal skin after keratinization occurs. What gestational age does this occur?**

Between 22 and 25 weeks gestation.

○ **When is amniotic fluid volume at its peak?**

34 to 36 weeks gestation.

○ **What is the average peak of amniotic fluid volume?**

1 L (1000 cc).

○   **What is the mean amniotic fluid volume at term?**
800 cc.

○   **What is the mean amniotic fluid volume at 42 weeks?**
250 cc.

○   **What is the composition of amniotic fluid in the first trimester?**
The electrolyte composition and osmolality are essentially the same as fetal and maternal blood.

○   **When does fetal urine first enter the amniotic sac?**
8 to 11 weeks.

○   **Is amniotic fluid hypertonic, isotonic, or hypotonic in the third trimester as compared with maternal plasma?**
Hypotonic.

○   **What is the pH of amniotic fluid?**
7 to 7.5.

○   **What is the pH of the upper vagina?**
3.8 to 4.5—this difference in pH aids in determination of rupture of membranes.

○   **What causes amniotic fluid osmolality to decrease as pregnancy progresses?**
Inflow of markedly hypotonic fetal urine.

○   **Under normal conditions, what is the average increase in amniotic fluid volume late in gestation?**
30 to 40 mL/day.

○   **What are the six major pathways that help to regulate amniotic fluid volume late in pregnancy?**
(1) Fetal urination.
(2) Fetal swallowing and reabsorption by the intestine.
(3) Secretion from the respiratory tract.
(4) Secretions from the fetal oral-nasal cavities.
(5) Intramembranous pathway.
(6) Transmembranous pathway.

○   **What are the three major determinants of amniotic fluid volume (when fetal anomalies are excluded)?**
(1) Movements of water and solutes within and across the membranes.
(2) Physiologic regulation by the fetus of flow rates such as urine production and swallowing.
(3) Maternal effects on transplacental fluid movement.

○ **Approximately what volume of amniotic fluid is swallowed daily by the fetus near term?**
200 to 500 mL/day.

○ **How many milliliters of fluid does the fetal lung secrete per day in the third trimester?**
300 to 400 mL/day.

○ **Over the course of 1 day, what is the net turnover volume of the amniotic fluid?**
95% of the total amniotic fluid volume is turned over daily.

○ **What is the source of meconium in the amniotic fluid?**
Fetal bowel movements associated with fetal stress and/or postmaturity (thought to be associated with maturation of nerves innervating the GI tract).

○ **What is the incidence of passage of meconium at?**
   a. <32 weeks?
   Rare.
   b. Term?
   10% to 15%.
   c. 42 weeks?
   25% to 35%.

○ **Why is the passage of meconium occurring with oligohydramnios of particular concern?**
It is thought that there may be an increase in the viscosity of the meconium, and therefore there may be an increased risk of aspiration pneumonia.

○ **How is amniotic fluid volume most commonly measured?**
Ultrasound.

○ **What are the two most commonly used objective methods to measure amniotic fluid volume via ultrasound?**
Measurement of the maximum vertical pocket (MVP) and calculation of the amniotic fluid index (AFI).

○ **How is the MVP obtained?**
Measurement of the vertical depth of the largest cord- and limb-free pocket of amniotic fluid.

○ **How is the AFI calculated?**
Summation of the depths of the largest vertical pocket in each of the four quadrants.

○ **When calculating the AFI, what anatomical landmarks are used to divide the uterus into quadrants?**
Linea nigra and umbilicus.

○ **How is the AFI calculated before 20 weeks' gestation?**
Summation of the two MVPs on each side of the linea nigra.

○ **How might the measurement of amniotic fluid volume be artificially increased?**

By not maintaining the transducer perpendicular to the floor.

○ **How might the measurement of amniotic fluid volume be artificially decreased?**

By applying excessive pressure on the maternal abdomen with the transducer.

○ **What is oligohydramnios?**

Less than normal or diminished amniotic fluid volume.

○ **What is the incidence of oligohydramnios?**

0.5 to 8% of all pregnancies.

○ **What MVP is consistent with oligohydramnios?**

<2 cm.

○ **What AFI is consistent with oligohydramnios?**

<5 cm, or less than 5th percentile for a particular gestational age.

○ **What AFI is consistent with severe oligohydramnios?**

<2 cm.

○ **What are some clinical findings pointing toward the possibility of oligohydramnios?**

- Fundal height less than estimated gestational age.
- Fetal parts easily palpated through maternal abdomen.
- Ultrasound examination demonstrates fetal crowding and poor visualization of fetal anatomy

○ **What subjective ultrasound criteria have been used to determine oligohydramnios?**

- Absence of fluid pockets throughout the uterine cavity.
- Crowding of fetal limbs.
- Absence of pockets surrounding the fetal legs.
- Overlapping of the fetal ribs (in severe cases).

○ **Name some causes of oligohydramnios.**

- Congenital anomalies, especially related to renal system dysfunction (eg, renal agenesis, polycystic kidneys, genitourinary obstruction, dysplastic multicystic kidneys, or posterior urethral valves in males).
- Chromosomal anomalies.
- Fetal anuria or oliguria due to decreased renal perfusion.
- Intrauterine growth restriction.
- Side effect of certain drugs [eg, indomethacin, NSAIDs, angiotensin-converting enzyme (ACE) inhibitors].
- Maternal dehydration.
- Severe preeclampsia.
- Postdate pregnancy.
- Ruptured membranes.

○ **What is the most common cause of oligohydramnios?**

Premature rupture of the membranes.

○ **What serious complications are associated with oligohydramnios occurring before 22 weeks?**

- Pulmonary hypoplasia.
- Amniotic band syndrome.
- Fetal compression syndrome.

○ **What is Potter sequence?**

A collection of physical features in addition to pulmonary hypoplasia resulting from oligohydramnios and fetal compression in utero. Physical features include skeletal malformation, typical facies (flattened nose, recessed chin, prominent epicanthal fold, low set ears), and cardiovascular malformations.

○ **What is the most common cause of Potter sequence?**

Bilateral renal agenesis.

○ **Why is the second trimester oligohydramnios associated with pulmonary hypoplasia?**

Amniotic fluid inspired at regular intervals, and the distending force it creates, is needed for proper terminal alveolar development.

○ **What is the most likely cause of second trimester oligohydramnios in the absence of ruptured membranes?**

Congenital anomalies.

○ **What is the most likely cause of third trimester oligohydramnios in the absence of ruptured membranes?**

Intrauterine growth restriction.

○ **What is the mechanism of oligohydramnios in fetuses with intrauterine growth restriction?**

Chronic hypoxia resulting in shunting of fetal blood flow from the kidneys, thereby decreasing glomerular filtration rate (GFR) and decreasing fetal urine output.

○ **A large bladder in the presence of oligohydramnios is associated with what cause for the oligohydramnios?**

Urethral obstruction.

○ **If a fluid-filled bladder is seen on ultrasound, what potential congenital abnormality is ruled out as a cause of oligohydramnios?**

Bilateral renal agenesis.

○ **What medications can cause oligohydramnios?**

Prostaglandin synthetase inhibitors and ACE inhibitors.

○ **What is the mortality rate of oligohydramnios in the second trimester?**

Fetal mortality rate has been reported as high as 80% to 90%. The earlier the diagnosis, the worse the prognosis.

○ **What is a common fetal heart rate tracing finding in patients with oligohydramnios?**

Variable decelerations.

○ **Why are variable decelerations more commonly seen with oligohydramnios?**

Cord compression due to lack of cushioning effect given by a normal amniotic fluid volume.

○ **What is the likely cause of oligohydramnios associated with asymmetric growth restriction?**

Uteroplacental insufficiency.

○ **What is the mechanism by which uteroplacental insufficiency might cause oligohydramnios?**

Chronic hypoxia causes shunting of fetal blood away from the kidneys to more vital organs, leading to decreased fetal urine output, thus decreasing amniotic fluid production.

○ **What is the likely cause of oligohydramnios associated with symmetric growth restriction?**

Chromosomal abnormalities.

○ **How does oligohydramnios make ultrasound assessment of the fetus more difficult?**

Amniotic fluid easily transmits sound waves; therefore, ultrasound visualization of fetal anatomy is impaired by less amniotic fluid.

○ **What can be done to improve the quality of diagnostic ultrasound in a pregnancy complicated by oligohydramnios?**

Intraamniotic placement of sterile saline (ie, amnioinfusion) may enhance visualization of the fetal anatomy.

○ **How does amnioinfusion help pregnancies complicated by oligohydramnios?**

Amnioinfusion decreases the incidence of variable decelerations and consequently decreases the cesarean delivery rate for nonreassuring fetal heart rate tracing.

○ **When might delivery be safely postponed in a term pregnancy complicated by oligohydramnios?**

In an otherwise uncomplicated pregnancy with an AFI close to 5 cm and otherwise reassuring fetal testing and an unfavorable cervix at 37 weeks gestation.

○ **What is polyhydramnios?**

Synonymous with hydramnios, means abnormally excessive amounts of amniotic fluid.

○ **What is the clinical definition of polyhydramnios?**

>2 L of amniotic fluid measured at time of delivery.

○ **What is the incidence of polyhydramnios?**

1% to 2% of all pregnancies.

○ **What MVP is consistent with polyhydramnios?**

>8 cm.

○ **What AFI is consistent with polyhydramnios?**

>25 cm, or greater than 95th percentile for a particular gestational age.

○ **What is one of the first clinical findings that might indicate a diagnosis of polyhydramnios?**

Fundal height greater than dates.

○ **What is the differential diagnosis for polyhydramnios?**

- Diabetes, gestational and insulin dependent.
- Congenital anomalies.
- Multiple gestation.
- Immune and nonimmune fetal hydrops.
- Idiopathic.

○ **What is the most likely etiology of polyhydramnios?**

Idiopathic; accounts for 66% of all cases of polyhydramnios.

○ **What specific congenital anomalies are associated with polyhydramnios?**

- Central nervous system anomalies (eg, anencephaly).
- Skeletal dysplasias (eg, achondroplasia).
- GI atresias (eg, esophageal, duodenal).
- Tracheoesophageal fistulas.
- Facial clefts.
- Neck masses (such as cystic hygroma) that may interfere with fetal swallowing.
- Cystic malformations of the lung.
- Diaphragmatic hernia.

○ **What five tests are included in the initial workup of a patient with polyhydramnios?**

- Glucola screen.
- Antibody screen.
- Screen for maternal hemoglobinopathies.
- Maternal viral titers (eg, parvovirus).
- Targeted ultrasound.

○ **Does excess fetal urine production play a major role in polyhydramnios?**

No.

○ **What percentage of patients with polyhydramnios in the second trimester have spontaneous resolution?**

40% to 50% of cases.

○ **What obstetrical complications are associated with polyhydramnios?**

- Maternal respiratory compromise.
- Preterm labor.
- Premature rupture of membranes.
- Fetal malposition.
- Umbilical cord prolapse and/or postpartum uterine atony (potentially leading to postpartum hemorrhage).

○   **What are two therapeutic options that might ameliorate polyhydramnios?**
- Therapeutic amniotic fluid drainage via amniocentesis.
- Maternal indomethacin administration.

○   **What is the mechanism of action of prostaglandin synthetase inhibitors in decreasing amniotic fluid?**

These medications stimulate fetal secretion of arginine vasopressin and facilitate vasopressin-induced renal antidiuretic responses as well as reduced renal blood flow, thereby reducing fetal urine flow. These medications may also impair production or enhance reabsorption of liquid in the lungs.

○   **What is the primary fetal concern with the use of indomethacin?**

Constriction of the ductus arteriosus.

○   **Why should rapid decompression of a gravid uterus with polyhydramnios be avoided?**

Rapid decompression may result in cord prolapse or placental abruption.

CHAPTER 19

The Placenta and Umbilical Cord

Chelsea Ward, MD

DEVELOPMENT

○ **What cell is the precursor of the placenta?**

Trophoblast.

○ **At what stage, does the trophoblast develop?**

Blastocyst—8 days.

○ **When does implantation occur?**

6 to 12 days postfertilization.

○ **What two cell types arise from the trophoblast?**

Syncytiotrophoblast and cytotrophoblast.

○ **What is the role of the cytotrophoblast?**

Form chorionic plate and chorion leave, invade and replace spiral arteries with uteroplacental arteries.

○ **What is the role of the syncytiotrophoblast?**

Transport of gases, nutrients, and waste products; synthesis of peptide and steroid hormones.

○ **What are the three distinct layers of the fetal membranes?**

Amnion, chorion laeve, and decidua capsularis.

○ **What placental hormone functions to maintain the corpus luteum in early pregnancy?**

human chorionic gonadotropin (hCG).

○ **When does the hCG level peak?**

9 to 10 weeks' gestation.

○ **When does the placenta become the major source of progesterone?**
7 to 9 weeks.

○ **What serves as the precursor for the placental progesterone?**
Maternal cholesterol.

○ **What enzyme activity is lacking in the placenta, limiting direct production of estrogen from cholesterol?**
17 α-hydroxylase.

○ **What precursor is used to make estrogen in the placenta, and from what source?**
Dehydroepiandrosterone (DHEA), from maternal and fetal adrenal glands.

○ **What other hormones are produced by placenta?**

Neuropeptide Y	Calcitonin	Parathyroid hormone-related protein (PTHrP)
Prolactin	Renin	Placental growth hormone (PGH)
Estrogen	Leptin	Human placental lactogen (hPL)
ACTH	Relaxin	Growth hormone variant (hGHV)
Inhibin	Activin	Hypothalamic-like releasing hormones

○ **What is hPL and what is its function?**
Human placental lactogen; promotes lipolysis, decreases maternal insulin, promotes mammary differentiation, and directs nutrients to the fetus.

○ **What is the name of the 10 to 30 lobes comprising the basal surface of a placenta?**
Maternal cotyledons.

○ **What is an accessory lobe called?**
Succenturiate lobe.

○ **What is its clinical significance?**
5% to 6% incidence. Infection or postpartum hemorrhage may result if retained in utero.

○ **What is the zone of fibrinoid degeneration between the invading trophoblast and the decidua basalis?**
Nitabuch layer.

○ **What are the fetal macrophages found within the chorionic villi called?**
Hofbauer cells.

MULTIPLE GESTATION

○ **Name the two types of twin placentation.**

Monochorionic and dichorionic.

○ **What zygosity is associated with each?**

Monochorionic placentas are always monozygotic twins. Dichorionic placenta can have monozygotic (DiMo) or dizygotic (DiDi) twins.

○ **What further differentiation can be made of monochorionic placentas?**

Monoamnionic versus diamnionic.

○ **Which type of twinning has the highest morbidity?**

Monoamnionic monochorionic.

○ **What feature of only monochorionic placentas leads to twin-twin transfusion syndrome?**

Arteriovenous anastomoses.

○ **What is the recommended method of delivery for mono-mono twins?**

Cesarean delivery.

○ **What is the biggest mortality risk of mono-mono twins?**

Cord entanglement.

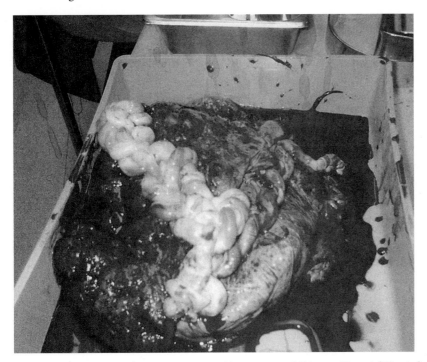

Cord entanglement seen with mono-mono twins. Photo courtesy of Abington Memorial Hospital, Abington, PA.

○ **What is different about the dividing membranes of DiMo versus DiDi twins?**

In DiMo the separating membrane contains only two amnions only. In DiDi, the membrane contains chorion (and thus blood vessels) as well.

○ **What early ultrasound finding is seen at the placenta-membrane junction with twin dichorionic placentas?**

Lambda sign or "twin peak" sign.

○ **What type of cord insertions is more common in twin placentas?**

Velamentous or marginal.

UMBILICAL CORD

○ **Name the types of cord insertion.**

Centric, accentric, marginal, velamentous, furcated, and circumvallate.

○ **What is the term used to describe an umbilical cord insertion at the margin of the placenta?**

Marginal insertion or "Battledore placenta."

○ **What is the incidence of marginal insertion?**

7%.

○ **What is a velamentous placenta?**

Insertion of the cord into the membranes. Approximately 1% of singleton deliveries.

○ **What complications can arise from a velamentous placenta?**

Vasa previa, thrombosis, rupture, and hemorrhage of vessels.

○ **What is a furcate cord insertion?**

A cord that begins its branching to major stem vessels before it inserts into the placenta and is not covered by Wharton jelly.

○ **What are some complications are associated with furcate cord insertion?**

Thrombosis and fetal hemorrhage.

○ **What is a circumvallate insertion?**

An incomplete covering of the basal plate of the placenta by the fetal membranes. A central depression and ring is formed at the attachment site of the membranes.

○ **What is significant about a circumvallate insertion?**

It is associated with abruption, hemorrhage, premature rupture of membranes (PROMs), and congenital malformations.

○ **What is the average length of the umbilical cord?**

60 cm.

○ **What length is defined as a short umbilical cord?**

<40 cm.

○ **What complications are associated with a short umbilical cord?**

Delivery: Avulsion of the cord, abruption, and uterine inversion.
Fetal: Congenital anomalies and CNS problems.

○ **What length is defined as a long umbilical cord?**

>70 cm.

○ **What complications are associated with a long umbilical cord?**

Cord prolapse, cord entanglement of the fetus, and true knots.

○ **What is the incidence of true knot in a cord?**

1.0%.

○ **What percentage of true knots are associated with intrauterine fetal demise?**

5% to 10%.

○ **What is the perinatal mortality rate with cord prolapse?**

5%.

○ **What are the risk factors for cord prolapse?**

Excessive cord length, malpresentation, low birth weight, grand multiparity, multiple gestation, obstetric manipulation (eg, artificial rupture of membranes), and polyhydramnios.

○ **What is the fetal heart tracing abnormality seen with cord prolapse?**

Sustained bradycardia or profound variable deceleration.

○ **What is the incidence of nuchal cord?**

25% overall, 21% with one nuchal cord, and 4% with two or more nuchal cords.

○ **What is the incidence of single umbilical artery?**

1%.

○ **What significance does a single umbilical artery have with congenital anomalies?**

15% of fetuses with congenital anomalies have a single umbilical artery. However, most infants born with a single umbilical artery have no known anomalies.

○ **Where is the preferred site for ultrasound-guided cordocentesis?**

The umbilical vein at its placental origin.

EVALUATION

○ **What time period denotes the third stage of labor?**

From delivery of the infant to delivery of the placenta.

○ **Name three signs of placental separation during the third stage of labor.**

Increased vaginal bleeding, lengthening of the umbilical cord, and changing of the shape of the abdominally palpated uterus to a more globular shape.

○ **What duration of time of the third stage of labor defines a retained placenta?**

>30 minutes.

○ **What are the complications of retained placenta?**

Infection and postpartum hemorrhage.

○ **What location of the placenta is associated with uterine inversion?**

Fundal.

○ **What characteristics of the placenta should be noted once the placenta is delivered?**

Time of delivery, cord insertion, number of vessels in cord, clinical evidence of infection or meconium staining, and completeness of the maternal surface and membranes.

○ **What information about the placenta should be noted on a routine second or third trimester ultrasound?**

Placental location, relationship to the internal cervical os, grade, and any evidence of abruption.

○ **Increasing placental maturity is associated with what ultrasound finding?**

Increased echogenicity secondary to increased calcium deposits.

○ **What conditions are associated with abundant placental calcifications prior to 36 weeks?**

Intrauterine growth restrictions (IUGR), oligohydramnios, maternal hypertension, diabetes, and smoking.

○ **What is the average weight of the term placenta?**

450 g.

○ **What defines placentomegaly?**

Weight >600 g, or ultrasound thickness >4 cm.

○ **What conditions are associated with placentomegaly?**

Maternal diabetes, maternal or fetal anemia, chronic infection, hydrops fetalis, and Beckwith-Wiedemann syndrome.

○ **What conditions are associated with small placentas?**

Maternal hypertension, preeclampsia, polyhydramnios, and fetal IUGR.

○ **What are the small white lesions that can be scraped away from the fetal placental surface?**

Desquamated skin cells: Amnion nodosum.

○ **What condition is amnion nodosum associated with?**

Long-standing oligohydramnios.

○ **What is the pathognomonic pathological finding of placental microabscesses?**

Listeriosis.

PLACENTAL COMPLICATIONS

○ **What is a vasa previa?**

Membranous cords in advance of the fetal presenting part, and often across the cervical os. Can occur with velamentous or marginal insertions, succenturiate lobes, and bilobed placentas.

○ **What is the incidence of vasa previa?**

Approximately 1 per 3000 deliveries.

○ **What is the perinatal mortality rate associated with vasa previa?**

60% if undiagnosed prenatally.

○ **Why is the perinatal mortality rate of vasa previa so high?**

Rupture of the membranes leads to rapid fetal exsanguination.

○ **How is the diagnosis of vasa previa made prior to delivery?**

By color flow Doppler techniques define placenta previa: Placenta covering the internal os of the cervix.

○ **What is the incidence of placenta previa at the time of delivery?**

0.5% (1 in 200).

○ **Name the factors that increase the risk of placenta previa.**

Advancing maternal age.
Multiparity.
Multiple gestation.
African or Asian ethnic background.
Smoking.
Cocaine use.
Prior previa.
Prior cesarean delivery.
Prior suction curettage or uterine surgery.

○ **What is the incidence of placenta previa in nulliparas at the time of delivery?**
1 in 1500.

○ **What is the incidence of placenta previa in grand multiparas at the time of delivery?**
Up to 1 in 20.

○ **What is the relative risk of previa for history of one cesarean delivery?**
4.5×.

○ **What is the relative risk of previa for history of four prior cesarean deliveries?**
45×.

○ **How are placental previas classified?**
Complete: The internal os is entirely covered by placenta.
Partial: The os is partially covered.
Marginal: The placenta edge just reaches the internal os.
Low-Lying: <2 cm from the internal os.

○ **What percentage of women with second trimester bleeding have a low-lying placenta diagnosed by ultrasound at that time?**
Up to 45%.

○ **What percentage of placenta previas diagnosed in the second trimester resolve by the time of delivery?**
>90%.

○ **What is the classic presentation of placenta previa?**
Sudden onset of painless vaginal bleeding in the second or third trimester.

○ **What is the most accurate method for diagnosing placenta previa?**
Transvaginal ultrasound.

○ **How has maternal mortality from placenta previa changed since the 1950s?**
From 25% to <1%.

○ **How has perinatal mortality from placenta previa changed since the 1950s?**
From 60% to <5%.

○ **What is the method of delivery for placenta previa?**
Cesarean delivery.

○ **What is the recommended timing of delivery for placenta previa?**
By 38 weeks (36–37 if fetal lung maturity is documented by amniocentesis).

○   **What are the complications of placenta previa?**

Longer hospital stay, cesarean delivery, abruptio placenta, postpartum hemorrhage, fetal malpresentation, disseminated intravascular coagulation (DIC), maternal death.

○   **What is placenta accreta?**

Trophoblastic invasion beyond the normal boundary established by Nitabuch layer.

○   **What is placenta increta?**

Placental invasion extends into the myometrium.

○   **What is placenta percreta?**

Placental invasion beyond the uterine serosa.

○   **What are the risk factors associated with placenta accreta?**

Placenta previa, prior uterine surgery, advanced maternal age, multiparity, Asherman syndrome, submucous leiomyoma, and anterior placenta.

○   **What is the frequency of placenta accreta?**

1 in 2500 deliveries.

○   **What is the risk of placenta accreta for placenta previa with no history of prior cesarean delivery?**

4% to 6%.

○   **What is the risk of placenta accreta for placenta previa and one prior cesarean delivery?**

10% to 25%.

○   **What is the risk of placenta accreta for placenta previa and two or more prior cesarean deliveries?**

>50%.

○   **What are the methods of diagnosing placenta accreta prior to delivery?**

Ultrasound and MRI.

○   **What gray-scale ultrasound findings have been associated with placenta accreta?**

Placental lacunae (lakes).
Loss of the retroplacental clear zone.
Uterine serosa-bladder line interruption.

○   **What is the standard of care treatment for placental accreta?**

Hysterectomy after delivery.

○   **What is the definition of abruptio placentae?**

Premature separation of the normally implanted placenta prior to the birth of the fetus, secondary to bleeding into the decidua basalis.

○   **What is the incidence of placental abruption?**

1%.

○   **What risk factors are associated with placental abruption?**

Maternal hypertension.

Advanced maternal parity and age.

Smoking.

PPROM managed expectantly.

Trauma.

Short umbilical cord.

Cocaine use.

Uterine anomalies or myomas.

Sudden decompression of the uterus (either by rupture of the membrane in a patient with polyhydramnios or by delivery of the first twin).

○   **When is the incidence of placental abruption highest?**

24 and 26 weeks.

○   **What are the classic signs and symptoms of placental abruption?**

Vaginal bleeding, abdominal pain, uterine contractions, and uterine tenderness.

○   **What is the characteristic uterine contraction pattern associated with placental abruption?**

High frequency and low amplitude, with increased baseline tone.

○   **What is a placental abruption without vaginal bleeding called?**

Concealed abruption.

○   **What percentage of placental abruptions are concealed?**

10% to 20%.

○   **How long should a patient be monitored after significant abdominal trauma late in pregnancy?**

4 to 6 hours if fetal heart rate tracing is reassuring and uterine contractions are absent.

○   **How long should a patient be monitored after significant abdominal trauma late in pregnancy with uterine activity present?**

At least 24 hours of continuous electronic fetal monitoring.

○ **What is the recurrence risk of placental abruption?**

5% to 16%; 25% if preceded by two consecutive abruptions.

○ **What is the sensitivity, specificity, and positive and negative predictive value of abruption via ultrasound?**

25%, 96%, 88%, and 53%.

○ **What laboratory studies are useful in the management of abruption?**

Hemoglobin and hematocrit, platelets, coagulation studies (PT, PTT, fibrinogen, and FSP).

○ **Abruptions account for what percentage of perinatal deaths?**

15%.

○ **What proportion of abruptions result in fetal death?**

4 in 1000 abruptions.

○ **What is the term used to describe abruption that leads to extravasation into and through the myometrium to the serosal surface of the uterus?**

Couvelaire uterus.

○ **What is the most common metastatic tumor of the placenta?**

Malignant melanoma.

○ **What are the most common benign tumors of the placenta?**

Chorioangiomas.

○ **What are placental site trophoblastic tumors?**

Very rare trophoblastic neoplasms characterized by absence of chorionic villi and proliferation of intermediate cytotrophoblast cells; they secrete beta hCG in amounts small in relation to tumor volume.

○ **Are placental site trophoblastic tumors sensitive to chemotherapy?**

No.

○ **What is the treatment of choice for placental site trophoblastic tumors?**

Hysterectomy, although D&C alone has cured some patients.

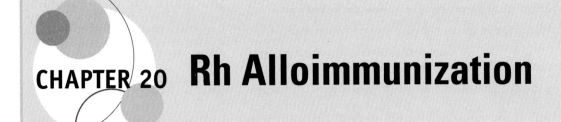

CHAPTER 20 Rh Alloimmunization

Jennifer Deirmengian, MD

○ **What is Rh factor?**

Rh refers to the immunogenic D antigen, an erythrocyte surface antigen of the rhesus (Rh) blood group system.

○ **What is alloimmunization?**

The development of antibodies in response to alloantigens, antigens present in other patients but not the patient who develops antibodies. This circumstance commonly occurs when a gravid patient develops antibodies to fetal red blood cell antigens.

○ **What type of maternal antibody can cross the placenta?**

Immunoglobulin G (IgG).

○ **What are the two systems of nomenclature for the Rh blood group system?**

Fisher-Race and Weiner.

○ **What is the Fisher-Race nomenclature with respect to Rh alloimmunization?**

The nomenclature assumes that there are three genetic loci with two major alleles each. The antigens produced by these alleles have a letter—C, c, D, E, and e (no "d" has been identified, but it is used to indicate an absence of an allele product). The most common genotypes are Cde/cde and CDe/Cde. The majority of Rh isoimmunization is caused by D antigen. Thus, Rh-positive has come to represent the presence of the D antigen and Rh-negative indicates the absence of D antigen on erythrocytes.

○ **On what chromosome is the genetic locus of the Rh antigen?**

Chromosome 1 (the short arm).

○ **What percentage of individuals are Rh-positive?**

Rh positivity varies by race.
Caucasians: 85%.
African Americans: 92% to 95%.
Asians and Native Americans: 98% to 99%.

○ **What percentage of Rh-positive individuals are heterozygous?**

Among whites, approximately 60% of Rh-positive individuals are heterozygous at the D locus.

○ **What must occur for Rh alloimmunization to develop?**

A patient must be Rh-negative. She must be exposed to RhD antigen. She must be able to produce antibody to the RhD antigen.

○ **How does Rh alloimmunization develop during pregnancy?**

An Rh-negative mother must be exposed to a sufficient amount of Rh-positive erythrocytes. The most common source is transplacental fetomaternal hemorrhage. Risk of fetomaternal hemorrhage increases with the duration of pregnancy. Other, less common causes of maternal Rh alloimmunization include transfusion with Rh-positive blood and injection with needles contaminated with Rh-positive blood.

○ **What is hemolytic disease of the fetus and newborn (HDFN)?**

HDFN occurs when maternal IgG antibodies to red cell antigens cross the placenta and bind the corresponding antigens on fetal red blood cells. This causes hemolysis of the fetal red blood cells, resulting in fetal anemia and occasionally fetal hydrops. HDFN has previously been known by the names hemolytic disease of the newborn (HDN) and erythroblastosis fetalis. Historically, the most common cause of HDFN was RhD alloimmunization. This has changed with routine use of anti-D immune globulin prophylaxis.

○ **Why are most first pregnancies unaffected by HDFN?**

The mother's antibody response mounts slowly (over 5–16 weeks). Exposure during pregnancy is mostly likely to occur after 28 weeks' gestation, meaning that a first child will likely be delivered before he or she is affected. In addition, transplacental fetomaternal hemorrhage is most common at delivery.

○ **Does a maternal antibody response occur in all cases of Rh incompatible pregnancies?**

No. Rh alloimmunization only occurs in approximately 15% of Rh-negative women who do not receive any anti-D immune globulin prophylaxis.

○ **What is the primary factor influencing severity of fetal anemia in Rh disease?**

Antibody concentration.

○ **How do fetal cells enter maternal circulation?**

Fetomaternal hemorrhage and transplacental passage of fetal red blood cells into the maternal circulation.

○ **When is fetomaternal hemorrhage most common?**

Fetomaternal hemorrhage is most common at the time of delivery.

○ **What percentage of fetomaternal hemorrhages at the time of delivery are thought to be sufficient to cause alloimmunization?**

15% to 20%.

○ **An estimated fetomaternal hemorrhage of >30 mL occurs in what percentage of cases?**

Approximately 1%.

○ **What are some common clinical factors associated with an increased risk of a substantial fetomaternal hemorrhage?**

Cesarean delivery, multiple gestation, manual removal of the placenta, placenta previa, placental abruption, and intrauterine manipulation.

○ **How frequently is a fetomaternal hemorrhage noted in the first trimester?**

Approximately 7%.

○ **How frequently is a fetomaternal hemorrhage noted in the second trimester?**

16%.

○ **What percentage of Rh-negative mothers become sensitized prior to delivery without Rh immune globulin prophylaxis?**

1% to 2%.

○ **How early does the Rh antigen develop?**

Rh antigens can be detected 38 days post conception.

○ **Can chorionic villus sampling performed on an Rh-negative patient result in sensitization?**

Yes.

○ **What are two mechanisms thought to impact the risk of sensitization?**

Approximately 10% to 20% of Rh-negative individuals are thought to be immunologic "nonresponders." ABO incompatibility exerts a protective effect against developing Rh sensitization.

○ **ABO incompatibility is associated with what risk of alloimmunization?**

1% to 2% (without Rh immune globulin prophylaxis).

○ **What combination of ABO incompatibility is associated with the most protective effect?**

Maternal blood type O, and fetal blood type A, B, AB.

○ **What is the definition of fetal hydrops?**

Fetal hydrops is defined as the presence of excess fluid within at least two compartments of the fetal-placental unit.

○ **The fluid collections used in the definition of hydrops include?**

Pericardial effusion, pleural effusion, abdominal ascites, scalp edema, polyhydramnios, or placentomegaly.

○ **What is the cause of fetal hydrops in the sensitized pregnancy?**

Severe anemia (hemoglobin 7 g/dL or less) leads to fetal hydrops. This could be a result of tissue hypoxia secondary to anemia causing increased capillary permeability.

○ **What process can lead to nervous system damage?**

Hyperbilirubinemia can lead to kernicterus. When levels of total serum bilirubin exceed 25 mg/dL, unconjugated bilirubin can enter brain tissue and cause apoptosis and necrosis. This leads to acute bilirubin encephalopathy that may result in permanent neurologic damage (kernicterus).

○ **0.1% to 0.2% of susceptible Rh-negative women still become alloimmunized despite recommendations for immunoprophylaxis. Why is this?**

(1) Failure to administer anti-D immune globulin at 28 to 29 weeks' gestation.

(2) Failure to recognize clinical events that place patients at risk of alloimmunization and administer anti-D immune globulin, when indicated.

(3) Failure to administer in a timely fashion anti-D immune globulin postnatally, when indicated.

○ **What amount of fetomaternal hemorrhage is necessary to cause alloimmunization?**

The exact amount varies. Alloimmunization may occur with exposure to as little as 0.1 mL of Rh-positive red cells.

○ **What is the associated risk of Rh alloimmunization in susceptible patients under the following circumstances: spontaneous abortion…induced abortion?**

Spontaneous first trimester abortion: 1.5% to 2%.
Induced abortion: 4% to 5%.

○ **What is the risk of fetomaternal hemorrhage under the following circumstances: chorionic villus sampling…amniocentesis…external cephalic version?**

Chorionic villus sampling: 14%.
Amniocentesis: 7% to 15%.
External cephalic version: 2% to 6%.

○ **What laboratory studies should every woman have at the first prenatal visit (with regard to alloimmunization)?**

ABO blood group.
Rh type.
Antibody screen.

○ **Who should be given Rh immune globulin during pregnancy?**

Rh-negative mothers with a negative antibody screen and a father of the pregnancy who is Rh-Positive or who has unknown status.

○ **When is Rh immune globulin given during an otherwise uncomplicated pregnancy?**

28 weeks (and within 72 hours of delivery if fetus is Rh-positive).

○ **What is the standard dose of Rh immune globulin used in the United States?**

300 μg.

○ **How does Rh immune globulin work?**

Rh immune globulin works by binding RhD antigen on fetal cells in maternal circulation. Because the fetal RhD antigens are "covered" by the Rh immune globulin, the mother does not develop her own antibodies to RhD.

○ **How is anti-D immune globulin obtained?**

It is collected by apheresis from RhD-negative male volunteer donors who are given multiple injections of RhD-positive red cells and thus have high titers of circulating anti-RhD antibodies. A search is currently underway for a synthetic anti-D immune globulin and some progress has been made on this front.

○ **Is Rh immune globulin indicated when a patient is already sensitized?**

No.

○ **How large a fetomaternal hemorrhage does the 300 μg dose of Rh immune globulin dose cover?**

30 mL of fetal whole blood or 15 mL of fetal red cells (only 1% of women have >5 mL of fetal blood in the maternal circulation after delivery).

○ **What test is used to QUANTITATE the volume of fetal red cells in the maternal circulation?**

Kleihauer-Betke (KB).

○ **What is the QUALITATIVE test for fetomaternal hemorrhage?**

Rosette test. If this test is negative, a standard dose of Rh immune globulin should be given. If this test is positive, further evaluation is recommended using the KB test to evaluate the percentage of fetal cells in maternal circulation.

○ **How is the dose of Rh immune globulin calculated if the volume of hemorrhage is estimated to be >30 mL of whole blood?**

When fetomaternal hemorrhage is >30 mL of whole blood, the KB is performed to quantitate the actual volume of hemorrhage. The percentage of fetal cells is multiplied by 50 (to account for estimated maternal blood volume of 5 L). This number is divided by 30 to determine the number of vials of Rh immune globulin (because each vial of 300 μg of Rh immune globulin neutralizes 30 mL of fetal whole blood). One additional vial of Rh immune globulin is always added to the number above as a precaution.

○ **Within what time limit should Rh immune globulin be given after delivery?**

The standard time interval for Rh immune globulin to be given is within 72 hours; however, this is just a by-product of how the original studies were performed because women had to return within 3 days. Rh immune globulin should be given before a primary immune response occurs, and it can be given up to 14 to 28 days after delivery.

○ **How long does the effect of Rh immune globulin last?**

The half-life of Rh immune globulin is 24 days, and a woman can be considered fully protected for 12 weeks after injection. There are scattered case reports of maternal sensitization from decreasing antibody concentrations.

○ **If standard antenatal anti-D immune globulin administration is given within 3 weeks of delivery, can the postnatal dose be withheld in the absence of excessive fetomaternal hemorrhage?**

Yes.

○ **What percentage of women have evidence of fetomaternal hemorrhage after delivery?**

75%.

○ **For which gestational events is Rh immune globulin indicated?**

Fetomaternal hemorrhage with ectopic pregnancy or abortion, chorionic villus sampling, amniocentesis, external cephalic version, significant antepartum bleeding, molar pregnancy (complete mole controversial), blunt abdominal trauma, fetal death in the second or third trimester, or multifetal reduction.

○ **Is threatened abortion before 12 weeks' gestation an indication for anti-D immune globulin prophylaxis?**

Controversial. The RhD antigen has been reported on fetal erythrocytes as early as 38 days of gestation, but alloimmunization rate is low in threatened abortions before 12 weeks.

○ **What dose of anti-D immune globulin, if indicated, should be given in the first trimester?**

50 μg.

○ **At what anti-D antibody titer is a patient considered to be sensitized?**

1:4.

○ **It has been suggested that severe erythroblastosis or perinatal death does not occur when antibody levels remain below a "critical titer." What is this critical titer level?**

1:16. This number may vary depending on the lab.

○ **In which situation is measuring maternal anti-D antibody titers not indicated?**

If a previous affected pregnancy included severe fetal anemia (perinatal loss or intrauterine/neonatal transfusion). In this situation, maternal antibody titers do not predict the degree of fetal anemia in the current pregnancy.

○ **If a mother has had a hydropic fetus, what is the recurrence risk?**

80%.

○ **What is the initial management for a subsequent pregnancy following an affected fetus/infant?**

First check the paternal genotype. If the father is a heterozygote, perform amniocentesis at 15 weeks' gestation to determine fetus' RhD status. If the fetus is RhD-negative, no further follow-up is needed. If the fetus is RhD-positive or the father is a homozygote, begin serial middle cerebral artery (MCA) Dopplers or amniocentesis (if Dopplers are not available) at 18 weeks.

○ **What noninvasive test is known to be the most accurate way to document fetal anemia in at-risk pregnancies?**

MCA Doppler studies.

○ **What are the sensitivity and specificity of MCA Doppler measurements?**

Up to 90% sensitive and 98% specific.

○ **What MCA Doppler measurement corresponds with severe fetal anemia?**

A MCA peak systolic velocity (PSV) >1.5 multiples of the median (MoMs).

○ **How often are MCA Dopplers performed during at-risk or affected pregnancies?**

Weekly.

○ **After what gestational age, do MCA Dopplers have a higher false-positive rate?**

34 to 35 weeks.

○ **How is amniotic fluid analysis used to estimate the degree of fetal red cell hemolysis?**

Bilirubin causes a shift in spectrophotometric density of the amniotic fluid, and the amount of shift from 450 nm (the ΔOD_{450}) is used to estimate the degree of fetal red cell hemolysis. The ΔOD_{450} value is plotted on a Liley curve (in the second and third trimesters) or a Queenan curve (early pregnancy). The Queenan curve has largely replaced use of the Liley curve at all gestational ages. It is useful to follow the trend of these results.

○ **If fetal hydrops is detected on an ultrasound, how low is the fetal hematocrit?**

Probably <15%.

○ **The Liley curve is divided into how many zones?**

Three zones.

○ **What does each zone of the Liley curve indicate?**

Zone I usually indicates mildly affected or unaffected fetus with a low risk of severe anemia.

Zone 2 indicates mild to moderate fetal hemolysis but low risk of severe anemia.

Zone 3 indicates severe anemia with high risk of fetal death within 7 to 10 days.

Lower zone expected hemoglobin is 11.0 to 13.9 g/dL; upper zone expected hemoglobin is 8.0 to 10.9 g/dL.

○ **Amniocentesis is performed and demonstrates results in Zone 1. When would the next amniocentesis be repeated?**

Every 10 days to 2 weeks.

○ **When describing the Liley curve, in addition to zones, what other information is needed to properly plot an amniocentesis result?**

Gestational age. The Liley curve is gestational age specific.

○ **In a preterm fetus with a value in Liley Zone 3, management would include what?**

Fetal blood sampling and intrauterine transfusion.

○ **What is the proper management of a fetus with severe Rh sensitization and absent lung maturity at 30 to 32 weeks' gestation?**

Controversial, but because of excellent outcomes with current neonatal intensive care, transfusion, and maternal steroid administration with delivery at 32 to 34 weeks may be considered.

○ **What is the proper management of mild fetal hemolysis and reassuring fetal testing?**

Delivery at 37 to 38 weeks' gestation or earlier if fetal lung maturity documented.

○ **Do the lungs of an infant with Rh sensitization mature more quickly or more slowly than an infant of the same gestational age?**

More slowly. Hydropic changes in the placenta may increase insulin production leading to delayed lung maturation as seen in diabetics.

○ **What ultrasound findings are suggestive of prehydropic fetal anemia?**

Polyhydramnios.

Placental thickness >4 cm.

Pericardial effusion.

Dilation of cardiac chambers.

Enlargement of spleen and liver.

Visualization of both sides of fetal bowel wall.

Dilation of the umbilical vein.

○ **For a fetus with evidence of hemolysis based on MCA Dopplers or amniotic fluid bilirubin analysis, what is the next best test to perform?**

Percutaneous umbilical blood sampling to determine fetal hematocrit.

○ **What routine tests, besides assessment of amniotic fluid bilirubin or umbilical cord hematocrit, are undertaken in cases of Rh alloimmunization?**

Antepartum fetal surveillance by nonstress test or biophysical profile is begun at 32 weeks' gestation.

○ **What are the two types of fetal transfusions?**

Intrauterine intraperitoneal (needle into peritoneal cavity of fetus).

Intrauterine intravascular (needle into umbilical vein).

○ **What are the advantages of intraperitoneal transfusions…intravascular?**

Intraperitoneal: Ease of placement and decreased dislodgement.

Intravascular: Ability to obtain fetal hematocrit prior to transfusion and after direct placement of red cells intravascularly.

Intravascular transfusion is generally preferred. However, intraperitoneal transfusion is considered if vascular access is difficult because of early gestational age or fetal position.

○ **What are the complications of transfusions, and which is the most common?**

Fetal bradycardia, infection, premature rupture of membranes, fetal death (4–9%), and need for emergent delivery secondary to fetal status (ie, fetal bradycardia).

Fetal bradycardia is the most common complication of fetal transfusion.

○ **What is the purpose of intrauterine transfusion?**

To correct fetal anemia that improves fetal oxygenation.

○ **What type of blood is used for the transfusion?**

Type O, leukocyte reduced, cytomegalovirus negative, and gamma irradiated packed erythrocytes that are cross-matched to a maternal blood sample.

○ **At what hematocrit level is transfusion considered in the fetus remote from term?**
<25%.

○ **At what gestation is intrauterine transfusion usually performed?**
Intrauterine transfusion is usually performed between 18 and 35 weeks' gestation.
After 35 weeks, delivery is generally considered safer than transfusion.

○ **Which antibodies to minor antigens have also been shown to result in fetal hemolytic disease?**
Anti-E, anti-Kell (K1), anti-c, anti-c + E, anti-Fy (Duffy).

○ **Of the above, which minor antigen is the most common?**
Anti-Kell (10% of people are Kell antigen positive).

○ **If a patient presents with anti-Kell antibodies, what two pieces of information should be obtained?**
(1) Paternal Kell status.
(2) Question the patient if she has ever had a transfusion (Kell status is not checked for in transfused blood).

○ **What is the management of patients with antibodies to minor antigens?**
Management is similar to Rh alloimmunization with measurement of maternal antibody titers, serial MCA Doppler measurement or serial amniocenteses after a critical titer is reached, and transfusion or delivery based on these results and gestational age. Because Kell sensitization causes suppression of fetal erythropoiesis as well as fetal hemolysis, the ΔOD_{450} is less predictive of the level of fetal anemia.

○ **What are the red blood cell surface antigens called that a fetus can inherit from the father?**
Private antigens (a mother may become sensitized at first pregnancy and future pregnancies may develop alloimmunization).

○ **What percentage of pregnancies are ABO incompatible?**
20 to 25%.

○ **What blood types (maternal and fetal) cause most cases of ABO incompatibility?**
O mother; A or B infant (mother has anti-A and anti-B IgG).

○ **Does ABO incompatibility require previous sensitization to affect the fetus?**
No. ABO hemolytic disease may affect the firstborn child.

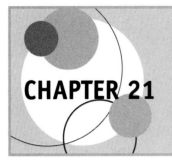

CHAPTER 21

Genetics for the Obstetrician

Amelia McLennan, MD and Jennifer McClarren, MS, CGC

○ **Meiosis begins with 46 chromosomes each consisting of two chromatids. At the end of meiosis I, how many chromosomes and chromatids are present? At the end of meiosis II, how may chromosomes and how many chromatids are present?**

Meiosis I—23 chromosomes and 46 chromatids.

Meiosis II—23 chromosomes and 23 chromatids.

○ **What is crossing over and when specifically does it occur?**

The exchange of genetic material between homologous chromosomes, a mechanism for increasing genetic variation. Occurs during Meiosis I (during Pachytene of Prophase I).

○ **When does female meiosis begin?**

At about 4 months' gestation.

○ **When is Meiosis I completed?**

At ovulation.

○ **When is Meiosis II completed?**

At fertilization.

○ **What is the most common trisomy in liveborn infants?**

Trisomy 21 (Down syndrome).

○ **What percentage of first trimester pregnancy losses have a chromosome abnormality?**

>50%.

○ **Monosomy for an entire chromosome is typically incompatible with life. What condition is an exception to this?**

45, X (Turner syndrome).

O   **What is the only etiologic factor conclusively linked to an increased risk of trisomy?**

Advanced maternal age.

O   **Chromosome analysis on your patient's husband revealed the following: 45,XY, der(14;21)(q10;q10). What would you discuss with this couple?**

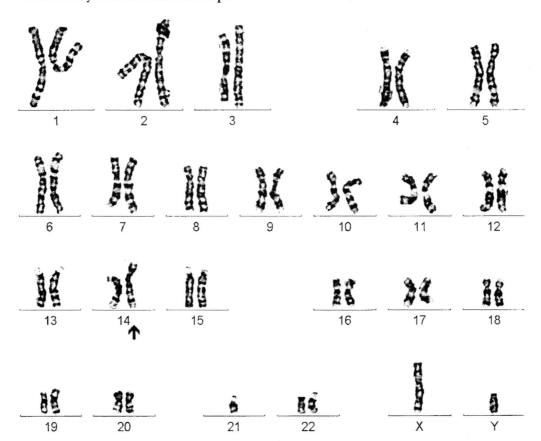

He is a carrier of a balanced 14:21 translocation. There is an increased risk of offspring with Down syndrome, recurrent pregnancy loss, decreased fertility, or uniparental disomy (UPD). Carriers of this translocation do not typically have developmental or phenotypic abnormalities.

O   **Your patient reports that her brother has a son with trisomy 21 and she is concerned about her risk to have a child with Down syndrome. What would you discuss with her?**

Her risk of Down syndrome would be greater than her age-related risk. Trisomy 21 is typically a sporadic occurrence (and is not inherited in families; however, you do not have documentation that it is a true trisomy; therefore, peripheral blood chromosomes need to be offered to rule out a familial translocation).

O   **What meiotic process is the major cause of aneuploidy?**

Nondisjunction.

O   **What percentage of fetuses with 45,X (Turner syndrome) spontaneously abort?**

>99%.

○ **Certain genetic disorders occur when both chromosomes of a pair are inherited from the same parent. What is the process called?**

UPD.

○ **What percentage of couples who have had two or more SABs will be found to have a chromosome abnormality?**

6% of these couples (or 3% of the individuals).

○ **What are the risks associated with advanced paternal age?**

Men who are 40 to 45 years of age or older, are at increased risk of new mutations, and associated with autosomal dominant conditions [eg, neurofibromatosis I (NF-1), achondroplasia, Marfan syndrome, and osteogenesis imperfecta].

○ **At a preconception visit, your patient and her husband disclose that they are first cousins. What would their offspring be at risk of?**

Birth defects, autosomal recessive conditions, and conditions that are more common in their ethnic background.

○ **What genetic test should be considered in women with unexplained ovarian failure or elevated FSH prior to 40 years of age?**

Fragile X carrier screening.

○ **A new patient reports that she suffers from depression and had a heart problem as a child. She seems to have difficulty following your conversation. Her mother, who accompanies her to the visit, has a scar over her upper lip. What genetic testing would your order on this patient?**

FISH for 22q11.2 deletion (DiGeorge).

○ **A patient of yours reports that her father has Marfan syndrome. What is her risk to have inherited the condition? What features would you look for in your patient and what consults would you recommend?**

50% risk.

Tall, thin body habitus, long, curved fingers (arachnodactyly), pectus, and striae.

Patient needs cardiology evaluation with echocardiogram, ophthalmology exam, and genetics evaluation.

○ **A patient reports that her brother died of Canavan disease. What is her risk to be a carrier?**

2/3.

○ **Chromosomes on the products of conception of your 38-year-old patient reveal a karyotype of 47,XX,+18. What is the likely etiology of this result, and what is her recurrence risk?**

The risk of trisomy increases with maternal age, and most trisomic conceptions spontaneously miscarry. Her recurrence risk after a fetus or child with autosomal trisomy ranges from 1.6 to 8.2 times the maternal age-related risk.

○ **A patient states that she was recently diagnosed with NF-1, following a diagnosis of NF-1 in her daughter. She tells you that her daughter has numerous café-au-lait marks, several neurofibromas, and learning difficulties. The patient herself appears clinically normal except for several café-au-lait marks. What genetic concept can explain this?**

Variable expressivity.

○ **What are the potential risks associated with selective serotonin uptake inhibitor (SSRI) use during pregnancy?**

Possible increased risk of congenital cardiac anomalies with first trimester exposure to Paxil. Exposure to SSRIs in late pregnancy can result in transient neonatal complications including persistent pulmonary hypertension.

○ **A patient reports that she and her partner are of Ashkenazi Jewish ancestry. Which screening tests would you offer and what inheritance pattern would you discuss with them?**

ACOG recommends screening for Tay-Sachs disease, Canavan disease, familial dysautonomia, and cystic fibrosis (CF). Additionally, this couple is at increased risk of Gaucher disease, Niemann-Pick disease, Fanconi anemia, Bloom syndrome, Mucolipidosis IV, glycogen storage disease 1A, Maple syrup urine disease, dihydrolipoamide dehydrogenase deficiency, familial hyperinsulinism, Usher Syndrome type IF, Usher syndrome type III, and nemaline myopathy. These conditions all have an autosomal recessive inheritance pattern.

○ **Besides the Ashkenazi Jewish population, what other ethnic backgrounds are at increased risk of Tay-Sach disease?**

French Canadian (1:30), Louisiana Cajun (1:30), and Celtic/Irish (1:50).

○ **Your patient is of Irish and German descent. What is her risk to be a carrier of CF? If she screens negative on the standard CF panel (23 mutations), what is her residual risk to be a CF carrier?**

1:25; 1:208.

○ **For which ethnic group is the detection rate for CF screening the lowest?**

Asian.

○ **An African American couple reports that they have a daughter with CF. Your patient's prenatal CF carrier screen is negative. What explanation can you give this couple?**

The standard CF panel looks for 23 mutations and has a 69% detection rate in the African American population (as compared with a 90% detection rate in the Caucasian population). There are over 1000 mutations in the CFTR gene; thus the patient may carry a mutation not screened for in the standard panel.

○ **A patient of yours has sickle cell trait and her partner's hemoglobinopathy evaluation revealed probable β-thalassemia trait. What are the risks to their offspring?**

25% carrier of hemoglobin S, 25% carrier of β-thalassemia, 25% noncarrier/unaffected, and 25% affected with sickle β-thalassemia.

○ **A patient's α-thalassemia DNA report shows she is a cis carrier of α-thalassemia; her husband is found to have one α-thalassemia mutation. What condition is their offspring at risk of?**

Hemoglobin H disease (--/α-)

○ **A pregnant patient with achondroplasia is under your care. Her husband is of typical stature. What is the inheritance pattern of this condition? What is the chance for this couple to have a child with achondroplasia?**

Autosomal dominant; 50%.

○ **Your patient is a fragile X premutation carrier. What is her risk to have an affected son?**

50%.

○ **Your patient is a fragile X premutation carrier and is pregnant with a female fetus. What are the clinical possibilities for this patient's daughter?**

She could be a premutation carrier (like her mother), the repeat size could expand to a full mutation (she could have some clinical symptoms of fragile X), or she could be "normal" if she receives the typical X from her mother.

○ **What analytes are utilized in first trimester screening?**

PAPP-A and beta hCG.

○ **At what gestational age, would you offer first trimester screening?**

Between 10 and 14 weeks (each center may have a slightly different range).

○ **What conditions are screened for by the first trimester screen?**

Trisomy 21 and trisomy 18 (some labs will report a risk of trisomy 13/trisomy 18 combined).

○ **If a patient has an increased nuchal translucency in the first trimester and a normal fetal karyotype on chorionic villus sampling (CVS), what other tests would you offer?**

Microarray and Noonan syndrome testing needs to be offered when there are normal chromosomes on CVS. Anatomy scan/level 2 ultrasound, fetal echocardiogram (due to increased likelihood of congenital cardiac anomaly), and MSAFP [as routine screen for open neural tube defects (ONTD)].

○ **If a cystic hygroma is seen on ultrasound, what is the likelihood of aneuploidy?**

60% to 75% (most of these will be 45X).

○ **When does ACOG recommend fetal microarray be offered?**

When there is abnormal anatomic findings and a normal conventional karyotype, or if there is a fetal demise with congenital anomalies and a karyotype cannot be obtained.

○ **What conditions are screened for by second trimester blood screening?**

Trisomy 21, trisomy 18, and ONTDs.

○ **What analytes are utilized for the quadruple screen?**

AFP, unconjugated estriol, dimeric inhibin A, and hCG.

○ **What are the potential causes of an elevated AFP level in a second trimester blood screen?**

Multiple gestations, IUFD, ventral wall defect, ONTD, incorrect dating of pregnancy, oligohydramnios, renal agenesis, and congenital nephrosis.

○ **What factors affect the interpretation of the quadruple screen?**

Maternal age, race, weight, maternal IDDM, gestational age, multiple gestations, and previous pregnancy with ONTD.

O   **What factors affect the interpretation of a first trimester screen?**

Maternal age, race, weight, multiple gestation, maternal IDDM, previous pregnancy with Down syndrome.

O   **If arthrogryposis is seen on ultrasound, what genetic syndromes should be considered?**

Spinal muscular atrophy (SMA) and myotonic dystrophy.

O   **What is the risk in the general population for your patient to be a carrier of SMA?**

Approximately 1/35.

O   **Your patient's SMA results come back showing that she has 2 copy number of the SMN1 gene. What does this mean?**

This means she has a decreased risk to be a carrier. The more copy numbers a patient has, the less likely she is to be a carrier. (If she had one copy of SMN1, then she would be a carrier.)

O   **Your patient's CVS results show 47, XY +21[3]/46, XY[17]. What does this mean for the patient's pregnancy? And what other tests, if any, should be offered?**

Possibilities with this result include true fetal mosaicism for Down syndrome, confined placental mosaicism (CPM)/normal fetus, and fetus with full trisomy 21. Amniocentesis should be offered to distinguish between these possibilities.

O   **How often does mosaicism occur in amniocentesis or CVS samples?**

0.25% amniocentesis and 1% CVS.

O   **An amniocentesis result reveals 46 total chromosomes with an inversion of chromosome 22. What follow-up testing on the parents should be recommended?**

Parental karyotype to determine if the results are de novo or inherited. If one of the parents has the same inversion and is clinically normal, there is a high probability that the fetus will be unaffected (like the parent).

O   **What is the risk of pregnancy loss from amniocentesis?**

1 in 300 to 500 if performed after 15 weeks' gestation.

○ **Chromosome analysis on your patient shows the following. What would be this patient's clinical picture?**

CB12-8738 B,M

3K

This patient has Turner syndrome. Features can include short stature, webbed neck, renal anomalies (eg, horseshoe kidney), cardiac anomalies (eg, coarctation of aorta), Mullerian abnormalities, and difficulty with visual-perceptual skills (overall intelligence is average or above).

○ **What genetic tests would you offer a patient for recurrent pregnancy loss?**

Factor V Leiden, prothrombin, antithrombin III, protein S, protein C, and parental chromosomes (on patient and partner). MTHFR and homocysteine levels are no longer recommended due to the lack of association with adverse pregnancy outcomes.

○ **On ultrasound a fetus has bilateral postaxial polydactyly with no additional findings. Neither parent reports a personal history of polydactyly, but the husband says that his father was born with an extra finger on each hand. What inheritance pattern is exhibited by this family history?**

Autosomal dominant inheritance with incomplete penetrance.

○   **What are the usual indications for prenatal diagnosis (eg, CVS, amniocentesis)?**

Advanced maternal age, abnormal maternal serum screen, ultrasound finding, parental or family history of genetic condition, or chromosome abnormality.

○   **What are the common chromosome abnormalities in humans?**

There are aneuploidies, polyploidies, and structural alterations. *Aneuploidy* refers to numeric abnormalities. These can be due to (i) nondisjunction: one pair of chromosomes fails to separate at anaphase resulting in one daughter cell having both parts of the pair and the other having none; (ii) anaphase lag: one chromosome of a pair moves slower during anaphase so its material is lost; (iii) polyploidy: the total number of chromosomes is duplicated more than once, for example, 69 chromosomes. *Structural alterations* include (i) deletion: losing a portion of a chromosome; (ii) duplication: there is an extra portion of a chromosome; (iii) insertion: a portion of a chromosome is attached to another; (iv) inversion: the order of placement of a genetic material is inverted in the chromosome; (v) translocation: portions of genetic material are removed from one chromosome and inserted onto another.

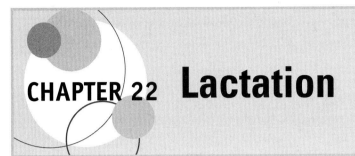

CHAPTER 22 Lactation

Jennifer Deirmengian, MD

○ **When do prolactin levels peak in pregnancy and postpartum?**

Prolactin levels peak at the time of delivery. The normal range varies, but in one study the mean value at term was 207 ng/mL. Baseline prolactin levels slowly decline after delivery, with levels of 35 ng/mL after 6 months postpartum. Prolactin levels increase by 80% to 150% with nipple stimulation.

○ **Why does lactogenesis, or actual lactation, not occur during pregnancy even though the prolactin levels are elevated?**

The receptor sites in the breast are competitively bound by estrogen and progesterone, preventing prolactin from activating lactation. When the placenta is delivered, these levels of estrogen and progesterone rapidly drop and the prolactin floods the receptors.

○ **Suckling produces a pulsatile release of what substance and where does it originate?**

Oxytocin, from the posterior pituitary.

○ **What is the letdown reflex?**

The letdown reflex describes the secretion of oxytocin in response to infant suckling or maternal clues related to nursing. The oxytocin causes myoepithelial cells in the breast to contract, resulting in ejection of milk.

○ **Does oxytocin have any other physiologic effects?**

Yes. It causes uterine contractions in the immediate postpartum period. This is thought to aid in uterine involution.

○ **What is the area of the breast that stores milk in preparation for the infant to extract? Where is this located? What is the clinical significance?**

The lactiferous sinuses are located just behind the areola. The lactiferous ducts, which drain from the alveolar sacs, empty into the sinuses. If the infant is not positioned such that his/her mouth is over the areola, the infant will suck only on the nipple and have to frequently regrasp the breast to suckle. This results in sore nipples and fissures, leading to possible mastitis.

○ **What term describes the maintenance of lactation over time after the initial episode of lactogenesis?**

Galactopoiesis. It is dependent on continued stimulation to the breast and on the presence of at least baseline levels of prolactin.

○ **When does complete involution of the breast occur?**

At menopause. Partial involution occurs at each weaning, but complete involution does not occur until withdrawal of all hormone stimulation. Women who receive postmenopausal hormone replacement will retard this process.

○ **For how long does the American Academy of Pediatrics (AAP) recommend breastfeeding?**

Exclusive breastfeeding is recommended for the first 6 months after birth, with continued breastfeeding until at least 1 year of age or longer as long as mutually desired by mother and infant.

○ **What are some important infant benefits of breastfeeding?**

Superior nutrition.
Prevention of infection (including otitis media, gastroenteritis, urinary tract infection).
Increased intelligence as adults.
Long-term reduction in obesity.
Reduction in the risk of childhood cancer.
Decreased risk of cardiovascular disease and type 1 diabetes mellitus.

○ **What are some important maternal benefits of breastfeeding?**

Improved uterine involution leading to decreased postpartum blood loss.
Enhanced postpartum weight loss.
Reduced risk of breast and ovarian cancer.
Decreased risk of cardiovascular disease.
Decreased cost (savings from formula, decreased expenditure for childhood illness).

○ **What are the some factors that promote success and longer breastfeeding duration?**

Nursing immediately following delivery
Rooming in
Skin-to-skin contact
Frequent demand feedings in the early postpartum period.

○ **What is the average weight gain on infants that are breastfed?**

Once breastfeeding is established, infants gain 15 to 40 g per day.

○ **What is colostrum?**

Colostrum is the milk secreted in the first 72 hours after delivery. It contains immunoglobulins and lactoferrin. It also contains macrophages, lymphocytes, and neutrophils. In addition to being a source of nutrients, colostrum bolsters neonates' immune systems.

○ **What is the caloric content of mature milk?**

Approximately 70 kcal/100 mL in a well nourished mother. Colostrum has a lower caloric content (58 kcal/100 mL).

○ **What is the primary carbohydrate in human milk?**

Lactose. Cow's milk is primarily sucrose. The lactose in humans is broken down into lactic acid, decreasing stool pH and giving the breastfed infant the characteristic loose stool. This should not be confused with diarrhea. Using a cloth diaper or smooth towel, the stool can be checked. If there is no ring of water around the stool, this is not diarrhea and should be considered normal.

○ **What are the major macronutrients of human milk?**

Lactose and oligosaccharides, milk fat (including triglycerides, cholesterol, phospholipids, and steroid hormones), proteins (including caseins, alpha-lactalbumin, lactoferrin, secretory immunoglobulin), and minerals (including sodium, potassium, chloride, calcium, magnesium, phosphate).

○ **How much milk should a breastfeeding woman drink?**

There is no minimum amount needed but she should have calcium supplements if she is not getting dairy products. A woman who drinks large quantities (>1 quart/day) of cow's milk runs the risk of sensitizing her infant to cow's milk protein, which can cross into her milk.

○ **Of an average 25-pound weight gain in pregnancy, what portion is considered to be lactation stores? What happens to this weight if the patient does not breastfeed?**

About 8 to 9 pounds or 3 to 4 kg. If she bottle feeds, she will have to diet it off—a great piece of propaganda to encourage someone to breastfeed!

○ **How long can breast milk be stored in the refrigerator?**

Approximately 48 hours, after which it should be frozen. Breast milk can be stored for up to 3 months in a daily-use freezer and for up to 6 months in a deep-freezer or chest freezer. Freezing will decrease the immunologic value, but not the nutritional component. Thaw under warm or hot running water or in a pan. Do not microwave.

○ **A mother calls you to say her pumped breast milk is "spoiling" in the refrigerator. What is wrong?**

The milk has separated! In our modern society, most people have only seen commercial homogenized milk. The separated milk (fat and water) can be reconstituted with gentle shaking.

○ **What is the term used to describe the presence of milky secretions from the breast of a newborn infant?**

Witch's milk. Can be found in both sexes and is due to the effect of maternal hormones on the fetal tissue. It generally disappears rapidly postpartum and no treatment is needed.

○ **What is the proper postpartum management of a mother who chooses not to breastfeed?**

A firmly fitting (but not binding) bra, ice packs as needed, and decreased stimulation to the nipples. Pharmacologic suppression is frequently ineffective because it is improperly prescribed and/or used. Bromocriptine is no longer indicated due to severe maternal side effects and should not be prescribed.

○ **What are the two major maternal illnesses in which breastfeeding is truly contraindicated?**

HIV infection and active untreated TB.

[Mothers with human T-lymphotropic virus type I or II (HTLV-I or HTLV-2) and untreated brucellosis should not breastfeed either, but these infections are less common.]

○   **In which infant illness is breastfeeding contraindicated?**

Galactosemia.

○   **Why is galactosemia an absolute contraindication to breastfeeding?**

Galactosemia is an inborn error of metabolism. Infants with this disorder are unable to utilize galactose, a component of the lactose sugar in human milk. Accumulation of galactose may lead to failure to thrive, liver dysfunction, cataracts, and mental retardation.

○   **What is the definition of tandem nursing?**

The nursing of two children of differing ages during the same time frame. This can be siblings (ie, a newborn and an older child) or could be adoptive nursing of an infant while nursing a biologic toddler. Of importance is that if both children are biologic, the newborn must be nursed first at any feeding time, as the milk produced will revert to colostrum just after delivery. Colostrum should be given to the newborn first to assure adequate nutrition and hydration. It is presumed that the older child receives most of its nutrition elsewhere and does not rely on the breast.

○   **Can a pregnant patient nurse her infant or toddler?**

Yes. In an uncomplicated pregnancy, a woman may continue nursing. However, her milk supply may decrease.

○   **Can an adoptive mother nurse her infant?**

Yes. If the mother has had a prior term pregnancy and lactated with that delivery, her success rate is highest. The breast of a woman who has never been pregnant can be primed with oral estrogen, and then given TRH to stimulate prolactin. If there is then mechanical stimulation and/or suckling, the breast will produce milk. The quantity in the latter circumstance may not be sufficient for total nutrition. The infant should be supplemented with formula.

○   **Your patient planned to breastfeed but delivers at 28 weeks. How do you counsel her?**

Encourage her to use an electric pump and take the milk to the NICU. This milk is rich in immunologic value. It is a way for the mother to be actively involved in her infant's care. Most insurance companies will reimburse for the pump rental. She should pump every 3 hours during the day and once at night to maintain a good supply.

○   **Should a baby with a cleft lip and/or palate be breastfed?**

Yes. It can actually be easier. The large surface area of the breast can help occlude the defect. In very large defects special devices may be needed.

○   **A 26-year-old patient is being treated during pregnancy for a microadenoma of the pituitary. She has had no tumor enlargement and no symptoms. She would like to breastfeed. How do you advise her?**

There is no contraindication to breastfeeding, but in some situations she may have a low milk supply. This is most common after surgery or prior radiation.

○   **Are the iron levels in breast milk affected in women who are anemic?**

No. They produce milk with normal iron levels.

○ **What are the three majors factors used to assess risk of maternal consumption of a drug to the breastfed infant?**

 (1) Dose consumed.

 (2) Oral bioavailability of the drug in both mother and infant.

 (3) Elimination route and timing in both mother and infant.

○ **A mother needs to be anticoagulated postpartum. What is your drug of choice?**

Coumadin is easiest for the mother and safe for the infant. Even though small quantities reach the infant, therapeutic levels are not reached. Heparin does not get excreted into the milk but is more complicated for mother to receive.

○ **What are the recommendations of ACOG regarding use of oral contraceptives while breastfeeding?**

ACOG cites that progestin-only pills and Depo-Provera do not impair lactation. Current recommendations are to start either progestin-only pills or Depo-Provera at 6 weeks postpartum. Combined oral contraceptives have historically not been recommended for breastfeeding women because of concerns about reduction in milk supply. However, combined hormonal contraceptives can be used once milk supply is well established.

○ **What is the lactational amenorrhea method?**

This method of family planning is advocated by the Population Council and other international groups, especially in areas where other methods of contraception are lacking. The method requires the presence of three criteria to reach 98% effectiveness: (1) no menses, (2) fully or nearly fully breastfeeding (ie, no solids or formula), and (3) infant <6 months of age. At 3 months, nearly 87% are anovulatory, but this drops to 57% by 6 months. If menses have not returned, it is felt that on the first ovulatory cycle the luteal phase is usually poor and would not sustain implantation, making it safe to wait for menses to return before using other contraception.

○ **Can a breastfeeding mother receive postpartum rubella vaccination?**

Yes.

○ **Your patient is an insulin-dependent diabetic. Can she breastfeed?**

Yes. Insulin does not cross. She must watch her diet carefully but can have a very successful experience.

○ **At 4 months postpartum, your patient has an emergency appendectomy and is separated from her infant for 1 week. Her milk supply is gone on return to home. Three weeks later she calls and says her infant is having an allergy to formulas and can she get her milk supply to return? How do you answer?**

You can have her use an electric pump until her supply returns. She can slowly reintroduce the baby to the breast in the meantime. The support of a lactation consultant during this process would be very helpful.

○ **Your patient is 2 months postpartum and has severe right lower quadrant abdominal pain? Can she have a CT scan with contrast?**

Yes. Iodinated contrast material and gadolinium-based contrast material enter breast milk at very low levels. It is estimated that <0.01% of maternal iodinated contrast and <0.0004% of gadolinium-based contrast are absorbed by the infant. If the patient is very concerned about exposure to her infant, she can pump and dump for 24 hours, but she should also be allowed to nurse. There are some agents with a long elimination half-life that can be excreted in breast milk. These should be avoided.

○   **What antihypertensives are considered most compatible with breastfeeding?**

Beta blockers such as propranolol, metoprolol, and labetalol.

Calcium channel blockers such as diltiazem, nifedipine, and verapamil.

○   **Which antihypertensives should be avoided during breastfeeding?**

Acebutolol and atenolol have been reported in cases of infant bradycardia and hypotension. ACE inhibitors should be used cautiously in the first few weeks of life because neonatal kidneys are very sensitive to these agents.

○   **What is the preferred medication for treatment of postpartum depression while breastfeeding?**

Sertraline (Zoloft).

○   **What are some drugs that should not be taken while breastfeeding?**

Cytotoxic agents (methotrexate, cyclophosphamide, doxorubicin).

Immunosuppressive agents (cyclosporine).

Lithium.

Chloramphenicol.

Isotretinoin.

Ergot alkaloids.

Amiodarone.

Radiopharmaceuticals.

○   **How long after a woman consumes alcohol is her breast milk free of the substance?**

A single drink (12 oz of beer, 5 oz wine, or 1 oz hard liquor) will clear from maternal circulation in 2 to 3 hours. Alcohol moves freely from maternal milk to plasma, so it is not necessary to express and/or discard milk after this time period in order to avoid infant exposure. Mothers can be advised to refrain from nursing until 2 to 3 hours after a single drink. They should refrain from nursing for an additional 2 hours for each additional drink.

○   **What is the most common cause of lactation failure?**

Inadequate stimulation is the usual cause of insufficient milk production to adequately nourish and satisfy an infant. This may be secondary to poor technique with inadequate contact with the breast or simply to not nursing frequently enough. The average newborn will nurse 8 to 10 times in 24 hours. True lactation failure not related to poor stimulation is very rare, and may be due to either anatomical defects such as hypoplasia (which may be unilateral) or to absence of prolactin. Other causes of inadequate intake include infant oral-motor or neurologic abnormalities.

○   **What are the most common misconceptions about breastfeeding that lead a woman to bottle feed? What arguments can you give to contradict these misconceptions?**

(1) I want to go back to work—upon returning to work, you can pump and save, or gradually wean down to only have milk during the hours you are home. Or you can nurse until you return to work and then wean. Even 2 to 3 weeks is valuable as it delivers colostrum and all its benefits.

(2) I am too embarrassed—discuss discrete techniques, availability of clothing just for nursing, and refer patient to supportive group.

(3) My husband does not want me to—common reasons are that he wants to feed the baby and that he fears sexual activity during lactation. Reassure him that an occasional bottle of pumped milk or even formula is fine after the first 2 to 3 weeks. Also let him know that sexual contact with the breast during lactation is not harmful. Letdown may occur, even during orgasm.

○ **When is the most common time for a breastfeeding mother to quit?**

In the first 2 to 3 weeks. This is the time of greatest adjustment. It also coincides with the first growth spurt at about 2 weeks, during which the baby may get fussy and nurse often to increase the supply. If she goes beyond 3 weeks, she will generally nurse for 4 to 6 months on the average.

○ **What are some factors that may interfere with successful breastfeeding?**

Hypoplastic breast tissue
Nipple abnormalities
Previous breast surgery.

○ **How may hypoplastic breast tissue effect lactation?**

Women without sufficient glandular tissue may have no breast enlargement during pregnancy and will produce little or no milk. As a result, their infants are at risk of early failure to thrive. One indication of the adequacy of breast tissue is noticeable breast growth during pregnancy.

○ **How does breast augmentation or reduction affect a woman's ability to breastfeed?**

Outcome cannot be predicted in individual cases, but circular incisions around the areola tend to cause the most damage to ducts, blood supply, and nerves and thus the most potential for difficulty with breastfeeding.

○ **What are Hoffman exercises?**

Inverted nipples can be everted if found early in the third trimester, in most cases. One technique is Hoffman exercises where the fingers are placed at 3 & 9 o'clock at the base of the nipple and is gently stretched, then this is repeated at 6 & 12 o'clock. The use of a perforated breast shell under the bra will also put pressure at the base of the nipple and help evert it.

○ **What is the most common cause of sore nipples in the immediate postpartum period?**

Improper positioning of the infant at the breast, resulting in abnormal friction or traction on the breast and the nipple. Poor latch-on by the infant can also cause nipple injury, leading to pain. Improved infant positioning and latch-on will help resolve this pain.

○ **What is the proper treatment of cracked nipples?**

Evaluate the positioning of the baby during nursing and check for pressure points. Vary the positions at each feeding (Madonna—across the chest, football—under the arm, and on the side). Check the infant's latch-on, correcting it if necessary. Evaluate the infant's oral cavity for abnormalities or ankyloglossia (tongue-tie).

○ **What is the most common cause of delayed nipple soreness?**

Yeast. Aggressive, simultaneous treatment of mother and baby is indicated, usually with an antifungal such as nystatin. During treatment, all objects such as pacifiers and toys that enter the baby's mouth must be washed between each use to avoid recontamination.

○ **A 2-week-old infant cries and wants to nurse every 1 to 2 hours around the clock. When at the breast, he nurses for about 5 minutes and falls asleep so the mother puts him down. She is now exhausted and thinking of bottlefeeding. What can you do to save this breastfeeding experience? What is wrong?**

This mother needs information, guidance, and reassurance. Her infant is not nursing long enough with each episode. The infant is only receiving the "foremilk," which is high in proteins, carbohydrates, and water. He falls asleep before getting the "hindmilk," which is high in fat and satiates the appetite and takes longer to digest. This infant should be stimulated when he dozes off, changed to the opposite breast, and not put down immediately. If this fails, the mother can pump or express the hindmilk at that time, and it can be given by another caregiver later so the mother can rest. This process is only a temporary measure as decreased contact time at the breast will ultimately lead to decreased milk production.

○ **What is breast engorgement?**

Engorgement refers to swelling of the breast and can occur early or late in the postpartum period. Early engorgement is secondary to edema, tissue swelling, and accumulated milk, while late engorgement is due solely to accumulated milk.

○ **What are some effective treatments of engorgement?**

Frequent breastfeeding with complete breast emptying at each feeding.

Warm compresses or shower prior to feedings.

Cold compresses after/between feedings to decrease swelling.

Acetaminophen or ibuprofen for pain control.

Pumping or expressing a small amount of milk prior to breastfeeding to improve latch-on.

Avoidance of pumping for longer than 10 minutes, as this can increase milk supply.

○ **How are plugged ducts distinguished from mastitis?**

Plugged ducts are localized areas of milk stasis with distention of mammary tissue. Symptoms include a palpable lump with tenderness. They are distinguished from mastitis by the absence of signs of systemic infection such as fever, erythema, or myalgia. Their etiology is unknown.

○ **How are plugged ducts treated?**

Plugged ducts are treated by frequent feedings that drain the affected breast entirely. Warm showers or compresses can be used to facilitate drainage. The affected area of the breast can be manually massaged to drain the duct.

○ **What is mastitis and what causes it?**

Mastitis is an infection of the breast. It typically presents as a hard, red, tender, swollen area of the breast associated with fever, myalgia, chills, malaise, and flu-like symptoms. Common etiologic agents include *Staphylococcus aureus*, *streptococcus*, and *Escherichia coli*.

○ **What is the proper management of a patient with postpartum mastitis?**

Antibiotics (dicloxacillin is the drug of choice), hydration, rest, and analgesics. It is also essential that the breast continue to be emptied regularly. If unable to nurse due to discomfort, she should pump or manually express milk. Warm compresses will aid the letdown and soothe the breast.

CHAPTER 23

Primary and Preventative Care

Cari Brown, MD

○ **At what age, does the American College of Obstetricians and Gynecologists (ACOG) recommend a first visit to an OB/GYN take place?**

Age 13 to 15.

○ **What are the five leading causes of mortality among teens age 13 to 18?**

(1) Accidents.

(2) Malignancy.

(3) Suicide.

(4) Assault/homicide.

(5) Diseases of the heart.

○ **What are the five leading causes of mortality of adults age 19 to 39?**

(1) Malignancy.

(2) Accidents.

(3) Diseases of the heart.

(4) Suicide.

(5) HIV.

○ **What are the five leading causes of mortality of adults age 40 to 64?**

(1) Malignancy.

(2) Diseases of the heart.

(3) Accidents.

(4) Chronic lower respiratory diseases.

(5) Cerebrovascular disease.

○ **What are the five leading causes of mortality of adults age 65 or older?**

  (1) Heart disease.

  (2) Malignancy.

  (3) Cerebrovascular disease.

  (4) Chronic lower respiratory diseases.

  (5) Alzheimer disease.

○ **What are the four important periodic vaccinations for teens?**

  (1) Tetanus-diphtheria-pertussis (once between 11 and 18 years of age).

  (2) Hepatitis B (if not previously vaccinated).

  (3) Human papillomavirus (HPV) (if not previously vaccinated).

  (4) Meningococcal (either given prior to starting high school, or if previously immunized, a booster at age 16).

○ **Which two vaccines are routinely recommended in pregnancy by ACOG and the CDC?**

  (1) Influenza-trivalent inactivated influenza vaccine is recommended annually.

  (2) Tdap-at greater than 20 weeks of gestation, if not given in the previous 10 years.

○ **Which vaccines are routinely recommended for women greater than 65 years of age?**

  (1) Influenza-trivalent inactivated annually.

  (2) Tetanus/diphtheria every 10 years, or Tdap if in contact with infants <12 months of age.

  (3) Zoster.

  (4) Pneumococcal.

○ **What four types of HPV does the Gardasil vaccination protect against?**

  HPV 6, 11, 16, 18.

○ **What percentage of American adults are overweight, obese, and morbidly obese, respectively?**

  Recent estimates indicate that 34% of Americans are overweight, 34% are obese, and 5.7% are morbidly obese.

○ **What recommendations should you be making to your patients regarding dietary changes?**

  A low-fat, high-fiber diet should be recommended since it has been shown to decrease the risk of coronary artery disease (CAD), type 2 diabetes mellitus, and several forms of cancer. It may be helpful to refer a patient to a dietician or nutritionist to help them to establish a healthy eating plan, especially if the patient has risk factors for CAD such as a sedentary lifestyle, obesity, or cigarette smoking.

○ **How is anorexia nervosa defined and how prevalent is it?**

  Anorexia nervosa is characterized by intentional and continued weight loss in a previously healthy person who perceives herself as overweight but is extremely thin. It is estimated that 0.5% to 1% of women suffer from this disorder; however, this is probably an underestimate because these women usually do not report it to their physicians.

○ **How should you screen for eating disorders?**

First calculate a body mass index (BMI) in every patient. Then inquire. Questions that may be helpful include:

Are you satisfied with your eating patterns?

Do you ever eat in secret?

Does your weight affect the way you feel about yourself?

Have any of your family members ever had an eating disorder?

○ **What is the lifetime risk of developing breast cancer?**

The average woman has a one in eight risk of developing breast cancer.

○ **What is the ACOG recommended screening schedule for breast cancer?**

A screening mammogram should be offered annually starting at age 40. Also, all women should have yearly clinical breast exams. (A study by the National Breast and Cervical Cancer Early Detection Program found that clinical breast examination detected 7.4 cancers per 1000 women with normal screening mammograms.)

○ **What screening schedule should be offered to patients who are at elevated (>20% in lifetime) risk of developing breast cancer?**

For women with a personal or first-degree relative with BRCA gene mutations, Li-Fraumeni syndrome, or other genetic cancer syndromes, as well as patients with a history of radiation to the chest between ages 10 and 30, patients should be offered screening starting at age 25, or 8 to 10 years after radiation therapy, whichever occurs later.

○ **What are appropriate options that you may offer a patient for colorectal cancer screening?**

Any of the following are acceptable:

(1) Colonoscopy every 10 years.

(2) Yearly patient-collected fecal occult blood test or fecal immunochemical testing.

(3) Flexible sigmoidoscopy every 5 years.

(4) Double-contrast barium enema every 5 years.

○ **When should you initiate cholesterol screening in women?**

Beginning at age 45, a lipid profile should be obtained and every 5 years thereafter. Earlier testing is warranted if the patient has a history of heart disease, diabetes, elevated cholesterol, is a smoker, or has a family history of CAD or hypercholesterolemia.

○   **Which test in the lipid profile is continuously correlated with the relative risk of developing CAD?**

Low-density lipoprotein (LDL) cholesterol.

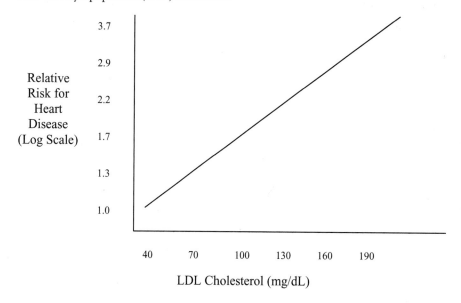

○   **What are the main side effects of the cholesterol lowering agents?**

Statins (HMG-CoA reductase inhibitors) → Myopathy, increased liver enzymes.
Bile acid sequestrants → Gastrointestinal (GI) distress, constipation, decreased absorption of other medications.
Nicotinic acid → Flushing, hyperglycemia, gout, upper GI distress, hepatotoxicity
Fibric acids → Dyspepsia, gallstones, myopathy.

○   **What are lifestyle factors that increase the risk of atherosclerosis?**

Inactive lifestyle, cigarette smoking, and obesity.

○   **How does exercise improve the lipid profile?**

Exercise increases the high-density lipoprotein (HDL) component.

○   **How does smoking affect the lipid profile?**

Smoking decreases the HDL component.

○   **At what age should one be screened for diabetes?**

Beginning at age 45, and repeated every 3 years, unless the patient is considered high risk.

○ **Who is considered high risk of diabetes and therefore warrants earlier screening?**

Overweight (BMI ≥25).

Family history of diabetes mellitus.

Habitual physical inactivity.

African American, Hispanic, Native American, Asian, Pacific Islander.

History of having a macrosomic baby or gestational diabetes.

Hypertensive.

HDL ≤35.

Triglycerides ≥250.

Polycystic ovary syndrome.

Vascular disease.

○ **What are the acceptable ways of diagnosing diabetes mellitus in nonpregnant adults?**

(1) If patient has the symptoms of diabetes and a casual plasma glucose of 200 mg/dL or greater. The classic symptoms include polyuria, polydipsia, and unexplained weight loss.

(2) A fasting plasma glucose of 126 mg/dL or greater.

(3) A 2-hour glucose tolerance test value of 200 mg/dL or greater. The 2-hour test uses a 75 g glucose load.

(4) Hemoglobin A_{1c} of ≥6.5%.

○ **How is hypertension in nonpregnant adults classified by the American Heart Association?**

	Blood Pressure (mmHg)	
Blood Pressure Classification	**Systolic**	**Diastolic**
Normal	<120	<80
Prehypertension	120–139	80–89
Stage I hypertension	140–159	90–99
Stage II hypertension	160–179	100–109
Hypertensive crisis	>180	>110

○ **What are the most important risk factors for osteoarthritis?**

Female gender, family history, obesity, and a history of joint trauma.

○ **How do the symptoms of osteoarthritis differ from those of rheumatoid arthritis?**

Osteoarthritis is typically exacerbated by exercise and relieved by rest, whereas rheumatoid arthritis is associated with morning stiffness and improvement with activity.

○ **At what rate do women experience bone loss in the first 5 years after menopause?**

Bone mineral density decreases by about 3% per year during this time frame, then it returns to 1% per year.

○ **Define osteopenia and osteoporosis.**

Osteopenia is classified as having a bone mineral density between 1 and 2.5 standard deviations below the mean value for a reference population of young women.

Osteoporosis is defined as a bone mineral density of 2.5 or more standard deviations below the mean for the reference population.

○ **When does ACOG recommend screening for osteoporosis?**

All women starting at age 65. Starting at age 60 for women with an increased risk of osteoporotic fractures, no more frequently than every 2 years. Risk factors include, white race, history of a fracture, family history, poor nutrition, smoking, low BMI, early menopause (prior to age 45), and inadequate physical activity.)

○ **What factor is predictive of 80% of a woman's peak bone mass?**

Genetics, with ethnic background also being highly predictive. Caucasian women are at highest risk of osteoporosis, followed by Asian women, Mexican women, and African American women.

○ **What type of exercise is most effective at slowing the rate of bone loss?**

Weight bearing exercise.

○ **What percentage of women is likely to have subclinical hypothyroidism?**

Up to 5%. The prevalence increases with age and is more common in white women than African Americans.

○ **What is the ACOG recommendation for screening for thyroid dysfunction?**

ACOG recommends checking a TSH every 5 years, beginning at age 50.

○ **A PPD is considered positive with what amount of induration in a given population?**

Millimeters of Induration	Populations
>5 mm	HIV positive
	Other immunosuppressed populations—ie, organ donor recipients
	Those in close contact with a person known to be infected with tuberculosis (TB)
	Those who have had TB in the past
	Patients with fibrotic changes on chest X-ray indicative of TB infection
>10 mm	Immigrants from high prevalence area within the past 5 years
	Intravenous drug users
	Residents and employees of prisons, homeless shelters, nursing homes, hospitals, or other long-term care facilities.
	Patients with medical conditions that increase their risk of TB, eg, diabetes, silicosis, or chronic renal failure.
>15 mm	Patients with no risk factors.

○ **What are the two most common reasons for a false-positive PPD?**

Infection with nontuberculosis mycobacteria and vaccination with Bacillus Calmette-Guerin (BCG).

○ **If a patient has a positive PPD and she tells you that she had the BCG vaccine as a child, is any further workup needed?**

Yes.

○ **What is the appropriate workup for a first-time positive PPD?**

A chest X-Ray should be performed and then based on the results treatment initiated.

○ **In 1997, what percentage of American women were using complementary or alternative medicine?**

49%—Most patients who use complementary and alternative therapies self-refer and do not tell their physicians.

○ **What is the BMI used for? What are the different categories?**

BMI is used as a screening tool to identify weight problems. The calculation is based on the patient's weight and height.

BMI	Category
<18.5	Underweight
18.5–24.9	Normal
25–29.9	Overweight
30–39.9	Obese
>40	Morbidly obese

○ **What is the recommendation of physical activity for adults by the CDC and the American College of Sports Medicine?**

(1) Adults should engage in moderate-intensity physical activities for at least 30 minutes on 5 or more days per week.

(2) Adults should engage in vigorous-intensity physical activities 3 or more days per week for 20 minutes minimum per activity.

○ **When are therapeutic interventions recommended for blood pressure management?**

When elevations in blood pressure readings are obtained with three measurements performed at different times over the course of several weeks.

○ **What are the nonpharmacologic interventions for blood pressure management? How long should these interventions be pursued before they are deemed ineffective?**

The nonpharmacologic interventions include weight reduction, exercise, dietary sodium restriction, decreased alcohol intake, decreased fat consumption, smoking cessation, and stress reduction. If no success after 3 months, drug therapy is recommended.

○ **What tests other than fasting lipid panel are used to evaluate dyslipidemia?**

Other tests include fasting blood glucose, liver function, thyroid function, renal function, and urinalysis to rule out secondary causes of dyslipidemia.

○   **What values are considered normal for LDL, HDL, triglycerides, and total cholesterol?**

LDL	<100
HDL	>40
Triglycerides	<150
Total cholesterol	<200

○   **Who does ACOG recommend screening for intimate partner violence?**

All women should be routinely screened for intimate partner violence at office visits. Pregnant women should be screened in each trimester.

○   **What types of behaviors constitute intimate partner violence?**

Intimate partner violence may include behaviors such as assault and coercion that includes physical injury, psychological abuse, sexual assault, progressive isolation, stalking, deprivation, intimidation, and reproductive coercion.

○   **In addition to physical injuries, how else might a woman experiencing intimate partner violence come to medical attention?**

Women experiencing intimate partner violence may also complain of somatic symptoms such as chronic headaches, sleep and appetite disturbances, palpitations, chronic pelvic pain, urinary frequency or urgency, irritable bowel syndrome, sexual dysfunction, abdominal symptoms, and recurrent vaginal infections.

○   **What is ACOG's recommended screening tool for at-risk drinking?**

T-A-C-E, which stands for:

T—Tolerance: How many drinks does it take to make you feel high?

A—Annoyed: Have you felt annoyed by criticism of your drinking?

C—Cut down: Have you ever felt you ought to cut down on your drinking?

E—Eye opener: Have you ever needed a drink in the morning to steady your nerves, or get rid of a hangover?

Yes to two or more of the above questions is considered a positive screen for at risk drinking.

The eye opener question is considered to be the most important of the four questions.

○   **Smoking increases a woman's risk of which chronic health problems?**

Smoking is the most prevalent cause of premature death in the United States, and increases risk of reproductive health problems, gynecologic and other cancers, vascular disease, chronic obstructive pulmonary disease, and osteoporosis.

○   **What is ACOG's recommended approach to encouraging patient smoking cessation?**

The five As:

(1) Ask about tobacco use.

(2) Advise patients to quit.

(3) Assess willingness to quit.

(4) Assist in quitting, offer medical quitting options, and/or counseling.

(5) Arrange follow-up, ask about smoking cessation at future visits, or by phone.

○   **How many attempts does the average smoker require to quit smoking and remain smoke free for 1 year?**

Seven.

CHAPTER 24
Functional and Dysfunctional Uterine Bleeding

Kristin Van Heertum, MD

○ **Define the normal menstrual cycle.**

The normal menstrual cycle is 28 days with a flow lasting 2 to 7 days. The variation in cycle length is set at 24 to 35 days.

○ **In a normal menstrual cycle, when does ovulation typically occur?**

Ovulation in a 28-day cycle occurs on day 14. The luteal (secretory) phase of the cycle is constant at 14 days. The estrogenic (follicular/proliferative) phase of the cycle can be variable.

○ **A woman normally has 32-day cycles. In this woman, when does ovulation occur?**

In this clinical situation, ovulation should occur on day 18. The luteal phase of the cycle should remain constant at 14 days.

○ **Name the hormones, and their source, that are involved in maintaining a normal menstrual cycle.**

From the ovary: Estrogen, progesterone, and inhibin A.

From the pituitary: Follicle-stimulating hormone (FSH) and luteinizing hormone (LH). Prolactin and thyroid-stimulating hormone (TSH) are also vital in maintaining a normal menstrual cycle.

From the hypothalamus: Gonadotropin-releasing hormone (GnRH).

○ **What are the three layers of the endometrium?**

(1) The pars basalis, (2) the zona spongiosa, and (3) the superficial zona compacta. The zona spongiosa and zona compacta make up the stratum functionalis, which is shed during menses.

○ **What vascular event triggers shedding of the endometrium?**

Spasm of the spiral arteries resulting in ischemia of the tissue and sloughing.

○ **Describe the effect of estrogen on the endometrium.**

Estrogen causes proliferation of the endometrium. The endometrial glands lengthen and the glandular epithelium becomes pseudostratified. Mitotic activity is present in both the glands and the stroma.

○ **What are the earliest histologic changes in the endometrium following ovulation and when do they occur?**

Progesterone causes mitotic arrest. The earliest histologic change that can be identified is the development of subnuclear vacuoles. Both mitotic arrest and subnuclear vacuoles are present by postovulatory day 3 (day 17, assuming a normal 28-day cycle).

○ **By which postovulatory day do the endometrial glands appear exhausted as it relates to the secretory phase?**

By postovulatory 6 (day 20, assuming a normal 28-day cycle).

○ **On which postovulatory day does the endometrium demonstrate peak endometrial stromal edema?**

Postovulatory day 8 (day 22, assuming a normal 28-day cycle).

○ **On which postovulatory day does predecidual change first begin to appear and where does it first appear?**

Postovulatory day 9 (day 23, assuming a normal 28 day cycle). Predecidual change (periarteriolar cuffing) first appears around the spiral arterioles. Predecidual cells contain glycogen.

○ **When does implantation of the fertilized ovum typically occur?**

At approximately postovulatory day 9 (day 23, assuming a normal 28-day cycle).

○ **How big is the dominant follicle at the time of ovulation?**

Approximately 20 and 26 mm.

○ **Define normal menstrual flow quantitatively.**

Approximately 30 cc.

○ **Define menorrhagia.**

Menses at regular normal intervals with excessive flow and duration.

○ **Define hypomenorrhea.**

Menses at regular intervals that is decreased in amount.

○ **Define menorrhagia quantitatively.**

Blood loss in excess of 80 mL.

○ **Define oligomenorrhea.**

Menses at intervals >35 days.

○ **Define polymenorrhea.**

Regular menses at intervals of 21 days or less

○ **Define metrorrhagia.**

Menses at irregular intervals.

○ **Define menometrorrhagia.**

Menses with heavy and irregular bleeding.

○ **Define primary amenorrhea.**

No menarche by age 16 in a female with normal growth and secondary sex characteristics; or, no menarche by age 13 without development of secondary sex characteristics.

○ **Define secondary amenorrhea.**

The absence of bleeding for at least three usual cycle lengths or 6 months in women who previously had menses.

○ **Define dysmenorrhea.**

Pain associated with menstruation.

○ **What is the incidence of dysmenorrhea?**

50% to 75% of women report that they have experienced dysmenorrhea.

○ **What are the main treatments of dysmenorrhea?**

NSAIDs, oral contraceptive pills (OCPs); alternatively GnRH agonist can be considered if first-line treatments fail.

○ **What percentage of patients present with chief complaint of abnormal vaginal bleeding?**

Approximately 12% of gynecology referrals are because of menorrhagia. Among women between ages 30 and 49, 5% consult physician for evaluation of menorrhagia.

○ **What percentage of women complaining of excessive or prolonged bleeding meet criteria for menorrhagia?**

40%.

○ **What is the percentage of women with menorrhagia that consider their periods as light or moderate?**

40%.

○ **What are the two direct (definitive) signs of ovulation?**

Pregnancy and visualization of follicle rupture either during laparoscopy or ultrasound.

○ **Broadly characterize the causes of abnormal uterine bleeding?**

Reproductive tract disease, systemic disease, trauma, pharmacologic alterations, anovulation, and ovulation.

○ **Define dysfunctional uterine bleeding (DUB).**

Bleeding that is not attributable to an underlying organic pathologic condition. DUB usually refers to anovulatory bleeding (90%).

○ **What are the components of the workup for abnormal uterine bleeding?**

A complete history, physical examination, laboratory studies, imaging studies, and tissue sampling.

O   **What is the first step in the evaluation of abnormal uterine bleeding following the history and physical examination in a woman?**

Hemodynamic status.

O   **What is the next step in the evaluation of abnormal uterine bleeding following the history and physical examination in a woman of reproductive age?**

A pregnancy test.

O   **What additional laboratory studies are important in the workup of abnormal uterine bleeding?**

CBC, PT/PTT, TSH, Prolactin levels, androgen levels, and testing for infection with *Chlamydia* and gonorrhea.

O   **What is the next step in the evaluation of a woman with abnormal uterine bleeding?**

Evaluation of the endometrial cavity by hysterosalpingography (HSG), sonohysterography (SHG), or hysteroscopy.

O   **In a woman after age 30 with abnormal bleeding what should be obtained next?**

Obtain a tissue biopsy. This may be in the form of endometrial biopsy or curettage.

O   **What is the advantage of curettage?**

In the woman with heavy bleeding, it may be therapeutic as well as diagnostic.

O   **What is the most important diagnosis to rule out in the postmenopausal woman?**

Cancer, primarily endometrial.

O   **Usual cause of abnormal genital bleeding in neonates?**

Withdrawal from maternal estrogens.

O   **What are the usual causes of abnormal genital bleeding in premenarchal patients?**

Foreign body, trauma including sexual abuse, infection, urethral prolapse, sarcoma botryoides, ovarian tumor, and precocious puberty.

O   **What are the usual causes of abnormal genital bleeding in patients early after menarche?**

Anovulation (hypothalamic immaturity), bleeding diathesis, stress (psychogenic, exercise induced), pregnancy, and infection.

O   **What are the usual causes of abnormal genital bleeding in reproductive years?**

Anovulation, pregnancy, cancer, polyps, fibroids, adenomyosis, infection, endocrine dysfunction (PCOS, thyroid, pituitary adenoma), bleeding diathesis, medication related.

O   **What are the usual causes of abnormal genital bleeding in perimenopausal women?**

Anovulation, polyps, fibroids, adenomyosis, and cancer.

○ **What are the usual causes of abnormal genital bleeding in postmenopausal women?**

Atrophy, cancer, and estrogen replacement therapy.

○ **What percentage of adolescents that require hospitalization for abnormal bleeding have an underlying coagulation disorder?**

Approximately 25%. The majority of these patients will have von Willebrand disease, problems with platelet count, or problems with platelet function.

○ **A 37-year-old woman, G2 P2 presents with a history of lengthening menses and acquired dysmenorrhea. This problem had been subtly going on for 2 years and now is a quality-of-life issue. Examination reveals a top normal size globular shaped uterus. What is the most likely diagnosis?**

Adenomyosis.

○ **What is the most common cause of postmenopausal bleeding?**

Atrophic endometrium and/or atrophic vaginitis.

○ **In what groups of patients other than postmenopausal women, can you find vaginal bleeding secondary to atrophic vaginitis?**

Premenarchal girls, postpartum lactating women, and women on chronic progestins.

○ **What are the most common bleeding patterns seen in a woman with cervical cancer?**

Intermenstrual and postcoital bleeding.

○ **What is the size of the normal uterus?**

7.5 to 9.5 cm in length (cervix to fundus), 4.5 to 6.5 cm in width (from cornua to cornua), and 2.5 to 3.5 cm in anteroposterior diameter. Uterine cavity averages 3.5 cm in length.

○ **What is the normal thickness of the myometrium?**

1 to 2 cm.

○ **What is the volume of a normal endometrial cavity in a woman of reproductive age?**

7 to 10 mL.

○ **How much blood blow does the nonpregnant uterus receive?**

Approximately 50 cc/min (as opposed to approximately 600 cc/min in the pregnant uterus).

○ **When in the cycle should an endometrial biopsy be performed?**

At or beyond day 18, because if it shows secretory endometrium, then it confirms that ovulation has occurred in that cycle.

○ **When should ultrasound be performed on premenopausal women for endometrium evaluation?**

Days 4 and 6, when endometrium is expected to be the thinnest.

○ **What is the normal endometrial thickness in women of reproductive age?**

Proliferative phase 4 and 8 mm and secretory phase 8 and 14 mm.

○ **Broadly characterize the major categories of DUB?**

Estrogen breakthrough bleeding, estrogen withdrawal bleeding, and progesterone breakthrough bleeding.

○ **What are the causes of estrogen withdrawal bleeding?**

Bilateral oophorectomy, radiation of mature follicles, and administration of estrogen to a previously oophorectomized woman followed by its withdrawal

○ **What is the cause of midcycle spotting or light bleeding?**

The decline in estrogen that occurs immediately prior to the LH surge.

○ **How does estrogen affect breakthrough vaginal bleeding?**

Low doses of estrogen cause intermittent spotting that may be prolonged. High levels of estrogen lead to amenorrhea followed by acute, often profuse bleeding.

○ **What are the causes of progesterone withdrawal bleeding?**

Removal of the corpus luteum, medically or surgically. Pharmacologically a similar event can be achieved by administration and discontinuation of progesterone or a synthetic progestin, provided the endometrium is estrogen primed.

○ **How can you narrow the differential diagnosis of uterine bleeding in patients of reproductive age?**

By establishing ovulatory status.

○ **How can you determine ovulatory status?**

Menstrual cycle charting, day 3 FSH, anti-Mullerian hormone levels, basal temperature monitoring, measurement of the serum progesterone concentration, monitoring of urinary LH excretion, and sonographic demonstration of periovulatory follicle.

○ **How can you determine ovulatory status based on menstrual history?**

If there are predictable cyclic menses, with duration of cycle 24 and 35 days, then most likely they are ovulatory. If the cycles vary in length by >10 days from one cycle to the next, then they are most likely anovulatory.

○ **If a single value of serum progesterone is low for the luteal phase, does it mean that the patient is not in the luteal phase?**

Not necessarily because it may be obtained between LH pulses, though a single level above 6 ng/mL is usually indicative of normal luteal phase.

○ **What are the systemic illnesses that may cause anovulatory bleeding?**

Hypo- and hyperthyroidism, chronic liver disease, chronic renal failure, Cushing disease, PCOS, prolactinoma, empty sella syndrome, Sheehan syndrome, adrenal and ovarian tumors, and tumors infiltrating the hypothalamus.

○ **What are the lifestyle elements that may cause anovulatory bleeding?**

Sudden weight loss, stress, and intense exercise.

○ **Decline in which hormone heralds the onset of menses?**

Normal menses occurs because of progesterone withdrawal.

○ **What is the life span of a normal corpus luteum in the absence of pregnancy?**

Approximately 14 days.

○ **What is Halban syndrome?**

It is the persistence of a corpus luteum. Patients commonly present with delayed menses, pelvic mass, and negative pregnancy test. Clinically, this is often confused with an ectopic pregnancy. Typically self-limited and usually does not recur.

○ **How does one measure the strength of a progestational agent?**

Delay of menses.

○ **In women of reproductive age, what is the most common cause of estrogen excess bleeding?**

Chronic anovulation associated with polycystic ovaries.

○ **What are the medications that can cause vaginal bleeding?**

Contraceptive medication [OCP, intrauterine device (IUD), Depo-Provera], hormone replacement therapy, anticoagulants, corticosteroids, chemotherapy, dilantin, antipsychotic medication, and antibiotics (eg, due to toxic epidermal necrolysis or Stevens-Johnson syndrome).

○ **What is the immediate objective of medical therapy in treating anovulatory bleeding?**

To stabilize the endometrium and control acute hemorrhage.

○ **How does progesterone work at the cellular level to control DUB when prescribed in pharmacologic doses?**

Progestins are powerful antiestrogens. They stimulate 17β-hydroxysteroid dehydrogenase and sulfotransferase activity. This results in conversion of estradiol to estrone sulfate that is rapidly excreted in the urine. Progestins also inhibit augmentation of estrogen receptors. Additionally, progestins suppress estrogen-mediated transcription of oncogenes.

○ **Failure of oral contraceptives to control bleeding when given twice daily for 5 and 7 days should prompt further evaluation. What are the most common diagnostic possibilities?**

Complications of pregnancy (incomplete abortion, ectopic pregnancy), endometrial polyps, and endometrial neoplasia (including hyperplasia).

○ **A 14-year-old female presents with her first menses. Her bleeding is profuse and her hemoglobin is 4 g/dL. The pregnancy test is negative and to the best of your ability a bleeding disorder is excluded. What would be your pharmacologic approach to this patient?**

Conjugated estrogens 25 mg intravenously (IV) every 4 hours until bleeding stops or for 4 doses (12 hours). Progestin treatment is started concurrently.

○ **What is the best medical treatment of severe acute menorrhagia related to anovulation?**

High-dose estrogens. IV conjugated equine estrogen (CEE) for up to 24 hours (25 mg IV/IM every 4 hours), followed with oral CEE (eg, 2.5 mg four times a day) for 21 to 25 days, with medroxyprogesterone acetate (10 mg per day) for the last 10 days to induce bleeding. A Foley catheter can be placed to tamponade bleeding temporarily. Antiemetics are required in 40% of patients.

○ **What are the risks of treatment with high dose estrogens?**

DVT and PE, particularly with IV estrogen. Nausea/vomiting, particularly with oral estrogen therapy.

○ **Can severe acute menorrhagia related to anovulation be treated with progestins only?**

Yes, but it is less effective. Treatment involves medroxyprogesterone acetate (20–40 mg per day in divided doses), or megestrol acetate (40–120 mg per day), or norethindrone (5–10 mg per day) for 5–10 days. A 2 to 3 weeks regimen may be prescribed to allow for an increase in the hemoglobin concentration of anemic patients.

○ **What is the best medical treatment of severe acute menorrhagia secondary to atrophic bleeding?**

Ethinyl estradiol (10–20 μg) for 2 to 3 weeks.

○ **A patient is taking a low-dose OCPs. She experiences repetitive spotting during the first week of therapy. How would you treat this?**

Estrogen therapy for 7 days in addition to her OCP. This could be as conjugated estrogens 1.25 mg or estradiol 2.0 mg. This is preferable to changing pills. May reassure patient that this is normal and wait for 3 cycles, as most of such symptoms resolve by that time, if not then may change the pill.

○ **What is the best pharmacologic approach to treat a woman with ovulatory cycles but heavy menses?**

A prostaglandin synthetase inhibitor (such as naproxen), beginning with the onset of symptoms.

○ **What percentage decrease in blood loss can be expected with the use of a prostaglandin synthetase inhibitor?**

Approximately 40% to 50%.

○ **What are the options for treatment of chronic or less severe acute menorrhagia?**

OCPs, IUDs, NSAIDs, antifibrinolytics: tranexamic acid, danazol, D&C, and hysteroscopic endometrial ablation (if completed child bearing).

○ **In what clinical situation is DUB best treated with a progestin containing IUD?**

Bleeding associated with chronic illnesses (such as renal failure).

○ **In what clinical situations is DUB best treated with a GnRH agonist?**

Renal failure, blood dyscrasia, or organ transplantation (especially liver transplantation).

○ **True or False: A woman with acute DUB having failed medical options and does not want a hysterectomy may benefit from interventional radiology uterine artery embolization (UAE) procedures.**

True, but only recommended if completed child bearing.

○ **What percentage of women develop amenorrhea following endometrial ablation?**

Approximately 60%.

○ **What percentage of women will develop improvement in their menstrual blood loss following endometrial ablation?**

Up to 90%.

○ **What percentage of patients after endometrial ablation require further procedures?**

Hysterectomy or repeat endometrial ablation is required in 20% to 40% of patients within 4 years.

○ **What is the most common reason for endometrial ablation to fail?**

Adenomyosis.

○ **In what clinical situations should estrogen be the initial choice of treatment for abnormal uterine bleeding?**

(1) When the bleeding has been heavy for many days, (2) when endometrial sampling yields minimal tissue, (3) when the patient has been on progestins and the endometrium is atrophic, and (4) when follow-up is uncertain, because estrogen will temporarily stop all categories of DUB.

○ **What is the role of curettage in the treatment of DUB?**

It is effective in controlling acute hemorrhage when hormonal therapy fails.

○ **What are common clinical conditions present when medical therapy fails to control menorrhagia?**

Submucous fibroids, endometrial polyps, hyperplasia, or cancer.

○ **How can one increase sensitivity and specificity of transvaginal ultrasound in assessment of endometrial cavity?**

By performing saline infusion sonography with instillation of sterile saline into the endometrial cavity. Sensitivity increases from 75% to 93%, specificity from 76% to 94%.

○ **What is the probability of endometrial cancer in a postmenopausal woman with vaginal bleeding with endometrial thickness <4 mm?**

0.5%.

○ **What is the probability of endometrial cancer in postmenopausal woman with vaginal bleeding after a negative hysteroscopy?**

0.4% to 0.5%.

○ **What is the probability of endometrial cancer in postmenopausal woman with vaginal bleeding with endometrial thickness >10 mm?**

10% to 20%.

○ **What are the diseases that may mimic vaginal bleeding?**

Urethritis, bladder cancer, urinary tract infection, inflammatory bowel disease, and hemorrhoids.

CHAPTER 25

Adenomyosis and Endometriosis

Rahil Malik, MD

○ **What is the prevalence of endometriosis?**

The prevalence of asymptomatic endometriosis is population dependent:

- 1% to 7% in women seeking elective sterilization.
- 12% to 32% among women of reproductive age with pelvic pain.
- 9% to 50% in infertile women.
- 50% among teens with chronic pelvic pain or dysmenorrhea.

The overall prevalence of endometriosis in reproductive-age woman probably is between 3% and 10%.

○ **The most common symptom of endometriosis is?**

Dysmenorrhea and pain throughout the menstrual cycle. (25–67% of women with endometriosis.)

Dyspareunia is found in 25% and associated with uterosacral involvement.

Dyschezia.

○ **Other common symptoms and signs of endometriosis are?**

Intraperitoneal bleeding, pelvic adhesions, pelvic pain, infertility, cyclic bowel and bladder symptoms, and inflammation.

○ **What risk factors/associations have been implicated with development of endometriosis?**

- Early menarche and short menstrual cycles—heavy consumption of alcohol and caffeine six to seven times more prevalent among the first-degree relatives of affected women than in the general population.

Protective factors

- Interestingly, the prevalence of endometriosis is inversely related to body mass index.
- Regular exercise and smoking may decrease the risk of endometriosis.
- Pregnancy has a protective effect that decreases with time; risk decreases with parity and prolonged periods of lactation.

○ **What proportion of patients has uterosacral and cul-de-sac nodularity?**

One-third of all patients with endometriosis.

○   **The mean age of diagnosis of endometriosis is?**

25 and 35.

○   **What is the best imaging technique for diagnosing endometriosis?**

Laparoscopy remains the optimal method, but MRI using the fat-saturation technique has a PPV of 95% and NPV of 50% with implants >4 mm.

○   **Does endometriosis have an ethnic predilection?**

The prevalence of asymptomatic endometriosis may be somewhat lower in Blacks and higher in Asians than in White women.

○   **True or False: The black powder lesions seen here in the posterior cul-de-sac should be biopsied to confirm the diagnosis of endometriosis.**

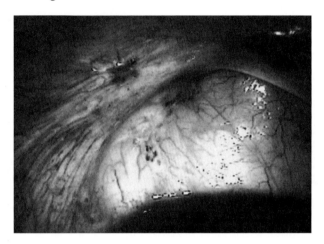

True. A biopsy is always recommended to confirm endometriosis on histology.

○   **What are the ultrasound findings consistent with endometriosis?**

Cystic structures with diffuse low-level internal echoes indicating a possible endometrioma.

○   **Does medical treatment of minimal-mild endometriosis increase fertility? How about surgical treatment?**

No. Surgical treatment may increase fertility rates; therefore, it is still recommended at time of laparoscopy.

○   **Does preoperative medical treatment assist in surgical treatment of endometriosis?**

Yes. It softens the endometrial implants for surgical removal.

○   **When does one achieve the highest pregnancy rates after surgical treatment?**

In the first year, success is inversely related to the severity of disease.

○   **What are the recurrence rates after surgical treatment and after medical treatment?**

For surgical tx: 10% in first year and 20% in 5 years.
For medical tx: 5% to 20% per year and 40% in 5 years.

○ **Is there any role for postoperative medical treatment?**

Yes. Medical treatment after surgical treatment can delay return of symptoms with at least 6 months postoperative medical treatment.

○ **What is the typical classification scheme of endometriosis?**

- Minimal endometriosis—Isolated superficial disease on the peritoneal surface with no significant associated adhesions.
- Mild endometriosis—Scattered superficial disease on the peritoneal surface and ovaries, totaling less than 5 cm in aggregate, with no significant associated adhesions.
- Moderate endometriosis—Multifocal disease, both superficial and invasive, that may be associated with adhesions involving the fallopian tubes and/or the ovaries.
- Severe endometriosis—Multifocal disease, both superficial and invasive, including large ovarian endometriomas, usually associated with adhesions, both filmy and dense, involving the fallopian tubes, ovaries, and cul-de-sac.

○ **What are the options for postoperative medical treatment?**

Gonadotropin-releasing hormone (GnRH) agonist.

Danazol.

Oral contraceptives.

Letrozole.

○ **How do oral contraceptive pills treat endometriosis?**

They suppress follicle-stimulating hormone (FSH) and luteinizing hormone (LH) secretion causing decreased estrogen production and reduced menstrual volume.

○ **Can tubal ligation be performed as a treatment of endometriosis?**

No. Some women even experience symptoms of endometriosis after hysterectomy.

○ **Can an intrauterine device (IUD) be used to treat endometriosis?**

Yes. The levonorgestrel IUD causes decidualization of the endometrium and decreased menstrual flow.

○ **True or False: A CA-125 level can predict active endometriosis.**

True, but controversial; CA-125 levels often correlate with the degree of disease; however, a normal level does not exclude the absence of disease.

○ **Name the three main theories for the pathogenesis of endometriosis.**

Coelomic metaplasia (Robert Meyer): Tissue from prenatal development transforms into endometrial cells.

Transplantation theory: Lymphatic, vascular, iatrogenic, retrograde menstruation (Sampson).

Induction theory: Possible substance in body that results in cellular transformation/differentiation.

○ **The familial nature of endometriosis has been reported in case reports and retrospective reviews. Simpson studied 123 patients with histologically demonstrated endometriosis. 5.9% of sisters and 8.1% of mothers were also affected. However, when the patient's husband's family history was looked at, only 1% of sisters and .8% of mothers had endometriosis. Propose a genetic mechanism for these findings.**

It can be polygenetic inheritance or a single mutant autosomal dominant or autosomal recessive gene, or lastly, a single mutant gene occurring in a small subset of patients with endometriosis. The most likely mode is polygenic and multifactorial.

○ **Name one characteristic of endometriosis that histomorphologically separates it from eutopic endometrium.**

Extensive stromal hemorrhage or dense stromal fibrosis.

○ **How is the immune system altered in patients with endometriosis?**

Macrophages that typically clear aberrant cells have been noted to be permissive in patients with endometriosis. In fact, cytokines and growth factors are secreted such that they promote endometriotic implants.

○ **Chronic progesterone therapy has what specific effect on endometriosis?**

Initial decidualization of endometrial tissue with eventual atrophy.

○ **What is the currently accepted rate of transformation of endometriosis to malignancy?**

<1%.

○ **Name at least three malignant neoplasms arising in endometriosis.**

Clear cell adenocarcinoma, adenoacanthoma, adenosquamous carcinoma, leiomyosarcoma, endometrial stromal sarcoma, mixed Mullerian tumor, or carcinosarcoma.

○ **You have seen a suspicious lesion at laparoscopy and biopsied the lesion. The pathology report indicates endosalpingiosis. What does this mean?**

The characteristics of the cells and stroma of the epithelial cells and the stroma of the biopsy specimen indicate tubal-type epithelium. Involvement of the canal of Nuck with endometriosis indicates the presence of a hernial sack of hydrocele to provide communication with the peritoneal cavity.

○ **Endometriosis of the cervix is well known. It usually is a result of cervical trauma. In retrospective study, what percentage of cases are associated with trauma?**

90%.

○ **With what tumor is endometriosis of the appendix associated with?**

Mucinous carcinoid.

○ **What is a catamenial pneumothorax?**

This is a rare condition that often involves endometriosis of the diaphragm, causing the lung to collapse during menses.

○ **Catamenial pneumothorax is associated with endometriosis what percentage of the time?**

25%.

○ **List three causes of pelvic pain associated with endometriosis.**

(1) Inflammatory factors.

(2) Scarring and retraction.

(3) Compression and stretching.

○ **Abnormal bleeding occurs in what percentage of women? (Specify a range).**

10% to 35%.

○ **State the macrophage hypothesis in endometriosis.**

The inflammatory response caused by endometriosis results in increased concentration of pelvic macrophages. This causes a decrease in fertility by phagocytosis of sperm and secretion of IL-1 that is shown to be toxic to mouse embryos.

○ **True or False: Spontaneous abortions are increased in women with endometriosis.**

False. There is no evidence that spontaneous abortion rate is altered in patients with this disease.

○ **True or False: Endometriosis is a risk factor for ectopic pregnancy.**

True. Management of endometriosis in adolescents.

○ **List two characteristics that increase the risk of endometriosis.**

Cycle lengths <27 days and menstrual flow >1 week.

○ **How do you choose medical treatment?**

By cost and side effect profile; no one medication has been shown to be more effective than any other.

○ **Name some side effects of danazol.**

Weight gain, fluid retention, fatigue, smaller breast size, acne, facial hair, atrophic vaginitis, hot flushes, muscle cramps, emotional lability, irreversible deepening of the voice, hepatocellular damage (check LFTS first), increase low-density lipoprotein (LDL), lower high-density lipoprotein (HDL), and in utero female pseudohermaphroditism.

○ **True or False: In premenopausal women, danazol lowers basal gonadotropin secretion.**

False. Danazol eliminates the midcycle LH and FSH surge, and inhibits steroidogenesis in the corpus luteum creating a high androgen, low estrogen state and amenorrhea.

○ **Name four currently utilized regiments in the treatment of endometriosis.**

Progestins, combination estrogen/progesterone pills (oral contraceptives), danazol, and GnRH agonists.

○ **What are the side effects of progestational agents?**

Weight gain, fluid retention, breakthrough bleeding, and depression.

○ **Name some side effects of GnRH agonists.**

Flare response, menopausal symptoms (hypoestrogenism), and bone loss (need add back therapy after 6 months of treatment).

○   **Name two goals of surgery for endometriosis.**

Restoration of normal anatomy and elimination of pelvic pain. Ninety percent of patients note some degree of pain relief with surgery.

○   **Total abdominal hysterectomy-bilateral salpingo-oophorectomy has generally been considered an excellent way to treat endometriosis definitively. If hormone replacement therapy is given, what is the expected rate of recurrence of endometriosis?**

8%.

○   **Endometriosis of the bladder has been reported in males. What treatment regimen are these men on?**

High-dose estrogen for prostate cancer.

○   **Presacral neurectomy is advocated for treating what condition associated with endometriosis?**

Dysmenorrhea; midline pain only (it is not a treatment for infertility).

○   **True or False: Provera at 30 mg/day was as effective as danazol in treatment of endometriosis.**

True.

○   **The Gilliam suspension utilizes which anatomic structure of the uterus?**

The round ligament.

○   **How would you diagnosis ovarian remnant syndrome?**

Check an FSH.

○   **To prevent adhesions after conservative surgery for endometriosis, name two parameters that must be satisfied.**

(1) Impeccable hemostasis.

(2) Lack of tissue necrosis.

○   **What is intercede?**

It is a physical barrier composed of oxidized regenerated cellulose.

○   **What is Seprafilm?**

Sodium hyaluronate-carboxy methyl cellulose absorbable adhesion barrier.

○   **What medication causes the estradiol level to be <20 pg/mL?**

Depo GnRH.

○   **Name a model that proposes a preexisting congenital or learned vulnerability that heightens the risk for chronic pain.**

The diathesis-stress model.

○ **Describe the diathesis-stress model.**

In the diathesis-stress model, a genetic vulnerability or predisposition (diathesis) interacts with the environment and life events (stressors) to trigger behaviors or psychological disorders.

○ **What class of medications has now supplanted narcotics as a treatment of chronic pelvic pain?**

Heterocyclic antidepressants.

○ **Based on a recent review of 500 consecutive cases by Shaw, what pelvic structure has a higher incidence of implants than the ovary?**

Uterosacral ligaments.

○ **As a woman with endometriosis ages, her endometriotic lesions change from clear papules to _____.**

Black.

○ **Who was the first person to describe adenomyosis in the medical literature?**

Rokitansky, in 1860.

○ **What is the definition of adenomyosis?**

The presence of endometrial glands and stoma within the myometrium with compensatory hypertrophy of the myometrium (most articles today used a depth of 3 mm, or 1 low-powered field, below the basal layer of endometrium as the required depth of invasion). It has an incidence of 31% to 61%.

○ **True or False: Adenomyosis appears equally in parous and nulliparous women.**

False. It has been correlated with increasing parity.

○ **What are the four theories of causality of adenomyosis?**

(1) Heredity.

(2) Trauma.

(3) Hyperestrogenemia.

(4) Viral transmission.

○ **Name the most common symptom in patients with adenomyosis.**

Abnormal uterine bleeding, secondary dysmenorrhea, and enlarged and tender uterus (but up to 35% may be asymptomatic).

O   **Name the imaging technology most likely to diagnose adenomyosis.**

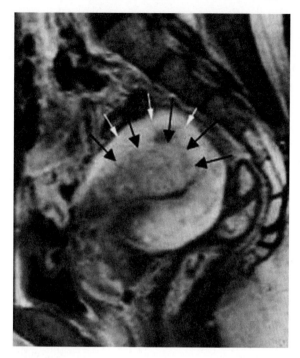

Magnetic resonance.

O   **What other condition is commonly associated with adenomyosis?**

Leiomyomata, up to 57% of the time.

Also frequently occurs in association with endometrial adenocarcinoma.

O   **What is the treatment of adenomyosis?**

Hysterectomy remains the first choice; bromocriptine and RU486 have been shown to suppress adenomyosis.

O   **True or False: Endometrioid carcinoma is of endometriosis origin.**

False. This designation is merely a description of the microscopic findings and has nothing to do with the etiology of the carcinoma.

O   **What are the ultrasound characteristics of adenomyosis?**

- Ill-defined hypoechoic areas.
- Heterogeneous myometrial echotexture.
- Small anechioc lakes.
- Asymmetrical uterine enlargement.
- Indistinct endometrial-myometrial border.
- Subendometrial halo thickening.

CHAPTER 26   Benign Disorders of the Upper Genital Tract

Kristin Van Heertum, MD

○ **What is the average weight of the mature woman's uterus?**

30 to 40 g.

○ **What is the normal length of the uterine cavity?**

3.5 cm.

○ **Approximately what percentage of uteri will be retroverted on examination?**

About one third. It is important to emphasize that this is a normal variant.

○ **What is a cystocele?**

The downward displacement of the bladder into the vagina.

○ **What is a cystourethrocele?**

A cystocele that includes the urethra as part of the prolapsing organ complex.

○ **What is uterine prolapse?**

The descent of the uterus and cervix down the vaginal canal toward the vaginal introitus.

○ **What is a rectocele?**

The protrusion of the rectum into the posterior vaginal lumen.

○ **What is an enterocele?**

The herniation of small bowel into the posterior cul-de-sac.

○ **What is the pelvic organ prolapse quantitative (POPQ)?**

An objective, standardized system for describing pelvic support in women. It allows for consistency between examiners and is the most commonly used pelvic support scoring system.

○   **How should physical examination be performed when using the POPQ system?**

The patient should be standing and performing a Valsalva maneuver to elicit maximum prolapse.

○   **What is the vaginal reference point for POPQ scoring?**

Hymen.

The following questions relate to POPQ.

○   **Define point Aa.**

A point located in the midline of the anterior vaginal wall 3 cm proximal to the external urethral meatus; the position of point Aa relative to the hymen can range from −3 to +3 cm.

○   **Define point Ba.**

Ba represents the most distal position of any part of the upper anterior vaginal wall from the vaginal cuff or anterior vaginal fornix to point Aa. By definition, point Ba is at −3 cm in the absence of prolapse.

○   **Define point C.**

C represents either the most distal (ie, most dependent) edge of the cervix or the leading edge of the vaginal cuff after total hysterectomy.

○   **Define point D.**

Point D represents the location of the posterior fornix (or pouch of Douglas) in a woman who still has a cervix. Point D is omitted in the absence of the cervix.

○   **Define point Bp.**

Point Bp is the most distal position of any part of the upper posterior vaginal wall from the vaginal cuff or posterior vaginal fornix to point Ap. By definition, point Bp is at −3 cm in the absence of prolapse.

○   **Define point Ap.**

A point located in the midline of the posterior vaginal wall 3 cm proximal to the hymen. By definition, the range of position of point Ap relative to the hymen is −3 (normal) to +3 cm (complete prolapse).

○   **What other landmarks are used in the POPQ 3 × 3 grid?**

Genital hiatus (gh): Measured from the middle of the external urethral meatus to the posterior midline hymen.

Perineal body (pb): Measured from the posterior margin of the genital hiatus to the midanal opening.

Total vaginal length (TVL) is the greatest depth of the vagina in centimeters when point C or D is reduced to its full normal position.

○ **How is POP staged according to the ordinal staging system?**

Stage 0: No prolapse is demonstrated. Points Aa, Ap, Ba, and Bp are all at –3 cm and either point C or D is between –TVL cm and –(TVL-2) cm.

Stage I: The criteria for stage 0 are not met, but the most distal portion of the prolapse is >1 cm above the level of the hymen.

Stage II: The most distal portion of the prolapse is ≤1 cm proximal to or distal to the plane of the hymen.

Stage III: The most distal portion of the prolapse is >1 cm below the plane of the hymen but protrudes no further than 2 cm less than the TVL in centimeters.

Stage IV: Essentially, complete eversion of the total length of the lower genital tract is demonstrated. The distal portion of the prolapse protrudes to at least +(TVL-2) cm. In most instances, the leading edge of stage IV prolapse will be the cervix or vaginal cuff scar.

○ **What is an alternative system to the POPQ for grading pelvic organ prolapse?**

Baden-Walker system—Grade 0–4.

Grade 0—No descent.

Grade 1—Descent halfway to introitus.

Grade 2—Descent to the introitus.

Grade 3—Descent halfway past the introitus.

Grade 4—Maximum possible descent.

○ **How common is POP?**

The Women's Health Initiative found that in women with a uterus 14% had uterine prolapse, 34% had a cystocele, and 19% had a rectocele. In women who had undergone hysterectomy, 33% had a cystocele and 18% had a rectocele.

○ **What factors are strongly associated with an increased risk of POP?**

Increased parity and obesity. Race also seems to play a role, as African American women have the lowest rates of POP, while Hispanic women have the highest rates.

○ **What is the course of the ascending limb of the uterine artery?**

It courses below the fallopian tube and eventually anastomoses with the ovarian artery.

○ **What are Mackenrodt ligaments?**

Also known as the cardinal ligaments, these are transverse fibrous bands that attach to the uterine cervix and to the vault of the lateral vaginal fornix, serving to stabilize the cervix.

○ **What three structures form the boundaries of the broad ligament?**

(1) The fold of peritoneum over the fallopian tube, (2) the infundibulopelvic vessels, and (3) the cardinal ligaments.

○ **What is the embryologic origin of the fallopian tube?**

Paramesonephric duct.

○ **What is the average length of the fallopian tube?**

10 to 12 cm.

○ **What is the largest and longest portion of the fallopian tube?**

The ampulla.

○ **What is the site of most ectopic pregnancies?**

The ampulla.

○ **Where do primitive germ cells originate?**

They originate in the dorsal part of the hindgut and then migrate to the gonad.

○ **What is the normal weight of the mature ovary?**

3 to 8 g.

○ **What is the location of the ovarian fossa?**

Below the external iliac vessel and in front of the ureter.

○ **What cell type covers the ovary?**

Germinal epithelium.

○ **What two ligaments support the ovary?**

The suspensory ligament at the tubal pole and the utero-ovarian ligament at the opposite pole.

○ **What is the name of the vestige of the mesonephric (Wolffian) tubule in the female?**

The epoophoron, which is an important potential source of cyst formation.

○ **What is the name of the vestige of the mesonephric duct in the female?**

The Gartner duct, which can course along the uterus, cervix, and vagina.

○ **What does the primordial follicle consist of?**

The primordial follicle consists of the oocyte with a layer of follicular cells surrounding it.

○ **What is the cumulus oophorus?**

A cluster of granulosa cells around the oocyte

○ **What action creates the corpus hemorrhagicum, and into what structure does it evolve?**

The formation of a clot at the site of follicular rupture, as the granulosa cells grow into this clot it becomes the corpus luteum.

○ **What is Halban syndrome?**

A persistent corpus luteum cyst that, prior to sensitive pregnancy tests, simulated an ectopic gestation because of pelvic pain, amenorrhea, and an adnexal mass.

○ **What functional ovarian cyst is most commonly associated with a hydatidiform mole?**

The theca lutein cyst is associated with up to 50% of molar gestations and 10% of choriocarcinomas. They are usually bilateral and produce moderate to massive enlargement of the ovaries. Theca lutein cysts may also be associated with ovulation induction or pregnancies where large placentas are produced (diabetes, twins, and Rh sensitization).

○ **What is the luteoma of pregnancy?**

A benign hyperplastic reaction of ovarian theca lutein cells that may cause virilization in the mother or female fetus, although most cases are asymptomatic.

○ **A 10-year-old girl presents with an adnexal mass. What is the most common etiology?**

Mature cystic teratomas (also known as dermoid cysts) develop from totipotential cells and are composed of well-differentiated ectodermal, endodermal, and mesodermal elements. They account for >50% of adnexal masses in the prepubertal period.

○ **A 6-year-old girl presents for evaluation of premature thelarche. Her workup reveals Tanner stage 4 breast development, numerous café au lait spots, and ovarian cysts. What is her most likely diagnosis?**

McCune-Albright syndrome is associated with an ovarian etiology of excess hormone production and is characterized by polyostotic fibrous dysplasia and café au lait spots. Patients have a genetic mutation in the G protein that results in polyglandular lesions involving the thyroid, pituitary, and gonads.

○ **What percentage of teratomas are bilateral?**

Fifteen to twenty percent of mature teratomas are bilateral whereas immature teratomas are almost always unilateral; however, there may be contralateral metastasis of an immature teratoma. The contralateral ovary should be inspected carefully at the time of surgery by visualization and palpation. The presence of a mature unilateral teratoma does not necessitate a wedge resection or bivalving of the contralateral ovary.

○ **What is the karyotype of a mature teratoma?**

The karyotype is 46 XX and arises from a single germ cell after the fist meiotic division.

○ **What are the most common complications of teratomas?**

Torsion occurs in nearly 15% of cases and is more common in younger women. Other complications include rupture, infection, hemorrhage, and malignant degeneration.

○ **What is the risk of malignant transformation in a mature teratoma?**

Malignant transformation occurs in <2% of mature teratomas, and >75% of the time this is in patients older than 40 years. Squamous cell carcinoma arising in ectodermal layers accounts for 80% of malignant transformations.

○ **What is struma ovarii?**

An ovarian mass (usually a teratoma) in which thyroid tissue is a major component. Thyroid tissue occurs in approximately 10% of teratomas. Patients usually present with a pelvic mass, and <5% of women with struma ovarii develop thyrotoxicosis. Struma ovarii occurs most often in women ages 40 to 60.

○ **What are the Rotterdam criteria for diagnosing polycystic ovary syndrome (PCOS)?**

Two out of three of the following:

- Oligo- and/or anovulation.
- Clinical and/or biochemical signs of hyperandrogenism.
- Polycystic ovaries by ultrasound.

Other etiologies must also be excluded.

○ **What percentage of patients with anovulation associated with PCOS do not have the expected reversal of the luteinizing hormone:follicle-stimulating hormone (LH:FSH) ratio?**

Between 20% and 40% of patients with PCOS will not have the expected reversal of the LH:FSH ratio. For this reason, it is not recommended to routinely measure FSH and LH levels in anovulatory patients and make the diagnosis on clinical presentation alone.

○ **What is the most common benign, solid ovarian tumor?**

The fibroma is the most common, with a malignant potential of under 1%. They are a type of sex cord stromal ovarian neoplasm. These are slow growing tumors with <10% occurrence of bilaterality. On cut section a homogeneous white or yellowish white solid tissue with a trabeculated appearance is seen.

○ **What is Meigs syndrome?**

The clinical triad of an ovarian fibroma, ascites, and pleural effusion (classically right sided). These clinical features are not specific to fibromas, and a similar clinical picture can be found with many other ovarian tumors. The ascites and hydrothorax are most likely caused by substances such as vascular endothelial growth factor (VEGF), which increases vessel permeability. Both the ascites and hydrothorax resolve after removal of the tumor.

○ **A benign ovarian tumor is removed from a 50-year-old. The pathology report makes note of pale epithelial cells with a "coffee bean" nucleus. What is the diagnosis?**

Brenner tumors are rare transitional cell ovarian tumors that usually occur in women from 40 to 60 years of age. They are rarely bilateral and <2% undergo malignant degeneration.

○ **What other neoplasms are frequently associated with Brenner tumors?**

Dermoid cysts or mucinous cystadenomas are often found in the same or contralateral ovary.

○ **A 43-year-old woman presents 5 years following a TAH/BSO for benign disease with a palpable pelvic mass and cyclical pelvic pain. An FSH level is in the premenopausal range. What is the most likely diagnosis?**

The ovarian remnant syndrome occurs in patients who have undergone bilateral oophorectomy usually complicated by endometriosis or pelvic inflammatory disease. This syndrome occurs when failure to skeletonize the infundibulopelvic ligament or incorrect clamp placement results in retention of a piece of ovarian tissue. Many patients present with cyclic pain and a mass. Sonography may aid in the diagnosis, as will FSH levels. CT/MRI may be useful in defining the relation of the ovarian remnant to surrounding structures.

○ **What is a fibroid/leiomyoma?**

These are benign smooth muscle tumors of the uterus. They are the most common tumor in the female pelvis.

○ **Do fibroids have hormone receptors on them?**

Yes. Estrogen and progesterone receptors are both present on leiomyomas. Leiomyomas actually have a great concentration of these receptors than either the endometrium or myometrium.

○ **What is the risk of malignant degeneration in a leiomyoma?**

Malignant degeneration in a preexisting leiomyoma is extremely rare, and occurs in <0.5%.

○ **What is leiomyomatosis peritonealis disseminata?**

A rare condition in which benign leiomyomatous nodules are spread out over the pelvic and abdominal peritoneum, simulating disseminated carcinoma. This usually occurs in young women and is associated with a recent pregnancy, estrogen secreting granulosa tumor, or oral contraceptive use.

○ **What are the clinical findings of leiomyoma?**

Abnormal uterine bleeding.
Pelvic pain.
Pressure effects (constipation, incontinence).
Infertility.
Spontaneous abortions.

○ **Leiomyomas undergo what types of benign degeneration?**

Atrophic, hyaline, cystic, calcification, septic, and carneous (red).

○ **What is the natural history of leiomyomas during pregnancy?**

Nearly three-fourths of all leiomyomas do not change size significantly during pregnancy; 5% to 10% undergo carneous or red degeneration, and may cause severe pain and peritoneal irritation. The larger the leiomyoma, the greater the risk of premature labor.

○ **What are the options for medical treatment of uterine myomas?**

Gonadotropin-releasing hormone (GnRH) agonist with add-back therapy (ie, addition of estrogen-progestin therapy).
GnRH antagonist.
Mifepristone (RU-486).
Danazol.
Raloxifene.
Levonorgestrel-releasing intrauterine device.

○ **What is the incidence of leiomyomas that are clinically apparent?**

25% to 50% of women have clinically apparent leiomyomas.

○ **What are the various possible locations of leiomyomas?**

Subserosal, submucosal, intramural, pedunculated, interligamentary, and parasitic.

○ **Which location is typically the most symptomatic?**

Submucosal.

○ **When using GnRH agonists to "shrink" leiomyomas, when does the maximum effect occur?**

Nonpulsatile GnRH agonist therapy has been shown to decrease leiomyoma size by 30% to 50% with the maximal effect noted in 2 to 3 months.

○ **For the symptomatic treatment of uterine leiomyomas, what is the rate of resolution of symptoms following abdominal myomectomy?**

Overall 81% with a range of 40% to 93%.

○ **What is the risk of reoperation following abdominal myomectomy?**

11% for a single myoma.

26% for multiple myomas.

18% overall risk of reoperation following abdominal myomectomy.

○ **What is the risk of undergoing unexpected hysterectomy at the time of abdominal myomectomy?**

<1% for the experienced surgeon, and higher rates appear for the inexperienced surgeon.

○ **What are side effects of uterine artery embolization (UAE)?**

Pelvic infection.

Premature menopause.

Vaginal expulsion of necrotic fibroids.

Severe pelvic pain requiring analgesia.

○ **Who is a candidate for UAE?**

Patients whose symptoms are directly related to fibroids.

Patients who have been ruled out for malignancy.

Absence of endometrial hyperplasia or neoplasm on pippelle for patients with intermenstrual bleeding.

○ **What are the contraindications to UAE?**

Pregnancy, pedunculated fibroid, active pelvic infection, active vasculitis, history of pelvic irradiation, evidence of pelvic malignancy, life-threatening contrast allergy, uncontrollable coagulopathies, and severe renal insufficiency.

○ **What percentage of patients undergoing UAE will pass fibroid sloughing through the vagina?**

5%.

○ **What percentage of patients undergoing UAE begin menopause following the procedure?**

5%.

○ **What is the success rate of UAE?**

85% to 94%.

○ **A 23-year-old woman presents for a primary infertility workup and is found to have a septate uterus. What treatments can be offered and what are their success rates?**

A septate uterus is associated with pregnancy wastage. Only 15% of patients without treatment achieve a term pregnancy. Most septums can be excised via hysteroscopy. Occasionally, a very large septum may necessitate a Jones (wedge) metroplasty. Term pregnancy rates of 75% are possible following repair.

○ **A 30-year-old woman presents 6 weeks postpartum from a vaginal delivery with mild uterine tenderness, heavy bleeding, and an 8-week size, boggy uterus. A serum pregnancy test is negative. What is the most likely diagnosis?**

Failure of the uterus to return to its normal size postpartum is referred to as "subinvolution." Microscopy of the placental site reveals retention of trophoblastic cells, enlarged vessels, and necrotic decidua. This may serve as a nidus for infection as well as cause delayed postpartum bleeding.

○ **What is the incidence of benign endometrial polyps?**

The reported incidence of polyps is nearly 25% of all uteri. They frequently present with abnormal uterine bleeding. This diagnosis should be considered especially when bleeding persists following D+C because the curette may miss small polyps.

○ **An endometrial biopsy is performed on a 36-year-old anovulatory, fertility patient and shows "tubal metaplasia." What does this mean?**

Ciliated cells are usually not seen in endometrial glands. The presence of a significant number of ciliated glandular cells is referred to as tubal metaplasia or ciliated cell change because of the resemblance to epithelium of the fallopian tube. This is a benign finding and reflects a mild degree of estrogenic stimulation. It may accompany endometrial hyperplasia.

○ **What is the first histologic sign on an endometrial biopsy that ovulation has occurred?**

The first sign of the secretory phase is the appearance of subnuclear intracytoplasmic glycogen vacuoles in the glandular epithelium. This is soon followed by active secretion into the endometrial cavity with a peak level reached about 7 days after ovulation—coinciding with the time of blastocyst implantation.

○ **What is the primary histologic feature of the endometrium at the time that implantation should occur?**

On days 21 to 22 of a normal cycle the predominant feature is stromal edema. This may be caused by an increased vascular permeability secondary to greater prostaglandin production.

○ **Which layer of the endometrium is responsible for the greatest increase in height during the menstrual cycle?**

The functionalis layer is primarily responsible for the increased height of the endometrium during the proliferative phase. After ovulation the height is generally fixed at approximately 6 mm by the growth restraining effects of progesterone.

○ **What is the risk of progression to malignancy with complex atypical hyperplasia of the endometrium?**

Approximately 25% of these cases progress to carcinoma without treatment. Only 2% of endometrial hyperplasia without atypia progresses this way.

○ **What percentage of adolescents with heavy dysfunctional uterine bleeding will have a coagulation defect?**

Although the most common cause is anovulation, as many as 20% of adolescents will have a coagulation defect—the most common being von Willebrand disease. Bleeding is usually a heavy flow with regular, cyclic menses. This is the same pattern seen in patients treated with anticoagulants.

○ **How much do oral contraceptive pills (OCPs) reduce menstrual flow?**

In normal uteri, OCPs reduce flow by 50% to 60% by limiting maximal endometrial growth and allowing orderly menses.

○ **What is adenomyosis?**

Adenomyosis is the presence of endometrial glands and stroma within the myometrium. It occurs most commonly in perimenopausal women and is present in approximately 15% of uteri. Some pathologists only use this term when the lower border of the endometrium and the adenomyosis are separated by at least one-half of a low-power field (about 2.5 mm).

○ **How is the diagnosis of adenomyosis made?**

Adenomyosis is primarily diagnosed postoperatively, upon histologic review of the uterus. Clinical suspicion is increased when a patient in her fourth or fifth decade presents with worsening dysmenorrhea and menorrhagia in the presence of a symmetrically enlarged, firm and tender uterus. MRI can make this diagnosis preoperatively with a high degree of accuracy. Curettage does not help in diagnosis or treatment.

○ **What is the embryological derivative of the hydatid cyst of Morgagni?**

This is the most common paramesonephric (Mullerian) cyst. Other paratubal cysts can arise from mesonephric (Wolffian) structures or mesothelial inclusions.

○ **What is salpingitis isthmica nodasa?**

These are outpouchings or diverticula of tubal epithelium in the isthmic region. Involvement is often bilateral and is associated with ectopic gestation and infertility. The etiology is unknown, although some evidence exists for a noninflammatory adenomyosis-like origin.

○ **Following tubal sterilization procedures, what is the rate of hysterosalpingogram documented "leak"?**

Hysterosalpingogram "leak rates" may reach 25% after Pomeroy or any of the other operations, but the actual fertility "failure rate" is much lower. Additional surgery on a fallopian tube found to leak dye does not guarantee permanent sterilization. Injection of dye under hydraulic pressure through the uterus may open a previously occluded fallopian tube.

○ **What are nabothian cysts?**

Nabothian cysts are retention cysts of endocervical columnar cells where a cleft has been covered by squamous metaplasia.

○ **What is the size of a nabothian cyst?**

It can vary from 3 mm to 3 cm.

○ **What are the symptoms of nabothian cysts?**

Nabothian cysts are asymptomatic.

○ **What is hematometra?**

Hematometra is a uterus distended with blood secondary to partial or complete obstruction of the lower genital tract.

○ **What are the causes of hematometra?**

In older women, this usually occurs at the cervical level (cervical stenosis, cervical fibroid, etc). In younger patients, this usually results from some congenital anomaly such as imperforate hymen and transverse vaginal septum.

○ **What are the acquired causes of lower tract stenosis?**

Senile atrophy of the endocervical canal, cervical stenosis associated with surgery, radiation, cryocautery or electrocautery, and malignant disease of the endocervical canal.

○ **What are the symptoms of hematometra?**

Primary and secondary amenorrhea and cyclic lower abdominal pain.

CHAPTER 27 Dysmenorrhea and Premenstrual Syndrome

Jacqueline Kohl, MD, MPH

○ **Define primary dysmenorrhea.**

Menstrual pain without pelvic pathology.

○ **What percentage of women are affected by dysmenorrhea?**

Between 50% and 90% of women, of which 10% may be incapacitated for 1 to 3 days each month. It is the most common reason women miss work, with 17% of women missing school or work.

○ **What are the risk factors for dysmenorrhea?**

Age <30 years, BMI < 20 kg/m^2, smoking, menarche prior to age 12, longer duration of bleeding, irregular or heavy bleeding, and prior sexual assault.

○ **What are the protective factors for dysmenorrhea?**

Younger age of first birth and higher parity.

○ **What is the cause of primary dysmenorrhea?**

Increased endometrial prostaglandin production. Prostaglandin levels increase threefold from the follicular to the luteal phase and further during menstruation.

○ **In what phase of the endometrium, are these compounds increased?**

The secretory endometrium.

○ **The fall of what hormone in the late luteal phase triggers the pathway that increases prostaglandin production?**

Progesterone.

○ **Name the compound that is the substrate for the release of prostaglandin.**

Arachidonic acid.

○ **Name the pathway through which prostaglandins are released.**

Cyclooxygenase pathway.

○ **What compound is responsible for dysmenorrhea?**

Prostaglandins F.

○ **Name another pathway that is not blocked by nonsteroidal anti-inflammatory drugs (NSAIDs) and produces leukotrienes.**

The lipoxygenase pathway.

○ **In primary dysmenorrhea, when is the typical onset in relation to the menstrual cycle?**

The pain usually begins a few hours prior to or just after the onset of menses. The pain may last as long as 48 to 72 hours.

○ **Describe the nature of the pain.**

It is colicky, with suprapubic cramping that may or may not be accompanied by back pain, nausea, vomiting, and diarrhea.

○ **How it is diagnosed?**

It is generally a diagnosis of exclusion, once underlying pathology has been excluded. There are no physical, laboratory, or imaging tests for primary dysmenorrhea.

○ **What is the treatment of choice?**

Prostaglandin synthase inhibitors (ie, NSAIDs).

○ **How should they be taken?**

Take the inhibitors just prior to or at the onset of pain and then continuously every 6 to 8 hours to prevent reformation of prostaglandin by-products.

○ **In what percentage of cases are prostaglandin inhibitors effective treatment?**
80%.

○ **Name a form of treatment that acts by decreasing endometrial proliferation, thus decreasing the production of prostaglandins.**

Birth control pills.

○ **What percentage of women with primary dysmenorrhea will have relief with birth control pills?**
90%.

○ **What other pharmacological agents may improve dysmenorrhea?**

Progestin therapies (pill, implant, depot, or intrauterine device), glyceryl trinitrate, magnesium, Ca antagonists, vitamin B, vitamin E, fish oil, and herbs.

○ **What other nonpharmacologic approaches may improve dysmenorrhea?**

Rest, heating pad to lower abdomen and back, regular nutritious diet, exercise, relaxation such as meditation or yoga, sexual activity with orgasm, transcutaneous electrical nerve stimulation (TENS), acupuncture/acupressure, and uterosacral nerve ablation/resection.

○ **How can severity of dysmenorrhea be classified?**

According to a verbal multidimensional scoring system, classification includes Grade 0 (unaffected), Grade 1 (rarely affected, with few needing treatment), Grade 2 (moderately affected, requiring therapy but without functional limitation), and Grade 3 (clearly inhibited, with poor treatment response).

○ **Define secondary dysmenorrhea.**

Menstrual pain with underlying pelvic pathology.

○ **Which patients should have a diagnostic evaluation of secondary dysmenorrhea?**

Those with onset after age 25, abnormal uterine bleeding, nonmidline pelvic pain, dyspareunia, dyschezia, progression of symptoms, or absence of other symptoms such as nausea, diarrhea, back pain, headache, or dizziness during menses.

○ **In relation to the menstrual cycle, when does the pain of secondary dysmenorrhea begin?**

1 to 2 weeks prior to menses. It will generally continue until a few days after the cessation of bleeding.

○ **What exam findings may be associated with secondary dysmenorrhea?**

Purulent cervical discharge, cervical motion or adnexal tenderness, uterosacral ligament nodularity, thickening or focal tenderness, lateral cervical displacement, cervical stenosis, adnexal masses, enlarged or irregularly shaped uterus, cervical or vaginal anomalies, and vulvar varicosity.

○ **Name the most common cause of secondary dysmenorrhea.**

Endometriosis, affecting approximately 5% of patients. This is followed by adenomyosis, infection (ie, intrauterine device or pelvic inflammatory disease) adhesions, and anatomic abnormalities.

○ **When should endometriosis be suspected?**

Patients who report pelvic pain related to menses and occurring without menses, dyspareunia, dyschezia, poor response to NSAID therapy, progressively worsening symptoms, or functional incapacitation.

○ **Name three causes of secondary dysmenorrhea that are a result of blockage of the outflow tract.**

Imperforate hymen, transverse vaginal septum, and cervical stenosis.

○ **Name five causes of secondary dysmenorrhea that are due to uterine causes.**

Endometrial polyps, uterine leiomyoma, adenomyosis, Asherman syndrome, pelvic congestion, and uterine anomalies.

○ **What is pelvic congestion syndrome?**

It is one of the etiologies of secondary dysmenorrhea and results from congestion of the uterus and engorgement of varicosities of broad ligaments.

O **What is the term for the cyclic appearance of a large constellation of symptoms (over 100) just prior to menses followed by a period of time entirely free of symptoms?**

Premenstrual syndrome or PMS.

O **Name the most common symptoms of PMS.**

Bloating, anxiety or tension, breast tenderness, depression, fatigue, irritability, and appetite changes.

O **How is the diagnosis of PMS made?**

It is a clinical diagnosis, often based on a cycle diary. However, the National Institute of Mental Health has suggested that PMS requires documentation of at least a 30% increase in the severity of symptoms in the 5 days prior to menses *and a symptom-free period starting sometime during the menses.*

O **What percentage of women suffer from PMS?**

It is actually difficult to ascertain, but up to 80% of women develop emotional and physical changes related to their cycles during the reproductive years.

O **How is the cognitive function of women with PMS changed during the luteal phase?**

Despite feelings of inadequacy, women with PMS show no deficit in memory, attention, or concentration.

O **Name six nonpharmacologic treatments that should be initial treatment of PMS.**

Elimination of caffeine.

Smoking cessation.

Regular exercise.

Adequate sleep.

Decrease stress.

Regular nutritious diet.

O **What dietary supplement has been associated with 48% reduction in symptom scores?**

Calcium (1200 mg daily).

O **Name the differential diagnosis of premenstrual dysphoric disorder (PMDD).**

Underlying psychiatric disorder, thyroid abnormalities, migraine, diabetes, asthma, epilepsy, irritable bowel syndrome, and autoimmune disorders.

O **What is PMDD?**

PMDD is considered a psychiatric disorder where women predominantly have emotional symptoms that are serious enough to disrupt their personal relationships and interfere with their daily lives.

O **How can PMS be distinguished from PMMD?**

PMS typically requires that women experience both physical and emotional symptoms, while PMMD can be purely emotional/behavioral. PMMD is more severe and tends to have predominance of anger, irritability, and internal tension.

◯   **Approximately what percentage of women suffer from PMDD?**

2% to 8%.

◯   **True/False: There is a strong hereditary component to PMDD.**

True.

◯   **What is the treatment of PMDD?**

Selective serotonin uptake inhibitors (SSRIs) are most effective in low doses taken during the luteal phase of the menstrual cycle.

◯   **Which patient group with PMDD may be recommended continuous SSRI therapy?**

Patients who have comorbid depressive or anxiety disorders are not adherent to dosing schedule or not able to tolerate intermittent therapy.

◯   **What other medications may relieve PMS symptoms?**

Oral contraceptives, diuretics, and danazol.

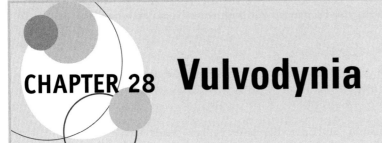

CHAPTER 28 Vulvodynia

Lisa Jambusaria, MD

○ **What is vulvodynia?**

Pain/burning persistently at the vulva or vagina that is not explained by a clear medical finding.

○ **What important information of social history should you elicit from a patient with vulvodynia?**

History of sexual abuse.

○ **What is the first-line medical treatment of different types of vulvodynia?**

Tricyclic antidepressants and anticonvulsants such as amitriptyline and gabapentin.

○ **What is vaginismus?**

Pain with insertion during intercourse causing spasm of the perineal muscles.

○ **What is the treatment of vaginismus?**

Vaginal dilators and perineal massage.

○ **What are other causes of pain with intercourse?**

Uterine fibroids, vaginal atrophy, vaginal infections, prolapse, and endometriosis.

○ **What is the name of point pain on entry/penetration at the introitus?**

Vestibulitis.

○ **What is the test for vestibulitis?**

The Q-tip test where a Q-tip is used to place pressure at 4 and 8 o'clock positions at the introitus to see if the pain is reproduced.

○ **What is the treatment of vestibulitis?**

Amitriptyline and/or gabapentin orally or topically, topical anesthetics, as well as pelvic floor physical therapy.

○ **What recurrent infection of the vagina has also been associated with vulvodynia development?**
Yeast infection.

○ **What should be sent for everyone with vulvar or vaginal burning pain before diagnosing vulvodynia?**
Yeast culture.

○ **What form of vulvodynia can antispasmodics and benzodiazepine vaginally treat?**
Vaginismus or myofascial pain.

○ **What other chronic pain syndromes can cause dyspareunia?**
Chronic bladder pain or spasms, chronic pelvic pain, irritable bowel syndrome, and interstitial cystitis.

○ **What last resort surgical treatment can you offer to a patient with vulvodynia?**
Vestibulectomy.

○ **What is the success rate of vestibulectomy?**
Approximately 50% will have improvement, 25% remain the same, and 25% have worsening pain.

○ **What is commonly found in patients with vulvodynia?**
Depression.

○ **What is the name for point pain at the clitoris?**
Clitordynia.

○ **What inflammatory disorders can cause vulvar pain?**
Atrophic vaginitis, desquamative vaginitis, lichen sclerosis, lichen simplex chronicus, lichen planus, and Behcet disease.

○ **What is the most common physical examination finding seen with someone who has vulvodynia?**
Erythema.

○ **What are theorized causes of vulvodynia?**
Increased urinary oxalates, immune factors, genetic factors, infection, inflammation, and neuropathic changes.

○ **If atrophic changes are noted with a patient reporting vulvar pain, what is the recommended treatment?**
Topical estrogen at area of pain or atrophic changes.

○ **Injectable treatment of focal vulvar pain include what?**
Trigger point injections with lidocaine or bupivacaine and steroid injections every 3 months.

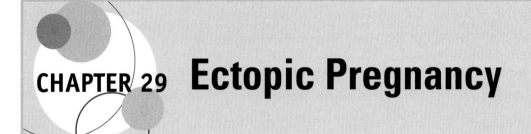

CHAPTER 29 Ectopic Pregnancy

Lindsay Curtis, MD

○ **What has happened to the rate of ectopic pregnancies in the United States during the past 10 years?**

The incidence of ectopic pregnancy has been relatively stable over the last 10 years. However, from 1972 to 1992 the rate did increase from 4.5 to 20/1000 pregnancies.

○ **What percentage of conceptions are ectopic pregnancies?**

About 2 in 100 women in the United States have an ectopic pregnancy (2%).

○ **Are ectopic pregnancies more common in multigravid or nulligravid women?**

Multigravid—only 10% to 15% of ectopic pregnancies are found in nulligravid women, while more than half occur in women who have been pregnant more than three times.

○ **What has happened to ectopic mortality since 1970?**

The rate of death has dropped 10-fold from 35 per 10,000 women with ectopic pregnancy in 1970 to 3.8 per 10,000 in 1989. Ectopic pregnancy remains the most common cause of maternal death in the first trimester and accounts for 4% to 10% of all pregnancy-related deaths.

○ **Are there racial discrepancies in the incidence and mortality rates from ectopic pregnancy in the United States?**

Yes. The incidence of ectopic pregnancy in nonwhite women is approximately 3% and the death-to-case rate is four times higher. Therefore, a pregnant black woman is about five times more likely to die of ectopic pregnancy than a white woman.

○ **What percentage of patients presenting to an emergency room with a positive pregnancy test and pelvic pain and/or vaginal bleeding will have an ectopic pregnancy?**

Approximately 7% to 20%.

○ **What is the most common cause of death in women with ectopic pregnancies?**

Acute blood loss accounts for over 85% of deaths.

○   **What can increase the likelihood of early diagnosis of ectopic pregnancy?**

Identification of risk factors, high index of suspicion, and transvaginal ultrasound.

○   **What is the most common risk factor for ectopic pregnancy?**

About half of ectopic pregnancies can be linked to a history of pelvic inflammatory disease (PID).

○   **Do chromosomal abnormalities increase the risk of ectopic pregnancy?**

Pregnancy associated with chromosomal abnormality does not increase the risk of having an ectopic pregnancy.

○   **What is the rate of ectopic pregnancy in women with a history of PID, as compared with the general population?**

A fivefold increase in ectopic pregnancy from 16.8/1000 is seen in women with a history of PID.

○   **List the high risk factors for ectopic pregnancy.**

Previous ectopic pregnancy.
Previous tubal surgery.
Tubal ligation.
Tubal pathology.
History of PID.
In utero DES exposure.
Current intrauterine device (IUD) use.

○   **List the moderate risk factors for ectopic pregnancy.**

Infertility.
Previous cervicitis (gonorrhea and *Chlamydia*).
Multiple sexual partners.
Smoking.

○   **List the low risk factors for ectopic pregnancy.**

Previous pelvic/abdominal surgery.
Vaginal douching.
Early age of intercourse (<18 years).
Advanced maternal age.

○   **What percentage of pregnancies after tubal ligation are ectopic pregnancies?**

The incidence depends on the type of tubal ligation; up to 50% of pregnancies after laparoscopic fulguration are ectopic pregnancies.

○   **Is there an association between ectopic pregnancy and endometriosis?**

Ectopic pregnancy is not increased in women with a history of endometriosis.

○ **What percentage of women with a previous ectopic pregnancy will conceive again?**

About 60% of women with a history of an ectopic pregnancy will conceive again; 25% will be another ectopic pregnancy. This may be dependent on age, history, prior infertility, and ectopic management.

○ **What is the best predictor of a successful intrauterine pregnancy in a woman with a history of ectopic pregnancy?**

The best predictor of another pregnancy is the condition of the contralateral tube.

○ **Is the rate of ectopic pregnancy higher or lower in women with an IUD?**

The rate of any pregnancy is much lower with an IUD, including ectopic pregnancies. IUDs, however, are more effective at preventing intrauterine pregnancy, making an ectopic pregnancy more likely if an IUD is in place. This varies with a copper device having a rate of 5%, while a progesterone IUD increases the risk to about 23% due to lowered tubal motility.

○ **Are ectopic pregnancies more or less likely during in vitro fertilization?**

Ectopic pregnancies are more likely, accounting for 3% of in vitro fertilization pregnancies, especially with tubal disease and very high hormone levels.

○ **Why do women who undergo clomiphene citrate or human menopausal gonadotropin ovulation induction have a higher incidence of ectopic pregnancy?**

Elevated levels of circulating estrogen or progesterone may alter the normal tubal contractility and delay transport of the embryo.

○ **Does therapeutic abortion increase the risk of an ectopic pregnancy in the future?**

When controlling for other variables, studies have found no association between elective abortion and subsequent ectopic pregnancy.

○ **What is the most likely site of an ectopic pregnancy within the tube?**

Over 80% of tubal pregnancies are ampullary; the next most common site is isthmic.

○ **Besides the tube, what is the most common location for an ectopic pregnancy?**

Although 98% of ectopics are found in the tube, 1.4% are in the abdomen. Less common are ectopics in the uterine cornua, cervix, and ovary.

○ **What is the incidence of ovarian pregnancy?**

Ovarian pregnancy occurs in 1/7000 pregnancies, or 1 in 200 ectopic pregnancies.

○ **What are the risk factors for ovarian pregnancy?**

It is a random event. History of PID or the use of an intrauterine contraceptive device does not increase the risk of ovarian pregnancy.

○ **Does a history of ovarian pregnancy increase the risk of recurrent ectopic pregnancy or infertility?**

There is no such association established.

○ **What is the source of an abdominal pregnancy?**

It is thought that most abdominal pregnancies were tubal abortions.

○ **What is the appropriate treatment for an abdominal pregnancy?**

Surgical removal of the fetus at the time of diagnosis is advised to prevent possible fatal hemorrhage. If possible the placenta should be removed; however, if it is adherent to vital structures or cannot be completely removed, it may be left to absorb over time.

○ **What is an interstitial pregnancy?**

A pregnancy implanted at the proximal segment, interstitial portion of the fallopian tube, which is embedded within the muscular wall of the uterus.

○ **How common are interstitial pregnancies?**

They account for only 2% to 4% of tubal pregnancies.

○ **What are the risk factors for interstitial pregnancy?**

Risk factors are the same as for other tubal pregnancies. However, ipsilateral salpingectomy is a risk factor specific for interstitial pregnancy.

○ **What is the mortality rate of interstitial pregnancies?**

2.5%, or seven times the rate of ectopic pregnancies in general

○ **What is the definition of a cornual pregnancy?**

A pregnancy implanted in the horn of a bicornuate uterus.

○ **What is a hysterotomy scar pregnancy?**

A pregnancy implanted at the previous hysterotomy (cesarean) scar.

○ **What is the incidence of hysterotomy scar pregnancy?**

6% of ectopic pregnancies among women with a prior cesarean delivery, 2% of all ectopic pregnancies.

○ **Is the incidence of hysterotomy scar pregnancies related to number of previous cesarean deliveries?**

No. Implantation occurs because the embryo migrates through a defect within the scar.

○ **How frequent are heterotopic pregnancies?**

About 1/4000 to 1/8000 pregnancies. The incidence increases to about 1/100 with assisted reproductive technologies.

○ **In a heterotopic pregnancy, how often will the intrauterine pregnancy survive after surgery for the ectopic pregnancy?**

About two-thirds of the intrauterine pregnancies survive following salpingectomy.

○ **How deep does the trophoblast invade into the tube?**

As there is no decidua to limit trophoblast growth, the pregnancy frequently grows through the muscularis of the tube.

○ **What percentage of women with ectopic pregnancy report "passing tissue"?**

Five to ten percent of women with ectopic pregnancy report passing tissue; women with ectopic pregnancy can pass the decidual cast, which can be misinterpreted as a spontaneous abortion.

○ **What are the most common symptoms of ectopic pregnancy?**

Pain, absence of menses, and irregular vaginal bleeding.

○ **What are some of the symptoms associated with tubal rupture and hemoperitoneum?**

Worsening pain, shoulder pain (due to diaphragmatic irritation), and dizziness/syncope.

○ **What is the most common location of pain with an ectopic pregnancy?**

Most commonly the pain is generalized over the abdomen; when localized the most common site is unilateral lower quadrant. Shoulder pain is also present in approximately one quarter of women with a ruptured ectopic pregnancy.

○ **What sign can distinguish an ectopic pregnancy from PID?**

Fever is rare with ectopic pregnancy (<2% of women).

○ **How often is an adnexal mass found in women with an ectopic pregnancy?**

Fifty percent of women with an ectopic pregnancy have an adnexal mass.

○ **How often is an ectopic pregnancy diagnosed the first time the patient presents?**

About half of patients are incorrectly diagnosed at least once prior to identification of the ectopic pregnancy.

○ **What are the most commonly used tools for establishing a diagnosis of ectopic pregnancy?**

Serial human chorionic gonadotropin (hCG) levels and transvaginal ultrasound are the most common tools for diagnosing ectopic pregnancy.

○ **What three patterns of hCG rise can be seen with an ectopic pregnancy?**

The hCG patterns associated with an ectopic pregnancy can be an abnormal rise (see previous question), a falling level, or a shift to the right (normal rise occurring later than expected based on menstrual dates).

○ **How is the hCG level used to diagnose ectopic pregnancy?**

Approximately 85% of women with ectopic pregnancy have serum hCG levels lower than those seen in women with intrauterine pregnancies at a similar gestational age. However, hCG levels alone cannot differentiate a normal pregnancy from an ectopic or spontaneous abortion. hCG levels should be monitored over at least a 48-hour period, and if the rate of rise or fall of the hCG is outside the established range, an ectopic pregnancy should be suspected. If the initial hCG level is low, a third level should be obtained to confirm the trend.

○   **What is the normal rate of rise of hCG in the first trimester?**

Ninety-nine percent of normal intrauterine pregnancies have an increase in hCG levels of at least 53% in 2 days. Newer hCG curves suggest using a cutoff of a rise of 35% to avoid misclassification of a normal intrauterine pregnancy as an ectopic pregnancy.

○   **What is the normal fall of hCG in spontaneous abortions?**

A minimal 2-day decline in hCG of 36% to 47% is present in 90% of spontaneous abortions.

○   **How do the hCG changes in ectopic pregnancies compare with those of viable intrauterine pregnancies or spontaneous abortions?**

Approximately 21% of ectopic pregnancies have a rise in hCG similar to an intrauterine pregnancy and 8% have a fall similar to a spontaneous abortion.

○   **Is culdocentesis helpful in the diagnosis of ectopic pregnancy?**

Historically, a culdocentesis was performed to evaluate for intraperitoneal blood. The presence of nonclotting blood (especially with a hematocrit >15%) was used to confirm ruptured ectopic pregnancy but may also be present with a bleeding corpus luteal cyst. The development of accurate ultrasounds has essentially replaced the need for this test.

○   **What progesterone level predicts a normal intrauterine pregnancy?**

A progesterone value >25 ng/mL suggests a normal pregnancy. There is no single level that will definitely confirm a normal pregnancy or rule out an ectopic.

○   **What progesterone level predicts an abnormal pregnancy?**

A progesterone level <5 ng/mL suggests an abnormal pregnancy; this does not distinguish between a spontaneous abortion and an ectopic pregnancy.

○   **At what hCG level, would an intrauterine pregnancy be seen by transabdominal pelvic ultrasound?**

An hCG level >6500 mIU/mL should show a gestational sac; the yolk sac and fetal pole may not be seen at this level.

○   **At what hCG level, would an intrauterine pregnancy be seen by transvaginal ultrasound?**

The discriminatory zone for detecting an intrauterine pregnancy by transvaginal ultrasound is an hCG level >1500 to 2000 mIU/mL. A higher discriminatory zone may be used for patients who are considered to be at high risk of multiple gestations, such as those patients undergoing assisted reproductive technology.

○   **List the significant ultrasound findings present in a normally developing intrauterine pregnancy according to gestational age.**

5.3 weeks: Gestational sac.

5.5 weeks: Yolk sac.

6 weeks: Fetal pole.

6.5 weeks: Cardiac activity.

In addition, an abnormal pregnancy is likely if there is absence of a fetal pole with a gestational sac of 2 cm and if no cardiac activity is seen with crown-rump length of >0.5 cm.

○ **If the hCG level is <3000 mIU/mL and rising abnormally, what diagnostic test(s) can be used to confirm the diagnosis of ectopic pregnancy?**

If the woman is not symptomatic, the options are as follows: continue to follow the hCG level until it reaches the diagnostic level and repeat the transvaginal ultrasound or perform a diagnostic dilation and curettage (D & C) to rule out an abnormal intrauterine pregnancy. If symptomatic, diagnostic laparoscopy can be performed.

○ **Does the presence of a thick endometrial stripe indicate an intrauterine pregnancy?**

The endometrium can be thickened due to the hormonal stimulation associated with either an ectopic or intrauterine pregnancy, so this is not a consistent sign of a normal pregnancy.

○ **Does the presence of a gestational sac always rule out an ectopic?**

Up to 15% of women with an ectopic pregnancy can have a "pseudosac" or fluid area (representing blood and mucus) within the cavity. Therefore, it is critical with women at high risk of an ectopic pregnancy to confirm an intrauterine pregnancy with a follow-up ultrasound. This ultrasound will identify the yolk sac ("double ring sign") or fetal pole within the gestational sac.

○ **Is Doppler flow ultrasonography useful in the diagnosis of ectopic pregnancy?**

Doppler flow may show variation in tubal blood flow in the case of a tubal pregnancy. It may also be useful in identifying the presence and location of a cervical pregnancy.

○ **At what gestational age, does tubal rupture most commonly occur?**

Rupture of an ampullary ectopic typically occurs at 8 to 12 weeks, allowing adequate time for early diagnosis and treatment prior to rupture in most cases. Isthmic ectopics may rupture earlier at 6 to 8 weeks.

○ **What type of ectopic pregnancy has the highest mortality rate?**

Although a rare site of an ectopic pregnancy, the highest mortality rate occurs with cornual pregnancies.

○ **Should women with ectopic pregnancies be given RhoGam?**

Most authors recommend administration of RhoGam with any failed pregnancy in an Rh-negative patient. A "mini" dose of RhoGam (50 μg) may be given up to 12 weeks or alternatively full-dose RhoGam (300 μg) may be given at any time.

○ **What are the indications for laparotomy in the treatment of ectopic pregnancy?**

Common indications for laparotomy include an unstable patient, large hemoperitoneum, and lack of appropriate surgical tools for laparoscopy. An interstitial pregnancy can most often be treated laparoscopically but occasionally will require laparotomy for resection. Some authors would also include a large ectopic (>6 cm) and fetal heart tones in the adnexa as indications of laparotomy.

○ **Is there an advantage in removing the ipsilateral ovary when the tube must be removed?**

In the past, the ovary was removed with the tube to promote fertility, but conception rates are not different if the ovary is removed or retained. Fertility is theoretically delayed, as ovulation occurs half the time on the side without a tube.

○ **What is the surgical treatment of choice for a patient with a nonruptured ectopic pregnancy who is desirous of future fertility?**

A laparoscopic linear salpingostomy is the most recommended surgical procedure. When performed correctly and compared with salpingectomy, the incidence of repeat ectopic pregnancy is no different, while the subsequent live birth rate is increased.

○ **What are the indications of conservative surgical therapy (conservation of the fallopian tube)?**

The tube can be conserved if the tube has minimal damage and the woman desires further fertility.

○ **List the possible techniques for conservative tubal surgery.**

Possible conservative techniques include salpingostomy, salpingostomy, fimbrial evacuation, and segmental resection (with future anastomosis of the tube).

○ **Which of the techniques listed in the previous question increase the risk of a future ectopic pregnancy?**

Fimbrial evacuation, with milking of the ectopic from the distal end of the tube, increases the risk of another ectopic pregnancy.

○ **When should salpingectomy be performed?**

With a severely damaged tube, recurrent ectopic in that tube, uncontrolled hemorrhage, or a desire for sterility especially after previous tubal ligation.

○ **If a salpingectomy is performed, what is the best predictor of future fertility?**

The best predictor is the degree of adhesive disease and the quality of the contralateral tube as well as a history of past fertility.

○ **What is the advantage of closing the salpingostomy site on the fallopian tube?**

There is no advantage to suturing the salpingostomy site. In fact, this may slow the return to normal function as subsequent pregnancy rates are decreased at 1 year when compared with salpingostomy.

○ **What follow-up is required for women undergoing linear salpingostomy?**

Serial hCG levels are necessary to rule out persistent trophoblastic tissue.

○ **What is the risk of persistent ectopic pregnancy with linear salpingostomy?**

About 5% to 10% of ectopic pregnancies treated by linear salpingostomy will have retained trophoblastic tissue and require further therapy.

○ **How is a persistent ectopic pregnancy treated?**

This can be treated with medical therapy or removal of the affected tube. Expectant management can be considered if the hCG levels are falling.

○ **When observing the tube at surgery, what is the most likely site of the ectopic pregnancy?**

The most likely site of implantation is proximal to the most dilated portion of the tube.

○ **What is the advantage of laparoscopy versus laparotomy for treatment of an ectopic pregnancy?**

The primary advantages are decreased hospital stay, decreased recovery, and decreased costs (over 20 million dollars/year if laparoscopy is performed primarily).

○ **What is the most common clinical presentation of cervical pregnancy?**

Profuse painless vaginal bleeding.

○ **What is the incidence of cervical pregnancy?**

1/9000.

○ **What is the treatment for hemodynamically stable patients diagnosed with cervical pregnancy?**

Systemic methotrexate and transcervical evacuation of the pregnancy after angiographic uterine artery embolization have been reported as successful methods to treat cervical pregnancy.

○ **What is the treatment of a patient with hemorrhage diagnosed with cervical pregnancy?**

Hysterectomy if there is uncontrolled hemorrhage (avoid if possible in cases of desired further childbearing). Dilation and evacuation with preoperative measures (such as transvaginal ligation of the cervical branches of the uterine arteries, Shirodkar cerclage, angiographic uterine artery embolization, or intracervical vasopressin injection) to reduce incidence of severe hemorrhage.

○ **What additional measures can be used to control the profuse bleeding in patient diagnosed with cervical pregnancy?**

- Foley catheter with a 30-mL balloon into the dilated cervix, with the tip extending into the uterine cavity for 24 to 48 hours in combination with a purse string suture around the external cervical os to prevent expulsion of the balloon.
- Placement of hemostatic sutures locally in the cervix.
- Angiographic embolization.
- Bilateral internal iliac artery ligation.
- Bilateral uterine artery ligation.

○ **What is the mode of action of methotrexate?**

Methotrexate is a folic acid antagonist. More specifically, it inhibits dihydrofolate reductase preventing the conversion of dihydrofolate to tetrahydrofolate, which is required for the production of purine nucleotides and the amino acids serine and methionine. Subsequently, this prevents DNA synthesis in the rapidly proliferating cells such as the trophoblast.

○ **The original methotrexate treatment regimens included multiple doses of methotrexate and alternate "rescue" treatments. What was given for "rescue"?**

Leucovorin also known as folinic acid.

○ **What short-term side effect can be seen with the dose of methotrexate used for ectopic pregnancy?**

Nausea, vomiting, stomatitis, mouth ulcerations, diarrhea, and fatigue have been reported. Thrombocytopenia, liver abnormalities, and neutropenia are rare.

○ **What instructions should be given to patients receiving methotrexate?**

Patients should be counseled to avoid folic acid supplements, NSAIDs, alcohol, and sunlight exposure. In addition, they should refrain from sexual intercourse or vigorous physical activity.

○ **What is the risk of early ovarian failure with methotrexate use?**

There does not appear to be an increased risk of ovarian failure with this chemotherapeutic agent.

○ **Single-dose methotrexate therapy (typically 50 mg/m² of body surface area) has what primary advantage over multiple treatment regimens?**

Fewer side effects are seen with single-dose treatment. The success rate is similar.

○ **What patients are reasonable candidates for medical treatment of an ectopic pregnancy?**

Hemodynamically stable patients with a confirmed or highly suspicious unruptured ectopic pregnancy who agree to comply with close follow-up care and do not have contraindications to methotrexate use.

○ **List the absolute and relative contraindications to methotrexate use.**

Absolute:

(1) Breastfeeding.

(2) Overt or laboratory evidence of immunodeficiency.

(3) Alcoholism, alcoholic liver disease, or other chronic liver disease.

(4) Preexisting blood dyscrasias, such as bone marrow hypoplasia, leucopenia, thrombocytopenia, or significant anemia.

(5) Known sensitivity to methotrexate.

(6) Active pulmonary disease.

(7) Hepatic, renal, or hematologic dysfunction.

Relative:

(1) Gestational sac larger than 3.5 cm.

(2) Embryonic cardiac motion.

○ **What lab values should be checked prior to giving methotrexate?**

Baseline hCG levels, liver function tests, platelet count, and white blood cell count should be checked before and after treatment. After treatment, hCG levels should be followed to zero.

○ **What criteria are used for assuring the success of methotrexate?**

With a single-dose therapy, the hCG levels should fall by 15% between days 4 and 7 after therapy and continue to fall weekly until undetectable.

○ **How common is pelvic pain following methotrexate therapy?**

Up to 30% of women will experience pain within 2 weeks of treatment.

○ **Does pelvic pain after methotrexate require surgery?**

Although these patients should be followed closely with ultrasound and CBCs, the pain often resolves without surgery.

○   **When is a second dose of methotrexate required?**

A second dose is required if the hCG level does not fall by at least 15% between days 4 and 7 of administration or if the levels subsequently plateau.

○   **What percentage of women require a second dose of therapy?**

About 6% of women getting single-dose therapy require a second dose.

○   **What percentage of women are successfully treated with methotrexate?**

Studies suggest that between 85% and 95% of women are successful with medical therapy.

○   **How does ectopic rate compare with medical versus surgical therapy?**

The rate of repeat ectopic pregnancy following medical therapy compares favorably with surgical therapy (8% vs. 15%).

○   **What percentage of patients treated with methotrexate rupture?**

10% depending on location and initial hCG titer.

○   **What percentage of ectopic pregnancies will spontaneously resolve?**

It has been estimated that up to 60% or more of ectopic pregnancies will resolve without therapy.

○   **What is the best predictor of spontaneous resolution of an ectopic pregnancy?**

The initial hCG is the most important factor. Approximately 88% of patients with an initial hCG level <200 mIU/mL will experience spontaneous resolution.

○   **If the hCG levels are falling, is surgery or medical therapy required in a patient with an ectopic pregnancy?**

Treatment is only required if the patient is symptomatic or the hCG levels do not continue to fall. Active treatment is indicated if compliance is a concern.

○   **What counseling should be provided to a woman with an ectopic pregnancy?**

Women need to be aware of the decreased fecundity associated with a history of an ectopic pregnancy, as well as the increased risk of another ectopic pregnancy. As with any pregnancy loss, supportive counseling should be offered.

○   **How should a woman with a history of an ectopic pregnancy be followed in a subsequent pregnancy?**

Early monitoring of the pregnancy with hCG levels and transvaginal ultrasound.

CHAPTER 30

Genital Tract Infections and PID

Lisa Jambusaria, MD

○ **What are some medical sequelae of pelvic inflammatory disease (PID)?**

Increased rate of ectopic pregnancy, chronic and acute pelvic pain, and infertility.

○ **What are some common organisms causing PID?**

The infection is usually polymicrobial, commonly included are *Chlamydia trachomatis*, *Neisseria gonorrheae*, cytomegalovirus (CMV), endogenous aerobic and anaerobic bacteria, and rarely genital *Mycoplasma* species.

○ **N. gonorrheae and C. trachomatis coexist in the same individual in what percentage of the time?**

25% to 50% of the time.

○ **What percentage of women with asymptomatic gonococcal cervical infection will develop acute salpingitis?**

15%.

○ **What is the incidence of infertility with one episode of PID?**

10%, and 25% with 2 and 40% to 60% with a third episode.

○ **What is Fitz-Hugh-Curtis syndrome?**

Syndrome characterized by perihepatic inflammation that occurs in 5% to 10% of patients with PID, likely from transperitoneal or vascular route of *N. gonorrheae* or *C. trachomatis*.

○ **What is the pathognomonic sign of Fitz-Hugh-Curtis syndrome?**

"Violin String" like filmy scar tissue at the RUQ from the liver to the anterior abdominal wall.

○ **What is the most common nonviral sexually transmitted disease?**

Chlamydia trachomatis. It is more common than *Neisseria* by as much as 10 to 1 in some studies.

○ **What warrants IV antibiotics or inpatient admission for findings of PID?**

Tubo-ovarian abscess (TOA), hemodynamic instability, poor compliance, high fevers, and severe pain requiring IV pain medication.

○ **What is the standard treatment of uncomplicated PID?**

Ceftriaxone IM 250 mg and doxycycline 100 BID for 14 days.

○ **What are the some risk factors for sexually transmitted disease?**

Age at first intercourse, number of sexual partners, and lack of contraception.

○ **What is the alternative to doxycycline for treatment of *Chlamydia*?**

Azithromycin 2 g one time dose.

○ **What is the incidence of adnexal abscesses in patients with acute PID?**

Approximately 10%.

○ **What are some options for drainage of tubo-ovarian complexes?**

Laparoscopy, interventional radiology, colpotomy, or laparotomy.

○ **Which organisms should be covered when considering antibiotic treatment of TOA?**

Anaerobic organisms, which are predominantly present between 60% and 100% of cases.

○ **How are TOAs treated?**

With IV broad-spectrum antibiotics until afebrile for 48 hours then with extended PO course antibiotics for up to 6 weeks with reimaging.

○ **When is a TOA treated with drainage in addition to antibiotics?**

When >9 cm size, when unresponsive to antibiotics alone and in postmenopausal patient.

○ **What is the infection most commonly associated with patients using an intrauterine device (IUD)?**

Actinomyces.

○ **What is the classic histologic finding of actinomyces israelii?**

The classic "sulfur granules" are observed along with gram-positive filaments.

○ **What are the predominant presentations of pelvic tuberculosis?**

Infertility and abnormal uterine bleeding.

○ **What is the gold standard for diagnosis of pelvic tuberculosis?**

Open biopsy, dilation and curettage or colposcopy guided histopathology showing caseating granulomas and TB culture.

○ **What is the classic finding in chronic endometritis?**

The presence of plasma cells on endometrial biopsy.

○ **What are the three most prevalent primary viral infections of the vulva?**

Herpes genitalis, condyloma acuminatum, and molluscum contagiosum.

○ **What are some treatments of choice for recurrent Bartholin duct cyst or abscess?**

Insertion of the Word Catheter or marsupialization of the Bartholin duct cyst.

○ **What is the organism responsible for syphilis?**

The spirochete *Treponema pallidum.*

○ **In pregnant patients with penicillin allergies, what is the treatment of syphilis?**

Desensitization protocol and then treat with penicillin.

○ **What are the confirmatory tests for syphilis?**

The fluorescent treponemal antibody absorption (FTA-ABS) or microhemagglutination assay for antibodies to *T. pallidum* (MHA-TP). The Venereal Disease Research Laboratories (VDRL) or rapid plasma reagin (RPR) are nonspecific and are only used for screening.

○ **What test is used to monitor successful treatment of syphilis?**

RPR titers decreasing.

○ **What is the classic skin lesion of primary syphilis?**

It is the chancre, a firm, painless ulcer that develops at a mucus or cutaneous site of entry of the spirochete.

○ **When does a serologic test for syphilis become positive after exposure?**

Generally 4 to 6 weeks after exposure.

○ **What percentage of women with primary herpes experienced systemic symptoms?**

70%. Primary herpes is much more severe than recurrent infection.

○ **How long can viral shedding occur after herpetic vulvar lesions appear?**

Up to 2 to 3 weeks.

○ **What is the benefit of acyclovir in the treatment of genital herpes?**

It reduces the duration of ulcerative lesions and the median duration of viral shedding, and decreases the recurrence rate when given prophylactically.

○ **What is the pathognomonic microscopic finding of granuloma inguinale?**

Donovan bodies, which are clusters of dark staining, bipolar-appearing bacteria in large mononuclear cells.

○ **What is lymphogranuloma venereum (LGV)?**

A chronic infection of lymphatic tissue produced by *Chlamydia trachomatis*, serotypes L1, L2, or L3.

○ **What is the classic clinical sign of LGV?**

A "groove sign," a linear depression between the inguinal and femoral groups of inflamed nodes.

○ **What is the treatment of LGV?**

Oral tetracycline or erythromycin (500 mg every 6 hours) for 21 days.

○ **What causes molluscum contagiosum?**

Poxvirus. It is acquired both through sexual and nonsexual contact.

○ **What is the difference between the ulcer of chancroid and syphilis?**

The lesion of chancroid is always painful and tender, whereas the chancre of syphilis is usually asymptomatic.

○ **What is chancroid caused by?**

Haemophilus ducreyi, a nonmotile, anaerobic, and small gram-negative rod.

○ **What is the treatment of pediculosis pubis?**

Topical application of lindane (Kwell) or 5% permethrin dermal cream (Nix). The organism responsible is the crab louse *Phthirus pubis.*

○ **How is scabies diagnosed?**

It is diagnosed by scraping of the papules, vesicles, or burrows and looking for the mite *Sarcoptes scabiei* under the microscope.

○ **What is the classic finding on wet smear of bacterial vaginosis?**

Clue cells, which are vaginal epithelial cells with clusters of bacteria covering their surfaces.

○ **What is the treatment of choice for bacterial vaginosis?**

Metronidazole 500 mg every 12 hours for 7 days. Alternatives included clindamycin or Augmentin.

○ **The appearance of a "strawberry cervix" is a classic sign of what infection?**

Trichomonas vaginalis.

○ **How is vulvovaginal yeast infection diagnosed?**

By wet mount or KOH mount finding of hyphae or yeast culture of vaginal wall.

○ **How often are hyphae seen on a wet mount with a person who has positive yeast cultures?**

30% to 50% of the time.

○ **If hyphae are not noted on wet mount, what other characteristic findings are noted with yeast infection?**

Swelling of the vagina and vulva, burning/pain with sex that stays afterward, and adherent white thick discharge at vaginal walls.

○ **What is the treatment of *Candida vaginitis*?**
Topical application of one of the synthetic imidazoles, terconazole, butonconazole, or oral fluconazole.

○ **What is the most practical method of diagnosing candidal vaginitis?**
Application of KOH on a wet smear and look for presence of mycelial and blastopore forms.

○ **What human papillomavirus serotypes usually cause genital warts?**
Types 6 and 11.

○ **What percentage of individuals infected with the human papillomavirus develop genital warts?**
3%.

○ **What are some treatment options for vulvar condyloma?**
Provider applied: Trichloroacetic acid, podophyllin, cryosurgery, laser ablation or 5-fluorouracil cream.
Patient applied: Imiquimod or podophyllin (Condylox gel or liquid).

○ **What are the criteria for hospitalization of patients with PID?**
A patient should be hospitalized when a surgical emergency cannot be excluded, pregnancy, the patient does not respond to oral antibiotic therapy, the patient is unable to follow or tolerate oral therapy, presence of TOA (see ultrasound below), and patients with severe illness, nausea, vomiting, or high fever.

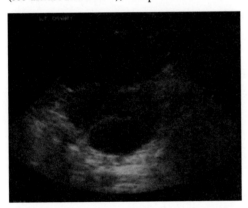

Ultrasound of TOA

○ **What is trichomonas vaginalis?**
A flagellated protozoan that infects the squamous epithelium of the urogenital tract. Its only host are humans. Always sexually transmitted.

○ **What is the treatment of choice for trichomoniasis?**
Metronidazole 2 g orally single dose or tinidazole 2 g orally single dose is the treatment of choice for trichomoniasis with one dose for partner as well.

○ **Which are the most specific criteria for the diagnosis of PID?**

Signs of infection with pain and fever combined with; Endometrial biopsy with histological evidence of endometritis, transvaginal ultrasound or MRI showing thickened fluid-filled tubes with or without free pelvic fluid, cystic mass on adnexa suspicious for abcess, or laparoscopic findings of PID.

○ **What is the most sensitive criterion for detection of PID?**

Pelvic motion tenderness on examination.

○ **Is a test of cure for *Chlamydia* routinely recommended?**

No, unless patient is pregnant, therapeutic compliance is in question, symptoms persist or reinfection is suspected. If indicated should be done 3 to 4 weeks after treatment is completed.

○ **What are the clinical criteria for bacterial vaginosis and how many do you need to make the diagnosis?**

Amsel criteria are used to make the diagnosis.

The diagnosis is made if at least three of the following criteria are present:

(1) Homogeneous, thin, white discharge that coats the vaginal walls.

(2) Clue cells on microscopic examination.

(3) Vaginal PH >4.5.

(4) Whiff test positive.

○ **What is the definition of recurrent vulvovaginal candidiasis (VVC)?**

Four or more episodes in 1 year.

○ **What is the first-line maintenance regimen for recurrent VVC?**

Oral fluconazole weekly for 6 months (100–150 or 200 mg weekly).

○ **What are the characteristics of complicated VVCs?**

Recurrent VVC, severe VVC, non-albicans candidiasis, women with uncontrolled diabetes, debilitation, immunosuppression, or pregnancy.

○ **When should the partner be treated when you made the diagnosis of chancroid?**

The partner should be treated if sexual contact occurs within the last 10 days preceding the symptoms.

○ **What is the most sensitive test for diagnosis of herpes simplex virus (HSV)?**

PCR.

○ **What other vaginal lesions can resemble HSV?**

CMV, hand-foot-mouth disease, and Behcet disease.

○ **What type of HSV causes genital tract lesions?**

HSV-2 has classically been linked with genital tract lesions but now HSV-1 has started to make up a larger fraction of genital ulcer cases.

○ **What can be done to prevent HSV outbreaks at time of delivery in pregnant women?**

Starting prophylactic valacyclovir or acyclovir at 36 weeks until delivery.

○ **What should be done on all women in labor with history of HSV?**

A speculum examination to evaluate for HSV lesions prior to allowing a vaginal delivery.

○ **What is the current recommendation for screening of *Chlamydia*?**

Annual screening should be performed in all sexually active female 25 or less years old or older if risk factors present including new sexual partner or multiple sexual partners.

○ **True or False: Suppressive therapy reduces the frequency of genital herpes recurrences by 70% to 80 % in patients with >6 recurrences per year?**

True.

○ **What is the recommended regimen for granuloma inguinale?**

Doxycycline 100 mg BID × at least 3 weeks and until all lesions are completely healed.

○ **When should the sexual partner be treated if you diagnosed a patient with granuloma inguinale?**

Within 60 days before the symptoms.

CHAPTER 31

Benign Vulvar and Vaginal Lesions

Lisa Jambusaria, MD

○ **What is the most common gynecologic problem of childhood?**

Vulvovaginitis.

○ **What are the two most common infectious causes of vulvovaginitis in children?**

Pinworms (*Enterobius vermicularis*) and *Candida*.

○ **What is the treatment of pinworm vaginitis?**

Albendazole.

○ **What is the most common benign condition affecting the external genitalia?**

Contact dermatitis.

○ **What condition does chronic vulvar contact dermatitis lead to?**

Lichen simplex chronicus.

○ **How do you treat lichen simplex chronicus?**

Avoid allergens including detergents, creams, fragrances and keep area dry with loose fitting clothes.

○ **What is hidradenitis suppurativa?**

A chronic occlusion of the follicular glands in the perineum, vulva, and/or perianal.

○ **How does hidradenitis suppurativa present?**

Ulcerated and draining sinuses with areas of abscess formation that causes pain, odor, and discomfort.

○ **How can recurrent episodes of hidradenitis suppurativa be prevented?**

Routine gentle cleansing, weight loss, avoidance of skin trauma, and shaving.

O **How are episodes of hidradenitis suppurativa treated?**

Short courses of antibiotic treatment with doxycycline are first line, antiandrogens, and surgery for more severe cases.

O **Why does hyperkeratosis occur?**

By disordered epithelial growth and nutrition that can be a result of chronic irritation, chronic inflammation, cancer, or precancer.

O **What is the treatment of squamous cell hyperplasia without atypia?**

Episodic mid to high potency topical corticosteroids.

O **What is lichen sclerosus characterized by histologically?**

Hyperkeratosis, thinning of the epidermis with acanthosis and elongation/flattening of the rete pegs; upper dermis is hyalinized with a band of lymphocytes below this region.

O **What is lichen sclerosis thought to increase the risk for?**

Squamous cell cancer of the vulva.

O **What other skin disease can also lead to white "patches" on the vulva?**

Vitiligo.

O **What is the appearance of vulvar lichen sclerosus?**

Thin white wrinkled skin classically characterized as "paper-like" with possible obliteration of normal anatomy including labia minora, clitoris, or urethra with scar tissue introitus may have yellow, waxy appearance.

O **What two vulvar diseases can obliterate normal vulvar anatomy?**

Lichen sclerosis and lichen planus.

O **When a lesion suspicious for lichen sclerosis is found what is the best first step in management?**

Biopsy.

O **What other lesions appear white on the vulva?**

Squamous cell cancer of the vulva.

O **How is lichen sclerosus treated in a child?**

It usually regresses, but tiny amounts of clobetasol (topical corticosteroid) for a longer period of time appear successful in young girls and maintenance therapy not always required; topical corticosteroids can arrest the process and the symptoms.

O **How is lichen sclerosus treated in the adult?**

High potency topical steroid, usually clobetasol 0.05% ointment or cream. The treatment is tapered over 4 to 6 weeks from initial BID/TID applications to a maintenance application of 1 to 3 times weekly. This is a chronic condition that usually requires indefinite therapy.

○ **What is second-line therapy for severe lichen sclerosis?**

Surgical lysis of adhesion/scar tissue with possible laser or cavitary ultrasonic surgical ablation (CUSA) ablation.

○ **What is intertrigo?**

Inflammatory condition of two closely opposed skin surfaces.

○ **In which patients is intertrigo of the vulva commonly found?**

Obese or diabetic women.

○ **What other skin discoloration causing darkened macular areas at the vulva is seen in diabetic women?**

Acanthosis nigricans.

○ **What is the common distribution of intertrigo?**

Axilla, inframammary folds, groin, perineum, intergluteal folds, toe webs, interlabial and intercrural folds.

○ **What causes labial agglutination?**

Chronic vulvar inflammation from any cause.

○ **What is the treatment of labial agglutination?**

If it is asymptomatic, no treatment is needed and often a girl's natural estrogen at the time of puberty will resolve the agglutination; if symptomatic, 2 to 4 weeks of topical estrogen may be used with manual separation.

○ **What symptom of labial agglutination requires prompt treatment of the agglutination?**

Inability to urinate.

○ **What is the most common cause of papillary lesions on the vulva?**

HPV.

○ **What characteristic of HPV explains the high rate of clinical relapse of treated warts?**

Viral latency.

○ **Which types of HPV are most commonly associated with malignancy?**

16 and 18.

○ **What cytotoxic agents are used in the treatment of HPV of the vulva?**

Podophyllin (mitotic poison), TCA (caustic agent), 5-FU (antimetabolite), Imiquimod (immune modulator), interferon alpha (immune modulator), and adefovir (nucleoside analog).

○ **What other techniques may be used in the treatment of HPV?**

Liquid nitrogen, electrocauterization, surgical excision, carbon dioxide laser, and CUSA.

○ **What is the duration of treatment of condyloma with 5-FU for vulvar and vaginal lesions?**

Two treatments of 5 to 7 days of consecutive nightly applications.

○ **Which treatment of vaginal condylomas is contraindicated in pregnancy?**

Podophyllin.

○ **What are the risk factors associated with vaginal condylomas and vaginal delivery?**

Trauma and heavy bleeding during delivery, and, infrequently, laryngeal papillomas in the newborn.

○ **What is the most common cystic lesion of the vulva?**

Epidermal inclusion cyst.

○ **What is an epidermal inclusion cyst?**

A cyst in which the cyst wall contains normal epidermis that produces keratin; most commonly these cysts arise from pilosebaceous ducts that have become occluded. A less common cause is traumatically buried skin fragments.

○ **What is the treatment of inclusion cysts?**

They need no treatment unless infected or for cosmetic reasons. If infected, they can be incised and drained after antibiotic treatment is instituted.

○ **What is the most common site of an inclusion cyst?**

The site of a previous laceration or episiotomy scar in the vagina or in the labia majora, especially the anterior half.

○ **What is a syringoma?**

A benign adenoma of the eccrine sweat gland, found most often around the eyelids and less commonly on the vulva, chest, or abdomen.

○ **How are Bartholin duct abscesses treated?**

A small stab wound is made in the abscess and a Word catheter is inserted and left in place for 4 to 6 weeks to allow epithelialization of a tract and permanent opening of the gland.

○ **How are recurrent Bartholin duct cysts treated?**

Marsupialization.

○ **How are Bartholin duct cysts treated differently in postmenopausal women?**

Malignancy must be ruled out; all or part of the Bartholin duct cyst should be removed for histologic evaluation when recurrent/persistent.

○ **What are the vulvovaginal cysts of embryonic origin?**

Mesonephric cysts, paramesonephric cysts, and urogenital sinus mucus cysts.

○ **What is a Skene duct cyst?**

Cystic dilatation of an occluded paraurethral duct, usually associated with infection in the duct.

○ **What is a complication of Skene duct cysts?**

Urinary obstruction due to enlargement.

○ **The Gartner duct arises from what structure?**

Vestigial remnant of the vaginal portion of the mesonephric duct (Wolffian duct).

○ **How do Gartner duct cysts usually appear?**

Multiple tiny cystic dilations, most commonly, or rarely as a large single cyst in the anterolateral vaginal wall.

○ **Where does endometriosis most commonly appear in the vagina?**

Posterior fornix as a result of penetration from the cul-de-sac.

○ **What is vaginal adenosis and what is it associated with?**

Presence of epithelial lined glands or their secretory products within the vagina and is associated with in utero exposure to DES.

○ **What are the examination findings of atrophic vaginitis?**

Vaginal mucosa is thin and pale with lack of normal rugae and often with visible blood vessels or petechial hemorrhages.

○ **What does a wet mount show with atrophic vaginitis?**

Small rounded parabasal epithelial cells with an increased number of PMNs.

○ **What other inflammatory condition are parabasal cells seen on wet mount?**

Desquamative inflammatory vaginitis.

○ **What are the symptoms of inflammatory desquamative vaginitis?**

Profuse purulent discharge, vaginal burning and pain, and dyspareunia.

○ **What is the treatment of desquamative inflammatory vaginitis?**

Clindamycin cream and hydrocortisone cream per vagina.

○ **What is a autoimmune disease causing ulcer like lesions in premenopausal women in the vagina and mouth?**

Behcet disease.

○ **What systemic disease can present with lacy macular rash with areas of ulceration on the vulva?**

Lichen planus.

○ **What does lichen planus look like?**

Violet, pruritic, polygonal papules or plaques (can also be bullous and ulcerate).

○ **What are common systemic lesions also seen in lichen planus?**

Skin lesions on extensor surfaces of arms and legs, oral lesions.

○ **What is a pathognomic finding of oral lichen planus?**

Lacey white pattern on the buccal mucosa referred to as Wickham's striae. Can also have painful ulcers/erosive lesions.

○ **What is lichen planus caused by?**

Unknown but is an auto immune response of activated T-cells to basal layer of keratinocytes.

○ **What is the treatment for lichen planus?**

Topical and oral steroids. Retinoids used for dermal manifestations as well.

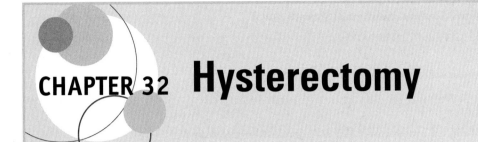

CHAPTER 32 Hysterectomy

Aroti Achari, MD

○ **How many hysterectomies are done each year in the United States?**

About 600,000 hysterectomies are performed annually in the United States, making hysterectomy the second most-commonly performed operation for women of reproductive age in the United States, after cesarean delivery.

○ **What are the most common indications of hysterectomy?**

From 2000 to 2004, approximately 3,100,000 hysterectomies were performed in the United States:
- 40.7% of them were done for symptomatic uterine fibroids.
- 17.7% for endometriosis.
- 14.5% for uterine prolapse.

○ **How do you determine the route and method of hysterectomy?**

Safety and cost-effectiveness.

○ **What is the correct terminology regarding hysterectomy?**

(1) Simple hysterectomy means removal of the uterus.

(2) Supracervical hysterectomy means removal of the uterine body while leaving the cervical portion of the uterus in place.

(3) Total hysterectomy is the removal of the uterus as well as the cervix.

○ **Describe the various surgical approaches to hysterectomy.**

(1) Abdominal hysterectomy is performed through an abdominal incision.

(2) Vaginal hysterectomy is performed through the vagina.

(3) Total laparoscopic hysterectomy is a hysterectomy where the uterosacral/cardinal ligaments are secured laparoscopically and the cervix is completely freed from the vagina.

(4) Laparoscopic-assisted vaginal hysterectomy (LAVH) is a hysterectomy performed primarily via the vaginal approach and the laparoscopic component is completed above the uterine vessels.

(5) Radical hysterectomy is the removal of the uterus, the upper 25% of the vagina, all of the uterovesical and uterosacral ligaments, and the entire parametrium on either side, as well as pelvic lymph node dissection.

(6) Robotic-assisted hysterectomy is performed with the aid of the da Vinci robot system.

○ **What percentage of hysterectomies are performed via each route?**

Abdominal 66%, vaginal 22%, and 12% laparoscopic.

○ **What is the safest and most cost-effective route of hysterectomy?**

Vaginal hysterectomy, if feasible.

○ **What are advantages of vaginal hysterectomy versus abdominal hysterectomy?**

Shorter duration of hospital stay, faster return to normal activities, fewer febrile episodes, or infections.

○ **What are advantages of vaginal hysterectomy versus laparoscopic hysterectomy?**

Shorter operating time.

○ **What is the mortality associated with hysterectomy?**

12 deaths per 10,000 procedures—for all surgical indications.

○ **What are alternatives to hysterectomy?**

Medical: NSAIDs, antifibrinolytics, hormonal, GnRH agonists, aromatase inhibitors, and Mirena IUD.
Surgical: D & C, endometrial ablation, UAE, myomectomy, MRI-guided focused US treatment.

○ **When is hysterectomy indicated in the management of abnormal uterine bleeding (AUB)?**

Hysterectomy may be indicated for women with AUB who have completed their childbearing, particularly if the bleeding is severe and/or recurrent, and unresponsive to hormonal therapy and endometrial curettage.

○ **Compare outcomes between endometrial ablation, endometrial resection, and hysterectomy in the treatment of AUB.**

Pinion et al. found that hysteroscopic ablation had fewer complications and a shorter postoperative recovery, but overall satisfaction was higher with hysterectomy.

○ **When is hysterectomy indicated for adenomyosis?**

Symptomatic patients who do not experience relief with D & C and hormonal therapy, and who have completed their childbearing, can be offered hysterectomy.

○ **What are nonsurgical options for uterine prolapse?**

Pessary.

○ **When is hysterectomy indicated in treating uterine prolapse?**

When the symptoms are, especially in the patient's view, severe enough to justify the risks of surgery. Hysterectomy does not necessarily need to be done as part of an operation to correct stress incontinence. A retropubic urethropexy may be done with the uterus left in place.

○ **What is the relationship of the ureter to cervix with uterine prolapse?**

The cervix descends farther than the ureter by a 3:1 ratio. For every 3 cm the cervix descends, the ureter drops 1 cm and the gap between the ureter and the cervix widens by 2 cm.

○ **When is hysterectomy indicated in the treatment of leiomyomata uteri?**

If the patient has no symptoms, treatment can often be expectant. In women who have completed their childbearing and who have symptoms related to myomas, hysterectomy represents the definitive cure.

○ **What are the ACOG guidelines for hysterectomy for leiomyomata?**

(1) Asymptomatic, but abdominally palpable, and of concern to the patient or

(2) Excessive uterine bleeding: With evidence of profuse bleeding with flooding/clots or repetitive periods lasting >8 days, or anemia or

(3) Pelvic discomfort: Acute and severe, chronic lower abdominal pain or low back pressure or bladder pressure with urinary frequency.

○ **When doing a hysterectomy for leiomyomata, what is the chance of discovering a leiomyosarcoma?**

About 0.2% to 0.3%.

○ **What are the indications of cesarean hysterectomy?**

• Uterine rupture.
• An unrepairable uterine scar.
• Laceration of major uterine vessels.
• Placenta previa or accreta, unreducible uterine inversion.
• Placental abruption.
• Uterine atony unresponsive to conservative management.
• Severe cervical dysplasia or early cervical cancer may prompt a planned caesarean hysterectomy.

○ **What are the major causes of morbidity associated with cesarean hysterectomy?**

Febrile morbidity and injury to the urinary tract are more common than in the nonpregnant patient, and blood loss is usually much greater because of the hypertrophy of the uterus and the vessels. Elective cesarean hysterectomy is known to carry an average blood loss of 1,500 mL and should therefore not routinely be done for sterilization or for trivial indications.

○ **What other obstetrical problems may require hysterectomy?**

Occasionally, septic abortion fails to respond to medical management and must be treated with hysterectomy. Abdominal, cervical, and interstitial pregnancies may also result in hysterectomy.

○ **When is hysterectomy indicated in pelvic inflammatory disease (PID)?**

Approximately 20% of patients with tubo-ovarian abscess will fail to respond to antibiotics and/or colpotomy drainage. These women are usually treated with total abdominal hysterectomy bilateral salpingo-oophorectomy (TAH-BSO). Ruptured tubo-ovarian abscess may also be treated with TAH-BSO. Hysterectomy may also be recommended for patients with chronic PID who have completed childbearing, or who are not interested in assisted reproductive technologies.

○ **When is hysterectomy indicated for cervical intraepithelial neoplasia (CIN)?**

If there is persistent CIN 2 or 3 on follow-up after LEEP or conization, then re-excision is indicated. If re-excision is found to be technically impractical, or if the woman has definitively completed childbearing, then hysterectomy is an option, but conization should be performed for frozen section prior to the hysterectomy to look for invasive cancer. If cancer is found by frozen section, radical hysterectomy may be appropriate; if no cancer is found, then simple hysterectomy is appropriate.

○ **What are the classifications of radical hysterectomy?**

- Class I: Extrafascial hysterectomy: incised pubocervical fascia allowing lateral deflection of ureter allowing for complete excision of cervix.
  - Indication: CIN/CIS cervix.
- Class II: Modified radical: Uterus, upper third of vagina, cervix, paracervical-parametrial tissue, lymph node dissection, washings, biopsies allowing for removal of paracervical tissue, while preserving blood supply to ureters and bladder.
  - Indication: Microinvasive cervical cancer.
- Class II: Meigs-Wertheim radical: Same as Class II but wider excision of parametrial/cervical tissue allowing uterine artery to be ligated at it's origin from the internal iliac artery.
  - Indication: Stage Ib and IIa cervical cancer.
- Class IV: Complete removal of periureteral tissue and ¾ of vagina while preserving the bladder.
- Class V: Removal of ureter (reimplantation-ureteroneocystostomy) and/ or bladder.

○ **When is hysterectomy indicated in the management of endometrial hyperplasia?**

Adenomatous hyperplasia with cytologic atypia is considered a precancerous lesion, and should be treated with hysterectomy except under very special circumstances. Less severe forms of hyperplasia, without cytologic atypia, can be managed medically. Hysterectomy for hyperplasia may be done vaginally or abdominally.

○ **What type of hysterectomy is done for endometrial cancer?**

Systematic surgical staging for endometrial cancer requires TAH with BSO, peritoneal washings, biopsies of any suspicious lesions, and pelvic +/− paraaortic lymphadenectomy. If papillary serous or clear cell carcinoma is present, then omental biopsy is required for full staging.

○ **What procedures are used in the treatment of uterine sarcoma?**

TAH, BSO, pelvic washings, and pelvic and paraaortic lymphadenectomy make up the appropriate surgical treatment and staging of uterine sarcoma. Postoperative radiation and chemotherapy may be of benefit, but this is an evolving area.

○ **When is hysterectomy used in the treatment of gestational trophoblastic disease (GTD)?**

In women who have completed their childbearing, hysterectomy performed during the first cycle of chemotherapy can reduce the total amount of chemotherapy required to achieve complete remission. Recurrence rates after successful treatment in these cases (with or without hysterectomy) are <5%.

Early hysterectomy is of no benefit in women with high-risk metastatic GTD with any of the following:

- hCG >40 k.
- Brain or liver metastases.
- Antecedent term pregnancy.
- >4 months since last pregnancy, or prior chemotherapy).

○ **Is hysterectomy always part of the surgical management of ovarian cancer?**

Systematic surgical staging and debulking is required for ovarian cancer. The staging procedure includes TAH, BSO, pelvic washings and cytology, inspection of all peritoneal surfaces with debulking of any visible tumor, bilateral pelvic and paraaortic lymphadenectomy, omentectomy, and peritoneal biopsies. In younger women desiring fertility who at the time of operation are found to have ovarian cancer that is low grade and confined to one ovary, the staging procedure may be modified to leave the uterus and uninvolved ovary in place.

○ **What workup should be done before recommending hysterectomy for chronic pelvic pain (CPP)?**

Other potential sources of chronic pelvic pain (CPP), many of them nongynecologic, should be ruled out. Psychiatric, musculoskeletal, gastrointestinal, and urinary tract sources are important to exclude.

○ **What preoperative testing should be done in patients scheduled for hysterectomy?**

- A thorough history and physical will reveal special needs as well as help in the evaluation of potential risks.
- Each patient should have normal cervical cytology or complete evaluation of abnormal cytology to exclude invasive malignancy.
- A complete blood count will give the opportunity to correct anemia and identify thrombocytopenia.
- A urine examination for blood and leukocytes is done.
- An EKG is generally done in healthy women over 35.
- A chest film is ordered for smokers and those with suspected pulmonary disease.
- Under special circumstances, intravenous pyelogram (IVP), computed tomography (CT) scan, mammogram, pulmonary function tests, colonoscopy, cystoscopy, or consultation from other medical specialists may be needed.

○ **When should IVP be done preoperatively?**

When the pelvic disease is extensive or located where the ureters may be compromised, such as with large adnexal masses or very large leiomyomata, or when extensive dissection is anticipated. Also, IVP should be done in women with Müllerian anomalies, since urinary collecting system anomalies are common in this group. If a previous pelvic operation may have injured the urinary tract, a pre-op IVP will help identify this.

○ **When should a "bowel prep" be done before hysterectomy?**

All hysterectomy patients should be instructed to eat light meals the day before surgery, and to remain NPO for 8 hours prior to surgery. Enemas may be given at home. A full mechanical bowel prep with electrolyte solution and antibiotics is reserved for those in whom bowel involvement is suspected: patients with bowel complaints, extensive endometriosis, or suspected ovarian cancer.

○ **What is the most frequent complication of hysterectomy?**

Infection. The most common organisms are those found in normal vaginal flora.

○ **Does pretreatment for bacterial vaginosis (BV) before hysterectomy reduce the rate of postoperative cuff cellulitis?**

No. Even though BV is associated with an increased risk of postoperative cuff cellulitis, pretreatment for BV does not appear to reduce this risk.

○ **What incisions are appropriate for abdominal hysterectomy?**

A midline vertical incision should be used in cases of suspected malignancy to facilitate access to the upper abdomen. For benign indications, a transverse Pfannenstiel incision is the most commonly used. A Maylard or Cherney incision may be used if exposure is difficult with the Pfannenstiel.

○ **When performing an abdominal hysterectomy, what should be done before making an incision?**

After induction of anesthesia, the bladder is emptied, and a pelvic examination is performed. The abdominal skin and vagina are then prepped and draped. Failure to perform an examination under anesthesia can result in the wrong incision being chosen, or an inappropriate operation being done.

○ **Which patients undergoing hysterectomy should receive perioperative antibiotic prophylaxis?**

All patients undergoing hysterectomy should receive antibiotic prophylaxis. The target in administering antibiotic prophylaxis is to have the antibiotic present in tissue prior to incision and then throughout the procedure. The antibiotic chosen should have a spectrum broad enough to cover the typical organisms found during the procedure—gram positive for skin and gram negative for abdominopelvic organisms.

○ **From a historical perspective, why are most abdominal hysterectomies total rather than supracervical and how has this changed?**

Before 1950, cervical carcinoma was the most common female genital cancer in the United States. Although this is still true worldwide, the incidence of cervix cancer in the United States has fallen dramatically. Cervical stump cancer is difficult to treat, and therefore carries a poor prognosis. Therefore, before widespread Pap smear screening, it was felt that the cervix should almost always be removed. Recently there has been renewed interest in supracervical hysterectomy because it is technically easier, and is associated with fewer surgical risks.

○ **What are contraindications for supracervical hysterectomy?**

Recent or recurrent cervical dysplasia, endometrial hyperplasia, or a gynecologic neoplasm.

○ **What percentage of women experience postoperative cyclical vaginal bleeding after a supracervical hysterectomy?**

5% to 20%.

○ **What is the percentage of women who have a reoperation for trachelectomy after a supracervical hysterectomy?**

1% to 3%.

○ **What is the role of LAVH?**

LAVH is associated with faster postoperative recovery and less pain than abdominal hysterectomy. However, LAVH offers no advantages over simple vaginal hysterectomy when vaginal hysterectomy can be done. LAVH has its chief utility in detecting and possibly correcting pelvic adhesive disease that would otherwise make vaginal hysterectomy more technically difficult and potentially dangerous. A further use of laparoscopic assistance is the ligation of the infundibulopelvic ligaments when they are technically difficult to reach via the vaginal approach.

○ **What are the disadvantages of laparoscopic hysterectomy?**

Longer operating times and higher genitourinary injuries.

○ **What are the advantages of laparoscopic hysterectomy?**

Shorter hospital stays, faster return to normal activity, lower EBL/smaller drop in hemoglobin, and fewer wound infections.

○ **When using a self-retaining retractor in a transverse incision, one must be aware of what potential nerve injury?**

The lateral femoral cutaneous nerve.

○ **Which ligament is divided first in performing abdominal hysterectomy?**

The round ligament. In cases where severe anatomic distortion or adhesions are found, the round ligament will almost always be identifiable, and can be followed to the uterus.

○ **If the adnexa are to be left in, where are the next clamps placed?**

On the tube and utero-ovarian ligament, as close to the uterus as possible. A window can be made in the peritoneum inferior to the fallopian tube; a clamp is then placed across the tube and the utero-ovarian ligament, just next to the uterus. This preserves the blood vessels located in the broad ligament as much as possible.

○ **What must be identified and located prior to clamping the infundibulopelvic ligament?**

The ureter. The most common site of ureteral injury is at the pelvic brim near the infundibulopelvic ligament and the most common procedure during which it is injured is abdominal hysterectomy.

○ **When is the ureter most likely to be injured?**

During attempts to obtain hemostasis.

○ **Why are the anterior and posterior broad ligament peritoneum incised prior to clamping the uterine vessels?**

This procedure, often referred to as "skeletonizing" the uterine vessels, aids in avoiding injury to the ureters and bladder, and provides a smaller pedicle that is less likely to slip out of a clamp.

○ **The blood supply to this organ crosses over the ureter 2 cm lateral to the cervix.**

Uterus.

○ **What is the purpose of incising the anterior leaf of the broad ligament?**

To facilitate dissection of the bladder from the lower uterine segment. In order to perform a TAH, the bladder must be completely mobilized.

○ **Where are the ureters located when the uterine vessels are being clamped?**

The ureter passes underneath the uterine artery ("water under the bridge") very close to the level of the internal cervical os. If the bladder has been mobilized, and the uterine vessels skeletonized, the ureter will be about 1 1/2 to 2 cm inferior and lateral to the uterine vessel clamps.

○ **Why are the uterine arteries usually doubly clamped abdominally, while they are only singly clamped during a vaginal hysterectomy?**

Double clamps are useful abdominally because there is a danger of tissue slipping out of a single clamp and the uterine artery retracting. Attempts at reclamping a retracted vessel may result in injury to the ureter. When operating vaginally, there is not enough room between the ureter and the uterine artery to safely apply two clamps. Curved Heaney clamps are designed to be used as single vascular clamps.

○ **What structures must be avoided when clamping the uterosacral ligaments?**

The pelvic portion of the ureter and the anterior rectal wall.

○ **What mistake in performing a TAH is most likely to result in a vesicovaginal fistula?**

Inadequate lateral and inferior mobilization of the bladder can result in unrecognized bladder injury and formation of a vesicovaginal fistula.

○ **What is an intrafascial TAH, and what are the advantages of this technique?**

An intrafascial hysterectomy is one in which the cervix is removed by placing the cardinal ligament clamps inside the pubovesicocervical fascia. This is done by making a V-shaped incision in the pubovesicocervical fascia anterior to the cervix just below the internal os. The fascia can then be reflected laterally. This is a safer technique since it avoids most bladder and ureteral injuries. It is appropriate only with benign disease.

○ **What is the purpose of suspending the vaginal cuff after removing the uterus?**

To avoid vaginal vault prolapse and enterocele formation later on.

○ **How is the vaginal cuff suspended after TAH?**

The posterior vaginal cuff is sutured to the uterosacral ligaments. In a patient with a deep cul-de-sac, a posterior cul-de-sac obliteration may also be performed using the Moschcowitz or Halban technique.

○ **At what point in abdominal hysterectomy do the most urinary tract injuries take place?**

During removal of the cervix.

○ **In addition to careful surgical technique, what can be done to reduce the risk of undiagnosed urinary tract injuries at the time of hysterectomy?**

Intraoperative cystourethroscopy is a low-risk, simple procedure that can identify undiagnosed injury to the urinary tract. Routine use of cystourethroscopy at the time of pelvic surgery is controversial, but should be considered for procedures in which the risk of urinary tract injury is 1% to 2% or greater.

○ **When performing a supracervical hysterectomy, at what point is the uterus amputated from the cervix?**

After ligation of the uterine vessels, the uterus is amputated just below the internal os.

○ **How is the cervical stump closed?**

A V- or conical-shaped portion of the cervical stroma is removed to facilitate closure. The remaining endocervix may be cored out or cauterized. Then the cervical stump is closed and suspended using the round ligaments. The cervix may be cauterized transvaginally at the end of the case.

○ **What factors influence route and method of hysterectomy?**

Vaginal/uterine size and shape, extent of extrauterine disease, need for concurrent procedures, hospital technology, and an informed patients preference.

○ **What factors are important for a successful vaginal hysterectomy?**

Adequate introitus, pubic arch >90°, uterine mobility (previous vaginal delivery or prolapse), and uterine size ≤12 weeks (280 g).

○ **What are relative contraindications for vaginal hysterectomy?**

Prior cesarean delivery, nulliparity, and adnexal mass.

○ **What are absolute contraindications for vaginal hysterectomy?**

Lack of descensus, extensive adhesions, and contracted pelvis.

○ **Is the risk of ureteral injury greater with abdominal hysterectomy or vaginal hysterectomy?**

Abdominal hysterectomy has a greater risk.

○ **Some surgeons inject a dilute solution of Pitressin into the vaginal mucosa just before beginning a vaginal hysterectomy. In whom must this be avoided?**

In hypertensives and patients with cardiac arrhythmias.

○ **What maneuvers during vaginal hysterectomy facilitate entry into the posterior cul-de-sac without injury to the rectum?**

Upward (anterior) and outward (caudad) traction applied to the cervix along with retraction of the posterior vagina places the cul-de-sac peritoneum on tension, making entry into the correct space easier.

○ **What should be done if the rectum is inadvertently entered during attempted entry into the cul-de-sac?**

The rectum should be repaired in layers at that time.

○ **What should be done if fluid is encountered when opening the posterior cul-de-sac?**

Approximately 75 to 100 mL of peritoneal fluid is a normal finding. However, if a much larger collection of fluid is encountered, the operator should carefully explore the exposed pelvis for findings that might necessitate an abdominal approach.

○ **What maneuvers can be used to help identify the anterior cul-de-sac?**

Moving the cervix up and down will help identify the point of attachment between the vagina and the cervix. Strong downward traction on the cervix helps identify the relatively avascular plane between bladder and cervix. A Foley bulb can help to identify the location of the bladder. Methylene blue can also be placed in the bladder. Often, a finger can be passed over the uterus from the posterior cul-de-sac to help identify the proper space. However, as long as the bladder is dissected off of the cervix, entry into the anterior cul-de-sac can be delayed.

○ **What should be done if the bladder is inadvertently entered while trying to enter the anterior cul-de-sac?**

The bladder should be closed at that point.

○ **How can ureteral injuries best be avoided while performing vaginal hysterectomy?**

By maintaining downward (outward) traction on the cervix, by carefully dissecting the bladder off the cervix, and by placing clamps as close to the cervix and uterus as possible.

○ **What maneuvers can be used vaginally to facilitate removal of a large uterine fundus?**

The size of the uterus can be reduced by coring, wedging, morcellating, or bisecting the fundus after the uterine arteries have been ligated. Care must be taken to avoid injury to a loop of bowel that may be adherent to the uterus.

○ **What is the most common reason for inadequate vaginal vault support after vaginal hysterectomy?**

Failure to recognize and repair an enterocele. An enterocele should always be checked for by placing a finger into the posterior cul-de-sac.

○ **What is the advantage of closing the peritoneum after vaginal hysterectomy?**

Peritoneal closure extraperitonealizes the pedicle stumps. Thus, postoperative bleeding is more likely to present vaginally and be recognized earlier than if it occurs intraperitoneally. Also, peritoneal closure can incorporate ligation of an enterocele sac.

○ **How should the vaginal vault be supported after vaginal hysterectomy?**

The uterosacral ligaments are used to support the vaginal vault. Often a modified McCall culdoplasty is performed. With uterine prolapse, the uterosacral ligaments may be attenuated, and need to be shortened in order to provide adequate support.

○ **How should the vaginal cuff be closed after vaginal hysterectomy?**

Longitudinally as it lengthens the vagina.

○ **Do the ovaries continue to function normally after hysterectomy?**

Yes. In almost all women undergoing hysterectomy prior to the natural menopause, the ovaries continue to produce normal levels of hormones in a cyclic fashion until the natural age of menopause.

○ **In women 40 to 64 years of age undergoing hysterectomy, how many undergo elective oophorectomy?**

50% to 66%.

○ **What does the term "incidental" oophorectomy indicate?**

Incidental oophorectomy refers to removal of the ovaries at the time of surgery performed for another indication, occurring by chance or without consequence. This is in contrast to prophylactic oophorectomy, when removal of the ovaries is performed for future benefit.

○ **When is a prophylactic BSO justified with a hysterectomy?**

Patient request, family history of ovarian cancer (only 5–10% genetic), and prevention of ovarian cancer (1.4% lifetime risks).

○ **What are downfalls of doing a prophylactic BSO with hysterectomy?**

Need for hormone replacement, possible re-operation for future de-novo ovarian cancer (0.1% risk of ovarian cancer after hysterectomy) increased risk of death from CAD and all nonovarian cancers, and osteoporosis.

○ **If premenopausal, what are the risk of prophylactic BSO at the time of hysterectomy?**

Increase risk of cognitive dysfunction (anxiety/depression, dementia, and Parkinson disease).

○ **In women undergoing prophylactic oophorectomy at the time of vaginal hysterectomy, in what percentage of patients can the ovaries be removed successfully?**

65% to 97%. Laparoscopic assistance can be used to facilitate the removal of the majority of the remainder.

○ **How often does ovarian cancer occur in hysterectomy patients with retained ovaries?**

Approximately 0.1% of these women develop ovarian cancer. This represents a relative risk of about 0.6 as compared with women who have not had a hysterectomy. Stated another way, of those women who develop ovarian cancer, between 4% and 14% have had an antecedent hysterectomy during which the ovaries were not removed.

○   **Why would hysterectomy reduce the risk of ovarian cancer?**

Several possibilities exist. These include the opportunity to examine the ovaries at the time of hysterectomy and remove the ones that are abnormal. Protection of the ovaries from environmental carcinogens, a possible reduction or alteration in ovarian blood flow, or more frequent prior use of oral contraceptives could also be mechanisms.

○   **After hysterectomy with ovarian conservation, how many patients will require a subsequent operation for ovarian or tubal pathology?**

Approximately 1% to 2%.

○   **If granulation tissue forms at the vaginal cuff, how should this be treated?**

This granulation tissue can be easily treated in the office by touching it with silver nitrate.

○   **How should prolapse of a fallopian tube be recognized and treated?**

This rare complication is usually recognized when suspected granulation tissue fails to go away with silver nitrate treatment, or when the "granulation tissue" seems to have a canal. This tissue can be excised vaginally, and the cuff then closed. Most often, this is done in the operating room.

○   **In the United States, what is the most common cause of GU tract fistula?**

While most fistulae worldwide are the result of obstetric trauma, the most common cause in the United States is pelvic surgery. Most follow an abdominal hysterectomy for benign disease.

REFERENCE

Pinion SB, Parkin DE, Abramovich DR. Randomised trial of hysterectomy, endometrial laser ablation, and transcervical endometrial resection for dysfunctional uterine bleeding. *BMJ*. 1994;309(6960):979–83.

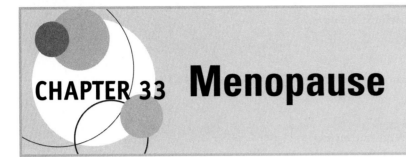

CHAPTER 33 Menopause

Kristin Van Heertum, MD

EPIDEMIOLOGY

○ **What is the definition of menopause?**

Cessation of menses for 12 months due to the loss of ovarian activity.

○ **What is the definition of perimenopause?**

The period of time immediately before and after menopause ending prior to completion of 12 months after the last menstrual period.

○ **Approximately how long is the perimenopausal period?**

Four years.

○ **What is the definition of the climacteric?**

The transition from the reproductive stages of life to the postmenopausal years, a period marked by waning ovarian function—this includes perimenopause and menopause.

○ **What is the mean age for menopause?**

51.4 years.

○ **What percentage of their lifetime will most women spend in postmenopausal life?**

30%. Given a life expectancy of 75 years and a median age of 51 for menopause.

○ **How much of the female population in the United States is currently postmenopausal?**

20%. This is increasing because life expectancy is also increasing.

○ **What causes earlier menopause?**

Smoking, low weight, some women who had hysterectomies, malnourishment, living at high altitudes, mosaic Turner's, and genetic predisposition. Age of menarche, race, family history, and parity do not influence age of menopause.

○ **How much earlier does menopause occur in smokers?**

About 2 years.

○ **What percentage of women will undergo premature menopause (before age 40)?**

1%.

○ **What percentage of women will undergo late menopause (after age 55)?**

5%.

○ **What percentage of women will undergo early menopause (between ages 40 and 45)?**

5%.

○ **What is the weight of the postmenopausal ovary?**

5 g.

○ **What histological changes occur in the ovary with menopause?**

Lack of follicles and a prominent stroma.

○ **What are the common changes associated with estrogen depletion?**

Menstrual cycle changes, cardiovascular disease, osteoporosis, genitourinary atrophy, vasomotor psychological, and sexual symptoms.

HORMONE PRODUCTION

○ **What happens to the menstrual cycle with age?**

Initially, the follicular phase and cycle decreases and then increases prior to menopause, and luteal phase defects may occur.

○ **What happens to gonadotropin levels in the premenopausal years?**

Follicle-stimulating hormone (FSH) increases (as a result of decreased inhibin production from granulosa cells) and luteinizing hormone (LH) remains the same.

○ **Why cannot FSH levels be suppressed in menopause?**

Inhibin production from granulosa cells is lost. Inhibin normally suppresses FSH levels prior to menopause. Inhibin is the hormone that starts to decline first in the climacteric.

○ **What FSH values are indicative of menopause?**

Levels >35 IU/L, but may vary based on laboratory.

○ **What are the expected changes in gonadotropin levels after menopause?**

FSH increases 10- to 20-fold and LH increases 3-fold, reaching a maximum 1 to 3 years after menopause.

○ **Which hormones decline as a result of menopause?**
Estrogen, androstenedione, and progesterone.

○ **Which hormones decline as a result of age?**
Dehydroepiandrosterone (DHEA), dehydroepiandrosterone sulfate (DHEA-S), and testosterone.

○ **What is the level of DHEA-S in a 70-year-old compared with peak levels in a 25-year-old?**
10% to 20% of peak.

○ **Where is most of the postmenopausal androstenedione produced?**
The adrenal gland.

○ **How much estradiol (E_2) is produced each day in postmenopausal women?**
6 μg/day, decreased from 80 to 500 μg/day in reproductive age women.

○ **How much estrone (E_1) is produced each day in postmenopausal women?**
40 μg/day, decreased from 80 to 300 μg/day in reproductive age women.

○ **What is the circulating estradiol (E_2) level in women after menopause?**
10 to 20 pg/mL (40 to 70 pmol/L).

○ **What is the primary source of estrogen in postmenopausal women?**
Peripheral conversion of adrenal and ovarian androgens by extraglandular aromatase in adipose.

○ **What is the predominant estrogen of the postmenopausal woman?**
Estrone (E_1).

○ **What is the biological potency of estrone compared with estradiol?**
It is only one third as potent as estradiol.

○ **What happens to progesterone production in menopause?**
Progesterone is no longer produced.

○ **What hormone is secreted more by the postmenopausal ovary than the premenopausal ovary?**
Testosterone; prior to menopause the ovary contributes 25% of circulating testosterone and in menopause the ovary contributes 40% of circulating testosterone.

○ **Why does the postmenopausal ovary produce more testosterone than the premenopausal ovary?**
Elevated gonadotropins stimulate the stromal tissue to secrete testosterone.

○   **Although the ovary produces increased testosterone in menopause, why is the total amount of testosterone not increased?**

Androstenedione is reduced, adrenal testosterone is reduced, and sex hormone binding globulin (SHBG) levels are reduced.

○   **Does serum testosterone change over the menopausal transition?**

No.

○   **What is the cause of mild hirsutism in menopause?**

Increased free androgen to estrogen ratio as a result of decreased SHBG and estrogen.

○   **What increases aromatization of androgens to estrogens?**

Age and weight. Aromatase activity increases twofold in the perimenopausal period and adipose tissue is a rich source of aromatase.

○   **In which tissues has aromatase been identified?**

Liver, fat, muscle, and certain hypothalamic nuclei.

CARDIOVASCULAR DISEASE

○   **What is the leading cause of death for women?**

Heart disease, followed by malignancies, cerebrovascular disease, and motor vehicle accidents.

○   **How many deaths are attributed to cardiovascular disease in women over 50?**

>50%.

○   **What is the risk of heart disease after menopause compared with premenopause?**

Twice the risk.

○   **What are the risk factors for cardiovascular disease?**

Hypertension, smoking, diabetes, hypercholesterolemia, obesity, and family history.

○   **Does the onset of heart disease occur at the same age in men as it does in women?**

No. Typically the onset of heart disease occurs 10 years later in women. Similarly, myocardial infarction and sudden death typically occur 20 years later in women than in men.

○   **What cholesterol fraction is associated with atherosclerosis in women?**

High-density lipoprotein (HDL) is more closely associated than low-density lipoprotein (LDL).

○   **How important are triglycerides in predicting coronary risk?**

Triglycerides are uniquely predictive in older women, especially at levels above 400 mg/dL.

○ **What contributes to cardioprotection in women?**

Higher HDLs, 10 mg/dL higher than in men, an effect of estrogen.

○ **What are the changes in cholesterol fractions at the age of menopause?**

HDL decreases, LDL increases, and the average cholesterol increases to levels higher than in men.

○ **What is estrogen's effect upon lipids and lipoproteins?**

It increases HDL and decreases total cholesterol and LDL.

○ **What lipoprotein-independent mechanisms of estrogen may protect against cardiovascular disease?**

Vasodilatation, decreased platelet aggregation, decreased smooth muscle cell proliferation of arterial vessels, direct inotropic actions on the heart, antioxidant activity, favorable impact on clotting mechanisms, inhibition of intimal thickening, inhibition of macrophage foam cell formation, improved glucose metabolism, and decreased insulin levels.

○ **Are estrogen and progesterone receptors present in the vascular tree?**

Yes. In the endothelium and smooth muscles of arterial vessels.

○ **How does estrogen exert a cardioprotective effect through the vasculature?**

Vasodilatation and decreased peripheral resistance.

○ **How does estrogen exert cardioprotection via endothelium-dependent mechanisms?**

Augmentation of nitric oxide and prostacyclin leading to vasodilation and decreased platelet aggregation.

○ **What direct effects does estrogen have on the heart?**

Increases left ventricular diastolic filling and stroke volume, delaying age-related decreases in compliance.

○ **What effect does acute administration of estradiol have on myocardial ischemia in women with coronary artery disease?**

Signs of ischemia on electrocardiograms are delayed and exercise tolerance is increased.

○ **How does estrogen decrease LDL levels?**

It increases hepatic LDL catabolism and increases LDL receptors.

○ **How does estrogen increase HDL levels?**

It inhibits hepatic lipase activity.

○ **How does estrogen replacement therapy exert an antioxidant cardioprotective effect?**

It inhibits LDL oxidation and resultant endothelial vasospasm.

○ **What other antioxidants may decrease the risk of coronary artery disease?**

Vitamin E and β-carotene (the prohormone of vitamin A).

O   **What effect does estrogen have on body fat distribution?**

It prevents the tendency to increase central body fat with aging.

O   **What is the relationship between truncal adiposity and coronary heart disease?**

An increased waist to hip circumference ratio is associated with an increased risk of coronary heart disease. Truncal adiposity is associated with an androgenic state, hypertension, insulin resistance, hyperinsulinemia, and an atherogenic lipid profile, all risk factors for coronary heart disease.

O   **What lipid profiles are correlated with women who have a central body fat distribution?**

Positive correlation with increases in total cholesterol, triglycerides, and LDL and negatively correlated with HDL.

O   **What effect does <u>oral</u> estrogen have on diabetes?**

The Nurses Health Study documented a 20% decreased risk of noninsulin dependent diabetes in current users of estrogen.

O   **Does postmenopausal estrogen replacement therapy adversely affect hypertension?**

No.

O   **What did the Postmenopausal Estrogen/Progestin Interventions (PEPI) trial demonstrate regarding hormone replacement therapy (HRT) and cardiovascular disease risk factors?**

Estrogen as well as estrogen progestin combinations had a favorable impact on cardiovascular risk factors, an increase in HDL, a decrease in LDL, as well as prevention of the age-related increase in fibrinogen.

O   **In the PEPI trial, which progesterone combined with conjugated equine estrogen had the most favorable effect on HDL?**

Cyclic micronized progesterone resulted in a significantly greater increase in HDL than either sequential or cyclic medroxyprogesterone acetate.

O   **What did the Women's Health Initiative (WHI) show regarding cardiovascular risk of HRT?**

An increase in coronary events with Prempro and no significant difference with Premarin.

OSTEOPOROSIS

O   **What is osteoporosis?**

A progressive, systemic skeletal disease characterized by low bone density and microarchitectural deterioration of bone tissue, leading to an increase in bone fragility and susceptibility to fracture (World Health Organization).

O   **In what type of bone is resorption more prevalent?**

Trabecular bone, which is the predominant type of bone in the spine, because it is most sensitive to changes in estrogen levels.

O   **What is the role of osteoclasts?**

They absorb and remove osseous tissue, forming lacuna.

○ **What is the role of osteoblasts?**

They deposit the osseous matrix called osteoid (*B* is for *build*).

○ **At what age does bone loss begin on most women?**

In the spine (trabecular bone), bone loss typically begins at age 20. However, the femur, which is made up of cortical bone, maximum density is typically in the late 20s.

○ **At what age does bone resorption exceed formation?**

40, by about 0.5%.

○ **After menopause, what is the percentage of bone loss per year?**

5% per year in trabecular bone, 1% per year total bone loss.

○ **What is the most important factor associated with bone loss?**

Age.

○ **What are the other risk factors for osteoporosis?**

Family history, early menopause (younger than 45), Caucasian or Asian race, low body weight, smoking, excessive alcohol use, sedentary lifestyle, low calcium intake, low vitamin D intake, poor health, impaired vision, natural menopause, surgical menopause, glucocorticoids, and caffeine intake.

○ **What medications are associated with bone loss?**

Corticosteroids, thyroid hormone, anticonvulsants, and heparin.

○ **What mechanisms contribute to osteoporosis?**

Menopause, thyrotoxicosis, glucocorticoid excess, hyperparathyroidism, multiple myeloma, leukemia or lymphoma, alcoholism, long-term heparin therapy, immobilization, and metastatic cancer.

○ **What preventive measures can be taken for osteoporosis early in life?**

Improved calcium intake, diet, weight-bearing exercise, avoidance of alcohol and smoking, and maintenance of normal menstrual cycles.

○ **What is the most common site of fractures in menopause?**

Vertebral fractures, they account for 50% of all fractures. 25% of women over age 70 will experience vertebral fractures.

○ **What is the expected loss in height as a result of vertebral fractures in untreated postmenopausal women?**

2.5 inches (6.4 cm).

○ **What percentage of patients will die within 1 year after hip fracture?**

20%, due to complications of prolonged immobilization.

○ **How does estrogen therapy help maintain bone mass?**

A direct effect on osteoblasts, improved intestinal absorption of calcium, and decreased renal excretion of calcium.

○ **What is the total calcium requirement to minimize bone loss in postmenopausal women <u>not</u> taking estrogen replacement?**

1500 mg.

○ **What is the total calcium requirement to minimize bone loss in women on estrogen replacement therapy?**

1200 mg.

○ **In addition to calcium, in women over the age of 70, what other supplementation should be included for osteoporosis fracture prevention?**

Vitamin D 800 IU, especially if in Northern latitudes.

○ **Does skim milk have less calcium than whole milk?**

No. Since calcium is water-soluble skim milk has more calcium than whole milk.

○ **What disease process can be unmasked with high calcium supplementation?**

Asymptomatic hyperparathyroidism.

○ **What other agents are known to reduce bone resorption?**

Calcitonin, fluoride, androgens and bisphosphonates (etidronate disodium, risedronate, alendronate), SERMS (selective estrogen receptor modulators such as raloxifene).

○ **Why is not calcitonin more widely used for osteoporosis?**

It is expensive and must be administered parenterally or nasally, and it is effective only against vertebral fracture reduction.

○ **How often are vertebral compression fractures asymptomatic?**

60% to 66% of the time.

○ **How many osteoporotic fractures occur each year in the United States?**

Approximately 1.3 million.

○ **How many of these are vertebral fractures?**

About 50%. Hip fractures account for another 25%.

○ **What percentage of Caucasian women will experience a hip fracture?**

20%.

○ **What percentage of bone is resting at any one time?**

88.

○   **What percentage of bone is remodeling (forming or resorbing) at any one time?**

12.

○   **What percentage of bone mass is formed in a young woman between the ages of 13 and 16?**

Almost 50.

○   **When does bone loss accelerate?**

After menopause, and the rapid loss continues for about 5 years. Accelerated bone loss has also been observed in women 2 to 3 years prior to the cessation of menstruation; the rate of bone loss was correlated to an elevation of FSH and bone turnover markers.

○   **What percentage of bone mass is lost in this time?**

20.

○   **Are osteoporotic fractures more common than heart attack, stroke, and breast cancer combined?**

Yes.

○   **What percentage increase in mortality is seen after hip fracture?**

24.

○   **What percentage of hip fracture survivors are incapacitated for an extended time?**

50.

○   **In women who have a vertebral fracture, what percentage will have another fracture within a year?**

19%. After one vertebral fracture, there is a fivefold increased risk of a second vertebral fracture and almost a twofold increased risk of a hip fracture.

○   **Does a hip fracture increase the risk of a second hip fracture?**

Yes.

○   **Which is more common, a fall causing a hip fracture or a fracture causing a fall?**

A fall causing a fracture is much more common.

○   **What are the secondary causes of osteoporosis?**

Low vitamin D intake, low calcium intake, irritable bowel syndrome, diabetes malabsorption syndromes, hyperparathyroidism, hyperthyroidism, malnutrition, liver disease, glucocorticoids, heparin, rheumatoid arthritis, and osteoarthritis.

○ **Who should have tests for bone mineral density (BMD) (DXA scan)?**

All women 65 years or older without risk factors.

All postmenopausal women younger than 65 with risk factors.

All postmenopausal women younger than 65 with a history of fracture.

All postmenopausal women considering therapy for osteoporosis.

All women on estrogen/progestogen therapy for a prolonged period (National Osteoporosis Foundation Guidelines).

○ **How is osteoporosis diagnosed? What is the most accurate technique available for measuring bone density?**

Using dual energy absorptiometry (DXA) measuring the hip and lumbar spine (central DXA). This is the most accurate technique available for measuring bone density. DXA scans are reported using a T score.

○ **What hip areas are routinely assessed for BMD using a DXA scan?**

The femoral neck, trochanter, Ward's triangle, and intertrochanter.

○ **What areas are most reproducible on DXA?**

A-P spine and femoral neck.

○ **What is the ideal screening interval for DXA?**

Every 2 years.

○ **Can a peripheral DXA (heel, finger, wrist) be used to diagnose osteoporosis?**

No. These are used to screen for osteoporosis. The diagnosis is made by central DXA.

○ **Can a peripheral DXA be used to predict fracture risk?**

Yes (NORA trial).

○ **What is the T score?**

A measurement of BMD that indicates the number of standard deviations above or below the average peak bone mass in a young woman.

○ **What does the T score indicate?**

A T score of −1.0 is one standard deviation below peak bone mass, and represents about a 10% loss in bone mass at the site measured.

○ **What is the Z score?**

This number indicates the number of standard deviations from average bone mass compared with a population the same age. If there is a significant variance, one should look for secondary causes of osteoporosis.

○ **Does the T score correlate with fracture risk?**

Yes. For each T score below normal the risk of fracture doubles at that site. (A T score of −1.0 doubles the fracture risk compared with a T score of 0.0.)

○ **How does age relate to fracture risk and T score?**

As age increases fracture risk increases at the same T score.

○ **Does the T score fully explain the fracture risk at one particular site?**

No. There are other characteristics that impact bone strength that are difficult to measure.

○ **What is the Fracture Risk Assessment tool (FRAX)?**

An online tool developed by the World Health Organization to predict an individual's 10-year fracture risk. It can be used with or without a bone mineral density result. It is used to help guide in treatment decisions.

○ **What impacts bone strength?**

Bone quality, bone turnover, and microarchitecture.

○ **Can you see a normal T score at one site and osteoporosis at another site in the same patient?**

Yes.

○ **What T score is considered normal?**

Above –1.0 (WHO).

○ **What T scores suggest low bone mass, or osteopenia?**

Between –1.0 and –2.5.

○ **What T score represents osteoporosis?**

Less than –2.5.

○ **What is severe osteoporosis?**

A T score of –2.5 or below with a previous fracture.

○ **When should treatment be started for osteoporosis?**

When the T score at the A-P spine or hip is –2.0 or lower without risk factors, or –1.5 or lower with risk factors (NOF Guidelines).

○ **What are biochemical markers of bone formation?**

Bone-specific alkaline phosphatase and osteocalcin.

○ **What are the biochemical markers for bone resorption?**

Pyridinoline, N-telopeptides, and c-telopeptides.

○ **Are biochemical markers usually used in individual patients to help diagnose osteoporosis?**

No. They are used more in research in large groups of patients to evaluate how effective a drug is regarding its effect on bone.

○ **What therapies are currently available to treat osteoporosis?**

Alendronate, risedronate, and ibandronate, which are bisphosphonates.

Raloxifene, a SERM.

Calcitonin nasal spray.

These are all antiresorptive agents—less bone resorbed by osteoclasts.

Another medication is teriparatide, a form of parathyroid hormone (PTH)—functions as an anabolic agent.

○ **What therapy is presently used only to prevent osteoporosis?**

Estrogen-progestin therapy.

○ **In the WHI trial, what effect did estrogen plus progestin have on fracture risk?**

There was a reduction in fractures of the spine and hip in patients who took estrogen plus progestin compared with placebo.

○ **Is it necessary to supplement an osteoporosis therapy drug with calcium and vitamin D to obtain maximal fracture protection?**

Yes.

○ **How important is it for a patient at risk of osteoporosis to exercise, specifically walking and upper body strengthening?**

Extremely important. This reduces the risk of falling and thus reduces the risk of fracture.

○ **Is long-term steroid use a risk factor for osteoporosis?**

Yes.

○ **How soon after starting steroids does one see significant bone loss?**

3 months.

○ **What percentage of patients taking prednisone 7.5 mg or greater develop an osteoporotic fracture?**

50.

○ **Can lower doses of steroids also increase risk of fracture?**

Yes.

○ **Does age or gender impact fracture risk if a person is on steroids?**

No.

○ **How do steroids affect bone?**

They cause a toxic effect on osteoblasts, which shortens their lifespan. Calcium absorption is blocked through the intestine. Calcium is also lost by the kidney, decreasing serum calcium. This causes PTH to be secreted, thereby increasing bone resorption.

○ **How soon after treatment is started should a repeat DXA be done?**

1 to 2 years. The sensitivity of DXA is such that it would take this long to see a meaningful change. One exception is a patient on steroids. In this situation, the DXA can be done as early as 6 months.

○ **What change would you expect to see after 1 to 2 years of treatment?**

The DXA should show stabilization or improvement in BMD.

○ **What if there is a significant loss (>4–5%) at 2 years?**

Check the Z score. If it is lower than expected, evaluate for secondary causes of osteoporosis.

○ **What logical steps can be suggested to a patient to prevent falls?**

Safeguard the home by removing electrical wires from the floor.
Remove throw rugs.
Improve lighting.
Evaluate the patient's vision.
Treat urinary incontinence—fewer nighttime awakenings and decrease urine leakage onto floor.

○ **Can smoking one pack per day throughout adulthood reduce bone density by as much as 10% by menopause?**

Yes.

○ **What percentage of patients with hip fractures have histological evidence of osteomalacia, the classic manifestation of vitamin D deficiency?**

30%.

○ **What is the largest source of dietary vitamin D?**

Milk.

GENITOURINARY CHANGES

○ **What genitourinary tissues are estrogen sensitive?**

The vagina, vulva, urethra, and trigone of the bladder.

○ **What vaginal symptoms are related to atrophy?**

Dryness, dyspareunia, and recurrent atrophic vaginitis.

○ **What causes dyspareunia in aging women?**

Decreased vaginal lubrication and elasticity.

○ **Is vaginal estrogen therapy more effective than moisturizers and lubricants?**

Yes.

○ **How much greater is the potency of vaginal conjugated estrogens than that of oral conjugate estrogens?**
Four times greater.

○ **What is the most common vulvar symptom of menopause relieved with estrogen replacement?**
Burning and pruritis secondary to atrophy.

○ **Pruritis is also the presenting complaint of vulvar dystrophies. What percentage of vulvar dystrophies are squamous cell carcinomas?**
5% on initial exam, another 5% may develop squamous cell carcinomas within 3–5 years after hypertrophic vulvar dystrophy is diagnosed.

○ **What is the most common cause of postmenopausal bleeding?**
Endometrial atrophy.

○ **Why does vaginitis increase during the postmenopausal years?**
Due to estrogen deficiency, the vaginal pH increases from 3.5–4.5 to 6.0–8.0, predisposing to colonization of bacterial pathogens.

○ **What cervical changes are associated with menopause?**
Stenosis, atrophy, erosion, and ulcers.

○ **What changes occur in the squamocolumnar junction and transformation zone?**
They migrate up into the endocervical canal.

○ **What urethral conditions can develop as a result of estrogen deficiency?**
Ectropion (urethral caruncle), diverticula, and urethrocoele.

○ **What is the most common problem in menopause related to urethral changes?**
Urethral syndrome, consisting of burning, frequency, hesitancy, nocturia, and urgency associated with sterile urine cultures.

○ **How is the urethral syndrome treated?**
Estrogen therapy.

○ **What urinary symptoms are associated with atrophy?**
Dysuria, urgency, and recurrent urinary tract infections.

○ **Does bacteriuria increase in menopause?**
Yes. The incidence of bacteriuria increases from 4% in reproductive age women to 7–10% in postmenopausal women. This is due to thinning of the urothelium, which predisposes to ascending infections, particularly with intercourse.

○ **Is urinary stress incontinence related to estrogen deficiency?**

Yes. Urethral shortening and decreased urethral closing pressures associated with atrophy may contribute to urinary incontinence.

○ **Can urge incontinence be treated with estrogen therapy?**

Yes.

○ **Can estrogen therapy improve urinary stress incontinence?**

There is conflicting data, but the best available evidence suggests estrogen therapy is not effective.

○ **What is the best initial therapy for urinary stress incontinence?**

Kegel exercises.

○ **What other treatments exist for urinary stress incontinence?**

Duloxetine (SNRI), collagen injections, and surgery.

VASOMOTOR AND PSYCHOLOGICAL SYMPTOMS

○ **What is a hot flash?**

Sudden onset of warmth and reddening of the skin beginning in the head spreading to the neck and chest, sometimes concluded by profuse perspiration, lasting a few seconds to several minutes. It is often accompanied by palpations and feelings of anxiety.

○ **What percentage of women experience hot flashes?**

75% to 85%.

○ **What is the physiology of the hot flash?**

It originates in the hypothalamus and represents thermoregulatory instability in response to estrogen fluctuation.

○ **How long do hot flashes typically continue?**

Typically 1 to 2 years, usually 5 years at most. The incidence of flashes is 80% at 1 year and 20% at 5 years.

○ **What physiologic changes are associated with the hot flash?**

An LH surge, an increase in body surface temperature, and skin conductance followed by a decline in core body temperature.

○ **What's the frequency of hot flashes?**

Usually several times a day. Can range from 1 to 2 daily to 1 per hour.

○ **Are hot flashes more common at night?**

Yes.

○ **What effect do "night sweats" (hot flashes at night) have?**

Interruption of sleep patterns and thus a decline in sleep quality and length.

○ **How does estrogen exert its effects on improving "quality of life" in postmenopausal women?**

Alleviation of hot flashes and improved quality of sleep leading to improved mood, memory, and quality of life.

○ **What alternatives to estrogen are partially effective in treating hot flashes?**

Clonidine, medroxyprogesterone acetate, methyldopa, SSRIs, gabapentin, and black cohosh.

○ **What alternatives to estrogen are <u>ineffective</u> in treating hot flashes?**

Bellergal, propranolol, vitamin E, and soy extracts.

○ **What alternatives to estrogen are currently recommended for the treatment of hot flashes?**

Transdermal clonidine 100 μg weekly, Effexor 37.5 to 75 mg qd, and black cohosh.

○ **Are there any safety data on black cohosh?**

Yes. For use up to 6 months.

POSTMENOPAUSAL BLEEDING AND ENDOMETRIAL CANCER

○ **What is the first diagnostic test recommended for postmenopausal bleeding if the uterus is normal?**

Endometrial biopsy.

○ **In the perimenopausal period, after exclusion of gynecological causes of dysfunctional uterine bleeding (DUB), what endocrine gland should be evaluated?**

The thyroid gland.

○ **What endometrial thickness on ultrasound requires biopsy in postmenopausal women?**

4 mm.

○ **How do you treat simple hyperplasia in <u>perimenopause</u>?**

Monthly oral progestin therapy, repeat biopsy in 6 months, if hyperplasia persists, D&C.

○ **How effective is monthly progestin therapy in treating simple hyperplasia?**

95% to 98% of the time.

○ **What is the incidence of endometrial hyperplasia after 1 year of unopposed estrogen (conjugated estrogen 0.625 mg or its equivalent)?**

20% incidence of hyperplasia, predominantly simple hyperplasia.

○ **When DUB in perimenopause is diagnosed, what are the treatment options?**

Observation, oral contraceptives, and progestational agents.

○   **What is the incidence of <u>adenomatous</u> or <u>atypical</u> hyperplasia in unopposed estrogen users?**
10% per year.

○   **What risks of progression to cancer are associated with the various types of endometrial hyperplasia?**

Simple hyperplasia without atypia	1%
Complex hyperplasia without atypia	3%
Simple hyperplasia with atypia	9%
Complex hyperplasia with atypia	30–50%

○   **What percentage of atypical endometrial hyperplasia will progress to cancer within 1 year?**
20% to 25%.

○   **What is the time required for endometrial hyperplasia to progress to cancer?**
5 years.

○   **What is the risk of endometrial cancer in postmenopausal women not on HRT?**
4 per 1000 (0.4%).

○   **What is the risk of endometrial cancer in postmenopausal women with abnormal uterine bleeding?**
20%.

○   **How much higher is the risk of endometrial cancer in patients on unopposed estrogen compared with the general population?**
2 to 10 times higher, depending on dose and duration of exposure.

○   **How long does the risk of endometrial cancer persist after discontinuation of estrogen?**
10 years.

○   **What characteristics of endometrial adenocarcinoma are present in patients on estrogen therapy?**
Most lesions are low grade and early stage, and associated with better survival.

○   **What is the 5-year survival rate in women whose uterine cancer was diagnosed while they were taking estrogen replacement therapy?**
95%.

○   **How does progesterone counter effect estrogen on endometrial growth?**
It decreases estrogen receptors, induces enzymatic conversion of estradiol to an excreted conjugate, estrone sulfate, and suppresses estrogen-induced oncogene transcription.

BREAST AND OVARIAN CANCER

○ **What are the top three types of cancer diagnosed in women?**

Breast cancer.

Lung cancer.

Colorectal cancer.

In men—Prostate (1), lung (2), and colorectal (3).

○ **What is the leading cause of cancer deaths in women?**

Lung cancer. Breast cancer is second.

○ **What is the leading gynecologic cancer in women?**

Endometrial cancer.

○ **What is the leading cause of gynecologic cancer deaths in women?**

Ovarian cancer.

○ **Is there an increased risk of breast cancer associated with estrogen replacement therapy?**

There may be a slightly increased risk of breast cancer especially with long duration of use (5 or more years in users of continuous combined therapy).

○ **Do estrogen users have improved breast cancer survival?**

Yes. This is probably as a result of earlier diagnosis but this is controversial after the results of the WHI.

○ **Does estrogen use affect breast cancer tumor differentiation?**

Yes. Women on estrogen develop better differentiated tumors.

○ **What is the diagnosis of an adnexal mass in menopause?**

Cancer, until proven otherwise.

○ **What type of adnexal mass may be managed conservatively, with serial ultrasounds?**

Clear fluid filled cysts without septations, <5 cm.

○ **What is the risk of breast and ovarian cancer in BRCA carriers?**

50% to 80% and 40% to 60%, respectively.

○ **Is the risk of breast cancer increased in all postmenopausal hormone users?**

Not according to WHI: not in users of Premarin.

○ **What is the recommended screening for colon cancer?**

Colonoscopy in women over the age of 50 every 10 years. Alternatives are yearly Hemoccults with sigmoidoscopy or barium enema every 5 years.

○   **Who should be offered genetic screening for BRCA mutation?**

Women with a history of a first-degree relative with premenopausal breast cancer or a family history of several women with breast and/or ovarian cancer or women with premenopausal breast or ovarian cancer.

○   **What can be recommended for BRCA protection for mutation-positive women?**

Prophylactic oophorectomy in the late 40s or use of oral contraceptive pill for long term.

○   **Is oophorectomy 100% protective in these women?**

No. About 2% to 3% of women get primary peritoneal cancer.

HORMONE REPLACEMENT THERAPY

○   **What dosages of the following estrogens are equivalent to conjugated estrogens 0.625 mg?**

Estrogen Medication	Equivalent Dose (mg)
Oral micronized estradiol	1
Transcutaneous 17 β-estradiol	0.05
Estrone sulfate	0.625
Esterified estrogen	0.625

○   **What type of estrogens is present in the following medications?**

Medication	Type of Estrogen
Premarin	Conjugated estrogens
Transdermal patch; Estrace	Estradiol
Ogen	Estropipate
Estratab	Esterified estrogens

○   **What are conjugated estrogens?**

Estrone, Equilin, and 17 α-dihydroequilin; they have hydrophilic side groups attached to them, such as sulfate.

○   **What is the daily dose of norethindrone equivalent to 2.5 mg medroxyprogesterone acetate?**

0.35 mg.

○   **Can intravaginal estrogen be absorbed and have systemic effects?**

Yes. Atrophic mucosa absorbs estrogen readily. If the patient has a uterus, she needs progesterone therapy as well.

○ **Is there an intravaginal estrogen therapy that is not systemically absorbed?**
Yes. Vagifem (vaginal estradiol) as well as vaginal estrogen ring.

○ **What herbs contain estrogen-like compounds?**
Ginseng, black cohosh, and red clover.

○ **What is the sequential method of hormone replacement administration?**
Estrogen on days 1 to 25 or 1 to 30 and medroxyprogesterone acetate 5 mg or norethindrone 0.5 mg for 13 days of estrogen administration per month.

○ **What is the recommended dose of micronized progesterone for sequential therapy?**
200 mg for 14 days every month.

○ **What is the continuous combined method of HRT?**
Daily estrogen and daily progestins, either medroxyprogesterone 2.5 mg, norethindrone 0.35 mg, or 100 to 200 mg micronized progesterone.

○ **What concentration differences of estrogen exist in the portal system versus the periphery after oral estrogen administration?**
The estrogen concentration is four to five times higher in the portal system.

○ **Does the first pass effect occur for transdermal estrogen administration?**
No.

○ **What are some of the adverse symptoms associated with the dose of progesterone in sequential HRT?**
Withdrawal bleeding, breast tenderness, bloating, fluid retention, and depression.

○ **What percentage of women on sequential hormone replacement will have progestin withdrawal bleeding?**
80% to 90%.

○ **What percentage of women will experience breakthrough bleeding on continuous HRT?**
40% to 60% in the first 6 months and 20% after 1 year.

○ **What is the origin of breakthrough bleeding in continuous HRT?**
Progestational dominance resulting in an atrophic endometrium.

○ **What evaluation should be performed for breakthrough bleeding in patients on continuous therapy?**
Observation for the first 6 months, then consider endometrial biopsy, or hysteroscopy and D&C to rule out fibroids and polyps.

○ **What are some conservative treatment alternatives to overcome breakthrough bleeding on continuous HRT?**
Observation, sequential therapy, or a progestin intrauterine device (IUD). A progestin IUD will suppress the endometrium.

○ **Is the addition of progestin required in women on estrogen replacement who undergo endometrial ablation?**

Yes.

○ **What are some causes of chronic estrogen exposure predisposing patients to a higher risk of endometrial changes?**

Obesity, DUB, anovulation and infertility, hirsutism, high alcohol intake, hepatic disease, diabetes, and hypothyroidism.

○ **When should endometrial biopsies be performed prior to initiating HRT?**

Patients at high risk of endometrial changes associated with chronic estrogen exposure and a history of previous unopposed estrogen therapy, or patients with abnormal bleeding.

○ **When is an endometrial biopsy recommended when breakthrough bleeding occurs on HRT?**

Women who have used unopposed estrogen in the past, an endometrial thickness >5 mm, or after 1 year of amenorrhea on HRT.

○ **How should women who take unopposed estrogen be followed?**

Endometrial sampling or vaginal probe ultrasound yearly.

○ **Why is the estrogen progesterone combination sometimes recommended in hysterectomized women with endometriosis?**

Adenocarcinoma has occurred in patients with endometriosis on unopposed estrogen.

○ **What are some of the potential benefits of androgen replacement?**

Improved well-being and sexual behavior.

○ **What negative effects does testosterone replacement therapy have?**

Hirsutism and adverse effects on lipids.

○ **Patients with what stage of endometrial cancer can safely take estrogen replacement therapy?**

Stage 1 grade 1, and low-grade adenocarcinoma.

○ **What conditions are not contraindications for HRT?**

Controlled hypertension, diabetes, and varicose veins.

○ **Does estrogen replacement therapy promote fibroid tumor growth?**

No.

○ **What gynecological malignancies are not contraindications to HRT?**

Ovarian, cervical, and vulvar.

○ **What effect does estrogen therapy have on colorectal cancer?**

It significantly decreases the risk of colorectal cancer.

○   **Does estrogen therapy improve visual acuity?**

Yes. Possibly due to the beneficial effect on lacrimal fluid and protection against lens opacities.

○   **What effect does estrogen therapy have on oral complaints common in menopause?**

It relieves oral discomfort, burning, bad taste, and dryness. It also decreases gingival inflammation, bleeding, and tooth loss.

○   **What effect does estrogen therapy have on skin?**

It prevents the age-related declines in skin collagen and thickness.

○   **What effect does estrogen therapy have on muscle strength?**

It prevents the age-related decline in handgrip strength.

○   **What are contraindications to estrogen therapy?**

Estrogen sensitive-cancers, chronically impaired liver function, undiagnosed genital bleeding, history of stroke, DVT or PE, neuro-ophthalmologic vascular disease, and known or suspected pregnancy.

○   **What disorders may be aggravated by estrogen?**

Seizure disorders, familial hyperlipidemias (high triglycerides), and migraine headaches.

○   **What effect does estrogen alone or in combination with progestin have on clotting factors in menopause?**

It prevents menopause-related increases in clotting factors (fibrinogen, factor VII, and plasminogen activator inhibitor) and does not alter antithrombin.

○   **When is a history of venous thromboembolism <u>not</u> a contraindication to estrogen therapy?**

A thromboembolic event related to trauma.

○   **Is there an increased risk of gallbladder disease with estrogen therapy?**

Estrogen therapy may increase the risk of gallbladder disease by 1.5- to 2.0-fold.

○   **How is estrogen believed to induce cholelithiesis?**

Estrogen alters bile salts leading to stone formation.

○   **What effect does <u>oral</u> estrogen replacement have on triglyceride levels?**

It increases triglyceride levels.

○   **What route of estrogen administration does not affect triglycerides?**

Transdermal.

○   **What complications can be precipitated by estrogen administration in women with elevated triglycerides?**

Pancreatitis and severe hypertriglyceridemia.

○ **How should estrogen be administered to women with triglyceride levels between 250 and 750 mg/dL?**

A nonoral route of estrogen with careful surveillance of triglyceride levels.

○ **How quickly do triglyceride levels increase after estrogen replacement administration?**

Triglycerides increase quickly and can be measured between 2 and 4 weeks.

○ **What triglyceride levels are an absolute contraindication to estrogen therapy?**

>750 mg/dL.

○ **What effect does estrogen have on Alzheimer disease?**

According to the NHS, Alzheimer disease is less frequent among HRT users, and cognitive function in affected individuals is improved; however, in WHI dementia is more frequent in HRT and ET users entering the study over age 65 although the difference is not statistically significant.

CHAPTER 34

Preoperative Evaluation and Preparation of Gynecologic Surgery

Lindsay Curtis, MD

○ **What is the purpose of the preoperative counseling of the patient?**

Provide informed consent, allows the patient to have questions answered, to work through emotions, and build trust.

○ **What material facts must a physician disclose in order to obtain effective informed consent?**

Informed consent must include the patient's diagnosis, proposed treatment, risks and benefits of the treatment, alternatives, and risks of refusal.

○ **A physician who fails to obtain informed consent prior to surgery may be accused of what legal charges?**

Battery actions and negligent nondisclosure.

○ **What four elements must be shown for a physician to be liable for negligent nondisclosure?**

Duty, breach of duty, injury, and causal relationship.

○ **What pertinent family history may play a role in the preoperative evaluation of a patient?**

A family history of bleeding disorders or malignant hyperthermia, which can be inherited as an autosomal dominant disorder, can be important.

○ **What laboratory evaluation should be performed on a routine preoperative workup?**

A complete blood count with hemoglobin level and platelet count is essential. Chemistries and/or coagulation studies are rarely helpful unless the patient has significant medical history.

○ **What is the anesthesiology classification of surgical risk?**

The Dripps-American Society of Anesthesiologists' Classification of surgical risk ranging from Class 1 (normal healthy patient) to Class 5 (moribund patient not expected to survive 24 hours with or without operation).

○ **The majority of gynecology procedures, including hysterectomy, dilation and curettage, and cesarean delivery, fall under what wound classification?**

Class II/clean-contaminated. This category includes any procedure that breeches the alimentary, genital, or urinary tracts under controlled conditions without unusual contamination.

○   **Preoperative prophylactic antibiotics are recommended for what commonly performed gynecologic surgeries?**

Hysterectomy, urogynecology procedures, hysterosalpingogram, or chromotubation, induced abortion or dilation, and evacuation. Antibiotics are generally not necessary in the case of operative hysteroscopy but may be considered for patients with a prior history of pelvic inflammatory disease (PID).

○   **Preoperative prophylactic antibiotics are not necessary for which gynecology procedures?**

Laparoscopy (diagnostic, operative, or tubal sterilization), laparotomy, intrauterine device (IUD) insertion, or endometrial biopsy.

○   **At what time, should preoperative antibiotics be administered?**

Antibiotics should be administered either shortly before or at the time of bacterial inoculation. It is therefore recommended they be given at the time of induction of anesthesia or within 1 hour of incision.

○   **When should surgical prophylactic antibiotics be redosed?**

Additional intraoperative antibiotics should be given at one to two times the half-life of the drug (3 hours for cefazolin) or when there is increased blood loss (>1500 cc). In addition, the initial dose should be increased in morbidly obese patients (BMI >35 or weight >100 kg).

○   **True or False: Antibiotics are necessary to prevent endocarditis in high-risk patients undergoing genitourinary procedures.**

False. The American Heart Association no longer recommends antibiotics solely for this purpose.

○   **How common are allergic reactions to penicillin?**

Allergic reactions occur in 0.7% to 4% of courses of treatment with penicillin. Anaphylactic reactions occur in only 0.2% and fatality in 0.0001%. Five to twenty percent of patients will report a history of reactions to β-lactam antibiotics.

○   **What is the most commonly used preoperative antibiotic in patients without allergies?**

Cefazolin is used most often due to its reasonably long half-life (1.8 hours) and low cost.

○   **True or False: Preoperative mechanical bowel preparation reduces the incidence of anastomotic leak and wound infection in patients undergoing large bowel resection.**

False. Historically this was believed to be true; however, randomized trials have shown the opposite.

○   **Is preoperative mechanical bowl preparation beneficial prior to advanced laparoscopic gynecologic procedures?**

Although one prospective study showed no difference, there is controversy as to whether its use improves visibility of the surgical field.

○   **What is the incidence of deep vein thrombosis (DVT) in patients undergoing major gynecologic surgery?**

In the absence of thromboprophylaxis, DVT may occur in 15% to 40% of patients. Use of appropriate prophylaxis may reduce this rate by 68% to 76%.

○ **How common is pulmonary embolism (PE) following DVT?**

PE occurs in 6% to 10% of cases following DVT in an upper extremity and 15% to 32% in a lower extremity.

○ **What is the timing and dosage of heparin for DVT prophylaxis?**

5000 units subcutaneously given 2 hours prior to surgery and continued every 8 to 12 hours postoperatively.

○ **Does prophylactic low-dose heparin affect the APTT or increase bleeding complications?**

Up to 10% to 15% of normal patients develop a prolonged APTT after 5000 u is given subcutaneously. Also, increase in bleeding complications and hematoma formation may occur.

○ **How do pneumatic compression stockings compare with heparin in the prevention of DVT?**

They are similar to heparin. The stockings must be placed intraoperatively, and particularly in patients with malignancy, should be maintained for 5 days.

○ **What food allergy may suggest an iodine allergy?**

Allergy to shellfish.

○ **How often do allergic reactions to radiologic contrast media occur during intravenous (IV) pyelogram?**

Overall, 5% to 8%, with life-threatening reactions occurring in 0.1%.

○ **If allergy to iodine is suspected, and yet an IV pyelogram is necessary, what can be done?**

Corticosteroid preparation help to prevent life-threatening anaphylaxis.

○ **Which patients scheduled for hysterectomy are at risk for abnormal IV pyelograms?**

Patients with PID, endometriosis, pelvic relaxation, lateral projections of uterine myomas, fixed adnexal masses, and prior abdominal surgery.

○ **What effect does preoperative nutritional preparation have?**

Optimizing nutritional, fluid, and electrolyte status leads to more rapid recovery, better wound healing, and less postoperative infection.

○ **What components are necessary to calculate the caloric needs of a surgical patient?**

Height, weight, sex, age, activity level, type of surgery, and extent of disease.

○ **In consideration of nutritional status, what variables are related to increased surgical morbidity and mortality?**

Generally, hypoalbuminemia (<2.5 mg/dL), and unintended weight loss (>10%).

○ **What are advantages and disadvantages of enteral nutritional supplementation?**

Advantages: easy and inexpensive. Disadvantages: high osmolarity can lead to vomiting or diarrhea, or electrolyte disturbances, and cannot be used with bowel obstruction.

○ **What is the most common side effect of peripheral parenteral nutrition?**

Phlebitis due to the high osmolarity solution.

○ **What is the most common complication associated with total parenteral nutrition?**

Catheter infection, which can be reduced with meticulous care of the catheter.

○ **What is the amount and distribution of total water in the average woman?**

Total water constitutes 50% to 55% of body weight with 40% to 66% in the intracellular compartment, and 20% to 33% in the extracellular compartment (one-fourth is in the plasma and three-fourth in the interstitium).

○ **What are the primary electrolytes contributing to the osmolarity in the extracellular fluid compartment?**

Sodium and chloride.

○ **How can one calculate the serum osmolarity?**

$2 \times Na + [Glucose (mg/dL)/18] + BUN (mg/dL)/2.8$.

○ **What conditions are associated with hyponatremia and extracellular fluid excess?**

Cardiac failure, liver failure, and renal dysfunction.

○ **What preoperative conditions predispose to hypokalemia?**

Significant gastrointestinal fluid losses, prolonged diuretic use, and prolonged parenteral potassium-free fluids.

○ **What risk factors place the hysterectomy patient at risk of postoperative infection?**

Low socioeconomic status, surgical duration >2 hours, malignancy, obesity, malnutrition, immunosuppression, and increased number of procedures performed.

○ **The Revised Cardiac Risk Index identifies what six independent predictors of major cardiac complications in patients undergoing elective major noncardiac procedures?**

(1) High-risk type of surgery (intraperitoneal, intrathoracic, or suprainguinal vascular surgery).

(2) History of ischemic heart disease (history of myocardial infarction or positive exercise test, significant angina, use of nitrate therapy, or ECG with pathological Q waves).

(3) History of heart failure.

(4) History of cerebrovascular disease.

(5) Diabetes mellitus requiring treatment with insulin.

(6) Preoperative serum creatinine >2.0 mg/dL.

○ **What physical examination findings are suggestive of cardiovascular disease?**

Hypertension, JVD, laterally displaced point of maximal impulse, irregular pulse, third heart sound, pulmonary rates, heart murmurs, peripheral edema, or vascular bruits.

○ **What is the predictive value of history in diagnosing coronary artery disease?**

90%.

○ **What is the sensitivity of stress test for coronary artery disease?**

75% to 80%.

○ **After a myocardial infarction, how long should gynecologic surgery be deferred?**

Usually at least 6 months to decrease reinfarction and mortality.

○ **What is the single most significant predictor of cardiac complications in the surgical patient?**

The presence of congestive heart failure.

○ **When are cardiac rhythm disturbances such as premature ventricular contractions associated with increased surgical risk?**

When accompanied by decreased left ventricular function.

○ **What is the most common perioperative time period for myocardial infarction?**

Postoperative day 3 to 4.

○ **What is the most common valvular abnormality of the heart?**

Mitral valve prolapse.

○ **Which arrhythmias are associated with mitral valve prolapse?**

Ventricular ectopic beats, atrial tachyarrhythmias, bradyarrhythmias, and rarely sudden death.

○ **How should patients with bioprosthetic valves be managed preoperatively?**

Coumadin should be stopped 2 days prior to surgery so that the prothrombin time decreases to 15 seconds; the Coumadin should be restarted as soon as it is deemed safe.

○ **What therapy do patients with Mobitz type I (Wenckebach) second-degree heart block need prior to surgery?**

No preoperative therapy needed.

○ **In patients with pacemakers, what preoperative preparation is advised?**

Demand pacemakers should be converted to fixed-rate mode by passing a magnet over the pacemaker.

○ **What is the classic history of a patient with severe aortic stenosis?**

Exercise dyspnea, angina, and syncope.

○ **What is the typical murmur of aortic stenosis?**

Systolic murmur at the right sternal border that radiates into the carotid arteries.

○ **What is the most common cause of death in the diabetic patient?**

Cardiovascular disease, which accounts for over half of deaths in diabetics.

○ **What are risk factors for postoperative mortality in diabetics?**

Serum creatinine >2.0 mg/dL, vascular disease, and onset of diabetes prior to age 40.

○ **What would be optimal preoperative insulin management for a diabetic patient in poor control?**

Admission 1 to 2 days prior to surgery for glucose control, likely by insulin drip. There is a threefold increase in morbidity and a doubling in mortality if an operation is performed in a diabetic patient with poor control.

○ **What is the most common etiology for hyperthyroidism?**

Graves disease.

○ **What anesthetic concerns arise in the hyperthyroid patient?**

Tracheal compression or deviation caused by the enlarged thyroid, tachycardia exacerbated by medications, and thyroid storm.

○ **Chronic glucocorticoid use prior to surgery may lead to what perioperative complications?**

(1) Hypothalamic-pituitary-adrenal (HPA) axis insufficiency resulting in intraoperative adrenal crisis.

(2) Impaired wound healing.

(3) Increased risks of bone fracture, infection, gastrointestinal hemorrhage, or ulcers.

(4) Increased friability of skin and superficial blood vessels resulting in an increased risk of subcutaneous hematomas and skin ulcerations.

○ **For which patients, should stress dose steroids be administered?**

Perioperative supplemental steroids should be given to patients with known adrenal insufficiency (Addison disease) or with recent significant steroid use. The HPA axis is suppressed in any patient who clinically has Cushing syndrome or uses the equivalent of 20 mg/day of prednisone for >3 weeks. The HPA axis is not suppressed in patients who use any dose of steroids for <3 weeks or who use the equivalent of 5 mg of prednisone each morning or less for any duration of time.

○ **How can one test for preoperative pituitary-adrenal axis insufficiency?**

An adrenocorticotropic hormone (ACTH) stimulation test can be performed. A cortisol level >18 μg/dL (497 nmol/L) 30 minutes after 250 μg ACTH stimulation predicts an adequate adrenal reserve during surgery with no need for glucocorticoid coverage perioperatively.

○ **How would one handle a patient with Addison disease or significant chronic steroid use?**

Hydrocortisone 100 mg intramuscularly (IM) on call to the OR, then 50 mg IV/IM in the recovery room, then give every 6 hours for 3 doses, then taper to a maintenance dose over the next 3 days.

○ **What potential complications may be caused by administration of stress dose steroids?**

Hypertension, hyperglycemia, fluid retention, and increased risk of infection

○ **What is the relationship between chronic hypertension and perioperative morbidity/mortality?**

No increased adverse results unless accompanied by cardiac disease.

○ **What is the greatest risk factor for the development of postoperative pulmonary complications?**

Chronic obstructive pulmonary disease (COPD).

○ **What is obstructive lung disease?**

A category of lung diseases that causes a reduction and prolongation of air flow during expiration.

○ **What are the three most common COPDs?**

Chronic bronchitis, emphysema, and asthma.

○ **What is restrictive lung disease?**

A category of disorders that limit lung expansion resulting in a decreased lung volume and increased work of breathing. This may be the result of either intrinsic pathology (such as pulmonary fibrosis or ARDS) or an extrinsic pathology (such as chest wall deformities, neuromuscular disorders, or diseases of the abdominal cavity that lower the thoracic volume).

○ **What is considered a normal forced expiration?**

Forced expiratory volume (FEV) in 1 second should be >75% of the predicted normal volume.

○ **What does high PCO_2 represent?**

Usually hypoventilation.

○ **What does low PaO_2 represent?**

Ventilation-perfusion mismatch, diffusion defect, or anatomical shunting.

○ **What is a confirmation that anatomical shunting is the cause of hypoxemia?**

By the inability to raise the PaO_2 above 55 mm Hg after breathing 100% oxygen for 30 minutes.

○ **What factor predisposes patients with COPD to postoperative pneumonia and atelectasis?**

The impaired ability for effective cough and clearance of secretions.

○ **What preoperative arterial blood gas findings are associated with postoperative pulmonary complications?**

PaO_2 values <70 mm Hg, and $PaCO_2$ values >45 mm Hg.

○ **What preoperative measures for patients with COPD help to minimize postoperative pulmonary complications?**

Chest physiotherapy, bronchodilators, and antibiotics for patients with positive sputum cultures.

○ **What FEV 1 value is correlated with postoperative pulmonary complications?**

An FEV1 value of <1 L.

○ **When should preoperative chest radiographs be performed?**

Age over 60; a history of smoking, pulmonary disease, surgery for malignancy to exclude pulmonary metastases, and patients who present with cardiac or pulmonary signs or symptoms.

○ **What percentage of the United States population is affected by asthma?**

Approximately 5%.

○ **Why has morbidity and mortality due to asthma increased in the recent years?**

This is probably due to under diagnosis and under treatment.

○ **What should be the preoperative workup of the asthmatic patient?**

Pulmonary examination, chest X-ray, and pulmonary function testing should be performed with and without bronchodilators (arterial blood gases in select cases).

○ **What role do corticosteroids have in the management of asthma?**

In curtailing the significant inflammatory component of asthma that is not treated by β-agonists.

○ **What is the single most significant reversible risk factor for pulmonary complications?**

Tobacco smoke that quadruples risk of pulmonary complications.

○ **What duration of smoking cessation is necessary to significantly lower the incidence of pulmonary complications?**

2 months.

○ **What screening test should be used when suspecting diabetes mellitus or glucose intolerance?**

A 2 hour 75 g glucose tolerance test.

○ **In what age group, is the highest incidence of major surgeries being performed?**

Between 60 and 69 years of age.

○ **What type of musculoskeletal evaluation should be performed in the preoperative phase?**

Back, hip, or lower extremity pathology should be assessed since often patients need to be in the dorsolithotomy position.

○ **What measures can be taken to avoid neurological injury to operative patients?**

Proper positioning and padding.

○ **What duration of gonadotropin releasing hormone agonist use has been associated with the maximum decrease of uterine leiomyomata size?**

3 months.

○ **How should patients with liver disease and elevated prothrombin time be prepared in the preoperative stage?**

The etiology of liver insufficiency should be investigated. Vitamin K 10 mg IM for 3 days should correct the prothrombin time. Electrolytes, LFTs, BUN, serum creatinine, platelet count, and PTT should be checked.

○ **How should a patient be evaluated when the platelet count is discovered to be <100,000/mm³?**

An etiology should be sought, and a bleeding time should be obtained.

○ **What is the most common inherited condition leading to platelet dysfunction?**

von Willebrand disease.

○ **What is the role for preoperative screening for coagulation defects?**

Only seriously ill patients and those with history of bleeding should be tested.

○ **What are the two most common causes of thrombocytopenia?**

Laboratory error and collagen vascular diseases.

○ **What medications have been shown to cause platelet dysfunction?**

Aspirin, amitriptyline, nonsteroidal anti-inflammatory agents, and high doses of penicillin and carbenicillin.

○ **When patients are noted to have increased bleeding times due to medications, what should be done in the preoperative period?**

The medications should be discontinued for 7 to 10 days before undergoing surgery.

○ **What is the most common method of diagnosing a platelet dysfunction?**

By history and physical examination (easy bruisability, sustained bleeding from cuts, bleeding with brushing teeth, petechiae on examination).

○ **How do platelet counts correlate with surgical hemorrhage?**

A platelet count above 100,000/mm³ is adequate for surgical hemostasis.

○ **What preoperative granulocyte count is associated with surgical morbidity?**

<1000/mm³.

○ **What are the most common etiologic factors leading to end-stage renal disease?**

Glomerulonephritis, hereditary factors (eg, polycystic kidney disease), and renovascular disease like diabetes and hypertensive disease.

○ **What type of anemia is the most common in patients with renal insufficiency?**

Normocytic normochromic.

○ **What measures may be employed for patients with renal insufficiency and anemia?**

Recombinant erythropoietin can help correct the anemia if surgery can be delayed for several weeks.

○ **What preoperative measures can reduce coagulation problems in patients with chronic renal insufficiency?**

Cryoprecipitate, desmopressin, and conjugated estrogen have been given to shorten the bleeding time.

○ **When should dialysis-dependent patients be dialyzed before surgery?**

Within 24 hours of surgery.

○ **What classification has been used to predict liver disease and risk assessment for surgery?**

The Child's classification taking into account serum bilirubin, albumin, ascites, encephalopathy, and nutritional status.

○ **In patients with ascites and hydrothorax, when should preoperative thoracentesis and paracentesis be considered?**

When massive ascites and hydrothorax cause marked pulmonary or abdominal symptoms.

○ **How does viral hepatitis affect timing of surgery?**

Perioperative morbidity approaches 12%, and mortality 9.5%. Thus surgery should be deferred until convalescence if possible.

CHAPTER 35 Postoperative Care of the Gynecologic Patient

Lindsay Curtis, MD

○ **How does postoperative stress affect sodium and water balance?**

Surgical stress can induce high levels of antidiuretic hormone (ADH) and aldosterone leading to water and sodium retention.

○ **How much fluid is usually sequestered in patients with a postoperative ileus?**

1 to 3 L.

○ **When in the postoperative period, does third spacing of fluid begin to resolve?**

Usually after 3 to 4 days, when the ADH and aldosterone levels normalize.

○ **What is the most common fluid and electrolyte disorder in the postoperative period?**

Fluid overload due to excess isotonic intravenous fluids.

○ **How much fluid should be replaced for insensible losses in patients with fever and hyperventilation?**

Up to 2 L of free water can be lost a day due to perspiration and hyperventilation. These losses are difficult to monitor, so trend in body weight can be useful.

○ **What is the most common acid-base abnormality encountered in the postoperative period?**

Alkalosis is common, caused by nasogastric suction, hyperventilation, and hyperaldosteronism.

○ **What is considered marked alkalosis, and what dangers does this entity pose?**

A pH >7.55 can induce seizures and cardiac arrhythmias, especially with hypokalemia.

○ **How does metabolic acidosis affect the cardiovascular system?**

It may cause a decrease in myocardial contractility, venodilation with hypotension, and a decreased responsiveness to defibrillation.

○ **What are the indications for bicarbonate administration in postoperative metabolic acidosis?**

A pH of <7.2 or severe cardiac complications due to the acidosis.

○ **What is the most common complication occurring in the postanesthesia care unit?**

Nausea and vomiting that occurs in 10% to 30% of patients after anesthesia.

○ **What common postoperative medication should be avoided in patients with QTc prolongation?**

Ondansetron (or any of the first-generation 5-HT3 antagonists) should be avoided as they may result in the potentially fatal cardiac arrhythmia torsades de pointes.

○ **What is the cause of postoperative hypothermia?**

Anesthetic-induced vasodilation and impaired thermoregulation in conjunction with the cold environment of the operating room.

○ **How can postoperative narcotic requirements be reduced?**

Administration of local anesthetics such as bupivacaine into the surgical wound, and administration of NSAIDs such as ketorolac may reduce overall narcotic use.

○ **Inadvertent injection of a local anesthetic into the vascular space may result in what complications?**

Systemic toxicity may result in tinnitus, metallic taste, agitation, and seizure. At higher doses cardiovascular complications may arise including bradycardia, vasodilation, AV block, ventricular arrhythmia, and cardiac arrest.

○ **What methods of postoperative pain control are most effective?**

Intraspinal anesthetics and/or narcotics administered in the epidural or intrathecal space; continuous subcutaneous infiltration of anesthetic solution via implanted catheter.

○ **What are the advantages of epidural rather than intrathecal analgesia?**

Epidural analgesia can provide extended pain relief (>24 hours), whereas intrathecal analgesia is limited to one dose due to the risk of CNS infection, the development of headaches, and respiratory depression.

○ **What is the most serious complication associated with epidural postoperative analgesia?**

Respiratory depression occurring in <1% of patients.

○ **How is a postdural puncture headache treated?**

A blood patch may be performed by injecting 10 to 20 cc of the patients own blood into the epidural space to form a clot over the dural leak.

○ **What is the mechanism of postoperative halothane-induced hepatitis?**

A halothane metabolite via an autoimmune process induces the hepatitis. Risk factors include familial history and obesity.

○ **When does halothane-induced hepatitis typically occur?**

Usually 1 to 2 weeks after the exposure to halothane.

○ **What is the definition of febrile morbidity in the postoperative patient?**

Temperature ≥100.4°F (38°C) on two separate occasions at least 4 hours apart excluding the first 24 hours.

○ **What are the causes of fever in the immediate postoperative period?**

Medications or blood products given during the perioperative period are the most common cause of early fever. Other causes may be due to trauma suffered prior to surgery or as part of surgery infections that were present prior to surgery; and rarely, malignant hyperthermia.

○ **When should blood cultures be obtained on the postoperative febrile patient?**

Blood cultures are of little value in immunocompetent patients unless the temperature is >102°F.

○ **How should the postoperative patient with costovertebral tenderness and fever be evaluated?**

The urine should be examined for evidence of infection. If infection is not evident, then an intravenous pyelogram should be considered to assess for ureteral damage or obstruction.

○ **Should prophylactic antibiotics be routinely used when patients have indwelling Foley catheters?**

Not unless the patient is immunocompromised.

○ **What is the most common postoperative site of infection?**

Intravenous catheter-related infections have a reported incidence of 25% to 35%. Urinary tract infections (UTIs) are much less frequent with the greater use of prophylactic antibiotics.

○ **When should a chest film be performed for the febrile postoperative patient?**

In the presence of pulmonary findings or risk factors for pulmonary complications.

○ **How often should intravenous catheters be changed?**

Every 72 hours, after which time the risk of catheter-related phlebitis increases greatly.

○ **What is the relationship between preoperative shaving and wound infection?**

Preoperative shaving increases the rate of wound infection.

○ **Does vaginal cuff cellulitis need antibiotics?**

It is present to some extent in most patients who have undergone hysterectomy, and is usually self-limited. However, when fever, leukocytosis, and pelvic pain are present, antibiotics are indicated.

○ **What are the most common bacteria isolated from pelvic abscesses in the postoperative patient?**

They are most often polymicrobial including *Escherichia coli*, *Klebsiella*, and *Bacteroides* species.

○ **What tissues are involved in necrotizing fasciitis?**

The dermis and subcutaneous tissue with necrosis of the superficial fascia, without muscle involvement.

○ **What are predisposing factors to the development of necrotizing fasciitis?**

Diabetes mellitus, trauma, alcoholism, immunocompromised state, hypertension, peripheral vascular disease, intravenous drug use, and obesity.

○ **What is the primary treatment of necrotizing fasciitis?**

Extensive surgical debridement down to the fascia.

○ **What bacteria are responsible for necrotizing fasciitis?**

It may be caused by any of the following: *Streptococcus pyogenes, Staphylococcus aureus (including MRSA), Clostridium perfringens, Bacteroides fragilis,* or *Aeromonas hydrophila.*

○ **What are the characteristics of a drug-induced postoperative fever?**

The patient appears well, without tachycardia, occasionally with eosinophilia.

○ **What is the biggest risk factor for the development of a postoperative UTI?**

The presence of an indwelling urinary catheter.

○ **What fraction of postoperative febrile morbidity is due to an infectious etiology?**

20%.

○ **What is the most common cause of postoperative fever in the first 48 hours?**

Atelectasis.

○ **What is the most common complaint associated with retained sponge or laparotomy pad?**

A tender infected pelvic mass.

○ **What is the etiology of pseudomembranous colitis?**

Broad-spectrum antibiotics such as clindamycin selects *Clostridium difficile* to predominate in the bowel. *C. difficile* releases an exotoxin.

○ **How is pseudomembranous colitis treated?**

Oral vancomycin *or* metronidazole.

○ **How can the spread of *C. difficile* be prevented?**

Hospital workers must wash hands with soap and water as alcohol-based hand rubs do not eradicate the spores of *C. difficile.*

○ **How long following laparotomy can a pneumoperitoneum normally be found?**

Up to 7 to 10 days following surgery.

○ **What is the incidence of postoperative ileus?**

Ileus has been reported to occur in 5% to 25% of patients undergoing gynecologic surgery and is most common after laparotomy.

○ **What are the causes of postoperative ileus?**

It is likely the result of a combination of neurogenic, inflammatory, and pharmacologic mechanisms.

(1) The acute phase is thought to be primarily neurogenic that results from the stimulation of afferent reflexes from direct peritoneal irritation.

(2) The prolonged phase is likely a stress response to tissue trauma that results in an inflammatory response.

(3) Use of perioperative opioids is the most common pharmacologic mechanism.

(4) All three mechanisms result in activation of the mu-opioid gastrointestinal receptors that inhibit the release of acetylcholine from the mesenteric plexus. This disrupts peristalsis by causing uncoordinated nonpropulsive contractions.

○ **True or False: There is no difference in the rates of aspiration pneumonia, wound dehiscence, or intestinal leakage with early versus delayed postoperative feeding.**

True. Early feeding does not appear to increase the rate of postoperative complications and can reduce the occurrence of postoperative ileus and length of hospital stay.

○ **Name five methods shown to reduce postoperative ileus.**

(1) Early feeding.

(2) Gum chewing.

(3) Bowel stimulation (with magnesium hydroxide, sodium phosphate, or bisacodyl suppositories).

(4) Use of Alvimopan, a mu-opioid receptor antagonist.

(5) Pain control with ketorolac—reduces total opioid use and may decrease the gastrointestinal inflammatory response.

○ **What is the most common cause of small bowel obstruction following surgery?**

Adhesions to the operative site.

○ **What findings indicate the need for immediate surgery for small bowel obstruction?**

Worsening symptoms, leukocytosis, acidosis, and fever that may indicate bowel ischemia.

○ **What is the most common cause of postoperative colonic obstruction in gynecological patients?**

Pelvic malignancy, most likely due to advanced ovarian cancer.

○ **What is the most common gynecological process associated with both bowel ileus and obstruction?**

Severe pelvic inflammatory disease.

○ **Which parts of the gastrointestinal tract recover first after intraperitoneal surgery?**

The small intestine recovers after several hours, the stomach after 24 to 48 hours, and the large intestine after 48 to 72 hours.

○ **When are the symptoms of postoperative small bowel obstruction most likely to present?**

5 to 7 days postoperatively.

○ **Where do most pulmonary emboli arise?**

The deep venous system of the legs.

○ **When do the majority of deep venous thromboses develop relative to surgery?**

Within the first 24 hours of surgery.

○ **How should a deep venous thrombosis be managed in the postoperative patient?**

Intravenous heparin for 7 to 10 days, then oral Coumadin for at least 3 months.

○ **What is the most definitive method of diagnosing pulmonary embolism?**

Pulmonary angiography.

○ **What is the most common sign associated with pulmonary embolism?**

Tachypnea, present over 90% of the time.

○ **What percentage of acute iliofemoral thrombosis will lead to pulmonary embolus?**

40% of these patients will develop pulmonary embolism.

○ **What is the initial procedure of choice for diagnosing deep venous thrombosis?**

Duplex ultrasonography.

○ **What is Virchow triad?**

Stasis, coagulability, and endothelial wall damage.

○ **How do intermittent compression devices help in preventing deep venous thrombosis?**

Decreasing venous stasis, and also decreasing coagulability (increasing fibrinolysis).

○ **How can postoperative pneumonia be differentiated from atelectasis?**

Pneumonia usually presents with a purulent productive cough, higher fever, and coarse rales over the infected area.

○ **How is adult respiratory distress syndrome (ARDS) distinguished from congestive heart failure or pulmonary edema?**

A Swan-Ganz catheter is helpful showing a low pulmonary capillary wedge pressure.

○ **Which blood product is the most volume efficient method of increasing fibrinogen?**

Cryoprecipitate has a volume of 40 mL versus fresh frozen plasma (200 mL).

○ **What is the most sensitive indicator of decreased volume status due to intraperitoneal hemorrhage?**

Decreased urine output, which precedes tachycardia and hypotension.

○ **What is the primary goal in the management of a patient in hypovolemic shock?**

Adequate oxygenation and ventilation, followed by fluid replacement.

○ **How much blood must be lost for a young woman to demonstrate signs of shock?**

At least 20% of blood volume.

○ **What are the risk factors associated with femoral neuropathy following gynecological surgery?**

Thin patient, self-retained retractor with deep blades, and a transverse skin incision.

○ **What is the best way to close a fascial dehiscence?**

A mass closure with through-and-through monofilament nylon or a Smead-Jones closure.

○ **What is the most common sign of wound disruption?**

Spontaneous serosanguinous fluid from the abdominal incision.

○ **When diffuse erythema surrounds a wound infection within the first 24 hours postoperatively, what is the most likely etiology?**

Beta-hemolytic streptococci, needing prompt intravenous antibiotics.

○ **How should granulation tissue at the vaginal vault apex following hysterectomy be treated?**

Chemical cautery, cryocautery, or electrocautery.

○ **In operative cases where the risk of wound infection is high, what measure can be used to decrease the risk?**

Delayed primary closure of the wound decreases wound infections from 23% to 2%.

○ **Where do rectovaginal fistulas usually occur following gynecological surgery?**

After hysterectomy, the fistula occurs in the upper third of the vagina; after a posterior repair, the fistula is usually in the lower third of the vagina.

○ **When do the majority of rectovaginal fistulas present in the postoperative period?**

7 to 14 days postoperatively.

○ **How is a prolapsed fallopian tube diagnosed?**

Watery discharge, postcoital spotting, coital pain, or lower abdominal pain within the first few months following hysterectomy. On speculum examination, a portion of tube may be visible at the vaginal apex.

○ **In what situations are suprapubic catheters useful?**

When prolonged drainage of the bladder is anticipated such as after a radical hysterectomy.

○ **What is the treatment of ARDS?**

Treatment of the underlying etiology, ventilatory support and PEEP, and careful fluid management.

○ **What is the treatment of cardiogenic pulmonary edema?**

Assessment of volume status and cardiac ischemia, oxygen, diuretics, and afterload reduction.

○ **What are the postoperative pulmonary changes that predispose patients to atelectasis?**

Decrease in vital capacity and functional residual capacity, discomfort from sighing and deep breathing, and impairment of the mucociliary clearing mechanism.

○ **What is the most common postoperative complication in patients with mitral stenosis?**

Pulmonary edema due to excess fluid administration.

○ **Why is sinus tachycardia to be avoided in postoperative patients with aortic stenosis?**

Decrease in ventricular filling in diastole exacerbating inadequate cardiac output.

○ **What is the most important aspect in diagnosing myocardial infarction in the postoperative patient?**

A high degree of suspicion, since only 50% of postsurgical patients have chest pain.

○ **What is the most sensitive indicator of postoperative myocardial infarction?**

The creatinine phosphokinase MB isoenzyme level.

○ **In patients with coronary artery disease, what constitutes significant hypotension, and puts the patient at risk of myocardial infarction?**

Decrease in systolic blood pressure of 33% to 50% for at least 10 minutes.

○ **What should be the management of patients who have been on beta-blockers in the intraoperative and postoperative period?**

Continuing these agents, since removal can lead to severe rebound with hypertension and angina.

○ **What precautions should be taken with patients with pacemakers?**

Electrocautery devices can trigger demand type pacemakers. Therefore, the electrode should be placed as far from the pacemaker as possible. Also, a magnet should be used to convert the pacemaker from the demand to a fixed pacing mode.

○ **How does intermittent positive pressure breathing (IPPB) therapy compare with incentive spirometry in the prevention of atelectasis in high-risk patients?**

Incentive spirometry is as effective, is cheaper, and has less complications.

○ **What glucose value is targeted in the postoperative diabetic patient?**

<180 to 240 mg/dL to prevent glucosuria, dehydration, and leukocyte inhibition.

○ **What are the indications of mechanical ventilation in the postoperative patient?**

Acute respiratory acidosis, ARDS, and progressive symptomatic hypoxemia unresponsive to oxygen supplementation.

○ **What is the difference between assist-control (AC) and intermittent mechanical ventilation (IMV)?**

With AC, the ventilator will provide assistance to any inspiration initiated by the patient; if necessary provide additional breaths so that the total number of breaths per minute meets the designated set rate. IMV provides only a set number of assisted ventilations and does not provide assistance to breaths initiated by the patient. IMV is useful in patients who hyperventilate or those being weaned from the ventilatory support.

○ **What is the most common renal problem in the postoperative patient?**

Oliguria as defined as <25 mL/hour urine output.

○ **How might postoperative prerenal oliguria be differentiated from acute renal failure?**

Prerenal azotemia tends to have a low fractional excretion of sodium, usually <1%. This is calculated by: (Urine sodium × Plasma creatinine) × 100/(Plasma sodium × Urine creatinine).

○ **What are the indications of dialysis in the postoperative patient who develops acute renal failure?**

Volume overload, hyperkalemia unresponsive to potassium binders, alteration in mental status, and a pericardial friction rub.

○ **How should hypertensive patients who have been taking diuretic medications be managed in the postoperative phase?**

Diuretics can cause volume and electrolyte disturbances, and usually are not needed in the first 2 postoperative days.

○ **What gynecological surgeries predispose to postoperative inability to void?**

Operations involving the urethra or bladder.

○ **What surgery is associated with the majority of vesicovaginal fistulas?**

Total abdominal hysterectomies for benign indications.

○ **How does a low albumin level reflect on nutritional status?**

A low albumin level reflects a depletion of visceral proteins of at least 3 weeks' duration.

○ **What protein level gives a more immediate picture of nutritional status?**

The transferrin level that has a half-life of 8 to 9 days provides a more recent protein assessment.

○ **What are the indications of total parenteral nutrition?**

No oral intake for 7 to 10 days, especially if nutritionally compromised.

○ **What is the most common etiology of postoperative hemorrhage arising from the vaginal vault following hysterectomy?**

Improperly ligated vaginal artery at the lateral vaginal angle.

○ **When does hemorrhage from cervical conization typically occur?**

Usually in the first 24 hours, or 7 to 14 days later when the cervical sutures lose their tensile strength.

○ **How much crystalloid should be administered per milliliter of blood loss in the initial treatment of hemorrhagic shock?**

3 mL of crystalloid per 1 mL of blood loss.

○ **What is the most common cause of shock in the perioperative period?**

Inadequate hemostasis related to hemorrhage.

○ **After intravascular fluid equilibration, what change in hematocrit usually corresponds to a blood loss of 500 mL?**

Usually a reduction in the hematocrit of 3% to 5%.

○ **What is the mechanism whereby hypogastric artery ligation helps in pelvic hemorrhage?**

Decrease in the pulse pressure, allowing a stable clot to form over the injured pelvic vessels.

○ **What flow of blood is required to visualize a bleeding vessel for angiographic embolization?**

At least 1 mL per minute.

○ **Which artery is most likely to be injured in performing a transverse muscle cutting incision (Maylard incision)?**

The inferior epigastric artery.

○ **Gynecologic procedures that carry a significant risk of postoperative infection include?**

Vaginal hysterectomy, abdominal hysterectomy, surgical treatment of pelvic abscess, pregnancy termination, or radical surgery of gynecologic cancers.

○ **Factors that place patients at risk of post hysterectomy infection include?**

Low socioeconomic class, duration of surgery >2 hours, presence of malignancy, and increased number of surgical procedures performed.

○ **A UTI is defined as?**

Growth of >10^5 organisms/mL of urine.

○ **Most UTIs are caused by the growth of which bacteria?**

E. coli, Klebsiella, Proteus, Enterobacter, and *Staphylococcus.*

○ **Symptoms of a wound infection most commonly occur after what postoperative day?**

Fourth.

○ **Standard therapy for intra-abdominal abscess?**

Surgical evacuation or drainage by interventional radiology combined with administration of intravenous broad-spectrum antibiotics.

○ **The organisms most likely to cause postabortive endometritis include?**

Neisseria gonorrheae, Chlamydia trachomatis, and *Streptococcus agalactiae.*

○ **What type of fascial closure technique has been shown to result in the lowest incidence of wound dehiscence and hernia formation?**

A loosely approximated mass closure using a slowly absorbable monofilament suture with a suture: wound length ratio of at least 4:1 (achieved by placing suture 1.5 cm from fascial edge with 1 cm between each placement).

○ **What are the four stages of wound healing?**

Inflammation

Epithelialization (migration)

Fibroplasia

Maturation

○ **What is the duration of each of these stages?**

Inflammation: completed within 3 days in absence of infection.

Epithelialization: completed within 48 hours of surgery.

Fibroplasia: collagen production begins on 2nd post op day, maximum rate at 5 days post op and continues for at least 6 weeks. Angiogenesis occurs during this stage.

Maturation: 80% or original tissue strength is restored by 6 weeks post op; appearance of normal skin at 180 days; remodeling continues for years.

○ **What is the most common complication following myomectomy?**

Fever, which may occur in up to 67% of patients. However, localizing symptoms are found in <15% of these patients when the fever occurs within the first 48 hours and may be related to hematoma formation and release of inflammatory markers from the uterine wall.

○ **How long after a myomectomy should a woman wait to conceive?**

3 to 6 months.

CHAPTER 36

Robotic Systems and Infertility Surgery

Brielle A. Marks, BA and
Larry I. Barmat, MD

○ **How do robotic surgeries differ from laparoscopic surgeries?**

Laparoscopies use a two-dimensional camera which projects an image on monitors that are in the operating room, the operation is done using instrumentation held by the surgeon, and the surgeon is at the bedside. Robotic surgeries use a three-dimensional camera and the surgeon is looking at the patient through the surgeon's console controlling the instruments using the robot.

○ **What are the advantages of robotic surgery over traditional open surgeries and laparoscopic surgeries?**

Open surgeries require a larger incision that results in increased scarring, longer inpatient stay, and increased morbidity. Laparoscopic surgeries have a lower presence of adhesions, decreased postoperative pain, decreased length of inpatient stay, quicker recovery time and return to normal activity, less scarring, and decreased blood loss. Robotic surgeries have a significant decrease in blood loss, decrease in complication rates, decreased length in inpatient stay, lower risk of infections, three-dimensional view, comfortable positioning of the surgeon in the surgeon's console, and wrist-like motion of the robotic arm; field of view is similar to the laparotomy, but the procedures were significantly longer than laparoscopies.

○ **What are the advantages of the Da Vinci robotic system?**

Three-dimensional vision, tremor filtration, immersive environment, motion-scaling, intra-abdominal articulation with most instruments, suturing, and tying of knots. For the surgeon, less fatigue, tremors, and frustration. For the patient, less inpatient hospital time, blood loss, and scarring.

○ **What are the disadvantages of the Da Vinci system?**

Lack of haptic feedback, bulky robotic arms (can lead to frequent collisions), limited instrumentation, inability to move the surgical table once the robotic arms are in place, difficulty for the surgical assistants to maneuver around the patient, and very costly (initial start-up for the system is approximately $1.5–2 million and each instrument is approximately $2,000 for 10 uses.), larger ports for robotic surgery.

○ **What are some improvements that can be made for the Da Vinci system?**

Haptic feedback, decrease the size of the surgical cart, cost, and the number of incisions.

○ **What are the differences between a passive robot and an active robot?**

A passive robot is used as a navigational aid and is turned on for positioning and then turned off. An active robot performs the surgery under the command of the surgeon by actually moving the tools.

○ **What are the three components of the Da Vinci system?**

Surgeon's console, video cart, and surgical cart.

○ **What are the similarities of the original Da Vinci S and the Da Vinci Si surgical system?**

Three-dimensional HD vision with digital zoom features and a high-intensity xenon light source, a motorized surgical cart with high-speed fiber optic connection as well as quickly guided instrument exchange, and extended arm range and an improved range of motion; the surgeon's console has ergonomic seated positioning, EndoWrist instrumentation, motion-scaling, and tremor filtration.

○ **What is the difference between the S and Si Da Vinci surgical system?**

The Da Vinci Si is more advanced than the S. The Si allows for two surgeons to perform a robotic procedure on one patient. The surgeon's console in the Si has the option to save setting preferences for the surgeon's comfort. The surgeon's console also has ergonomic settings and touchpad controls. The finer controls allow for repositioning of the rolling camera focus. The Si is manufactured to accept upgraded instruments.

○ **How much does the S-Type Da Vinci cart weigh and how is it maneuvered?**

544 kg; it is maneuvered on a wheelbase.

○ **What does the robotic cart consist of?**

Four robotic arms and a monitor.

○ **What is the function of the buttons at each joint of the arms of the robotic cart?**

The buttons act as a clutch. Releasing the button locks the arm in place.

○ **What does the central robotic arm house?**

The central robotic arm houses a 12-mm telescope. This telescope consists of two separate 5-mm telescopes that allow for a three-dimensional view.

○ **What are the parts of the camera system?**

Dual lens with two three-dimensional chip cameras that are spatially separated in a 12-mm casing.

○ **Why are there two complete optical systems in the camera?**

To represent the left and right eye.

○ **What are the components of the robotic video cart?**

The video cart contains two video camera control boxes, two light sources, and a synchronizer.

○ **How are the images projected through this camera into the surgeon's console?**

The images are projected to the surgeon's eyes in the binocular viewer; this allows for true three-dimensional imaging in the console.

○ **What are the other three arms used in the surgical cart?**

The other three arms attach to 8-mm metal ports that are supplied with both blunt and sharp trocars.

○ **How many times can the robotic instruments be used before they need to be replaced?**

10.

○ **What is the EndoWrist?**

The EndoWrist is an instrument that mimics the degrees of freedom of the human wrist.

○ **What are the advantages of the EndoWrist?**

Provides precise movement, decreases rotation through the operative ports of the abdominal wall, allows for seven degrees of freedom, and assistance in knot tying and suturing.

○ **What are the seven degrees of freedom of the EndoWrist?**

Four movements found in the traditional laparoscopy (pitch, yaw, roll, and grip) three endocorporeal movements by the EndoWrist technology (insertion, pitch, and yaw).

○ **What does the surgical console consist of?**

Binocular viewer, instrument controllers, system setup, control panels, and 5-foot control pedals.

○ **The console hardware and software are equivalent to what type of processor?**

5 Pentium 300 Processor.

○ **How does the surgeon's console control image magnification?**

Adjusting the depth of camera insertion in the operative field.

○ **How is the surgeon positioned in the console?**

The surgeon is seated in a comfortable, ergonomic position. The elbows rest on a padded arm bar and the thumb and index finger of each hand are placed in adjustable loops that are attached to the master controllers. The surgeon's forehead is placed against a padded bar and eyes set comfortably in the binocular viewer.

○ **What happens if the surgeon removes their head from the binocular viewer?**

An infrabeam detects the surgeon has removed their head from the viewer and locks all the robotic arms.

○ **What is the purpose of the clutch pedal?**

The purpose of the clutch pedal is to disengage the instruments from the controllers. This allows for the relocation of the controllers without changing the position of the instrument.

○ **How does the camera pedal work?**

To engage the camera, the surgeon applies continues pressure on the camera pedal. The camera pedal locks the three robotic operative arms and allows the master finger controls to freely move the robotic arm housing the telescope.

○ **What are the functions of the pedals in the Da Vinci S-type and Si-type systems?**

S: 4 pedals, 1 clutch, 2 cameras, 3 dead, 4 monopolar

Si: 1 camera, 2 bipolar, 3 monopolar, clutch to the left of pedal 1

○ **Where are the control panels found?**

They are found on the surgeon's console.

○ **What do the control panels do?**

The left side of the console controls the camera, motion-scaling, and endoscopic calibration. The right side of the console controls the system start control, emergency stop, and system standby.

○ **What happens when the emergency stop button is pressed?**

The master controllers are immediately locked.

○ **How can the emergency stop button be reengaged?**

The emergency stop button can be reengaged by pressing the fault override button.

○ **In a case of conversion to laparotomy, how can the system be rapidly disengaged?**

The system can be placed on standby mode, removing the instruments, and releasing the arms from the ports. Once the instruments are removed and the arm ports are released, the cart can then be wheeled away from the field.

○ **Approximately how long does it take to disengage the robot to convert to laparotomy?**

2 to 4 minutes.

○ **What other features are included in the surgical console?**

Endoscopic cardiac stabilizer, ultrasonic instrumentation, and Gyrus plasma kinetic dissector.

○ **What is the role of the bedside surgical assistant?**

They are used for irrigation, presentation, and retrieval of suture material and general surgical assistance.

○ **What types of gynecologic surgeries are most commonly performed robotically?**

Hysterectomy (simple and radical), sacrocolpoplexy, myomectomy, tubal ligation reversal, severe endometriosis, reconstructive pelvic surgery, and lymphadenectomy.

○   **What is the reported conversion rate from robotic surgery to laparotomy during myomectomy?**

8.6%.

○   **What are the advantages of robotic surgery of colpohysteropexy?**

Increased visualization, dissection of presacral space, positioning of the mesh, and intracorporeal suturing.

○   **What are the advantages for robotic surgery of a vesicouterine fistula?**

Ability to manipulate fine tissue, visual improvement in the operative field, faster recovery, shorter hospital stay, and prevention of fistula reoccurrence.

○   **True or False: Robotic surgery in patients with cervical cancer has resulted in more lymphocysts, lymphoceles, and decreased risk of postoperative infection.**

False. Robotic surgery in patients with cervical cancer has resulted in fewer lymphocysts and lymphoceles.

○   **Identify the procedure below.**

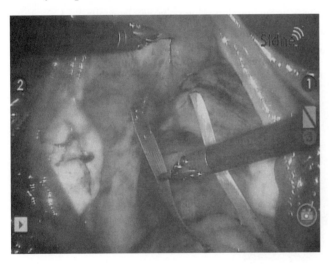

The image is a robotic trans-abdominal cerclage.

○   **Where is the cerclage placed during a transabdominal cerclage and what is used to hold the cerclage?**

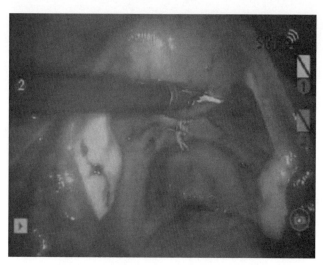

The transabdominal cerclage is placed at the cervioisthmic junction using polypropylene tape.

○   **Identify the image below and the surgical technique to correct it.**

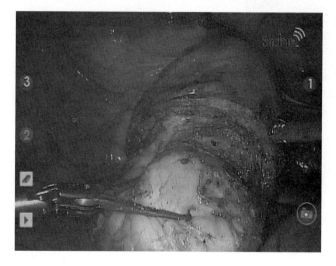

The above image is an intramural myoma. The procedure used to correct the intramural myoma is a robotic myomectomy.

○   **Where is the incision made and what is the surgical technique below?**

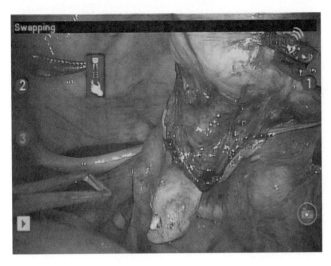

The incision is made in the peritoneum of the broad ligament. The technique is a broad ligament myomectomy.

○   **Where is the location of the myoma?**

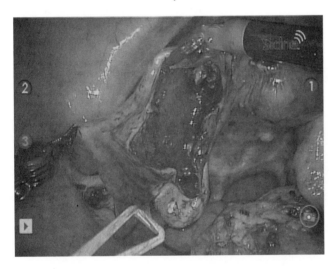

The location of the myoma is in the broad ligament.

○   **Where is the suture being placed during the tubal reanastomosis?**

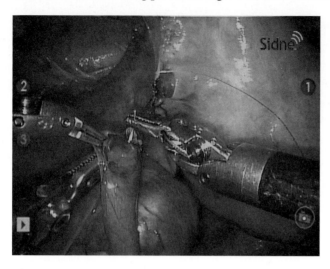

The suture is going into the muscularis of the fallopian tube.

CHAPTER 37

Lower Urinary Tract Injuries During Gynecologic Surgery

Vincent Lucente, MD, MBA and Cristina M. Saiz, MD, FACOG

○ **What is the overall incidence of urologic injury during gynecologic procedures?**

Injury to the lower urinary tract (LUT) occurs during 1% to 2% of all major gynecologic procedures. Given the absence of routine cystoscopy during benign gynecologic procedures, the overall incidence of lower urinary tract injuries (LUTI) is most likely underestimated.

○ **What urologic organ is most commonly injured?**

Bladder injuries outnumber ureteral injuries, with a ratio of 5.3:1. A recent review (Gilmour, 2006) that included 47 studies and over 120,000 patients estimated the incidence of bladder and ureteral injury to be 2.6/1000 and 1.6/1000, respectively.

○ **What is the best way to prevent injuries to the LUT during surgery?**

The most successful prevention method, as well as cost-effective, is the surgeon's profound knowledge of pelvic anatomy and the use of proper surgical dissection techniques.

○ **Is preoperative ureteral stent placement a good method to prevent LUT injuries?**

The usefulness of preoperative lighted ureteral stent placement has been questioned in that it does not secure avoidance of the injury and it is not a cost-effective measure.

○ **What is the most important step to avoid long-term sequelae after LUT injuries?**

Intraoperative detection and immediate repair is the single most important step in decreasing long-term complications such as fistula formation. Several studies have demonstrated the usefulness of routine cystoscopy in order to detect unsuspected LUTI during benign gynecologic surgery, although a recent study evaluating the routine use of cystoscopy after hysterectomy supported its selective rather than universal use.

○ **What is the major cause of urethral injuries?**

Urethral injury is rare. Formerly, obstructed labor or instrumented deliveries were the major causes of urethral injury resulting in fistula in the United States and are still in the developing countries. In the United States, most urethral injury resulting in fistula results from complications after excision of a diverticulum, including failed repair, hematoma, or infection. Urethral injury may occur during anterior colporrhaphies, pubovaginal sling procedures for urinary incontinence or related to traumatic catheterization, especially if a rigid catheter is used.

○ **What is the leading cause of bladder injury resulting in vesicovaginal fistula?**

Hysterectomy.

○ **What is the most frequently damaged organ during routine hysterectomy?**

The bladder is the most frequently damaged organ during routine hysterectomy, abdominal route being more often than during vaginal approach.

○ **Can you describe the proper steps of bladder dissection during hysterectomy?**

Blunt dissection into the vesicocervical space, and more specifically surgical entry into the vesicovaginal space during caudal mobilization of the bladder, increases the risk of injury and can also damage the autonomic innervation to the detrusor muscle. Although there is variation in the supravaginal septum that separates the vesicocervical space from the vesicovaginal space, it is more appropriate to surgically transverse the septum with careful sharp dissection rather than blunt maneuvers. In addition, failure to adequately mobilize the bladder will create the risk of incorporation of the bladder serosa, and potentially the muscularis as well, into the vaginal cuff closure.

○ **True or False: An abdominal hysterectomy has a lower risk of ureteral injury than a vaginal hysterectomy.**

False. Seventy-five percent of ureteral injuries occur during abdominal hysterectomy, and 25% during vaginal hysterectomy. The rate of ureteral injury during abdominal hysterectomy is 0.5% to 1%, and during vaginal hysterectomy is 0.1%.

○ **What is the leading cause of ureteral injury?**

Abdominal hysterectomy for benign causes. Gynecologic surgery accounts for 75% of ureteral injuries.

○ **What is the ureteral injury incident during hysterectomies?**

The overall incidence is somewhere between 0.4% and 2.5% and the rate of injury is higher during laparoscopic hysterectomies (13.9 per 1000) versus vaginal hysterectomies (0.2 per 1000).

○ **How often are ureteral injuries recognized at the time of hysterectomies?**

Only one-third of the injuries are recognized at the time of the surgery. *It is not a sin to injure the ureter. However, it is a great sin not to recognize the injury.*

○ **Mention six signs that make you suspect a LUTI.**
   • A defect that can be seen grossly after a laceration or transection of a ureter or a cystotomy.
   • Bladder catheter is seen in the operative field or the bladder mucosa is visualized.
   • Ureter is noted in close proximity to a clamp, suture, or staple.
   • The appearance of urine in the operative.
   • The appearance of blood in the urine output from the bladder catheter.
   • In laparoscopic surgery, gas may be visible in the bladder catheter output.

○ **At what times during an abdominal hysterectomy is the bladder at greatest risk?**

(1) Incising the parietal peritoneum

(a) Failure to drain the bladder before entering the peritoneal cavity increases this risk.

(2) Entering the vesicouterine fold

(b) If the fold is entered too low, the dome of the bladder may be injured.

(3) Separating the bladder from the uterine fundus, cervix, or upper vagina

(c) Adhesions from previous surgery, endometriosis, irradiation, or pelvic inflammatory disease can cause the bladder to be densely adherent to the lower uterus and upper vagina. Sharp dissection with Metzenbaum scissors pointed away from the bladder will decrease this risk.

(4) Entering the anterior vagina and suturing the vaginal vault

(d) Vagina or grasping the edges of the vaginal cuff in preparation for repair will prevent bladder injury here. In addition, suturing the vaginal cuff in an anterior to posterior direction will decrease the risk of bladder injury.

○ **Where is the most common location of a bladder injury during entry into the peritoneal cavity?**

Bladder dome.

○ **What is the most common location of a bladder injury during vaginal hysterectomy?**

Supratrigonal portion of the bladder base.

○ **How is the correct plane between the bladder and the cervix recognized during vaginal hysterectomy?**

Firm downward traction on the cervix with gentle countertraction of the bladder with a right-angled retractor should reveal the correct plane, which is *white and relatively avascular.*

○ **Once a bladder injury is suspected, how is it diagnosed?**

Use a Foley catheter to instill 400 to 600 cc of sterile milk or sterile water and methylene blue into the bladder and watch for this colored fluid in the surgical field.

○ **How should a bladder injury be repaired?**

The bladder can be damaged at the trigone, the base, or the dome. The size, nature (thermal, sharp laceration, or crush), and location of the injury will determine the most appropriate management. Careful assessment of the extent of injury with intraoperative cystoscopy should be performed. Intravenous (IV) indigo carmine should be administered to assure ureteral patency and absence of damage to the ureters. Several key surgical principles must be followed to ensure a successful repair; the repair should be tension free, water tight, and hemostatic. Adequate mobilization in order to achieve a tension-free closure must be performed. Repair should include a multilayer closure with delayed absorbable sutures (typically 3-0) because permanent suture may cause stone development. Small perforations of <1 cm, such as those following trocar injuries, usually require no repair. Prolonged bladder drainage may be useful in cases of injury over dependent areas of the bladder and ureteral catheterization could be required if the injury involves the trigone or is in close proximity to the ureteral orifices.

○ **What should the postoperative management of a cystotomy repair include?**

Bladder decompression for 7 to 10 days. Consider prophylactic antibiotic suppression. Performing a voiding cystourethrogram to assure that the bladder is completely healed prior to removing the indwelling catheter is recommended by some authors; however, care should be taken as to not over distend the bladder during the study. Ureteral catheterization is not necessary for injuries at the dome that do not involve the ureters.

○ **What injury to the urinary tract is the most difficult to recognize?**

Injury to ureter.

○ **What injury to the urinary tract produces the most serious complications?**

Injury to ureter.

○ **Where is the most common site of ureteral injury?**

Approximately 80% to 90% of all ureteral injuries occur in the distal portion of the ureter from the uterine artery to the ureterovesical junction.

○ **At what sites is the ureter at greatest risk?**

Understanding of pelvic anatomy is essential to avoid injuries to the ureter. There are several danger zones encountered as the ureter travels through the pelvis.

- Bifurcation of the iliac vessels as the ureter enters the pelvis and runs medial to the branches of the anterior division of the internal iliac artery. Injury can occur during oophorectomy, lymphadenectomy, or hypogastric artery ligation.
- At the level of the cardinal ligaments as the ureter passes under the uterine artery.
- Vaginal fornices as the ureter passes medial to them in order to enter the bladder trigone.
- Uterosacral ligaments during culdoplasty, endometriosis ablation, or while performing high uterosacral ligament suspension vaginally.

○ **What types of ureteral injury can occur?**

(1) Crushing injury from misapplication of surgical clamps, (2) ligation with suture, partial, or complete transection, (3) angulation with partial or complete obstruction, (4) ischemia from stripping of the adventitia and decreased blood supply to that part of the ureter, and (5) resection of a segment of ureter intentionally or unintentionally.

○ **What pelvic conditions may predispose to ureteric injury?**

Lateral displacement of the cervix by tumors or large fibroids, masses adhering to the peritoneum overlying the ureter, intraligamentary tumors, retroperitoneal tumors, abscesses in the broad ligament, and cervical cancer.

○ **What technique should be used to mobilize masses that may involve the ureter?**

Open the retroperitoneal space lateral to the mass, identify the ureter, and dissect the mass away from the ureter under direct visualization.

○ **Where does ureteral injury most often occur during abdominal surgery?**

Where the ureter crosses beneath the uterine artery lateral to the cervix. This happens most often when trying to gain hemostasis.

○ **True or False: Using ureteral stents prevents intraoperative injury to the ureters.**

False.

○ **What techniques protect against ureteral injury at the time of vaginal hysterectomy?**

Ureteral injury occurs rarely in vaginal hysterectomy, despite the fact that downward traction on the uterus pulls the ureter downward. Clamping the uterine vessels at a right angle to the vessel and as close to the uterus as possible will decrease the risk of ureteric injury.

○ **What percentage of ureteral injuries are recognized at the time of surgery?**

20% to 30%.

○ **What should be done when ureteral injury is suspected?**

Administer 5 mL or indigo carmine IV, followed by cystoscopy to verify bilateral excretion of dye from each ureteral orifice.

○ **What should be done when a ureteral injury is diagnosed?**

Severe or complicated injuries will often require urologic consultation and possible stent placement. The location of the injury will dictate the type of repair (distal, middle, or proximal third). Most gynecologic surgical injuries occur in the distal ureter, although some may occur in the middle portion of the ureter. Injury to the proximal ureter is rare. Distal injuries may be repaired with an ureteroneocystostomy.

○ **What is the most common cause of ureterovaginal fistula?**

Unrecognized clamp injury or suture ligation of the ureter.

○ **What should be done if the ureter is included in a clamped or ligated vessel?**

The clamp should be removed and the ureter inspected. If the damage is minor, the area of injury should be drained extraperitoneally. A suture should simply be removed. If after removal of a clamp or suture the ureter appears pale, ureteral catheterization for 7 to 10 days should be performed to allow revascularization.

○ **How should a partially transected ureter be managed?**

Repair with several interrupted sutures of 4-0 delayed absorbable sutures over a ureteral stent with retroperitoneal drainage.

○ **How should a total transected ureter be managed?**

Management of a total transection depends on location. If the transection occurs within 5 cm of the vesicoureteral junction, ureteroneocystostomy (direct reimplantation of the ureter into the bladder wall) should be performed. If the transection is higher and the ureter will not reach the bladder without tension, a psoas hitch is performed. The bladder is mobilized and secured to the psoas muscle, and a tension-free ureteroneocystostomy is performed. If the ureter is transected above the pelvic brim, a ureteroureterostomy is performed. Both ends of the ureter are spatulated for 5 mm and approximated without tension over a silastic catheter with interrupted 4-0 delayed absorbable suture. The stent should be left in place for 2 to 3 weeks. The repair should be drained extraperitoneally.

○ **What is a patient at risk of after ureteroneocystostomy, and how can this be prevented?**

Vesicoureteral reflux. This can be prevented by tunneling the ureter in the submucosa of the bladder (Politano and Leadbetter technique).

○ **What postoperative symptoms are associated with ureteral injury?**

Flank pain or tenderness, fever, sepsis, ileus, abdominal distension, unexplained hematuria, urine leakage through the vagina or skin, urinoma, oliguria or anuria, and elevated serum creatinine.

○ **What should be done if ureteral injury is suspected postoperatively?**

IVP.

○   **What should be done if IVP shows obstruction or hydronephrosis?**

Attempts to pass a ureteral catheter past the point of obstruction should be made. If successful, the catheter should be left in place for 14 to 21 days. Follow-up IVP should be performed after catheter removal.

○   **What should be done if a catheter cannot be passed past the ureteral obstruction?**

Immediate ureteral repair or percutaneous nephrostomy. If percutaneous nephrostomy is performed, the injury may resolve spontaneously, thus definitive surgery should be deferred for 8 weeks. However, when unintentional ureteral ligation is performed in a healthy patient and is discovered within 10 to 14 days of surgery, immediate repair consisting of ureteroneocystostomy can be performed.

○   **How long can an obstructed, uninfected kidney survive?**

7 to 158 days.

○   **What is a common cause of litigation in gynecology?**

Failure to recognize a urinary tract injury. Patients do quite well with intraoperative urinary tract injury repair, but suffer tremendously when these repairs go undiagnosed.

REFERENCE

Gilmour DT, Das S, Flowerdew G. Rates of urinary tract injury from gynecologic surgery and the role of intraoperative cystoscopy. *Obstet Gynecol.* 2006;107(6):1366–72.

CHAPTER 38 Pelvic Organ Prolapse

Lisa Jambusaria, MD

○ **Pus expressed through the urethral meatus on palpation of the urethra may indicate the presence of what defects?**

Infected urethral diverticulum or infected Skene glands.

○ **What is the most common compartment for pelvic organ prolapse?**

The anterior compartment (commonly known as a cystocele).

○ **What is the most common compartment for prolapse recurrence after surgical repair?**

The anterior compartment.

○ **What defect of pelvic support is due to a weakened cul-de-sac of Douglas?**

Enterocele.

○ **What standardized measurement system is used to describe pelvic organ prolapse?**

Pelvic Organ Prolapse Quantitation System or the POPQ giving measures at different compartments and a stage of prolapse based on the measure of the leading edge of prolapse.

○ **What point on the Pelvic Organ Prolapse Quantification System (POP-Q) is not measured after a hysterectomy?**

Point D at the posterior fornix.

○ **What is the other commonly used system for describing prolapse?**

The Baden Walker Scoring System.

○ **How does the Baden Walker Halfway Scoring System describe prolapse?**

The Baden Walker Halfway Scoring System describes position of the leading edge of prolapse being halfway to the hymen, to the hymen, halfway past the hymen or fully everted out of the vault:
- Grade 0: Normal position for all anatomical markers.
- Grade 1: Descent half way to the hymen.
- Grade 2: Descent to the level of the hymen.
- Grade 3: Descent half way past the hymen.
- Grade 4: Maximum possible descent at all markers.

○ **When describing the stage of pelvic organ prolapse, what is actually being described?**

The leading edge of prolapse in relation to the hymenal ring.

○ **What is the benefit of describing prolapse using the POPQ system versus only describing the stage of prolapse or using the Baden Walker Halfway score?**

The POPQ system is a validated reproducible tool that quantifies measurements and is generally utilized for research purposes. It also outlines the degree of prolapse in anterior, apical and posterior compartments of the vagina.

○ **What four compartments does the POPQ system measure?**

Anterior, apical, posterior and cul-de-sac support areas.

○ **What are the measurements of the POPQ system?**

All measurements are in reference to the hymen level. Measurements above the hymen are recorded as negative numbers, while measurements beyond the hymen are designated at positive values.

Measurements are of the following:
- Point Aa: Midline anterior wall, 3 cm proximal to urethral meatus.
- Point Ba: Most proximal part of anterior vaginal wall, anterior fornix.
- Point Ap: Midline of posterior vaginal wall.
- Point Bp: Furthest and the most dependent in the posterior vaginal wall.
- Point C: Anterior cervix, most dependent in anterior wall.
- Point D: Deepest point in the posterior fornix (uterosacral ligament level).
- TVL: Total vaginal length is the distance from hymen the point D (without prolapse).
- Genital hiatus (gh): distance from mid-urethra to posterior hymen.
- Perineal body (pb): distance from posterior hymen to mid anus.

○ **What are the risk factors for pelvic organ prolapse?**

Caucasian race, older age, obesity, vaginal delivery, family history, smoking, and hysterectomy.

○ **What structures are most important in prevention of posthysterectomy enterocele formation?**

Uterosacral-cardinal ligament complex and rectovaginal fascia.

○ **The contents of an enterocele may include omentum but always include what structure?**

Small intestine.

○ **What is the classification of the leading edge of prolapse at the introitus or hymen for the Baden Walker and POP-Q System?**

Grade 2 or Stage II.

○ **Although ulcers of the vagina associated with complete prolapse are rarely malignant, they should be biopsied. What is the most common cause?**

Stasis and abrasion with garments. Vaginal atrophy found in post menopausal women also likely plays a role.

○ **What are conservative therapies for POP?**

Pessaries and Kegel exercises.

○   **What conditions may mimic a urethrocele?**

Urethral caruncle, urethral diverticulum or inflamed Skene's gland.

○   **What forms the intermediate layer of the pelvic floor between the endopelvic fascia and the urogenital diaphragm?**

Levator ani.

○   **What structure is located on the pelvic sidewall approximately halfway between the pubic bones and the sacrum?**

Ischial spine.

○   **What two band of fibrous tissue are located on the pelvic wall between the spines and pubic bones?**

Arcus tendineus fasciae pelvis and arcus tendineus muscularis levator ani.

○   **What muscle overlies the sacrospinous ligament?**

Coccygeus muscle.

○   **Trunks of what nerve cross the surface of the piriformis muscle?**

Sciatic nerve.

○   **The cardinal ligaments arise from what region?**

Greater sciatic foramen.

○   **The uterosacral ligaments originate from what region?**

Second, third, and fourth sacral vertebrae.

○   **What muscles support the pelvic viscera?**

Pubococcygeus and iliococcygeus.

○   **What are three common apical attachment points used in pelvic organ prolapse repair?**

The sacrum, uterosacral ligaments and sacrospinous ligaments.

○   **Vesical neck support is provided by what structure and its attachment to the fascial arch (arcus tendineus musculi levatori ani)?**

Pubovesical fascia.

○   **What are the most frequent symptoms of uterine prolapse?**

Fullness of the vagina, sensation of something "falling out," or a protrusion/bulge at the introitus. At times vaginal bleeding maybe the first complaints if the bulge rubs against clothing.

○   **Marked degrees of uterine prolapse may compress the ureters resulting in what abnormality of the ureters?**

Hydroureter.

○ **True or False: Pain is a common symptom of pelvic organ prolapse?**

False, pain should alert a further workup for cause. Extremely rarely, severe prolapse can become incarcerated, causing pain.

○ **Name four medical conditions that make worsen or lead to pelvic organ prolapse?**

Smoking, chronic cough, obesity and chronic constipation.

○ **Name two urological findings that are contraindications to expectant management of uterine prolapse.**

Hydroureter and hydronephrosis.

○ **What is the most successful procedure for high-grade prolapse in postmenopausal women who are not sexually active?**

Colpocleisis.

○ **What is a colpocleisis procedure or colpectomy?**

Skinning of the vaginal wall and suturing the vaginal wall mucosa together.

○ **What is a partial colpocleisis or Le Fort procedure?**

This an obliterative prolapse surgery done on candidates for colpectomy who still have their uterus and cervix, where two canals are left at either side of the closed vagina to allow discharge to pass through.

○ **What is the gold standard reconstructive surgical procedure for high-grade apical pelvic organ prolapse?**

Transabdominal sacral colpopexy.

○ **What type of mesh is commonly used in sacral colpopexy?**

Type I macroporous mesh, synthetic.

○ **What is a sacral colpopexy?**

Transabdominal placement of Y-shaped mesh from longitudinal sacral ligament to anterior and posterior vaginal wall.

○ **What are the risks of abdominal sacral colpopexy?**

Mesh exposure, mesh erosion, bowel perforation, bleeding/injury to presacral plexus, and rarely osteomyelitis.

○ **The standard Le Fort procedure or colpectomy is contraindicated in the postmenopausal patient with a desire to preserve what function?**

Coital function.

○ **What did the January 2012 FDA statement of vaginal mesh warn consumers about?**

The FDA statement addressed the use of vaginal for reconstruction as being associated with safety risks and being of unknown efficacy. It did not include the use of mesh transabdominally for sacrocolpopexy or the use of transvaginal mesh as sling for urinary incontinence procedures.

○ **What is commonly associated with pelvic organ prolapse that is revealed after surgery?**

Urinary incontinence.

○ **What is the CARE trial?**

Colpopexy and Urinary Reduction Efforts study. This study randomized women to have abdominal sacral colpopexy with and without incontinence surgery. Study showed that the group with the incontinence procedure, a Burch colposuspension, had clinically significant lower rates of SUI postoperatively thus proposing the performance of Burch procedure at time of abdominal sacrocolpopexy.

○ **What is the OPUS trial?**

The OPUS trial looked at performance of slings at the time of sacral colpopexy procedures for incontinence and did not come to clear conclusions except that urodynamics prior to sacral colpopexy procedure with prolapse reduced may help triage patients requiring incontinence surgery concomitantly.

○ **What is a McCall's Culdoplasty?**

The attachment of the vaginal cuff to bilateral uterosacral ligaments at the level of the ischial spine. Usually performed at time of vaginal hysterectomy to prevent post hysterectomy vaginal vault prolapse.

○ **Failure to recognize and repair what defect results in prolapse of the vaginal vault after hysterectomy?**

Failure to suspend vaginal cuff with cardinal and uterosacral ligaments complex.

○ **The need to "splint" the vagina to defecate is indicative of what defect?**

Rectocele or posterior compartment prolapse.

○ **The need to "splint" the vagina to fully void is indicative of what defect?**

Cystocele or anterior compartment prolapse.

○ **Most women with a rectocele have a concomitant defect of what structure?**

Perineal body.

○ **What surgical treatment is standard care of lone posterior compartment prolapse or rectocele?**

Posterior colporraphy specifically midline plication has been shown to have the lowest recurrence rate after repair, but site specific repair is also commonly performed.

○ **What is the drawback of anterior colporrhaphy for anterior compartment prolapse repair?**

High rate of prolapse recurrence with anterior native tissue repair alone versus lower recurrence rate with posterior compartment native tissue repair.

○ **Disorders of what sacral nerves may be responsible for uterine prolapse?**

S1-S4.

○ **Inflatable, Gellhorn, Smith-Hodge, donut and ring are types of what device used in pelvic organ prolapse?**

Pessaries.

○ **What is the name of the operation combing anterior and posterior colporrhaphy with amputation of the cervix and use of the cardinal ligaments to support the anterior vaginal wall and bladder?**

Manchester-Fothergill.

○ **The Miya Hook is an instrument commonly used in what procedure?**

Sacrospinous ligament fixation.

○ **Femoral hernias are more common in which gender?**

Females.

○ **Inguinal hernias are more common in which gender?**

Males.

○ **Intraoperative injury to what nerve results in the patient experiencing foot drop?**

Common peroneal.

○ **Injury to the sciatic nerve presents what clinical picture?**

Weakness during knee flexion.

○ **A patient who experiences pain in the medial groin, inner thigh, or labia after bladder suspension may have entrapment of what nerve?**

Ilioinguinal.

○ **Saphenous nerve injury is manifested by what symptoms?**

Pain, burning, or aching in the calf.

○ **What nerve injury results in weakness of the thigh on adduction?**

Obturator.

○ **Quadriceps weakness and gait impairment may be indicative of injury to what nerve?**

Femoral.

○ **Rectal prolapse is more common in multiparous or nulliparous women?**

Nulliparous.

○ **What is the name of the defect that is present when the pubocervical fascia separates from its attachment to the fascia covering the obturator internus and levator ani muscles?**

Paravaginal defect.

○ **A hernia through the canal of Nuck may be confused with what cystic lesions?**

Gartner duct cyst or Bartholin cyst.

◯ **What complication of ovarian malignancy can cause a cystocele?**
Ascites.

◯ **Name a group of women more likely than Asian women to develop prolapse?**
Caucasian.

◯ **The anterior separation between the levator ani is known by what term?**
Levator hiatus.

◯ **McCall sutures have what purpose?**
Posterior cul-de-sac obliteration to prevent enterocele formation.

◯ **If the uterosacral-cardinal ligament complex is too attenuated to use for vaginal suspension, what other structures can be used?**
Higher uterosacral ligament bite or sacrospinous ligaments.

◯ **During repair of the perineal body constriction of the posterior fourchette may result in what patient complaint?**
Dyspareunia.

◯ **What should be the basic principle in the management of pelvic organ prolapse?**
Individualization.

◯ **As pelvic organ prolapse is thought to be in many instances a result of vaginal delivery, it is best to defer surgical treatment until when?**
Childbearing is complete.

◯ **Name three problems apart from infection and hemorrhage that may be the result of ventral suspension of the vagina.**
Urethral or ureteral kinking and enterocele development.

◯ **Name two approaches to paravaginal repair.**
Abdominal (open or laparoscopy) and vaginal.

◯ **What is the gold standard procedure for stress urinary incontinence?**
Tension free suburethral vaginal sling placed at the midurethra, either retropubic or transobturator.

◯ **What vaginal complication results from excessive trimming of vaginal mucosa in an anterior colporrhaphy?**
Vaginal shortening or stenosis.

◯ **Anterior colporrhaphy is indicated for correction of a cystocele caused by what type of vaginal wall defect?**
Anterior midline.

○ **The Moschcowitz or Halban techniques although different are used to accomplish what?**

Cul-de-sac obliteration to prevent enterocele.

○ **To what structure is the distal posterior wall of the vaginal fused?**

Perineal body.

○ **What procedure done at time of posterior compartment repair can cause dyspareunia?**

Levator Ani plication.

○ **Name two defects resulting from anterior vaginal prolapse.**

Cystocele and cystourethrocele.

○ **Patient with symptoms of pelvic organ prolapse should be evaluated in what positions?**

Sitting, standing, and lithotomy.

○ **Name three urologic complications of anterior colporrhaphy.**

Incontinence, ureteral injury, cystotomy, vesicovaginal fistula, and urethral injury.

○ **Wide sheets of anterior and posterior vaginal epithelium are removed and the denuded walls are then approximated in what procedure?**

Le Fort.

○ **What is the common name of the arcus tendineus fascia pelvis?**

White line.

○ **What are the three goals in the management, whether operative or nonoperative, of genital prolapse?**

Relief of symptoms, restoration of anatomy, and preservation or restoration of normal function.

○ **What is the most common defect in cystocele?**

Paravaginal defect.

○ **Describe supporting system of vagina.**

Apex of the vagina is suspended with cardinal-uterosacral ligament complex, majority of mid vagina is attached with white line of fascia pelvic up to the level of ischial spine, and base of the vagina is fused with perineal body and pubic bone.

○ **Name the muscle groups of the pelvis.**

Iliopsoas, obturator internus, piriformis, ischicoccygeal, iliococcygeal, puborectalis, coccygeus, and urogenital diaphragm.

○ **What is the specific defect seen in prolapse of the vaginal vault after hysterectomy?**

Failure of vaginal cuff suspension with cardinal-uterosacral ligament complex.

○ **What is the specific defect seen in enterocele?**

Disruption of cervical ring between pubocervical fascia and rectovaginal fascia.

○ **What other condition beside prolapse of pelvic organ should be evaluated before corrective surgery?**

Urinary incontinence.

○ **What is Occult Stress Urinary Incontinence?**

Stress urinary incontinence revealed with reduction of prolapse during urodynamic testing, usually performed prior to surgical correction of prolapse.

○ **What material makes up these commonly used permanent sutures in pelvic organ prolapse surgery; Prolene, Ethibond and Gore-tex?**

Polypropylene, polyester and expanded polytetrafluoroethylene (PTFE), respectively.

○ **What is the best position for examination?**

Supine position with heels in stirrups with full Valsalva. Standing position with straining can be attempted as well. In women with pessaries, remove pessary first. Following a standard examination, always perform a single blade examination, which allows site-specific evaluation.

For enterocele detection the best position is a standing position with one leg elevated while performing a rectovaginal examination.

○ **Does estrogen have a role in treatment or prevention of prolapse?**

No.

○ **What are the considerations in selecting synthetic meshes?**

Pore size and subsequent rates if infection, vaginal versus abdominal approach, and degree of mesh erosion and presence of chemical coating and subsequent failure rates.

○ **What type of mesh have studies found to be more effective for the treatment of apical prolapse at time of abdominal sacrocolpopexy; allograft, autograft, xenograft or synthetic?**

Synthetic mesh in the form of polypropylene has been shown to be the most durable.

○ **What is the most common sit of prolapse?**

Anterior vaginal wall prolapse (40% of evaluated prolapse).

○ **Is there a relationship between prolapse and incontinence?**

Not direct relationships, but it is found that up to 40% of patients with prolapse will develop incontinence. Upon evaluation in office, always reduce prolapse and evaluate for different types of incontinence (beneficial for patient to consider two procedures at the same time.)

○ **What are some of the factors physicians should discuss with patient when deciding surgical versus medical therapy?**

Desire to have intercourse

Durability

Recovery time

Type of complications rate

Surgical candidacy?

Foreign body risks

○ **In a patient with apical defect, is there a benefit of vaginal sacrospinous l suspension versus abdominal sacrocolpopexy?**

There are no clear studies. Recently various small randomized trials have been done, showing similar patient satisfaction at a distant follow-up care, although, objective findings of anatomical prolapse outcome are more superior with the abdominal approach. Each patient must be evaluated individually and have a full disclosed discussion of all possible treatment regiment and true long-term success rates.

○ **What is the success rate of sacrospinous ligament suspension?**

63 to 97%.

○ **What are the complications of sacrospinous ligament suspension?**

Pudendal hemorrhage, bowel/bladder injury, and possible entrapment of the sciatic nerve causing sever pain in the posterior leg/gluteal area (upon diagnosis needs to remove stitches immediately).

○ **What are the possible treatments in hemorrhage from middle sacral artery/venous plexus during sacral colpopexy?**

Sterile thumbtacks, ligation (if vessel is visualized,) bone wax, various thrombogenic materials (Gelfoam, FLOSEAL, Surgicel, thrombin, and Arista), and finally abdominal packing with VAC closure and reexploration in 48 hours.

○ **Is fecal incontinence a symptom of posterior wall prolapse?**

No.

○ **Which pessary is specifically designed to correct rectoceles?**

Gehrung pessary.

○ **What are possible complications of pessary use?**

Urinary retention, vaginal irritation, new onset urinary incontinence, vaginal ulceration, recurrent UTIs, and abnormal d/c (foreign body reaction).

○ **What can local vaginal estrogen be used for?**

Prevention of ulcers and discomfort with pessary use, increase lubrication for sexual intercourse, treating vaginal dryness, and preventing recurrent UTIs in postmenopausal patients.

CHAPTER 39

Urinary Incontinence and Urodynamics

Lisa Jambusaria, MD and Vincent Lucente, MD, MBA

○ **What is urinary incontinence?**

The International Continence Society defines urinary incontinence as the "demonstrable involuntary loss of urine that is socially or hygienically unacceptable to the patient or detrimental to her physical well-being."

○ **What is the prevalence of urinary incontinence?**

One of the risk factors for developing urinary incontinence is age, thus, as the population ages, the prevalence of incontinence will increase. The prevalence of incontinence also depends on the population under study. Studies have reported overall rates ranging from 8% to 41%, and in the nursing home population, the prevalence is as high as 70%.

○ **What risk factors predispose someone to the development of urinary incontinence?**

Sex: Urinary incontinence is 2 to 3 times more common in women than in men.

Age: The prevalence of urinary incontinence increases with age, with a 30% greater prevalence for each 5-year increase in age.

Childbirth: The risk of developing stress incontinence increases with parity. Urge incontinence is not related to parity. Close to 50% of women who have had vaginal deliveries will develop some form of incontinence.

Menopause, smoking, and obesity are also risk factors for the development of urinary incontinence.

○ **There are four main types of established urinary incontinence in women. What are they?**

Genuine stress incontinence

Detrusor overactivity/also known as urge incontinence (formerly know as detrusor instability)

Mixed incontinence

Overflow incontinence

○ **What is the most common type of incontinence?**

Stress urinary incontinence.

○ **What is genuine stress urinary incontinence (GSUI)?**

The involuntary loss of urine secondary to increases in intra-abdominal pressure (coughing or bearing down) without a bladder contraction or when leakage of urine occurs when intra-abdominal pressure exceeds urethral closure pressure, with no bladder contraction.

○ **What is detrusor overactivity incontinence?**

Detrusor overactivity is also known as overactive bladder (OAB) or urge incontinence. It is the involuntary loss of urine following a strong urge to void. Detrusor overactivity associated with the urge to void without associated incontinence is also called "dry" urge incontinence.

○ **What is urge urinary incontinence?**

It is the involuntary loss of urine following a strong urge to void. Detrusor overactivity is also known as OAB.

○ **What is mixed urinary incontinence?**

Urinary urge incontinence (UUI) and GSUI occurring together in the same patient.

○ **What is overflow incontinence?**

The involuntary loss of urine secondary to bladder over distension. The hydrostatic pressure within the bladder rises above the urethral pressure and a "decompression" of pressure occurs often leaving a high-volume residual as there is no detrusor contraction.

○ **What are some causes of overflow incontinence?**

Bladder atony (postepidural, diabetic neuropathy)
Outflow obstruction (pelvic mass, pelvic organ prolapse, gravid uterus with extreme retroversion)

○ **What type of incontinence is associated with urinary retention?**

Overflow incontinence.

○ **What are three rare causes of urinary incontinence?**

Ectopic ureter
Fistulas
Urethral diverticulum

○ **What should always be ruled out when a patient presents with complaints of incontinence?**

Reversible causes of incontinence.

○ **What are the reversible causes of incontinence?**

Remember the mnemonic "DIAPPERS":
Delirium
Infection (lower urinary tract)
Atrophic vaginitis
Psychological (depression, dementia)
Pharmaceutical (including alcohol, caffeine)

Excessive urine output (eg, from hyperglycemia)
Restricted mobility
Stool impaction

○ **What should be included in the basic evaluation of a patient with incontinence?**

A detailed history including description of incontinence episodes (including precipitating or preceding events—for example, urine leakage with exertion suggests genuine stress incontinence, leakage preceded by urgency suggests OAB), frequency of incontinent episodes, amount of urine loss, intake of bladder irritants (such as caffeine and alcohol), voiding dysfunction symptoms, pelvic organ prolapse symptoms, prior pelvic surgery or radiation therapy, current medications and physical examination including neurological evaluation, assessment of urethral mobility, pelvic floor support, urinalysis with culture if indicated and simple cystometry. For those patients with any voiding dysfunction symptoms, a postvoid residual should also be obtained.

○ **How is urethral mobility assessed?**

The "Q-tip test" is an office-based assessment of urethral mobility (which is a risk factor for stress incontinence). A cotton swab is placed in the urethra to the level of the vesical neck and the measurement of the axis change with strain is performed with a goniometer. Hypermobility is defined as a change in angle with Valsalva of >30 degrees.

○ **What is simple cystometry?**

Simple cystometry is the evaluation of bladder filling. It examines the pressure-volume relationship during filling. It is a "single channel" measurement in that only bladder pressure is being measured. It can be done without urodynamic equipment using a "hand held" system. A 50-mL syringe without its piston or bulb is attached to the catheter and held above the bladder. The bladder is then gradually filled by gravity in 50-mL increments and the patient's first sensation of filling (normal values vary, usually the patient senses this when asked), first sensation of urgency (normal range 150–250), and maximum bladder capacity (normal 300–500) are noted. Any rise in the column of water in the syringe may be due to inappropriate bladder contractions (the patient inadvertently bearing down may also cause this). The standing stress test may then be performed, after the patient's catheter is removed.

○ **What is the standing stress test and how is it performed?**

The cough stress test involves filling a patient's bladder to at least 300 mL or symptomatic fullness and having the patient cough while standing when the urethral meatus is visualized. If urine leakage is observed, the test is positive. This test is an indicator of stress incontinence.

○ **What is intrinsic sphincter deficiency (ISD)?**

It is the most severe form of stress urinary incontinence. It is defined by the following urodynamic parameters: leak point pressure of <60 cm H_2O and/or maximal urethral closure pressure of <20 cm H_2O.

○ **How is ISD diagnosed?**

By complex multichannel cystometry (urodynamic testing, UDT). GSUI in the absence of urethral hypermobility (failure of extrinsic support) is most often considered by definition due to ISD. Maximum urethral closure pressure (MUCP) <20 cm H_2O and/or Valsalva leak point pressures <60 cm H_2O. A positive empty stress test (stress test done after patient has emptied her bladder) is also a sign of ISD.

○ **What are the risk factors for ISD?**

Women of advanced age, a history of previous radiation, previous failed incontinence procedure, or spinal cord injury.

○   **Why is the distinction between GSUI and ISD important?**

There is a higher failure rate with midurethral transobturator pubovaginal sling procedures in patients with ISD. These patients should be treated with retropubic suburethral slings or bulking agents.

○   **What type of suburethral sling is more effective for patients with ISD?**

Retropubic slings are the most effective type of midurethral pubovaginal slings for patients with ISD.

○   **When is UDT?**

Urodynamic testing is a global term referring to various quantitative metrics regarding both filling/storage of the urinary tract and the emptying phase. This includes uroflowmetry, cystometrogram, pressure voiding studies, urethral pressure profiles, and measurement of postvoid residual volume.

○   **When is UDT indicated?**

Newer research demonstrates that UDT is not indicated for uncomplicated/direct diagnosis of SUI but maybe indicated for patients with suspected ISD or mixed UI.

○   **What is complex cystometry?**

Multichannel cystometry is a more sophisticated method of measuring filling cystometrography. With this technique, intravesical pressure (P_{ves}), intra-abdominal pressure (P_{abd}), detrusor pressure (P_{det}), and maximum flow rate (Q_{max}) are recorded simultaneously.

Usually, the patient feels the first sensation as the bladder begins to fill with 100–200 mL of water. As the bladder nears capacity, 300–400 mL, the patient may begin to feel uncomfortable, and a true urge to void will. An average adult bladder capacity is approximately 450–500 mL. During the test, provocative maneuvers (eg, coughing and straining) may help to unveil bladder instability or demonstrate genuine stress urinary incontinence.

A pressure-flow study simultaneously records the voiding detrusor pressure and the rate of urinary flow. Voiding cystometrography is the only test able to provide information about bladder contractility and the extent of a bladder outlet obstruction.

○   **What are the classic findings on UDT with stress incontinence?**

On Valsalva, there is an increase in abdominal and vesical pressures, the detrusor pressure remains the same (no increase), and there is urinary leakage. Urethral pressure may increase slightly, but it is less than the vesical pressure, thus the urethral closure pressure is negative, allowing urinary leakage.

○   **What are the classic findings on UDT with detrusor overactivity?**

On filling the bladder with fluid, there is an increase in vesical pressure, and abdominal pressure has little or no increase in pressure. The true detrusor pressure (vesical pressure-abdominal pressure), therefore, is positive (represented by an increased pressure curve on the tracing). This increase in pressure is usually associated with a sense of urgency. If there is associated incontinence, then the diagnosis of detrusor overactivity incontinence or urge incontinence is made. The urethral pressure should stay the same or may increase if the patient attempts to suppress the urge to void.

○   **What are treatment options for patients with OAB?**

Anticholinergic medications are first line as well as behavior modifications. Patients who are refractory to these modalities can be candidates for Botox and electrical nerve stimulation devices.

○ **What is the gold standard treatment of SUI?**

Midurethral tension-free vaginal sling.

○ **What are the risks/benefits of the midurethral transobturator pubovaginal sling?**

Risks: Higher incidence of groin and inner thigh pain postoperatively, higher incidence of dyspareunia due to the proximity of the sling to the anterolateral vaginal sulcus, and decreased efficacy in patients with ISD.

Benefits: Decreased incidence of both bladder and bowel injuries as well as decreased incidence of voiding dysfunction.

○ **What are the risks/benefits of the retropubic midurethral pubovaginal sling?**

Risks: Higher incidence of bowel and bladder perforations, slight higher incidence of voiding dysfunction and blood loss, with higher risk of developing a hematoma.

Benefits: Less incidence of neuropathic complications (such as groin pain), less incidence of postoperative dyspareunia, and higher success rates for patients with ISD.

○ **What is the treatment option for women who continue with SUI after surgical intervention or are not candidates for surgery?**

Periurethral injection of bulking agents.

CHAPTER 40 Pediatric and Adolescent Gynecology

Marlesa R. Moore, DO and
Stephen G. Somkuti, MD, PhD

○ **What is the most frequent gynecologic disease of children?**

Vulvovaginitis. In children, symptoms usually involve the vulva rather than the vagina.

○ **What are two types of vulvovaginitis?**

(1) Nonspecific vulvovaginitis.

(2) Specific infectious vulvovaginitis.

○ **What are some common causes of nonspecific vulvovaginitis?**

(1) Chemicals (detergents, soaps).

(2) Tight-fitting clothing.

(3) Poor hygiene and allergens.

○ **List three reasons why children are more susceptible to nonspecific vulvovaginitis than adults.**

(1) Nonestrogenized state.

(2) Proximity of anus to the vagina.

(3) Lack of pubic hair.

○ **Adhesive vulvitis does not require treatment unless what condition occurs?**

Voiding is compromised.

○ **What conditions are included in the differential diagnosis of persistent or recurrent vulvovaginitis?**

(1) Foreign body.

(2) Pin worms.

(3) Primary vulvar skin disease.

(4) Ectopic ureter.

(5) Child abuse.

○ **Name three common organisms that cause prepubertal vulvitis.**

(1) Candida.

(2) Pinworms.

(3) Group A β-hemolytic streptococcus.

○ **What is the classic symptom of *Enterobius vermicularis* infestation?**

The classic presentation of pinworm infestation is nocturnal itching of the vulvar and perianal areas.

○ **What medication is used to treat pinworms?**

Mebendazole.

○ **What is the most common foreign body found in the vagina of a child?**

Toilet paper.

○ **List the differential diagnosis of persistent vaginal bleeding in a preadolescent female.**

(1) Neoplasia.

(2) Precocious puberty.

(3) Ureteral prolapse.

(4) Trauma.

(5) Sexual assault.

(6) Vulvovaginitis.

(7) Exposure to exogenous estrogen.

(8) Shigella infection.

(9) Group A & Beta hemolytic streptococcal infection.

(10) Foreign body in vagina.

○ **List five indications of vaginoscopy in a female child.**

(1) Recurrent vulvovaginitis.

(2) Persistent bleeding.

(3) Suspicion of foreign body.

(4) Suspicion of neoplasm.

(5) Congenital anomalies.

○ **What strategies could be employed if a bimanual examination could not be performed in a child or adolescent?**

(1) A rectal-abdominal examination in the dorsal lithotomy position.

(2) Inserting a cotton-tip swab in the vagina to evaluate for agenesis or a transverse septum.

(3) Ultrasonography.

○ **List five ways in which the vagina of a child is different from the vagina of an adult.**

    (1) Thinner epithelium.

    (2) Neutral pH.

    (3) Lack of glycogen.

    (4) Lack of lactobacilli.

    (5) Insufficient level of antibodies to help resist infection.

○ **What is the initial endocrinologic change associated with the onset of puberty?**

The occurrence of episodic pulses of luteinizing hormone (LH) occurring during sleep.

○ **What is the last endocrinologic event of puberty?**

The activation of the positive gonadotropin response to increasing levels of estradiol, which results in the mid cycle gonadotrophic response.

○ **What is the relationship between the age of menarche and the onset of ovulatory cycles?**

Adolescents with an early menarche at <12 years of age achieve ovulatory cycles sooner, with 50% of cycles being ovulatory within a year of menarche. Women with later onset of menarche could take 8 to 12 years before their cycles become fully ovulatory.

○ **When is the normal length of the menstrual cycle established?**

The normal cycle length is usually established by the 6th year after menarche.

○ **What is a useful way to group the various causes of primary amenorrhea?**

Based on the presence or absence of secondary sexual characteristics and female internal genitalia.

○ **List several differential diagnosis of primary amenorrhea in a patient with absent breast development and a present uterus.**

    (1) Chromosomal abnormalities: 45X, 46X, mosaicism.

    (2) 17 alpha hydroxylase deficiency with 46XX karyotype.

    (3) Hypothalamic failure.

    (4) Pituitary failure.

○ **List several differential diagnosis of primary amenorrhea in a patient with present breast development and an absent uterus.**

    (1) Androgen insensitivity.

    (2) Uterovaginal agenesis (Mayer-Rokitansky-Küster-Hauser syndrome).

○ **List one differential diagnosis of primary amenorrhea in a patient with absent breast development and an absent uterus.**

17 alpha hydroxylase deficiency with 46XX karyotype.

○ **List several differential diagnosis of primary amenorrhea in a patient with absent breast development and an absent uterus.**

 (1) Anatomic causes (imperforate hymen).

 (2) Ovarian causes (primary ovarian failure).

 (3) Hypothalamic/pituitary causes (exercised-induced, stress, drugs).

○ **What is the differential diagnosis of irregular menses and/or secondary amenorrhea in an adolescent?**

 (1) Pregnancy.

 (2) Endocrine: Diabetes, PCOS, Cushing syndrome, thyroid disease, premature ovarian failure, and late onset congenital adrenal hyperplasia.

 (3) Tumors of the ovaries, adrenals, or a pituitary prolactinoma.

 (4) Acquired disorders: Stress-related hypothalamic dysfunction, exercise-induced amenorrhea, and eating disorder.

○ **What is the differential diagnosis of a patient presenting with vaginal agenesis?**

 (1) Müllerian agenesis.

 (2) Congenital absence of vagina with present uterine structures.

 (3) Androgen insensitivity.

 (4) 17-hydroxylase deficiency.

 (5) Low transverse vaginal septum.

 (6) Imperforate hymen.

○ **Describe the characteristics of a patient with Müllerian agenesis.**

 (1) Normal breast development.

 (2) Normal secondary sexual characteristics and body proportions.

 (3) Presence of body hair.

 (4) Present hymenal tissue.

 (5) Normal ovarian hormonal and oocyte function.

 (6) 46 XX karyotype.

○ **What tests are useful in differentiating Müllerian agenesis from androgen insensitivity in a pubertal female?**

 (1) Serum testosterone is in the male range in androgen insensitivity.

 (2) Ultrasound studies show ovarian tissue in Müllerian agenesis.

 (3) The karyotype is 46 XY in androgen insensitivity.

○ **What is the role of MRI in the evaluation of Müllerian agenesis?**

About 2% to 7% of patients with Müllerian agenesis have active endometrium present in the Müllerian structures. MRI is useful in assessing the presence of functional endometrium if the ultrasound is equivocal in a patient presenting with chronic or cyclical abdominal or pelvic pain.

○ **What is the role of laparoscopy in vaginal agenesis?**

Laparoscopy is useful in evaluating patients with cyclic abdominal pain. It is useful in identifying the presence of obstructed hemiuteri, and in the surgical removal of these structures.

○ **What congenital anomalies are associated with Müllerian agenesis?**

(1) Inguinal hernia.

(2) Renal agenesis.

(3) Pelvic kidney.

(4) Scoliosis.

○ **What is the first-line approach to the creation of a neovagina?**

The nonsurgical creation of a neovagina using dilators in a recumbent position is the primary approach. Many patients report dilation using the bicycle seat stool to be awkward and uncomfortable. Adherence to the treatment protocol is improved by providing the patient with a "buddy" who has successfully had vaginal dilation.

○ **Describe the steps in the creation of a neovagina using the Abbe-McIndoe operation.**

(1) Dissection of the space between the bladder and the rectum.

(2) Placement into the space of a mold covered with split-thickness skin graft.

(3) Regular postoperative use of vaginal dilators, until regular coitus is assured.

○ **Name the important components of an annual examination of patients after the creation of a neovagina.**

Examination for vaginal strictures or stenosis.
Screening for sexually transmitted disease (STD) when appropriate.
Inspection for malignancies for both bowel and skin neovaginas.
Inspecting bowel neovaginas for colitis or ulceration.

○ **When is it appropriate to initiate cervical screening in adolescents?**

Cervical cancer screening should begin at 21 years of age, regardless of age at first sexual intercourse. The rate of infection with human papillomavirus (HPV) in adolescent and young women is high; however, most HPV infections resolve spontaneously within 1 to 2 years. Only 0.1% of cervical cancers occur in women under the age of 21.

○ **What HPV genotypes cause 70% of all cases of cervical cancer?**

Genotypes 16 and 18.

○ **What HPV genotypes cause 90% of all cases of genital warts?**

Genotypes 6 and 11.

○ **Describe the two FDA-approved vaccines shown to be effective at preventing HPV infection.**

(1) A quadrivalent HPV vaccine that protects against HPV infections due to HPV genotypes 6, 11, 16, and 18. This vaccine is effective at providing protection against cervical cancer and vulvar, vaginal, and cervical dysplasia, as well as genital warts caused by these strains.

(2) A bivalent HPV vaccine that protects against HPV infections due to HPV genotypes 16 and 18. This vaccine is protective against cervical cancer and vulvar, vaginal, and cervical dysplasia, but not offer protection against genital warts infection.

○ **How should the HPV vaccine be administered?**

Given intramuscularly as three separate 0.5 mL doses. All doses should be given within 6 months of the first dose. Dose #1, give at chosen date; dose #2, give 1 to 2 months after the first dose; dose #3, give 6 months after the first dose.

○ **Who should receive the HPV vaccine?**

The vaccine is approved for girls and women aged 9 to 26 years old. The vaccine is also approved for boys and men aged 9 to 26 years old; however, routine vaccination for boys and men is not yet recommended. The vaccine is most effective if given before the onset of sexual activity. After initiation of intercourse, the vaccine may still be given; however, the vaccine will not protect against genotypes of HPV that a person has already been exposed to. While the HPV vaccine is categorized as a class B drug, more research is needed regarding the administration of the vaccine during pregnancy. Women who are known to be pregnant should not be vaccinated. Lactating women may be vaccinated.

○ **What is the most common gynecologic complaint among adolescents?**

Dysmenorrhea is the most common complaint among adolescent girls. It is also the leading cause of repeated short-term absences from school in this age group.

○ **What is the most common cause of dysmenorrhea in adolescents?**

Most cases of dysmenorrhea in adolescents have no underlying pelvic pathology, and are thought to be due to the uterine release of prostaglandins during menstruation. The remaining 10% have an underlying pathology, which is most commonly endometriosis. Other causes are obstructing Müllerian anomalies and pelvic inflammatory disease.

○ **What is the usual presentation of endometriosis in adolescents?**

Pelvic pain is the primary reason adolescents with endometriosis seek medical attention. This presents as an acquired, progressive dysmenorrhea, usually with both cyclic and acyclic components.

○ **Describe the appearance of endometriotic lesions on laparoscopy, in an adolescent.**

Endometriotic lesions in adolescents are usually red, clear, or white, in contrast to the powder-burn lesions commonly seen in adults.

○ **What are the treatment guidelines for endometriosis in adolescents?**

(1) NSAIDs and continuous combination hormone therapy is considered first-line treatment.

(2) Gonadotropin-releasing hormone (GnRH) agonists with add-back is reserved for failure of hormonal treatment, because of concern over its potential to retard bone growth.

(3) Surgery should be used to preserve fertility.

(4) A multidisciplinary pain management service should be provided, including support groups.

○ **What is the role of empiric treatment with GnRH agonists for endometriosis in adolescents?**

A trial of a GnRH agonist is reasonable in adolescents aged 18 years or older who do not have an ovarian mass or tumor. In younger adolescents, a diagnostic or therapeutic laparoscopy is the preferred first step in treatment if pain persists despite medical therapy.

○ **Which infections are diagnostic of sexual abuse in infants and children?**

Gonorrhea, *Chlamydia*, HIV, and syphilis are considered diagnostic for sexual abuse. The presence of *Trichomonas*, condyloma, or herpes is considered highly suspicious for abuse. Conversely, bacterial vaginosis is considered inconclusive.

○ **What situations indicate the need for STD testing in children?**

(1) Signs and symptoms consistent with STD, such as vaginal discharge or pain, genital itching or odor, urinary symptoms, genital ulcers or lesions, even if there were no suspicion for abuse.

(2) A suspected assailant is known to have an STD or high-risk behavior.

(3) Evidence of genital, oral, or anal penetration.

(4) The patient or a parent requests testing.

○ **What is the treatment of choice for gonorrhea in infants and children?**

Ceftriaxone IV/IM is the agent of choice for infants; however, exudates must be cultured and tested for antibiotic susceptibilities. Spectinomycin is also suitable for children. Fluoroquinolones are not recommended due to concern over potential damage to cartilage.

○ **What percentage of sexually active adolescents report consistent condom use?**

45%.

○ **Who is eligible to purchase emergency contraception without a prescription?**

Women age 17 or older may purchase emergency contraception without a prescription.

○ **What clinical evaluation is needed prior to prescribing or dispensing emergency contraception?**

None. Emergency contraception should be made available to any woman who believes she is at risk of an undesired pregnancy. Clinical examination and/or pregnancy testing is not necessary.

○ **What is the effect of over-the-counter availability of emergency contraception though the pharmacy on the frequency of its use among adolescents?**

A study of 2117 patients from San Francisco aged 15 to 24 showed that pharmacy access did not improve the frequency or promptness of emergency contraceptive use overall, when compared with clinic access. However, condom users were twice as likely to use emergency contraception if they could obtain it over-the-counter, possibly because a high proportion of women in this subgroup did not have an established relationship with a clinic doctor.

○ **What is the effect of access to emergency contraception on the sexual behavior of adolescents?**

Adolescents as a group are more likely to rely on condoms rather than hormonal methods for contraception, and are more likely to engage in unprotected intercourse than adults. Adolescents with access to emergency contraception were more likely to use it more frequently; however, their behavior in terms of the rates of unprotected intercourse, condom use, STD acquisition, and pregnancy was similar to those adolescents who did not have access to emergency contraception.

○ **What are the components of proper STD counseling for adolescents?**

(1) Discussing what constitutes responsible and consensual sexual behavior.

(2) Saying that abstinence is the only effective way of preventing pregnancy and STD.

(3) Reinforcing correct and consistent condom use.

○ **What are the risk factors in adolescents that make them more susceptible to STD infection?**

(1) Cervical ectropion presenting a large area of exposed columnar epithelium.

(2) Immature local immunity.

(3) Lack of foresight to understand the consequences of sexual acts.

(4) Need for peer approval.

(5) Use of alcohol or drugs.

(6) Presence of tattoos or body piercings.

○ **Forty percent of all <u>Chlamydia</u> cases present in sexually active adolescents aged 15 to 19 years. What is the incidence of infection in this population?**

1 in 10.

○ **What are the indications of annual screening for HIV and syphilis in adolescents?**

(1) Diagnosis of a STD.

(2) Multiple partners, or a high-risk partner.

(3) Engaging in sex for drugs or money.

(4) Recreational IV drug use.

(5) Admission to jail or a detention facility.

(6) Residing in an area of high prevalence for HIV or syphilis.

○ **What are the important components of the initial examination of an adolescent victim of sexual assault?**

(1) Gonorrhea and *Chlamydia* testing from penetration sites.

(2) Wet mount or swab culture for *Trichomonas, Candida,* or bacterial vaginosis.

(3) Serum tests for HIV, hepatitis B, and syphilis.

○ **When is it appropriate to repeat serologic testing for HIV in adolescent victims of sexual abuse?**

Repeat evaluation is recommended at 6 weeks, 3 months, and 6 months after the assault if the initial testing is negative, but HIV infection in the assailant cannot be ruled out.

○ **What is the appropriate prophylaxis given to adolescent victims of sexual assault?**

(1) Postexposure vaccination for hepatitis B, without hepatitis B immune globulin.

(2) Empiric antibiotics for gonorrhea, *Chlamydia, Trichomonas,* and bacterial vaginosis; ceftriaxone, metronidazole, azithromycin, or doxycycline are all appropriate agents.

(3) Emergency contraception.

○   **Under what circumstances is it indicated to give post-exposure prophylaxis for HIV?**

 (1) High-risk behavior in the assailant.

 (2) Multiple assailants.

 (3) Mucosal lesions on the assailant.

 (4) Vaginal or anal penetration.

 (5) Ejaculation on mucous membranes.

○   **What is the most common cause of breast asymmetry in an adolescent?**

Normal variation in the development of the breasts is the most common cause of asymmetry, with 25% of cases persisting to adulthood. Biopsy should almost always be avoided in prepubertal girls or during early puberty, to avoid causing potentially irreversible damage to the breast bud.

○   **What is the usual presentation of mastalgia in an adolescent?**

Cyclic breast pain that is often most severe during the luteal phase of the menstrual cycle. Symptoms might also include mild breast swelling or palpable nodularity in the upper outer quadrants, consistent with fibrocystic changes.

○   **What are the characteristic findings in benign mammary ductal ectasia in an adolescent?**

 (1) Bloody or dark-brown nipple discharge.

 (2) Dilation of mammary ducts.

 (3) Periductal fibrosis and inflammation.

 (4) Breast mass.

○   **Describe the four types of female genital cutting or circumcision.**

 (1) Type I: Excision of the prepuce with or without removal of all or part of the clitoris.

 (2) Type II: Removal of the clitoris and part or all of the labia minora.

 (3) Type III: Removing part or all of the external genitalia and sewing together the remaining edges to leave a small neo-introitus (infibulation).

 (4) All other forms, such as burning, pricking or scraping.

○   **What are the criteria that would allow an Institutional Review Board to waive the requirement for parental permission in research involving adolescents?**

 (1) Only minimal risk is involved.

 (2) Waiving parental permission does not adversely affect the welfare of the adolescent.

 (3) Research could not practically be done without a waiver.

 (4) Subjects will be provided with pertinent information after participation.

○   **In which areas of adolescent research may parental permission be waived?**

 (1) STDs.

 (2) Birth control use.

 (3) High-risk sexual behavior.

 (4) HIV prevention.

 (5) Pregnancy.

 (6) Family planning.

○ **What is the most frequent gynecologic disease of children?**

Vulvovaginitis.

○ **What percentage of all neoplasms in premenarcheal children are ovarian tumors?**

1%.

○ **Seventy-five percent of ovarian neoplasms in children that necessitate surgery are found to have what pathologic diagnosis?**

Benign teratoma.

○ **Precocious puberty is defined as the appearance of any sign of secondary sexual maturation at age of more than how many standard deviations below the mean?**

2.5 standard deviations.

○ **Which type of precocious puberty involves premature maturation of hypothalamic pituitary ovarian axis and includes normal menses, ovulation, and the possibility of pregnancy?**

GnRH-dependent precocious puberty.

○ **Which type of precocious puberty involves premature female sexual maturation and uterine bleeding but without associated ovulation?**

GnRH-independent precocious puberty.

○ **Breast hyperplasia is a normal physiologic phenomenon in the neonatal period and may persist for how many months?**

Up to six months of age.

○ **Anatomically, most central nervous lesions associated with precocious puberty are located in what region of the brain?**

Hypothalamus in the region of the third ventricle, tuber cinereum, or mammillary bodies.

○ **What blood tests would be appropriate in the evaluation of a female child with precocious puberty?**

Serum level of follicle-stimulating hormone (FSH), LH prolactin, TSH, estradiol, testosterone, dehydroepiandrosterone sulfate (DHEAS), hCG, androstenedione, 17-hydroxyprogesterone, triiodothyronine, and thyroxine.

○ **In childhood, what percentage of ovarian neoplasms necessitating surgery are benign?**

75% to 85%

○ **What percentage of cases of true precocious puberty are secondary to a life-threatening central nervous system disease?**

30%.

○ **What percentage of precocious puberty is caused by idiopathic (constitutional) development?**

70%.

○ **What are the goals of medical therapy in precocious puberty?**

(1) Reduce gonadotropin secretion.

(2) Reduce or counteract peripheral actions of sex steroids.

(3) Decrease the growth rate to normal.

(4) Slow skeletal maturation.

○ **What percentage of all cases of sexual abuse of children involve a family member as the perpetrator?**

80%.

○ **What nonhormonal diagnoses should be in the differential for heavy bleeding at menarche?**

(1) Blood dyscrasias (von Willebrand disease, prothrombin deficiency).

(2) Platelet dysfunction (leukemia, idiopathic thrombocytopenic purpura, hypersplenism).

○ **If a pediatric patient has an asymptomatic transverse vaginal septum, what condition might occur at the time puberty?**

Hematocolpos or hematometrium.

○ **If a pediatric patient has an asymptomatic imperforate hymen, what condition might occur at the time of puberty?**

Hematometra and hematosalpinx, causing a menstrual blood bulge behind the imperforate hymen.

○ **What complaints might a pubertal patient with an imperforate hymen describe?**

Cyclic cramping but no menstrual flow.

○ **You are examining a neonate. Labial fusion is noted. What other portion of the physical examination may most likely assist you in your analysis of this condition?**

Groins and labial folds should be palpated for evidence of gonads.

○ **What is the most common cause of labial fusion?**

Congenital adrenal hyperplasia. The most common form is caused by an inborn error of metabolism involving 21 hydroxylase.

○ **Name a rare variant of embryonal rhabdomyosarcoma that most often presents in infancy and adolescence.**

Sarcoma botryoides is a rare tumor of the vagina that most often presents before 8 years of age, although cases have been reported among adolescents. The tumor grossly forms multiple polypoid masses resembling a cluster of grapes. Histologically, they appear as malignant pleomorphic cells in a loose myxomatous stroma and occasional "strap cells," eosinophilic rhabdomyoblasts with characteristic cross striations. To confuse matters further, there is a benign entity called pseudosarcoma botryoides found in infants that resembles sarcoma botryoides. Grossly, these polyps do not have a grape-like appearance, and histologic examination demonstrates an absence of strap cells.

○ **List the criteria for the diagnosis of anorexia nervosa in an adolescent female.**

(1) Refusal to maintain normal weight for age and height (<85% recommended level).

(2) Morbid fear of becoming fat.

(3) Disturbance of body image.

(4) Absence of menstruation for three consecutive cycles.

○ **List some of the laboratory findings found in anorexia nervosa.**

(1) Prepubertal levels of FSH and LH.

(2) Diminished response toGnRH.

(3) Postmenopausal levels of estrogen.

(4) Absence or reversal of normal circadian rhythm of plasma cortisol.

(5) Reduction in metabolic clearance rate of cortisol.

(6) Incomplete suppression of adrenal corticotropin and cortisol by dexamethasone.

○ **List the criteria for the diagnoses of bulimia nervosa.**

(1) Uncontrolled binge eating at least twice weekly for at least 3 months.

(2) Recurrent inappropriate compensatory behavior to prevent weight gain, such as, self-induced vomiting, laxatives or diuretics, strict dieting or fasting, or vigorous exercise averaging at least twice weekly for 3 months.

(3) Over concern with weight and body shape.

○ **List three physical findings that may be present in a patient with bulimia nervosa.**

(1) Erosion of dental enamel.

(2) Calluses on dorsal aspects of the hands.

(3) Parotid hypertrophy.

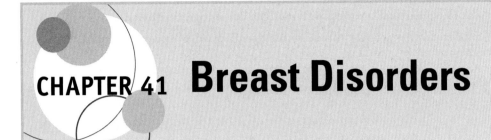

CHAPTER 41 Breast Disorders

Lauren Abern, MD

○ **What is Mondor disease?**

A painful string-like thrombophlebitis within a cutaneous vein of the chest wall or breast. A tender cord is usually palpable and visible in the lateral aspect of the breast.

○ **What is the treatment of Mondor disease?**

Warm compresses, elevation of the breast in a well-fitting bra, and use of anti-inflammatory medications.

○ **What is the most common cause of nipple discharge in the nonlactating breast?**

Fibrocystic changes.

○ **What are other causes of nipple discharge in the nonlactating breast?**

Intraductal papilloma, duct ectasia, galactorrhea, and, rarely, carcinoma.

○ **What is the most common cause of bloody nipple discharge?**

Intraductal papilloma, which is a benign process. Carcinoma can also cause bloody discharge.

○ **When do patients typically present with symptoms of an intraductal papilloma?**

When they are perimenopausal.

○ **What is the most important histopathologic feature that distinguishes a benign papilloma from a papillary carcinoma?**

The presence of a myoepithelial layer.

○ **Is there an increased risk of carcinoma in a patient with a single, central intraductal papilloma?**

No.

○ **Is there an increased risk of carcinoma in a patient with multiple intraductal papillomas?**

Yes. They may be also associated with concurrent atypical ductal hyperplasia (ADH), ductal carcinoma, in situ (DCIS), or invasive carcinoma.

○ **What condition most commonly causes a greenish nipple discharge?**

Ductal ectasia

○ **What is ductal ectasia?**

Periductal mastitis, which is characterized by duct dilatation, fibrosis, and lymphoplasmacytic inflammation.

○ **What is seen on ultrasonography with ductal ectasia?**

Dilated ducts with thickened walls in the central breast.

○ **Nonpuerperal mastitis is most commonly seen when?**

After trauma. Other causes include foreign body and malignancy.

○ **What are contraindications to breastfeeding?**

Those who take street drug or alcohol abuse, infant with galactosemia, HIV positive, active, untreated tuberculosis, breast cancer treatment or radiation therapy, human T-cell lymphotropic virus type I or type II, and use of certain medications, such as antiretrovirals or cancer chemotherapy agents.

○ **Does hepatitis B infection preclude breastfeeding?**

No. With appropriate immunoprophylaxis, including hepatitis B immune globulin and vaccine, breastfeeding poses no additional risk for the transmission of the virus.

○ **What are the complications of lactation?**

Mastitis, breast abscess, nipple excoriation, tenderness, and galactocele formation.

○ **What condition may result from severe intrapartum or early postpartum hemorrhage?**

Sheehan syndrome (pituitary failure).

○ **What are the signs and symptoms of Sheehan syndrome?**

Failure of lactation, amenorrhea, breast atrophy, hypothyroidism, and adrenal cortical insufficiency.

○ **Which vitamin is absent in breast milk?**

Vitamin K.

○ **What is galactorrhea?**

The pathologic secretion of milky fluid without associated pregnancy and lactation. It is frequently associated with amenorrhea and may be caused by a host of endocrine disorders or be a consequence of a medication.

○ **What is the most common cause of galactorrhea?**

Hyperprolactinemia.

○ **How should galactorrhea be investigated initially?**

Serum prolactin levels.

○ **How can galactorrhea be treated if caused by a pituitary adenoma or persistent lactation?**

Bromocriptine.

○ **Breast hypoplasia is generally associated with what conditions?**

Gonadal dysgenesis and Turner syndrome.

○ **A 9-year-old patient presents with a complaint of unilateral breast lump and tenderness. What is the proper management?**

Reassurance. This mass represents the breast bud's initial development at thelarche.

○ **What is the preferred radiographic technique to diagnose breast abscess?**

Ultrasound.

○ **What is the workup of a 25-year-old patient with a palpable breast mass?**

A complete history and physical examination is initially performed. The next step is an ultrasound of the lesion. Fine needle aspiration or core needle biopsy is the final step.

○ **What are the initial imaging studies for a breast mass during pregnancy and lactation?**

Ultrasound.

○ **What is the cause of axillary swelling and pain during late pregnancy?**

Ectopic axillary breast tissue.

○ **How is swelling from ectopic axillary breast tissue treated?**

The condition is initially treated with reassurance and observation. The swelling will usually resolve with the cessation of nursing and lactation. When swelling is persistent and causes discomfort or cosmetic dissatisfaction, ectopic axillary breast tissue can be removed by a subcutaneous resection.

○ **When is core needle biopsy preferred over fine-needle aspiration?**

Core needle biopsy is preferred for solid lesions. Fine-needle aspiration is preferred for cyst aspirations.

○ **What is the average radiation exposure during a routine mammogram?**

The FDA limits radiation dose for a mammogram to 300 mrad for an average thickness breast per exposure.

○ **Which lymph node groups are most likely to be affected by breast cancer metastases?**

Axillary, supraclavicular, internal mammary, and cervical lymph nodes.

○ **Ductal proliferation is dependent on what hormone?**

Estrogen.

○ **Lobuloalveolar development depends on what hormone?**

Progesterone.

○ **What is the average number of lobes in the mature breast?**

Each breast contains milk glands: 15 to 20 subdivided lobes of glandular tissue surrounded by fatty or fibrous tissue.

○ **A patient with bronchogenic carcinoma may present with what symptom relative to the breast?**

Galactorrhea.

○ **How does a lactational breast abscess present?**

It typically presents with pain, fever, and localized redness or warmth of the overlying skin. It is often difficult to distinguish from mastitis. Clinical palpation will disclose focal tenderness with induration or a palpable mass.

○ **What is the most common infecting organism found in a lactational breast abscess?**

Staphylococcus aureus.

○ **How is a lactational breast abscess treated?**

Broad-spectrum oral antibiotic. The patient should be encouraged to continue nursing from both breasts and to apply warm compresses to the tender area several times daily. An ultrasound examination of the breast should be performed if there is no improvement by 48 to 72 hours after starting antibiotic treatment. Consideration should be given to prompt surgical incision and drainage or ultrasound-guided percutaneous drainage if necessary.

○ **What are the most common locations of an abscess in a lactating breast?**

The central and subareolar areas.

○ **What structure supports the breast tissue?**

The skin ultimately supports the breast tissue along with a framework of fibrous, semielastic bands of tissue called Cooper ligaments.

○ **What is the name of the staging system for breast development?**

Tanner Stage 1 (prepubertal)—Papilla elevation only.
Tanner Stage 2—Breast buds palpable and areolae enlarge at age 10.9 years (8.9–12.9 years).
Tanner Stage 3—Elevation of breast contour; areolae enlarge at age 11.9 years (9.9–13.9 years).
Tanner Stage 4—Areolae form secondary mound on the breast at age 12.9 years (10.5–15.3 years).
Tanner Stage 5—Adult breast contour and areola recesses to general contour of breast (>15.3 years).

○ **What glands are present under the areola?**

Montgomery glands.

○ **What is the purpose of the Montgomery glands?**

These glands secrete lubricating substances and IgA that protect the nipple and areola during nursing.

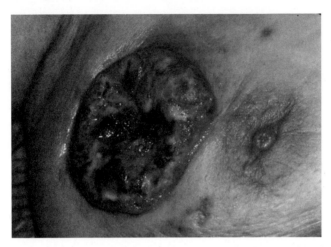

Figure 41.1 *A locally advanced phyllodes tumor with ulceration through the skin.*

○ **What are the main characteristics of phyllodes tumor?**

A circumscribed round to oval nodular mass with a gray-white appearance. They typically present as palpable masses in the breast. Shiny, stretched, and attenuated skin with varicose veins can overlie a phyllodes tumor as it pushes against the skin. Skin ulcerations can develop from ischemia secondary to the stretching.

○ **Where do phyllodes tumors metastasize?**

Metastasis is uncommon. When it does occur, it can spread to the lungs, and less frequently, liver and bones.

○ **What is the most common benign breast neoplasm?**

Fibroadenoma.

○ **What stimulates the growth of a fibroadenoma?**

Estrogen.

○ **What are the management recommendations for fibroadenomas?**

As transformation into cancer is rare and regression is frequent, current management recommendations are conservative. Enlarging fibroadenomas or those >2 cm should be excised.

○ **What can happen after menopause in someone with fibroadenomas?**

After menopause, fibroadenomas can atrophy from the lack of estrogen causing calcifications in a clustered arrangement within a round or elliptical mass on mammogram. This appearance can mimic breast carcinoma and require biopsy.

○ **What is the image modality of the management of a premenopausal patient that presents with a palpable breast mass?**

Ultrasound. Masses may be further evaluated by mammogram, especially if the woman is 30 years of age or greater.

○ **What is the image modality of a postmenopausal patient with a palpable breast mass?**

Mammogram. Ultrasound or compression and magnification views to clarify the mammographic image can be ordered if deemed necessary.

○ **What malignant component is rarely found in fibroadenomas?**

Atypical hyperplasia of both ductal and lobular types may be found in <1% of the cases. Very rarely, lobular carcinoma in situ (LCIS), DCIS, invasive ductal carcinoma (IDC), or invasive lobular carcinoma (ILC) has been observed in association with a fibroadenoma.

○ **In general, what criteria do you use to evaluate the malignant potential of a cyst aspirate?**

Clear or straw-colored fluid is generally considered benign, while hemorrhagic fluid has a higher malignant potential.

○ **What is the treatment of severe mastodynia?**

In addition to avoidance of dietary methylxanthines and adhering to a low-fat diet, patients should be instructed to wear a well-supporting bra and avoid physical activities that exacerbate pain from breast motion. Evening primrose oil at a dose of 3 g/day has been associated with improvement in mastalgia. Androgen therapy should be considered a last resort measure.

○ **What is the only androgen approved for the treatment of mastalgia?**

Danazol.

○ **What is the dose of Danazol when treating mastalgia?**

Initially 100 mg twice daily. The dose may be doubled if no improvement occurs after 2 months.

○ **What are side effects of Danazol?**

Oily skin, acne, hirsutism, lowered vocal pitch, hot flashes, abdominal cramps, increased libido, dyspareunia, headaches, nervousness, depression, and venous thromboembolism.

○ **How common is breast cancer?**

One in nine women will develop the disease.

○ **What is the most common congenital abnormality of the breast?**

Polythelia (supernumerary nipples).

○ **Where are supernumerary nipples located?**

They are identified at birth as 2 to 3 mm pigmented spots that lie on the embryonic milk lines (mammary ridges) that extend from the axilla to the groin on each side of the thoracoabdominal skin.

○ **What conditions are associated with polythelia?**

There is a slight increased association with renal anomalies, vertebral anomalies, and cardiac rhythm abnormalities.

○ **What is microscopically lacking in the male breast to distinguish it from the female breast?**

Lobules.

○ **What conditions are associated with gynecomastia?**

Puberty, medications, cirrhosis, malnutrition, primary or secondary hypogonadism, testicular tumors, hyperthyroidism, renal disease, or idiopathic.

○ **What medications can cause gynecomastia?**

Estrogens, antiandrogens, ketoconazole, metronidazole, cimetidine, omeprazole, ranitidine, methotrexate, alkylating agents, amiodarone, captopril, digoxin, diltiazem, enalapril, nifedipine, spironolactone, verapamil, diazepam, haloperidol, tricyclic antidepressants, reglan, phenytoin, and theophylline.

○ **What are the most common types of breast masses in premenopausal women?**

Fibroadenomas, fibrocystic changes, cysts, abscesses, and carcinomas.

○ **What factors affect fibrocystic change?**

The changes are believed to be associated with ovarian hormones since the condition usually subsides with menopause and may vary in consistency and symptomatic intensity during the menstrual cycle.

○ **What is the incidence of fibrocystic change?**

The incidence is estimated to be over 60% of all women and is lower in women taking birth control pills.

○ **Is there an increased risk of subsequent development of cancer in fibrocystic change?**

The risk of development of carcinoma is related to the degree and type of epithelial hyperplasia present. Proliferative or atypical fibrocystic changes increase the risk of breast carcinoma.

○ **What histologic pattern of the epithelial component of phyllodes tumor is useful in differentiating it from a fibroadenoma?**

The epithelial component in phyllodes tumor is characteristically "leaf-like" with a branching pattern. The stroma in phyllodes tumor is also more cellular and mitotically active and has more atypical cells, including multinucleated cells.

○ **What are some risk factors for the development of carcinoma of the breast?**

Increasing age, female gender, genetic factors (BRCA1/2, ataxia-telangiectasia, CHEK-2, Li-Fraumeni syndrome), family history, personal history, Caucasian race, previous chest irradiation, early menarche, late menopause, exposure to diethylstilbestrol (DES), nulliparity, and hormone replacement therapy (HRT).

○ **What is the recommended screening for breast cancer in average-risk patients?**

Yearly mammograms are recommended starting at age 40 and continuing for as long as a woman is in good health. Clinical breast examination should be performed every 3 years for women in their 20s and 30s, and every year for women 40 and over.

○ **What is the recommended screening for breast cancer in high-risk patients?**

Women at increased risk should start screening 10 years younger than the age of the youngest affected first-degree relative when they were diagnosed with breast cancer. These women may be screened with mammography, ultrasound, or MRI as appropriate. They should perform breast self-examinations monthly and have clinical breast examinations every 6 months.

○   **What mammographic features are most worrisome for the possibility of a breast malignancy?**

Any density that is new or increasing in size in comparison to prior mammographic studies, clusters of calcifications, especially very fine or linear calcifications, or a stellate or spiculated density.

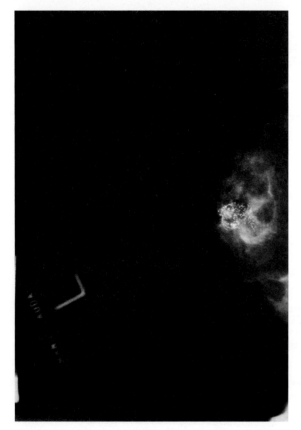 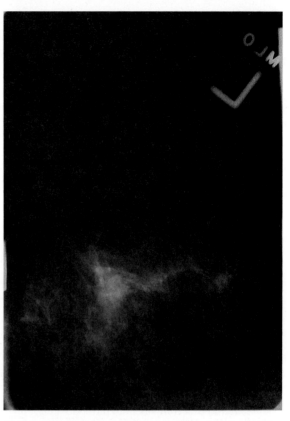

Figure 41.2 *Craniocaudal (CC) view mammogram showing subareolar calcifications. Note the linear, irregular nature of the calcifications, typical of ductal carcinoma in situ (DCIS).*

Figure 41.3 *Medial-lateral oblique (MLO) mammogram. Note the asymmetric mass with an irregular, spiculated appearance. This lesion is worrisome for breast carcinoma.*

○   **What is the most ominous sign seen on mammography?**

A stellate or speculated density, especially if associated with clustered calcifications.

○   **What unusual diagnostic difficulties are associated with infiltrating lobular carcinoma?**

These tumors arise from a small focus of tumor that permeates extensively throughout the breast without an associated concentrically enlarging central mass. This makes recognition difficult or impossible on mammogram.

○   **Does papillary carcinoma have a generally good or bad prognosis?**

Good prognosis.

○ **Based on a pathological classification, how are benign breast disorders divided?**

Nonproliferative lesions.

Proliferative lesions without atypia.

Atypical proliferative lesions.

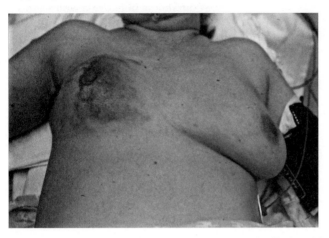

Figure 41.4 *A 54-year-old woman with locally advanced infiltrating lobular right breast carcinoma exhibiting inflammatory and peau d'orange skin changes. Note the foreshortening and retraction of the right breast.*

○ **What is the risk of subsequent development of invasive carcinoma in patients with nonproliferative and proliferative breast disorders?**

These lesions carry no increased risk of development of carcinoma as long as the patient does not have a strong family history of breast cancer. Included in this category are fibroadenomas, duct ectasia, cysts, apocrine metaplasia, and mild ductal epithelial hyperplasia.

○ **What is the risk of subsequent development of invasive carcinoma in patients with proliferative breast disorders without atypia?**

The risk is 1.5 to 2 times normal.

○ **What is the risk of subsequent development of invasive carcinoma in patients with atypical proliferative breast disorders?**

The risk is increased by about 4 times normal.

○ **What is the relative risk of development of invasive carcinoma of the breast in a patient with ADH?**

4 to 5 times.

○ **What is the relative risk of development of invasive carcinoma of the breast in a patient with hyperplasia (mild)?**

1.5 to 2 times.

○ **What is the relative risk of development of invasive carcinoma of the breast in a patient with atypical lobular hyperplasia (ALH)?**

Four to five times.

○   **What is the risk of developing breast cancer for a person with LCIS?**

These patients have a rate of development of invasive carcinoma of about 1% to 2% per year, with a lifetime risk of 30% to 40%.

○   **Is there an increased relative risk of development of invasive breast carcinoma in patients with sclerosing adenosis?**

1.5 to 2 times.

○   **What two genes account for the vast majority of inherited breast cancers?**

BRCA1 and BRCA2.

○   **What percentage of breast cancer is genetic?**

5% to 10%.

○   **Where are BRCA1 and 2 located?**

BRCA1 is found on chromosome 17q21, and BRCA2 is found on chromosome 13q12.

○   **Is there a risk of development of other types of malignancies in patients with mutations involving BRCA1 and BRCA2?**

Yes. BRCA1 mutations are associated with a pronounced increased risk of development of ovarian cancer (up to 60% by age 70), prostate cancer, and colon cancer. BRCA2 is associated with the development of male breast cancer, ovarian cancer, and cancer of the bladder, prostate, and pancreas.

○   **What is the risk of development of breast cancer in a patient who has two first-degree relatives with breast cancer?**

4 to 6 times.

○   **Do the majority of women with a family history of breast cancer have the BRCA1 and 2 genes?**

No, <10% do.

○   **How significant is the risk of development of breast cancer in a patient with Cowden disease?**

These patients have up to 50% risk of development of breast carcinoma by the time they reach age 50.

○   **What initial receptors in carcinoma cells should be determined at the time of initial biopsy?**

Estrogen, progesterone, and human epidermal growth factor receptor 2 (HER-2/neu).

○   **How common is the presence of estrogen receptors in carcinoma cells?**

About half of the cases contain estrogen receptors.

○   **Why is it important to determine the presence or absence of estrogen and progesterone receptors in the cytoplasm of tumor cells?**

They are of proven value in determining adjuvant therapy and therapy for patients with advanced disease.

○ **How does the status of HER-2/neu affect the prognosis in breast cancer?**

It is associated with decreased survival when overexpressed in tumor cells.

○ **What percent of breast cancers are HER-2/neu positive?**

20%.

○ **What is HER-2/neu and where is it located?**

It is a proto-oncogene found on chromosome 17q21-22, and it has structural similarity to the epidermal growth factor receptor.

○ **What drug can be used as a single agent or can be added to first-line chemotherapy in HER-2/neu receptor positive to improve outcome?**

Herceptin (trastuzumab), which is a recombinant, humanized monoclonal antibody directed against the HER-2/neu product.

○ **What is the most significant side effect of Herceptin?**

Cardiotoxicity.

○ **What is the risk of developing breast cancer in association with caffeine consumption and cigarette smoking?**

There is no substantial data to prove a causative effect of either substance.

○ **What structure within the breast gives rise to all carcinomas?**

The terminal duct lobular unit.

○ **What is the most common type of in situ carcinoma and invasive carcinoma?**

Ductal carcinoma accounts for 80% of the in situ lesions and 80% of the invasive lesions.

○ **What are the various treatment options for a patient with breast carcinoma?**

- Breast conservation therapy, which consists of lumpectomy plus radiation or mastectomy.
- Radiation is indicated after mastectomy for tumors >5 cm, chest wall invasion, and/or 4 or more positive lymph nodes.
- Chemotherapy is used in patients with tumors >1 cm, positive lymph nodes, young age, and aggressive tumor factors.
- Herceptin is used if the tumor is positive for the HER2/neu receptor.
- Antiestrogens are used if the tumor is ER/PR+.
- In premenopausal women, tamoxifen is used.
- In postmenopausal women, either tamoxifen or aromatase inhibitors are used.

○ **What is required to qualify for breast conservation therapy?**

The tumor should be <5 cm, without any associated inflammatory carcinoma, skin nodules, or ulcerations, and with a favorable ratio of breast size to tumor size such that the patient would have a good cosmetic result.

○ **What nerve injuries can occur after a mastectomy?**

The long thoracic nerve innervates the serratus anterior muscle, and injury results in winged scapula. The thoracodorsal nerve can be injured causing paresis of the latissimus dorsi muscle. Injury to the intercostal brachial nerve causes numbness, tingling, or pain on the upper, medial aspect of the ipsilateral arm.

○ **What is the best single indicator of breast cancer prognosis?**

The extent of nodal involvement.

○ **What is the characteristic histologic invasion pattern of infiltrating lobular carcinoma?**

These tumors classically invade in a single file fashion and exhibit a "targetoid" or concentric ring formation around normal ducts.

○ **What is the prognosis of medullary carcinoma?**

It has an excellent prognosis with 10-year survivals of up to 90%.

○ **What is the prognosis for tubular carcinoma?**

It is the best of all invasive carcinomas with a 5-year survival rate approaching 100%.

○ **What is the prognosis for mucinous (colloid) carcinoma of the breast?**

It has a 10-year survival of up to 90% for the typical mucinous carcinoma.

○ **How common are axillary lymph node metastases in tubular carcinoma?**

<10% of cases.

○ **What is the maximal tumor measurement for a stage I breast carcinoma?**

2 cm or less.

○ **What is the maximal tumor measurement for a stage II breast carcinoma?**

5 cm or less.

○ **How does the presence or absence of hormone receptors in a tumor affect prognosis?**

Tumors with high numbers of hormone receptors have a slightly better prognosis than those without.

○ **How does mammary Paget disease differ from extramammary Paget disease?**

While it is uncommon to have underlying adenocarcinoma in extramammary Paget disease, Paget disease of the nipple is characterized by the presence of intraepidermal malignant cells from an underlying invasive ductal carcinoma or DCIS.

○ **What is the clinical presentation of mammary Paget disease?**

Erythema, thickening, crusting, and/or itching of the nipple-areolar complex.

○ **Is there an association with the BRCA1 and BRCA2 genes in male breast cancer?**

There is an association with BRCA2 in some familial breast cancers in males but not BRCA1.

○ **What is the characteristic histologic feature of mucinous (colloid) carcinoma?**

It is characterized by pools of mucin within which groups of tumor cells "float."

○ **What does the term "metaplastic carcinoma" describe in breast cancer?**

These are tumors with "sarcomatoid" features or a mixture of malignant epithelial and mesenchymal elements.

○ **What is the most common pure sarcoma to occur in the breast?**

Angiosarcoma.

○ **What is the mean age of development of angiosarcoma of the breast?**

Approximately 40 years.

○ **What factors are associated with the development of angiosarcoma?**

Lymphatic obstruction and radiation.

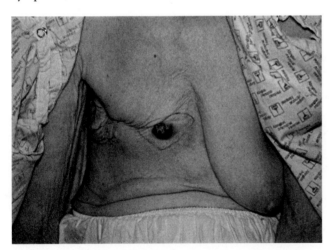

Figure 41.5 *A 85-year-old patient with a 15-year prior right-sided mastectomy and chest wall radiotherapy for locally advanced carcinoma now exhibits a raised, nodular, purplish mass that is angiosarcoma.*

○ **What is the prognosis of angiosarcoma of the breast?**

There is a 5 yr survival rate of 8% to 50%.

○ **Where does recurrence of angiosarcoma of the breast occur?**

Recurrence usually is local, although hematogenous dissemination may occur. Dissemination usually involves the lungs, skin, contralateral breastbone, liver, brain, and ovary, in decreasing frequency.

○   **What are the odds for a response of metastatic angiosarcoma of the breast to chemotherapy?**

Approximately 35%, with rare complete responses. If metastases are amenable to surgical extirpation, surgery should be attempted first for cure, and chemotherapy and radiation should be reserved for either the immediate postoperative period or for the next failure.

○   **Does non-Hodgkin lymphoma occur in the breast?**

Yes. Many believe this condition to be a part of the lymphomas related to mucosa-associated lymphoid tissue (MALT).

○   **What is the typical age at presentation for male breast cancer?**

The median age is 67 years.

○   **In general terms, what is the prognosis of male breast cancer?**

The prognosis is the same for males and females with breast cancer, although men tend to present at later stages than women.

○   **What is the most important aspect of treatment for fibromatosis of the breast?**

The initial wide excision of the lesion.

○   **What characteristics differentiate a granular cell tumor?**

Abundant eosinophilic granular cytoplasm, immunoreactivity with S-100 protein, and oval to round cells.

○   **What is the definition of microinvasive carcinoma of the breast?**

This refers to a carcinoma that is almost exclusively in situ. However, there are one or more separate foci of early invasion by tumor. In order to qualify as microinvasion, the foci cannot measure >1 mm in diameter.

○   **What are some immunohistochemical markers associated with the tumor cells in Paget disease of the nipple?**

The tumor cells will react with low-molecular weight cytokeratin, epithelial membrane antigen, and HER2/neu.

○   **What condition can present after trauma to the breast?**

Fat necrosis.

○   **Breast cancer accounts for what percentage of all new cases of cancer diagnosed in women?**

27%.

○   **What is a woman's lifetime risk of developing breast cancer?**

12% or 1 in 8.

○   **What are the components of breast cancer screening?**

Breast imaging, clinical breast examination, and patient self-screening

○ **When is ultrasonography found to be useful?**

It aids in evaluating inconclusive mammographic findings, women with dense breast tissue, and differentiating a cyst from a solid mass.

○ **When should an MRI be recommended for screening?**

In women with a 20% or greater lifetime risk of developing cancer.

○ **Who is considered to have a 20% or greater lifetime risk of developing cancer?**

Women with a history of radiation therapy to the chest between the ages of 10 and 30 years have a known BRCA1 or BRCA2 mutation, a first-degree relative with a BRCA1 or BRCA 2 mutation that have not been tested themselves, and other genetic syndromes.

○ **What genetic syndromes increase one's risk of breast cancer?**

Li-Fraumeni, Bannayan-Riley-Ruvalcaba, and Cowden syndrome,

○ **What screening is recommended for women with BRCA1 and BRCA2?**

Twice yearly clinical breast examinations, annual mammography, annual breast MRI, and instruction in breast self-examinations

○ **What screening should be implemented in women who received thoracic irradiation between the ages 10 and 30?**

Annual mammography and MRI.

CHAPTER 42

Ethics, Psychosocial, and Psychiatric Pearls

Alison B. McGrorty, MD

○ **What are the principles of medical ethics?**

Autonomy, beneficence, nonmaleficence, justice/fairness, and confidentiality.

○ **What is an ethical dilemma?**

When two or more ethical principles are in conflict with each other.

○ **What is mental competency/capacity?**

Sufficient understanding and memory to generally comprehend the situation in which the patient is currently in, including the nature, purpose, and consequence of any act or transaction that the patient may enter.

○ **What condition should always be evaluated before declaring competency?**

Depression.

○ **What is an advance directive?**

An advance directive is the formal mechanism by which a patient may express her values regarding her future health status. It may take the form of a proxy directive and/or an instructional directive.

○ **What is power of attorney?**

The durable power of attorney for health-care designates a surrogate to make medical decisions on behalf of the patient who is no longer competent to express his/her choices. The terms durable power of attorney, health-care proxy, health-care agent, and surrogate are all interchangeable.

○ **What is a living will?**

A living will is an instructional directive that focuses on the types of life-sustaining treatments that a patient would or would not choose in various clinical circumstances (ie, CPR and intubation).

○ **A fully coherent, adult Jehovah's Witness is having a massive lower GI hemorrhage and is refusing transfusions. Is the physician legally bound to administer blood products due to the imminence of death if a transfusion is not performed?**

No. The principle of autonomy dictates that this patient may refuse blood products even if it results in his/her death.

○ **True or False: A patient with stage I bronchogenic carcinoma has pulmonary edema requiring mechanical ventilation. You explain this to the patient and he agrees with proceeding with intubation and mechanical ventilation. His wife refuses. The physician should not intubate the patient.**

False. The principle of autonomy declares that each individual is the ultimate arbiter of his or her own health care.

○ **When can confidentiality be broken?**

Confidentiality can be broken at the patient's request, in the case of abuse (child or elder), court mandate, reportable diseases (HIV, gonorrhea, chlamydia, etc), and in instances of a patient being a danger to themselves or others.

○ **Is it ethical to release information to insurance companies?**

Yes. However, this information should be limited to processing an insurance claim.

○ **May a physician disclose the content of a medical record to another health-care professional in the regular course of treatment?**

Yes. As long as the other physician is participating in the care of the patient.

○ **May a physician disclose the content of a medical record under a court order?**
Yes.

○ **May a physician disclose the content of a child's medical record to school officials who request it?**
No.

○ **In what circumstances do minors *not* need consent from a parent/guardian?**
(1) When receiving care for sexually transmitted diseases (STDs).
(2) When receiving treatment/care for pregnancy (NOT including abortion).
(3) When receiving treatment related to drugs and alcohol.
(4) When prescribing OCPs or receiving condoms in a clinic setting (rules are different in other settings).

○ **True or False: Testing may be performed on a patient at the request of the patient's partner, family members, employers, or health insurers without the consent of the patient.**

False. Testing may only be performed when the patient understands the risks and benefits of a test and has given their consent

○ **When is partner consent needed for a woman to participate in a clinical research trial?**
(1) The partner is a subject of the trial himself.
(2) The partner will be exposed to an investigational agent, which has a potential for greater than minimal risks.
(3) The partner's acceptance of the treatment, or the impact of his acceptance on the woman, will be collected as data.
(4) If characteristics of the partner are listed as inclusion or exclusion criteria.

○ **True or False: When it comes to testing that may have certain medical and/or psychosocial ramifications for a patient (ie, HIV testing and genetic testing) that may require comprehensive explanations and possible counseling, a physician must be the person that portrays this information to the patient.**

False. Physicians may need to refer some patients for comprehensive counseling if time constraints or lack of specialized expertise make it difficult to offer appropriate counseling in a particular practice.

○ **Do patients need to be informed prior to testing if the results of the test must be reported (ie, HIV testing and STDs)?**

Yes. Patients must be told before being tested if their tests results must be reported.

○ **Are physicians obligated to perform every test a patient requests?**

No. Physicians are not ethically obligated to perform every test a patient requests.

○ **Is there an ethical difference between *withholding* and *withdrawing* life-support measures?**

No. Ethical principles underlying the decision apply equally in these two measures.

○ **What is the definition of medical futility?**

(1) The patient has a lethal diagnosis or prognosis of imminent death.*

(2) Evidence exists that the suggested therapy cannot achieve its physiologic goal.*

(3) Evidence exists that the suggested therapy will not or cannot achieve the patent's or family's stated goals.

(4) Evidence exists that the suggested therapy will not or cannot extend the patient's life span.*

(5) Evidence exists that the suggested therapy will not or cannot enhance the patient's quality of life.*

○ **Does the concept of medical futility apply only to the cases of patients with terminal illnesses?**

No. The concept of medical futility can apply to any clinical situation in which a proposed treatment offers virtually no chance of achieving a desired result.

○ **In artificial insemination by donor, where the recipient of the insemination is married, who is considered the legal father?**

The husband of the woman receiving the insemination is considered the legal father.

○ **In order for surgical sterilization (tubal ligation) in a female to be performed, who needs to consent for the procedure?**

Although it is highly recommended that a woman consults with her significant other before the procedure is performed due to the possible effects it may have on them, only the women undergoing the procedure needs to consent prior to being performed.

○ **True or False: Consent is not required when sterilizing a woman/man with mental disabilities.**

False. Consent is still required and can often require the assistance of an individual who is trained in communicating with mentally disabled individuals. However, in situations where there is disagreement among patient's caregivers and consultants, court approval may be obtained.

---

*Imminent death, physiologic goal, life span, and quality of life do not have established definitions and are often a point of contention between patients and physicians and even amongst medical professionals.

○ **Can pre/postfertilization techniques for sex selection be used when requested by patient for the purpose of family balancing or for religious reasons?**

No. The ACOG Committee of Ethics supports the practice of offering patients procedures for the purpose of preventing serious sex-linked genetic diseases. However, the Committee opposes meeting requests for sex selection for personal and family reasons (ie, family balancing and cultural or religious beliefs).

○ **Should a physician withhold telling a patient the sex of a fetus when a test is being performed for another indication that will subsequently reveal the sex in an effort to avoid unwitting participation in sex selection?**

No. When a medical procedure is done for a purpose other than obtaining information about the sex of a fetus but will reveal the fetus's sex, this information should not be withheld for any reason from the pregnant woman who requests it.

○ **Are physicians obligated to perform a reduction procedure in a multifetal pregnancy if a pregnant patient requests it?**

No. Physicians are not mandated to perform fetal reductions if they believe that such a procedure is morally unacceptable; however, they should still be knowledgeable about the procedure and be prepared to react in a professional and ethical manner when patients request information/services.

○ **Can embryos abandoned by the donors of the gametes or somatic cells used in its creation be used for research?**

No. Donors of gametes or somatic cells used in the creation of an embryo must give consent in order for an unused embryo to be used for research. Further, donation of embryos for stem cell research requires specific consent.

○ **Can a physician have a sexual or romantic relationship with a current patient if the relationship is consensual by both parties?**

No! Mere mutual consent is rejected as a justification for sexual relations with patients because the disparity in power, status, vulnerability, and need makes it difficult for a patient to give meaningful consent to sexual contact or sexual relations.

○ **Can a physician have a sexual or romantic relationship with a former patient if the relationship is consensual by both parties?**

Sexual contact or a romantic relationship with a former patient may be unethical under certain circumstances. However, the issue still remains that there may be the potential for misuse of physician power or exploitation of patient emotions derived from the former relationship.

○ **True or False: The terms "rape" and "sexual assault" should be used in a medical record when doing an evaluation of a potential victim.**

False. "Rape" and "sexual assault" are legal terms, and should be avoided when documenting in medical records. Instead, the physical findings of the evaluation should be described as "being consistent" with the reported assault.

○ **What efforts can be made on the part of a sexual assault victim to aid in better collection of evidence?**

The victim should avoid bathing, changing her clothes, douching, urinating, defecating, washing out her mouth, cleaning her fingernails, smoking, eating, or drinking.

○ **What are the most common STDs reported in sexual assault victims?**

Trichomoniasis, gonorrhea, and *Chlamydia trachomatis.*

These are also the most common STDs overall in the general public.

○ **What health concerns have been found to be more prevalent in lesbians than in heterosexual females?**

Depression and drug and alcohol abuse.

○ **True or False: It is not necessary to test lesbian females for STDs because these infections are only transmitted between a man and a woman.**

False. Lesbians should still be routinely tested for STDs because female-to-female transmission is possible for many infections. Lesbians are particularly susceptible to bacterial vaginosis, candidiasis, herpes, and HPV.

○ **Should lesbians be tested for HIV?**

Yes. Although there are no documented cases of HIV transmission between two lesbians, female-to-female transmission is feasible and should still be tested.

○ **What are the potential dangers with the use of two-dimensional or three-dimensional ultrasonography for nonmedical purposes, such as keepsake photographs or videos?**

(1) Possibly adverse effects of ultrasonography cannot be totally ruled out, thus such imaging should be limited to medical indications only.

(2) A false reassurance of fetal well-being may be implied by an aesthetically pleasing sonogram and can be misinterpreted as a diagnostic test.

(3) Abnormalities, if detected, may create an undue sense of alarm if the personnel performing the scan are not trained to discuss their implications.

(4) Abnormalities detected may be lost to follow-up when the scan is performed outside an integrated prenatal care delivery system.

○ **What is the 5-A approach to smoking counseling for pregnant women?**

(1) ASK about smoking status in multiple choice format:
   (a) never smoked?
   (b) smoked before pregnancy but not now?
   (c) smoked after discovering pregnancy but not now?
   (d) smokes now but less than before pregnancy?
   (e) smokes now with the same number of cigarettes as before pregnancy?

(2) ADVISE about the benefits of quitting and the impact of smoking and quitting on the woman and her fetus.

(3) ASSESS the willingness to quit within 30 days.

(4) ASSIST by providing skills and methods, as well as support groups, for smoking cessation.

(5) ARRANGE for follow-up evaluation of smoking status and the impact of the proposed interventions.

○ **What is the prevalence of alcoholism in the United States?**

10% to 15% lifetime prevalence.

○ **What laboratory changes are suggestive of alcoholism?**

2:1 ratio of AST to ALT.

○ **What is the consequence if a glucose solution is administered to an alcoholic patient before thiamine has been administered?**

Wernicke encephalopathy.

○   **What is Wernicke encephalopathy?**

A syndrome due to thiamine deficiency most often seen in alcoholics.
Consists of:

(1) Ataxia

(2) Ophthalmoplegia

(3) Nystagmus

(4) Confusion

(5) Impairment of short-term memory

○   **What is the temporal order of the symptoms of alcohol withdrawal (time since last drink)?**

(1) Autonomic hyperactivity → 6 to 8 hours

(2) Hallucinations → 24 hours

(3) Delirium tremens → 24 to 72 hours

○   **What is the only medication approved for the treatment of opioid dependence that may be dispensed in an office-based setting?**

Buprenorphine. This drug is a partial agonist of the opioid receptors and is approved for use during pregnancy. Unlike methadone, buprenorphine can be prescribed in an office setting by a credentialed physician.

○   **What medication should never be used to treat the tachycardia found in cocaine intoxication? Why?**

B-blockers. Allow for unopposed alpha-adrenergic activity thus increasing hypertension, reducing coronary blood flow, and reducing cardiac output.

TABLE 42.1 Signs, Symptoms, and Treatment of Substance Intoxication and Withdrawal

	Intoxication		Withdrawal	
	Signs and Symptoms	**Treatment**	**Signs and Symptoms**	**Treatment**
Alcohol	Slurred speech, disinhibition, ataxia, emotional lability, memory and judgment impairment, blackouts, coma	Supportive measures, thiamine, multivitamin, folic acid	Tremor, tachycardia, hypertension, seizures, delirium tremens, death	Benzodiazepines
Opiates	Euphoria, apathy, pupillary constriction, CNS depression, constipation, respiratory depression (possibly life threatening)	Naloxone	Nausea, vomiting, mydriasis, diarrhea, anorexia, piloerection, yawning, abdominal pain, muscle spasms, and leukocytosis	Methadone
Cocaine	Psychomotor agitation, pupillary dilation, euphoria, impaired judgment, tachycardia, hypertension, hallucinations, possible sudden death	Haloperidol, symptom-specific treatment, and supportive measures	Hypersomnolence, depression, severe cravings/increased appetite, malaise, suicidality, nightmares	Supportive measures

○ **What is dementia?**

Disturbed cognitive function that results in impaired memory, personality, judgment, or language.

○ **What is delirium?**

"Clouding of consciousness" that results in disorientation, decreased alertness, and impaired cognitive function.

TABLE 42.2 Delirium Versus Dementia

	Delirium	**Dementia**
Causes	Infection, substance use/withdrawal, metabolic and endocrine disturbances, hypoxia, toxins, and heavy metals	Most often due to neurodegenerative diseases (Alzheimer, Parkinson, Huntington, Creutzfeldt–Jakob diseases, etc),
Onset	Acute	Gradual
Course	Fluctuating from hour to hour	Progressive deterioration
Level of attention	Impaired	Intact
Hallucinations	Often present	Present in only about 30% of patients with advanced disease
Prognosis	Reversible	Most often irreversible. However, up to 15% of cases can be attributed to treatable cause, and thus can be reversed.

○ **What is the most common cause of dementia?**

Alzheimer disease—it accounts for 70% to 80% of all dementia cases.

○ **What are some examples of treatable causes of dementia?**

Uremia, syphilis, depression, hypothyroidism, and vitamin B12 deficiency.

○ **What conditions may mimic dementia in the elderly?**

Hypothyroidism
Depression – referred to as pseudodementia

○ **What are the characteristics of normal bereavement?**

The following characteristics are those of normal bereavement, and can last up to 6 to 12 months (beyond 12 months, evaluation of major depression should be performed):

(1) Uncomplicated grief

(2) Crying

(3) Decreased appetite

(4) Weight loss

(5) Decreased concentration

(6) Guilt

(7) Auditory and visual hallucinations of the deceased individual

○ **What are the diagnostic criteria for major depression?**

Five or more of the following symptoms that have been *present for 2 weeks* and at least one of the symptoms is depressed mood or loss of interest:

(1) Marked diminished interest or pleasure in all.

(2) Weight loss or weight gain.

(3) Insomnia or hypersomnia.

(4) Psychomotor agitation or retardation.

(5) Decrease energy.

(6) Feelings of worthlessness.

(7) Inability to concentrate.

(8) Suicidal ideation.

○ **What is the lifetime prevalence of major depression?**

15%.

○ **What is the name given to a common, transitory, mild depression that occurs in the first week after delivery? What is the treatment?**

Postpartum blues. This condition is self-limited and requires supportive care only.

○ **What are the criteria for diagnosing postpartum depression?**

The criteria for major depressive disorder and postpartum depression are the same ("*Five or more* of the [aforementioned] symptoms that have been *present for 2 weeks...*"). The difference being that postpartum depression occurs, as appropriately named, during the postpartum period.

○ **What disorder is often mistaken as postpartum depression in the postpartum female? How do you rule out this condition?**

Hypothyroidism. If hypothyroidism is suspected, check serum TSH and T4.

○ **Who is more likely to complete an attempt at suicide, men or women?**

Males are more likely to be successful in their attempts at suicide compared with women (3:1); however, women attempt suicide about three times more often than men.

○ **Why are men more likely to complete suicide as compared with women?**

Men tend to use more aggressive approaches to their attempts (ie, use of handguns and hanging), whereas women tend to use more "slowly effective" or "ineffective" approaches to suicide such as ingestion of pills or wrist cutting.

○ **What potentially detrimental effect on the fetus is most often seen in patients with preexisting mental disorders (ie, bipolar, schizophrenia, and depression)?**

Complications due to noncompliance with prenatal care.

○ **What is the difference between low potency and high potency neuroleptics?**

Low potency neuroleptics have greater sedative, postural hypotensive, and anticholinergic effects. High potency neuroleptics have greater extrapyramidal effects.

○ **What are the autonomic side effects of antipsychotics?**

Dry mouth, urinary retention, orthostatic hypotension, and sedation.

○ **What are the extrapyramidal side effects of antipsychotics?**

Dystonia, akathisia, Parkinsonism, tardive dyskinesia, and neuroleptic malignant syndrome (NMS).

○ **What is the timeframe for the occurrence of extrapyramidal side effects with the use of antipsychotics?**

(1) Dystonic Reaction → hours to days

(2) Akathisia → weeks

(3) Parkinsonism → months

(4) Tardive dyskinesia → years

○ **What treatment is used in the case of dystonic reactions when using antipsychotics?**

Benadryl or anticholinergics (benztropine/*Cogentin* or trihexyphenidyl).

○ **What is NMS?**

A life-threatening neurological disorder characterized by hyperthermia, rigidity, and an increase in creatinine phosphokinase (CPK) caused by the use certain neuroleptics (haloperidol, chlorpromazine, etc). It can occur at any time during the use of neuroleptics.

○ **What is the treatment of NMS?**

Treatment includes discontinuation of antipsychotic, aggressive IV hydration, and dantrolene.

○ **What options are available for chemical restraint?**

(1) Benzodiazepines

    (a) Lorazepam—*Ativan*

    (b) Midazolam—*Versed*

    (c) Diazepam—*Valium*

(2) Sedative hypnotics

    (a) Haloperidol—*Haldol*

    (b) Droperidol—*Inapsine*

○   **True or False: Benzodiazepines and sedative hypnotics should never be combined when being used as chemical restraints.**

False. Benzodiazepines may be given in combination with sedative hypnotics (specifically the ones listed in the previous question) to both hasten and potentiate each other's effect. Ultimately, titrate to effective dose and monitor appropriately.

○   **What may occur when ethanol is combined with a benzodiazepine?**

Severe respiratory depression, possibly leading to death.

○   **In a patient with bipolar disorder who now presents with polyuria, what medication is the patient most likely taking?**

Lithium. Long-term use can result in nephrogenic diabetes insipidus.

○   **What is Munchausen syndrome?**

A factitious disorder in which the patient fabricates their symptoms or causes injury to themselves in order to achieve the 1° gain of the "sick role."
Commonly seen in health-care workers.

○   **What is Munchausen syndrome by proxy?**

A factitious disorder with the same characteristics as Munchausen syndrome, but instead of the patient playing the "sick role," he/she projects this role onto an individual that he/she is caring for. This is considered a form of abuse.

○   **What is somatization disorder?**

Multiple, chronic somatic symptoms from different body systems including GI, neurologic, pain, and sexual complaint that do not have a medical explanation; seen more often in women. The complaints are very real to the patients, and they have no control over these symptoms (no 1° gain).
Criteria:

(1) Eight or more symptoms

(2) At least four pain symptoms

(3) At least one gynecologic/sexual complaint

○   **A 30-year-old woman complains of calf pain, a headache, shooting pain when flexing her right wrist, epigastric pain and bloating, and irregular menses. The physician is unable to find a medical condition to explain this constellation of symptoms. What is a possible diagnosis?**

Somatization disorder.

○   **What are the four phases of the female sexual response cycle and possible abnormalities of each of them?**

(1) Excitement phase → Hypoactive sexual desire disorder

(2) Plateau → Female sexual arousal disorder

(3) Orgasmic phase → Female orgasmic disorder

(4) Resolution phase → Postcoital dysphoria/Postcoital headache

○   **What is dyspareunia?**

Painful sexual intercourse due to medical/psychological cause.

○ **What is vaginismus?**

Inability to engage in any form of vaginal penetration (intercourse, tampon use, gyn examinations) due to involuntary muscle contractions in the vagina.

○ **True or False: Sexual trauma such as rape can cause vaginismus.**

True.

○ **What are paraphilias? Are they ever considered normal?**

Paraphilias are abnormal expressions of sexuality (exhibitionism, fetishism, pedophilia, etc), and are never considered to be normal variants of sexual expression.

○ **What psychiatric medications are absolutely contraindicated during pregnancy?**

Estazolam (Prosom), flurazepam (Dalmane), quazepam (Doral), temazepam (Restoril), and triazolam (Halicon).

○ **What treatment of bipolar disorder has yet to be linked to major fetal anomalies and is an option for treatment during pregnancy?**

Lamotrigine (Lamictal).

○ **What side effects have been observed in infants born to mothers using carbamazepine during pregnancy?**

Transient cholestatic hepatitis and hyperbilirubinemia; however, these side effects are rare. Carbamazepine has been declared as "probably safe" during pregnancy.

○ **What side effect is seen in infants born to mothers using benzodiazepines shortly before delivery?**

Floppy infant syndrome.

Symptoms consist of hypothermia, lethargy, poor respiratory effort, and feeding difficulties.

TABLE 42.3 Teratogenic Effects of Certain Psychiatric Medications

Drug	Effect on Fetus
Carbamazepine	Spina bifida, craniofacial defects, fingernail hypoplasia
Benzodiazepines	Cleft lip, cleft palate
Lithium	Ebstein anomaly
Valproic acid	Neural tube defects, craniofacial and cardiovascular abnormalities, IUGR, cognitive impairment

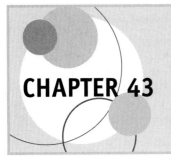

CHAPTER 43 Cervical Lesions and Cancer

Janos L. Tanyi, MD, PhD

○ **When the Pap smear examinations should be initiated?**

The American College of Obstetricians and Gynecologists (ACOG) revised their recommended cervical cancer screening schedule for women in 2009. The new recommendation is that all women should have their first Pap smear at age 21.

○ **What is the recommended schedule of Pap smears?**

In 2009, the ACOG revised their recommended cervical cancer screening schedule for women. They recommend start at age 21. Women in their 20s should have a Pap smear every 2 years (revised from previous recommendations that it should be done annually). Women in their 30s who have had three consecutive normal Pap smears should undergo one screening every 3 years. Women 65 to 70 who have had three consecutive normal Pap smear results and no abnormal findings in the previous 10 years can discontinue screenings altogether if they choose. Women who have undergone a total hysterectomy due to a noncancerous condition and have not had previously abnormal Pap smears can also discontinue screenings.

○ **How frequently should a Pap smear be performed on an HIV-infected woman?**

Women infected with HIV should have cervical cytology screening twice in the first year after diagnosis and annually thereafter

○ **How frequently should a Pap smear be performed in a woman with history of CIN 2–3?**

Women treated in the past for CIN 2, CIN 3, or cancer remain at risk of persistent or recurrent disease for at least 20 years after treatment and after initial post treatment surveillance and should continue to have annual screening for at least 20 years.

○ **Is human papillomavirus (HPV) transmitted through vaginal intercourse alone?**

No. HPV can be acquired through same-sex and nonpenetrative sexual contact.

○ **Should all women who have <u>not</u> undergone hysterectomy have Pap smears performed annually?**

After initiation of screening, American Cancer Society recommends cervical screening be done annually with conventional cervical cytology smears or every 2 years using liquid-based cytology. ACOG recommends every 2 years screening regardless of the type of Pap performed. After age 30, women who have had three consecutive, technically satisfactory normal cytology results may be screened every 3 years (unless DES history, HIV positive, or are immunocompromised).

○ **How effective have Pap smears been in reducing the incidence of cervical cancer?**

Since the development of cytological screening in the 1940s, the incidence of cervical cancer in the United States has fallen by almost 80%. In contrast, cervical cancer remains the major cause of cancer-related deaths among women in many third world countries where Pap smears are not routinely performed.

○ **What type of cervical cancer is caused by HPV 18 infections?**

Most of the squamous cell carcinomas.

○ **What type of cervical cancer is caused by HPV 16 infections?**

Most of the cervical adenocarcinomas.

○ **What is the false-negative rate for conventional Pap smears?**

Up to 30% to 40%.

○ **The quadrivalent HPV vaccine should be given to females in what age group?**

The FDA approved the vaccine for administration to girls and women between 9 and 26 years of age.

○ **The quadrivalent HPV vaccine should be given to males in what age group?**

The FDA did not approve the vaccine for administration to boys and men in any age group.

○ **The HPV vaccine is effective against the oncogenic types 16 and 18. What percentage of cervical cancers is caused by these two types of HPV?**

HPV types 16 and 18 are responsible for about 70% of all cervical cancers.

○ **What is the most common presenting symptom for patients with cervical cancer?**

The classic symptoms are intermittent painless metrorrhagia or spotting. Up to 80% of patients present with abnormal vaginal bleeding, most commonly postmenopausal. Only 10% note postcoital bleeding. Less frequent symptoms include vaginal discharge and pain. Late symptoms or indicative for more advanced disease are pain referred to flank or leg, dysuria, hematuria, and rectal bleeding.

○ **What is the most appropriate management for a gross cervical lesion discovered during a routine examination?**

Biopsy. Specimens from ulcerated lesions should be obtained from their center.

○ **What is the next appropriate step in management of an ASCUS Pap test in a patient whose reflex HPV testing is positive for high-risk HPV subtypes?**

Colposcopy including cervical biopsy and endocervical curettage.

○ **If high-grade squamous intraepithelial lesions are left untreated over a period of several years, what percentage will progress to invasive cancer?**

Approximately 20%.

○ **What is the relative frequency of the two major histologic subtypes of cervical cancer?**

Approximately 80% of cervical cancers are squamous cell carcinoma, and 15% are adenocarcinomas.

○ **What is the most common stage at diagnosis of cervical cancer?**

Approximately half of patients with cervical cancer present with stage I disease.

○ **What epidemiologic risk factors have been identified for the development of cervical cancer?**

Women in lower socioeconomic status, young age at first intercourse, multiple sexual partners, high parity, HIV infection, and history of other sexually transmitted infections.

○ **What other modifiable risk factor has been clearly linked to an increased risk of cervical cancer?**

Exposure to cigarette smoke. The relative risk of cervical cancer is increased two- to fourfold among cigarette smokers compared with nonsmokers.

○ **A carcinoma 5 cm in diameter and clinically confined to the cervix is assigned what International Federation of Gynecologists and Obstetricians (FIGO) stage?**

According to the 2009 FIGO staging modifications, lesions clinically confined to the cervix and ≤4 cm in diameter are designated stage IB1. Lesions >4 cm are classified as stage IB2.

○ **A carcinoma 3 cm in diameter and extended to the upper third of the vagina is assigned what FIGO stage?**

According to the 2009 FIGO staging modifications, lesions with clinical involvement of the upper two-thirds of the vagina, without parametrial invasion, <4 cm in greatest dimension are designated stage IIA1.

○ **A carcinoma 5 cm in diameter and extended to the upper third of the vagina is assigned what FIGO stage?**

According to the 2009 FIGO staging modifications, lesions with clinical involvement of the upper two-thirds of the vagina, without parametrial invasion, >4 cm in greatest dimension are designated stage IIA2.

○ **How do para-aortic lymph node metastases detected by computed tomography (CT) scan and confirmed by thin-needle sampling affect staging?**

This information helps to direct therapy, but it does not affect staging that is clinically assigned.

○ **What radiographic study has the highest sensitivity to detect para-aortic lymph node metastases?**

Lymphangiogram, CT scan, and ultrasound were prospectively evaluated by the Gynecologic Oncology Group. Sensitivities were 79%, 34%, and 19%, respectively. Specificities were 96%, 73%, and 99%, respectively.

○ **What diagnostic methods are accepted in the staging of cervical carcinoma?**

Physical examination, colposcopy, cystoscopy, routine radiographs (chest X-ray), intravenous pyelogram (IVP), proctoscopy, sigmoidoscopy, and barium studies of the large bowels. Other imaging or diagnostic methods such as magnetic resonance imaging (MRI), computed tomography (CT), venography, arteriography, hysteroscopy, laparoscopy or laparotomy, are NOT acceptable for staging determination.

○   **Examination under anesthesia reveals a 3 cm in diameter cervical carcinoma with left parametrial involvement not extending to the pelvic wall. The remainder of the staging evaluation is unremarkable. To what stage is this patient's tumor assigned?**

Stage IIB. According to the 2009 FIGO staging modifications, lesions with clinical involvement of the parametrium but not reaching the sidewall is stage IIB.

○   **For the above patient, if her IVP had revealed hydronephrosis, to what stage would her tumor is assigned?**

Stage IIIB classified as either tumor extension to the pelvic sidewall or hydronephrosis or a nonfunctioning kidney.

○   **If this patient's cystoscopy had identified bullous edema, what should her stage have been?**

It would remain stage IIIB. Bullous edema without pathologic confirmation of malignancy does not permit assignment to stage IVA.

○   **Are cystoscopy and proctoscopy necessary in the staging of all patients with cervical cancer?**

They may be omitted in the staging of asymptomatic patients with early disease (typically IIA or lower) for whom these studies are rarely abnormal.

○   **What is the incidence of pelvic and para-aortic lymph node metastasis for stage IB cervical cancer?**

Approximately 15% to 20% and about 2%, respectively.

○   **For stage I cervical cancer, how does tumor size >4 cm affect the incidence of pelvic lymph node metastasis?**

When compared with smaller lesions, an approximately threefold increase has been demonstrated.

○   **What lymph node group is most frequently involved with metastatic cervical cancer?**

In most series, the external iliac group is most commonly involved followed next by the obturator group.

○   **A colposcopically directed cervical biopsy from a 25-year-old G0P0 reveals a small focus of microinvasive squamous cell carcinoma. The resection margin is positive for carcinoma in situ. What is the next step in this patient's management?**

Cervical cone biopsy to establish the full extent of invasion.

○   **A patient underwent conization with a FIGO stage IA1 squamous cell cancer and Society of Gynecologic Oncologists (SGO) criteria for microinvasion but with surgical margins are free of cancer. Does she need any further treatment?**

Patient with FIGO stage IA1 and SGO criteria for microinvasion could be treated conservatively with simple hysterectomy, or of continued fertility is desired conization only, provided surgical margins are free of cancer.

○   **For the above patient, final pathology shows invasion extending 2 mm below the basement membrane with a width of 4 mm. No lymphovascular space involvement is present, and the margins are free of involvement. What is this patient's stage, and what are her therapeutic options?**

Stage IA1. The SGO defines microinvasion as stromal invasion of 3 mm or less below the basement membrane without lymphovascular space involvement. For patients who desire preservation of fertility, most authorities agree that the risk of recurrence is very low, and that no additional therapy is necessary. If fertility is not desired, simple hysterectomy is recommended.

○ **What is the incidence of pelvic lymph node metastasis for squamous cell carcinoma of the cervix invading 1 to 3 mm and for lesions invading 3 to 5 mm?**

<1% and 4%, respectively.

○ **What is the possibility of lymph metastasis in stage II disease?**

The prevalence of lymph node disease correlated well with the stage. Lymph node involvement in stage II is between 25% and 40%; in stage III, it is assumed that at least 50% have positive nodes.

○ **For stage IB1 and early stage IIA disease, which therapy is more effective, radical hysterectomy, or radiation therapy?**

For these stages, the two modalities are considered equivalent therapeutically. Choice of therapy is dependent on a wide variety of factors.

○ **What is the 5-year survival for stage I cervical cancer?**

Approximately is 90% overall. Five-year survival when nodes are negative is often >90%. When nodes are involved, survival ranges from 20% to 75% depending on the number, size, and location of the positive nodes.

○ **The cardinal ligaments are exposed during a radical hysterectomy when what two pelvic spaces are developed?**

The paravesical space anterior to the cardinal ligament and the pararectal space posteriorly.

○ **Ureterovaginal and vesicovaginal fistulas occur in what percentage of patients undergoing radical hysterectomy?**

1% to 2% and <1%, respectively.

○ **What is the difference between modified radical (class II) and radical hysterectomy (class III)?**

The purpose of the class II hysterectomy is to remove more paracervical tissue while still preserving most of the blood supply to the distal ureters and bladder. The uterine artery just ligated medial to the ureters. The class III procedure is a wide radical dissection of the parametrial tissues. The uterine artery is ligated at its origin on the internal iliac artery so lateral from the ureters.

○ **Define the reference points A and B used in radiation treatment planning for cervical cancer.**

Point A: 2 cm lateral and 2 cm superior to the external cervical os, approximating the location where the uterine artery crosses the ureter.

Point B: 3 cm lateral to point A, corresponding to the pelvic wall.

○ **The standard unit for measuring absorbed radiation is the gray (1 joule/kg). How many rads are equivalent to 1 Gy?**

100 rads equal to 1 Gy.

○ **What dosage of radiation is required to sterilize microscopic disease?**

4000 to 5000 cGy will sterilize over 90% of occult tumor deposits.

○ **What dosage of radiation is required to sterilize clinically apparent disease?**

>6000 cGy.

○ **How many cGy given in 200 cGy fractions are required to produce ovarian failure?**

1000 cGy will cause ovarian failure in 50% of women.

○ **What organ is most radiosensitive in the pelvis?**

Rectum.

○ **What is the incidence of small bowel obstruction following radiation used as primary therapy for cervical cancer?**

1% to 4%. The terminal ileum is most commonly involved due to its fixed position and limited blood supply. The majority of patients will present within 2 years of therapy. Recurrent disease must be ruled out.

○ **What radioisotopes are most commonly used in intracavitary radiation applicators?**

Cesium (Cs) for the traditional low-dose rate brachytherapy and iridium (Ir) for high-dose rate therapy.

○ **When radiation is used as primary therapy, what doses are delivered to points A and B?**

7000 to 8500 cGy to point A and 6000 cGy to point B with individualization by lesion and treatment center.

○ **What are the radiation tolerances for the rectum and bladder?**

Approximately 6000 and 7000 cGy, respectively.

○ **What are the advantages of radical hysterectomy relative to radiation therapy for stage I cervical cancer?**

- Ovarian preservation possible.
- Unimpaired vaginal function.
- Extent of disease established.

○ **How does lesion size affect therapy for cervical carcinoma confined to the cervix?**

Though controversial, many consider lesion size >4 cm to be a contraindication to radical hysterectomy. Radiation therapy is used with some recommending a simple hysterectomy following radiation.

○ **For locally advanced (stage IIB-IVA) cervical cancer, what treatment has become the standard of care?**

Concurrent cisplatin-based chemotherapy with radiation therapy.

○ **List pathologic findings following radical hysterectomy that indicate a high risk of recurrence.**

- Lymph node metastasis.
- Surgical margin involvement.
- Parametrial invasion.

○ **What is the incidence of para-aortic lymph node metastasis for stage IIB and III disease?**

Approximately 19% and 30%, respectively.

○ **What is the 5-year survival for stage IIB and III disease?**

Approximately 65% and 45%, respectively.

○ **What is the most common site of distant metastases of cervical cancer?**

Lung. Twenty-one percent of distant metastases of cervical cancer are found in the lung.

○ **What are the usual borders used for whole pelvic external beam radiation therapy?**

- Superiorly, the midvertebral level of L5.
- Inferiorly, the inferior aspect of the obturator foramina or at least 2 cm below the most distal vaginal tumor.
- Laterally, 1 cm lateral to the margins of the bony pelvis.

○ **How is the external beam treatment field altered when the para-aortic nodes are included?**

A 10 cm wide portal extends from the pelvic field up to the T12-L1 interspace.

○ **What percentage of cervical cancers occur in women during reproductive years?**

10% to 15%.

○ **What is the incidence of cervical cancer during pregnancy?**

Approximately 1.2 per 10,000 pregnancies.

○ **What is the most frequent female genital cancer during pregnancy?**

Cervical cancer.

○ **How does pregnancy affect survival for patients with cervical cancer?**

When prognostic factors are controlled for, survival is not affected by pregnancy.

○ **What is the incidence of supraclavicular lymph node involvement when the para-aortic nodes contain metastatic disease?**

5% to 30%. The left side is more commonly involved (entry of portal for the thoracic duct).

○ **What percentage of cervical cancer recurrences will be detected within 1, 2, and 5 years of follow-up?**

50% of recurrences will be detected within the first year, 75% within 2 years, and 95% within 5 years.

○ **How do survival rates of patients with adenocarcinoma of the cervix compare with those of squamous cell carcinoma?**

Controlling for prognostic factors such as stage, volume of disease, and lymph node metastasis and survival appears to be similar.

○ **When invasive cervical cancer is incidentally discovered following a simple hysterectomy, what is the most common preoperative diagnosis?**

Cervical dysplasia.

○ **A simple hysterectomy is performed and invasive cervical cancer is incidentally discovered. What are the therapeutic options?**

Patients who are good candidates of radical surgery and who had small lesions with uninvolved surgical margins can be treated with radical parametrectomy, upper vaginectomy, and pelvic lymphadenectomy. All others should receive chemoradiation therapy.

○ **Is conservation of the ovaries appropriate for young patients undergoing radical hysterectomy for stage IB adenocarcinoma of the cervix?**

Yes. If the ovaries appear grossly normal. The incidence of ovarian metastasis is <2%.

○ **What is the incidence of vesicovaginal fistula formation following radiation therapy for cervical cancer with bladder invasion?**

4% with 5-year survival up to 30%.

○ **What procedure is often considered prior to initiating radiation therapy for locally advanced cervical cancer complicated by a rectovaginal fistula?**

A diverting colostomy is often recommended to avoid sepsis.

○ **What is the 1-year survival rate following cervical cancer recurrence?**

Approximately 15%.

○ **What is the therapy of choice for an isolated vaginal cuff recurrence following radical hysterectomy?**

External beam radiation therapy followed by brachytherapy. Exenteration is generally reserved for patients who have previously received radiation.

○ **What criteria should be met prior to surgically exploring a patient for an exenteration?**

- Central pelvic disease without evidence of extension to the pelvic wall.
- No evidence of distant disease.
- A physically and emotionally fit patient.

○ **What clinical triad is strongly indicative of surgically unresectable recurrent cervical cancer?**

- Unilateral leg edema.
- Sciatic pain.
- Ureteral obstruction.

○ **What percentage of patients explored for an exenteration will be found to have unresectable disease?**

Approximately half. This is in part due to the limitations of the pelvic examination when radiation fibrosis of the parametria is present.

○ **What is the 5-year survival rate of patients undergoing pelvic exenteration for recurrent cervical cancer?**

With careful patient selection, up to 50%.

○ **What is the incidence of long-term response to cisplatin when used for advanced or recurrent cervical cancer?**

Overall response to cisplatin is 25%. However, long-term response is generally not seen.

○ **Match the following characteristics to the appropriate histologic subtype of cervical cancer.**

(1) Histologically similar to oat cell cancer of the lung   Clear cell carcinoma (c)

(2) Radiation may induce a more malignant transformation   Small cell neuroendocrine tumors (a)

(3) Associated with DES exposure   Verrucous carcinoma (b)

(4) Associated with Peutz–Jeghers syndrome   Minimal deviation adenocarcinoma (adenoma malignum) (d)

CHAPTER 44 Endometrial Hyperplasia and Carcinoma

Janos L. Tanyi, MD, PhD

○ **The World Health Organization classifies endometrial hyperplasia based on what two factors?**
   (1) Simple or complex glandular/stromal architecture.
   (2) The presence or absence of cytologic atypia.

○ **What is the best predictor that endometrial hyperplasia will progress to endometrial carcinoma?**
   The presence or absence of cytologic atypia.

○ **What is the endocrinologic milieu for the development of endometrial hyperplasia?**
   Unopposed estrogen.

○ **What other common risk factors have been correlated to the development of endometrial hyperplasia?**
   • Polycystic ovary (PCO) syndrome
   • Obesity
   • Diabetes mellitus
   • Late menopause (after age 55)
   • Nulliparity

○ **Which ovarian steroid hormone promotes growth of the endometrium?**
   Estrogen.

○ **Which ovarian steroid hormone promotes differentiation of the endometrium?**
   Progesterone.

○ **What percentage of women with atypical hyperplasia have coexistent endometrial cancer at the time of hysterectomy?**
   Up to 43%.

○ **In the absence of cytologic atypia, what percentage of endometrial hyperplasia will progress to endometrial carcinoma?**

Approximately 1% to 3%.

○ **What percentage of complex atypical hyperplasia will progress to endometrial cancer?**

29%.

○ **Why is endometrial hyperplasia more common at the extremes of reproductive life, near puberty, and the perimenopause?**

At both extremes anovulatory cycles are more common.

○ **In the postmenopausal woman, what is the main circulating estrogen and what is its source?**

Estrone. It arises from the peripheral conversion of adrenal and ovarian androstenedione. In a slender woman this amounts to 40 μg/day. In an obese woman it may exceed 200 μg/day.

○ **What are the most common presenting symptoms of endometrial hyperplasia in a woman of reproductive age?**

(1) Metrorrhagia.

(2) Menometrorrhagia.

○ **What is the most common presenting complaint in a postmenopausal woman with endometrial hyperplasia?**

Postmenopausal vaginal bleeding.

○ **Can endometrial hyperplasia be accurately diagnosed by transvaginal ultrasonography?**

No. Endometrial hyperplasia is a histologic diagnosis. An endometrial sample is necessary to exclude adenocarcinoma. A thickened endometrial stripe in excess of 10 mm in a woman with abnormal uterine bleeding may suggest endometrial hyperplasia but is not diagnostic.

○ **What type of ovarian neoplasm is most commonly associated with endometrial hyperplasia?**

Granulosa cell tumor, as it secretes estradiol.

○ **In a postmenopausal woman, what sign on pelvic examination should suggest an elevated endogenous estrogen level?**

The absence of vaginal atrophy. The presence of a vagina with multiple rugal folds suggests an estrogen effect.

○ **What percentage of perimenopausal and postmenopausal women will have endometrial hyperplasia on an endometrial biopsy performed for abnormal or postmenopausal bleeding?**

8% to 9%. In women under the age of 40, only 1% to 2% will have endometrial hyperplasia diagnosed on endometrial biopsy.

○ **What is the gland-stromal ratio in simple hyperplasia?**

The gland stromal ratio in simple hyperplasia favors the glands. In a normal proliferative endometrium, the gland stromal ratio favors the stroma.

○ **What are the earliest signs of cytologic atypia?**

- Enlarged round nuclei.
- Fine and evenly dispersed chromatin.

○ **What differentiates complex atypical hyperplasia from well-differentiated adenocarcinoma?**

The presence of stromal invasion defined as a desmoplastic stromal response or a complex proliferation exceeding half of a low power microscopic field, approximately 2.1 mm.

○ **In what type of hyperplasia there is back-to-back glandular crowding without cytologic atypia?**

This is the definition of complex hyperplasia.

○ **What is the value of mitotic activity in the diagnosis and prognosis of endometrial hyperplasia?**

It has none.

○ **Is there any difference between the biologic behavior between simple and complex hyperplasia?**

No. Neither has cytologic atypia and both have a low incidence of progression to cancer.

○ **What characterizes the endometrial hyperplasia that is most likely to progress to endometrial carcinoma?**

A complex architectural pattern and a moderate degree of cytologic atypia.

○ **What factors influence the treatment of endometrial hyperplasia?**

- Age.
- Amount and duration of vaginal bleeding.
- Associated anemia.
- Desire for future childbearing.
- The presence or absence of cytologic atypia.
- The degree of cytologic atypia.

○ **What medical therapeutic options exist for treating endometrial hyperplasia in women who do not desire pregnancy at this time?**

- Progesterone.
- Oral contraceptive pills (OCPs).
- Gonadotropin-releasing hormone (GnRH) analogs.
- A progesterone-containing IUD.

○ **What surgical options are currently available for the treatment of endometrial hyperplasia?**

- Curettage for acute bleeding.
- Hysteroscopy to exclude polyps and carcinoma.
- Hysterectomy, particularly if cytologic atypia is present.

○ **What nonmedical, nonsurgical lifestyle changes are important in counseling the woman with endometrial hyperplasia?**

Dietary counseling and weight loss, screening for diabetes mellitus, and discontinuing exogenous unopposed estrogen.

○ **What are the common side effects of depo-medroxyprogesterone therapy for endometrial hyperplasia?**

Spotting, breast soreness, weight gain, fluid retention, nervousness, irritability, and bloating.

○ **What are common side effects of GnRH analog therapy for endometrial hyperplasia?**

Menopausal symptoms: hot flashes, vaginal dryness, changes in the serum lipid profile, effects on the coronary arteries, and bone loss.

○ **What is the recommended follow-up for a woman with a histologic diagnosis of simple or complex hyperplasia without cytologic atypia?**

In addition to medical therapy, follow-up endometrial sampling is recommended in 6 months.

○ **What is the failure rate of medical therapy for simple and complex hyperplasia?**

Approximately 20%.

○ **What is the recommended follow-up for a woman with a histologic diagnosis of atypical hyperplasia treated conservatively?**

In addition to medical treatment, repeat endometrial sampling in 3 months; however, more recent evidence suggests that intervals up to 6 months may be necessary to establish hormonal conversion.

○ **What is the most common gynecological malignancy in the United States?**

Endometrial cancer, of which 80% are the endometrioid adenocarcinoma type. Endometrial cancer accounts for 6% of all cancers in women.

○ **In 2012, approximately how many new cases and deaths from endometrial cancer occurred?**

Endometrial cancer is the most common invasive gynecologic cancer in US women, with an estimated 47,130 new cases expected to occur in 2012. This disease primarily affects postmenopausal women at an average age of 60 years at diagnosis. In the United States, it is estimated that approximately 8010 women will die of endometrial cancer in 2012. Incidence rates of endometrial cancer have been increasing by an average of 1.1% per year from 2004 to 2008. Death rates from cancer of the uterine corpus have been increasing by an average of 0.3% per year from 1998 to 2007.

○ **What is the estimated prevalence of endometrial cancer in asymptomatic postmenopausal women?**

Approximately 24.1 per 100,000 for women in the United States.

○ **What is the 5-year survival rate for women with a diagnosis of endometrial carcinoma confined to the uterus at the time of surgical staging?**

>80%.

○ **What is the effect of cigarette smoking on the endometrium?**

Cigarette smoking significantly reduces the incidence of endometrial cancer. Endometrial atrophy, even in women on estrogen replacement therapy, is common in smokers, particularly if they are thin.

○ **Describe the screening test for endometrial cancer.**

There is no screening test for endometrial cancer; however, the American Cancer Society recommends annual endometrial biopsy starting at age 35 for all women at risk of hereditary nonpolyposis colorectal cancer (HNPCC).

○ **What are the risk factors associated with the development of endometrial carcinoma?**

Obesity, nulliparity, early menarche, and late menopause. Women 21 to 50 pounds over ideal body weight increase their risk of developing endometrial carcinomas threefold. Women in excess of 50 pounds over ideal body weight increase their chance of developing endometrial carcinoma 10-fold.

○ **What is HNPCC Lynch syndrome type II?**

A hereditary predisposition to the development of colon, breast, ovarian, and endometrial cancer. In approximately one-half of cases of affected women, endometrial and ovarian cancers precede colon cancer.

○ **What is the most frequent mismatch repair gene that is associated with the accumulation of endometrial cancer cases in HNPCC families?**

MSH6

Although MSH2 and MLH1 are also associated with endometrial cancer, the highest accumulation of endometrial cancer cases was observed in families with MSH6 mutation.

○ **Women who are at risk of HNPCC have what percentage risk of developing endometrial and ovarian cancers?**

40% to 60% risk of developing endometrial cancer and 12% risk of ovarian cancer.

○ **What other than colon, endometrial, and ovarian cancers are seen in HNPCC families?**

Gastric, urologic, and small bowel cancers.

○ **The Breast Cancer Linkage Consortium reported that elevated number of endometrial cancer was due to the mutation of which BRCA gene?**

Among BRCA1 carriers, the risk of endometrial cancer was reported to be 2.6 times higher than expected (95% CI 1.7 to 4.2). But the penetrance of BRCA1 mutations or endometrial carcinoma is low and the hereditary fraction is small. No elevated number of endometrial carcinoma was detected due to BRCA2 mutation.

○ **What rare dominant skin disease syndrome is associated with endometrial, thyroid, and breast cancer?**

Cowden syndrome. Inherited constitutional mutation of phosphatase and tensin homolog (PTEN) is the reason of Cowden disease. Somatic mutation in PTEN is also common in endometrial cancer.

○ **Which hereditary syndrome increases the risk of endometrial cancer?**

HNPCC with MHS6, MLH1, and MSH2 mismatch repair gene mutations. Women with HNPCC syndrome have a markedly increased risk of endometrial cancer compared with women in the general population. Among women who are HNPCC mutation carriers, the estimated cumulative incidence of endometrial cancer ranges from 20% to 60%. Mildly increased incidence was detected with BRCA1 mutations and in Cowden syndrome (PTEN mutation).

○ **Name four medical conditions that increase the risk of developing endometrial cancer because of excess endogenous estrogen.**

(1) Women with chronic anovulation (PCO).

(2) Women with estrogen secreting ovarian neoplasms, most commonly granulosa cell and theca cell tumors.

(3) Obese postmenopausal women.

(4) Women with severe liver disease.

○ **Explain why PCO syndrome, obesity, estrogen secreting ovarian tumor, or liver disease can increase the risk of developing endometrial carcinoma?**

The unopposed estrogen effect can be related because of the absence of progesterone effect, the overproduction of estrone or estradiol, and the increased free-biologically active fraction of estrogen because of the decreased level of steroid hormone binding globulin (SHBG) produced by the liver.

○ **In whom should a diagnosis of endometrial cancer be excluded?**

(1) All patients with postmenopausal bleeding.

(2) Postmenopausal women with a pyometra.

(3) Asymptomatic postmenopausal women with endometrial cells on a Papanicolaou smear.

(4) Perimenopausal women with intermenstrual bleeding or increasingly heavy menses.

(5) Premenopausal women with abnormal uterine bleeding, particularly if they are anovulatory.

○ **The background endometrium in a uterus with typical endometrioid endometrial adenocarcinoma histologically represents what process?**

Endometrial hyperplasia of varying types (asynchronous proliferative pattern).

○ **What effect does the prior use of OCPs have on the development of endometrial cancer?**

Women who use combination OCP for at least 12 months have a relative risk of endometrial cancer of 0.6. This protective effect persists for at least 15 years after cessation of OCP use.

○ **Epidemiologically how many types of endometrial cancer are there?**

Two:

(1) Type I is estrogen related and occurs on a background of endometrial hyperplasia. This type occurs in younger women and has a good prognosis.

(2) Type II occurs predominantly in older women, appears to arise de novo, and is unassociated with estrogen excess. The histologic grade is high and histopathologic types associated with aggressive behavior (clear cell, papillary serous) are common. The prognosis is poorer.

○ **What is the most common presenting complaint of a woman with endometrial cancer?**

Postmenopausal bleeding (or abnormal uterine bleeding in the premenopausal woman).

○ **What is the most common cause of postmenopausal bleeding?**

Atrophy

○ **Describe the indicated office evaluation of a woman whose history is suspicious for endometrial cancer.**

Pelvic examination, Pap smear, biopsy of any abnormal cervical or vaginal lesion, and endometrial biopsy.

○ **What percentage of endometrial carcinomas will shed abnormal cells that can be seen on a cervicovaginal cytology?**

25% to 35%.

○ **After which day of the menstrual cycle is the presence of endometrial cells a cause for concern?**

After day 14. Some authors would use day 10. During menses and immediately thereafter the presence of endometrial cells in a Pap smear is normal.

○ **What histologic findings would be expected if atypical endometrial cells are identified on a routine Pap smear?**

- Adenocarcinoma 20%.
- Hyperplasia 11%.
- Polyps 11%.

Thus over 40% of women with atypical endometrial cells identified on a Pap smear will have abnormal histology on an endometrial biopsy.

○ **In what clinical circumstances is a pelvic and abdominal computed tomography (CT) scan helpful in evaluating patients with endometrial cancer on biopsy?**

(1) Abnormal liver function tests.

(2) Clinical hepatomegaly.

(3) Palpable upper abdominal mass.

(4) Palpable extrauterine pelvic disease.

(5) Clinical ascites.

○ **How does endometrial carcinoma spread?**

(1) Direct extension to adjacent structures.

(2) Transtubal passage of exfoliated cells.

(3) Lymphatic dissemination.

(4) Hematogenous dissemination.

○ **Why do younger women have a better prognosis when they have endometrial carcinoma in compared with older women?**

Young women tend to have lower grade tumors with less myometrial invasion.

○ **How is endometrial cancer staged?**

Surgically and includes TAH/BSO, selective pelvic, and para-aortic node sampling.

○ **What is the role of the peritoneal washing and cytology in the staging of endometrial carcinoma?**

Nothing. The revised International Federation of Gynecologists and Obstetricians (FIGO) staging for endometrial adenocarcinoma (2009) removed the peritoneal washing and cytology as component of the staging.

○ **What percentage of women with endometrial cancer are diagnosed while in stage I?**

72%.

○ **Are postmenopausal women taking tamoxifen at higher risk of developing endometrial cancer than are age-matched controls?**

Yes. The increased relative risk of developing endometrial cancer for postmenopausal women taking tamoxifen is two to three times higher than that of age-matched controls.

○ **A neoplasm that histologically has <5% solid areas and invades approximately one-third of the myometrial thickness is what grade and stage? There is no other evidence of gross or microscopic disease.**

Grade 1, stage 1A. Grade 1 has <5% solid areas. Stage 1 disease is limited to the uterine corpus, and stage 1A can have invasion of up to 50% of the myometrium.

○ **A neoplasm that histologically has >50% solid areas and invades approximately three-fourth of the myometrial thickness is what grade and stage? There is no other evidence of gross or microscopic disease.**

Grade 3, stage 1B. Grade 3 has >50% solid areas. Stage 1 disease is limited to the uterine corpus, and Stage 1B has invasion of >50% of the myometrial thickness.

○ **A neoplasm that histologically has >50% solid areas and invades for approximately 3/4 of the myometrial thickness is what grade and stage if the para-aortic nodes are positive for disease?**

Grade 3, stage III C2. Grade 3 has >50% solid areas. Disease extension beyond the uterus is stage III. Involvement of the para-aortic lymph nodes is stage III C2. Based on the new 2009 revised FIGO staging, the stage IIIC diseases are separated to IIIC1 if pelvic lymph nodes are positive, and stage IIIC2 if para-aortic lymph nodes are positive.

○ **How does the presence of cervical glandular involvement modify the stage of endometrial cancer?**

It does not. The cervical glandular involvement was the part of the 1988 FIGO staging but it is not used in the new 2009 FIGO staging. The new 2009 revised staging excludes glandular involvement and counts only stromal cervical invasion as stage II cancer.

○ **A woman has a diagnosis of well-differentiated adenocarcinoma (histologic grade 1) from a curettage specimen. If surgical staging is performed within 1 month how often will (a) the histologic grade be higher and (b) will there be deep myometrial invasion?**

(1) Approximately one-third of neoplasms will be grade 2 or 3 (13% to 50%).

(2) Approximately 25% of uteri will have deep myometrial invasion.

○ **How does the presence of squamous change influence the prognosis of endometrial adenocarcinoma?**

Squamous change is typically nonmalignant and occurs in as many as 25% of endometrial adenocarcinomas. The overall prognosis is unchanged for those tumors known as adenoacanthomas. The histologic grade is assigned based on the glandular element within the neoplasm.

○ **How does significant nuclear (cytologic) atypia affect the grading of an architectural grade 1 endometrial adenocarcinoma?**

Significant nuclear atypia, otherwise inappropriate for the architectural grade, increases the tumor grade by 1. This commonly occurs in papillary serous and clear cell endometrial carcinomas.

○ **What is the incidence of pelvic and para-aortic node involvement when the neoplasm appears grossly confined to the endometrium?**

Approximately 6% to 7% of patients will have pelvic node metastases and 2% to 3% will have para-aortic node metastases.

○ **What is the local and distant recurrence for typical endometrial adenocarcinoma?**

20% to 30% recur in the pelvis, 55% to 65% recur at distant sites, and 5% to 10% recur in both sites.

○ **What are the estrogen receptor (ER) status and the progesterone receptor (PR) status in papillary serous endometrial adenocarcinoma and clear cell endometrial adenocarcinoma?**

Papillary serous and clear cell endometrial carcinomas are usually negative for both ER and PR.

○ **What is the effect of race on the prognosis of endometrial carcinoma?**

Compared with white Americans, endometrial cancer incidence is lower in Japanese Americans [relative risk (RR) = 0.6; 95% confidence interval (CI), 0.46–0.83] and in Latinas (RR = 0.63; 95% CI, 0.46–0.87), but not in African Americans (RR = 0.76; 95% CI, 0.53–1.08) or in native Hawaiians (RR = 0.92; 95% CI, 0.58–1.46). Higher mortality from endometrial cancer in African Americans is at least partly attributable to lower socioeconomic issues that impair access to care.

○ **What is the effect of gross cervical involvement in the prognosis of endometrial cancer?**

Gross cervical involvement is associated with a poorer prognosis. When treated with intracavitary application of cesium followed by extrafascial hysterectomy, the mean survival time in women without gross cervical disease was 94.2 months, compared with 29.1 months for women with gross cervical disease.

○ **What are the two best prognostic indicators of endometrioid endometrial adenocarcinoma?**

Histologic grade and depth of myometrial invasion.

○ **What are the differences in frequency and 5-year survival between surgical stage 1 typical endometrioid adenocarcinoma and papillary serous carcinoma of the endometrium?**

Typical endometrioid adenocarcinoma accounts for approximately 80% of endometrial adenocarcinoma. Papillary serous carcinoma accounts for approximately 8% of all endometrial adenocarcinomas.

The 5-year survival for stage 1 typical endometrioid adenocarcinoma is 88% and that of stage 1 papillary serous carcinoma is 63%.

○ **Is the quantity of ER and PR higher or lower in endometrial carcinoma as compared with normal cycling endometrium?**

The concentration varies, but with adenocarcinoma the concentration is usually less than normal cycling endometrium.

○ **What is the significance of ER and PR status in the prognosis of women with a diagnosis of endometrial carcinoma?**

ER status does not correlate well with prognosis. The absence of PRs is associated with a poor prognosis.

○ **Which factors or interventions decrease the incidence of endometrial cancer?**

Factors that have been associated with a decreased incidence of endometrial cancer include parity, lactation, use of combined oral contraceptives, a diet low in fat and high in plant foods, and physical activity.

○ **What percentage of women with endometrial carcinoma clinically confined to the uterus will develop recurrent disease?**

Approximately 16%.

○ **What is the average time from diagnosis to recurrence in endometrial carcinoma?**

2.2 years.

○ **When endometrial carcinoma recurs, what percentage of recurrence are detected within the first and the second year?**

34% and 70%, respectively.

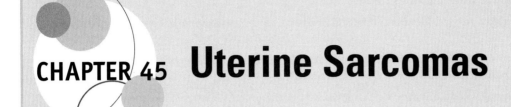

CHAPTER 45 Uterine Sarcomas

Maria A. Suescum, MD and Justin Chura, MD, MBA

○ **What is the incidence of uterine sarcomas?**

Sarcomas account for 3% to 8% of all uterine malignancies. The annual incidence is approximately 2 cases per 100,000 women.

○ **Define the following terms that Ober used to classify uterine sarcomas according to cell type and origin.**

Pure/Mixed.
Homologous/Heterologous.
Pure sarcoma—Virtually all are homologous coming from mesenchymal type cells.
Mixed—More than one cell type present, usually malignant mesenchymal and epithelial elements.
Homologous—Cell types are indigenous to the uterus (ie, leiomyosarcoma, stromal sarcoma, and angiosarcoma).
Heterologous—Cell types are foreign to the uterus (ie, rhabdomyosarcoma, chondrosarcoma, and osteosarcoma).

○ **List the four major groups of uterine sarcomas by decreasing incidence.**

Carcinosarcomas (previously known as MMMT)—50%.
Leiomyosarcoma—40%.
Endometrial stromal sarcoma (ESS)—8%.
Adenosarcoma—<2%.

○ **Prior pelvic irradiation is associated with the development of which type of uterine sarcoma?**

Approximately 10% of patients with carcinosarcoma have a prior history of pelvic irradiation.

○ **What histologic criteria are used when diagnosing a benign endometrial stromal nodule?**

Endometrial stromal nodules are characterized by a proliferation of uniform, normal-appearing stromal cells with a well-circumscribed, noninfiltrative margin. Lymphvascular space involvement is absent, and the mitotic count is usually <5 per 10 high-power fields.

○ **How are endometrial stromal nodules treated?**

Hysterectomy is recommended. However, successful treatment using myomectomy has been reported.

○ **Worm-like extension of tumor into lymphatic and vascular channels, occasionally with extensive extrauterine extension, is seen in which type of sarcoma?**

ESS, formerly known as endolymphatic stromal myosis. At operation, this may resemble intravenous leiomyomatosis or a broad ligament leiomyoma, but frozen section analysis can usually make the distinction.

○ **Why is removal of the ovaries recommended for patients undergoing surgery for a endometrial stromal sarcoma?**

These tumors often have high levels of estrogen and progesterone receptors, and their growth may be stimulated by estrogen. High-dose progesterone has been demonstrated to be therapeutically active.

○ **What percentage of stage I ESS cases recur?**

Approximately 50% recur at a median of 3 years following diagnosis.

○ **What is the most common uterine tumor in reproductive-aged women?**

Benign leiomyomata.

○ **What is the incidence of discovering a leiomyosarcoma following surgery for presumed benign leiomyomata?**

Approximately 0.2% to 0.3%.

○ **How does the origin of leiomyosarcomas differ from that of other uterine sarcomas?**

Leiomyosarcomas originate in the myometrium; all others originate in the endometrium.

○ **What histologic criteria are used to classify a leiomyosarcoma?**

Hypercellularity, moderate to severe nuclear atypia, mitotic index >15 mitoses total per 10 high-power field, and coagulative tumor cell necrosis.

○ **What is the average age for patients with leiomyosarcomas?**

53 years of age.

○ **What are the most frequent presenting symptoms for patients with leiomyosarcomas?**

Abnormal uterine bleeding, which occurs in over three quarters of patients. Pelvic pain and rapid uterine enlargement can be other presenting symptoms.

○ **How reliable is the preoperative diagnosis of a rapidly enlarging uterus in predicting the presence of a leiomyosarcoma?**

A recent study found only one leiomyosarcoma among 371 patients undergoing hysterectomy for a rapidly enlarging uterus.

○ **A preoperative diagnosis of leiomyosarcoma is made in what percentage of cases?**

15%, despite up to one-third of the tumors being submucous.

○ **What therapy is recommended for disseminated peritoneal leiomyomatosis?**

This is a benign condition often associated with oral contraceptive use or pregnancy. No specific therapy is required, though discontinuation of oral contraceptives or resolution of a pregnancy often results in regression.

○ **How does the development of a leiomyosarcoma within a benign leiomyoma affect prognosis?**

This is considered to be a favorable prognostic feature.

○ **Are leiomyosarcomas generally solitary or multifocal lesions?**

Unlike leiomyomata, they are usually solitary lesions.

○ **What prognostic feature best predicts recurrence-free interval for early stage leiomyosarcomas?**

Mitotic index.

○ **What is the effect of adjuvant radiation therapy on early stage leiomyosarcomas?**

Though not demonstrated in all studies, pelvic recurrences are reduced by almost 50%. Pelvic radiation does not prevent distant recurrences and has yet to be shown to improve survival.

○ **What are the most active chemotherapeutic agents in leiomyosarcomas?**

Adriamycin has an overall response rate of 25%.
Combination therapy with gemcitabine and docetaxel has also shown to have efficacy.
Smaller studies have found efficacy with aromatase inhibitors.

○ **What two histologic components must be present to make the diagnosis of a carcinosarcoma?**

Carcinosarcomas are composed of an admixture of malignant epithelial (carcinoma) and stromal (sarcoma) components, hence the name carcinosarcoma.

○ **How does an adenosarcoma differ histologically from a carcinosarcoma?**

The epithelial component of an adenosarcoma is benign.

○ **How does race affect the incidence of carcinosarcoma?**

The relative risk is greater for black women as compared with white women and rises at a disproportionately greater rate with advancing age.

○ **What is the most common epithelial histologic subtype in a carcinosarcoma?**

Approximately 60% are endometrioid followed in order of decreasing frequency by adenosquamous, serous, and clear cell histologies.

○ **What proportion of carcinosarcomas contains heterologous stromal elements?**

Approximately 50% of cases.

○ **What is the most common heterologous stromal component in a carcinosarcoma?**

Rhabdomyosarcoma followed by chondrosarcoma and osteosarcoma.

O **Initial metastases from carcinosarcomas are usually of epithelial or stromal origin?**

Epithelial.

O **How is the prognosis for patients with carcinosarcomas affected by the presence or absence of heterologous elements?**

Recent studies have shown no prognostic difference.

O **The triad of pelvic pain, postmenopausal bleeding, and what physical finding is highly suggestive of a carcinosarcoma?**

Tissue protruding through the cervical os.

O **Surgical staging will upstage what percentage of patients with carcinosarcoma clinically confined to the uterus?**

25% to 50%. Risk of extrauterine disease is related to depth of myometrial invasion, lymphvascular space involvement, and cervical extension.

O **What is the 5-year survival rate for each type of uterine sarcoma?**

Carcinosarcoma (MMMT) → 35%.
Leiomyosarcoma → 25%.
ESS → 60%.

O **Which chemotherapeutic agents have demonstrated activity against carcinosarcomas?**

Combination therapy with either paclitaxel and ifosfamide or paclitaxel and carboplatin are the current regimens of choice for treating carcinosarcoma.

O **Which chemotherapeutic agent is recommended for leiomyosarcoma?**

Doxorubicin currently is considered first line therapy. However, treatment with the combination of gemcitabine and docetaxel currently has the highest proven response rate (36%).

O **What is the frequency of pelvic lymph node metastases in uterine carcinosarcomas and leiomyosarcoma?**

15% for uterine carcinosarcoma and 3% for leiomyosarcoma.

O **What is STUMP (smooth muscle tumor of uncertain malignant potential)?**

Tumors that show some worrisome histologic features, such as necrosis or nuclear atypia, but cannot be diagnosed reliably as benign or malignant based on generally applied criteria fall into this category.

O **At which stage is leiomyosarcoma most frequently diagnosed at?**

Stage 1 68% of the cases.

O **Describe the differences between endometrial stromal nodule and ESS.**

Nodules are benign, characterized by a well-delineated margin, and composed of neoplastic cells that resemble proliferative-phase endometrial stromal cells. Grossly, the tumor is a solitary, round or oval, fleshy nodule measuring a few centimeters. Histologically, they are distinguished from ESS by a lack of myometrial infiltration.

○ **How does staging differ for a leiomyosarcoma versus a carcinosarcoma?**

Early stage disease refers to stage 1 (tumor confined to the uterus) and stage 2 (tumor extends to the pelvis). Surgery is the best treatment via staging laparotomy.

With uterine leiomyosarcoma, all patients should undergo a hysterectomy, if feasible. A modified radical or radical procedure may be occasionally required if there is parametrial infiltration. In the absence of other gross disease, fewer than 5% will have ovarian or nodal metastases. Ovarian preservation is therefore an option for premenopausal women. In addition, lymph node dissection should be reserved for patients with clinically suspicious nodes.

For uterine carcinosarcoma, hysterectomy and BSO are mandatory.

Lymph node metastases will be found in up to one-third of patients with clinical stage I disease, and thus, comprehensive lymphadenectomy should be performed. Omentectomy is usually performed as part of surgical staging for carcinosarcoma as well.

○ **How do you follow patients after surgical staging?**

Physical examination every 3 months for the first 2 years and then at 6- to 12-month intervals thereafter. Most recurrences will be distant, and thus Pap tests are not part of routine surveillance according to guidelines of the Society of Gynecologic Oncology.

○ **What is the most independent variable associated with survival for sarcomas?**

International Federation of Gynecologists and Obstetricians (FIGO) staging.

○ **Describe the differences in patterns of spread of leiomyosarcoma versus carcinosarcomas.**

Leiomyosarcomas have a propensity for hematogenous dissemination. For example, lung metastases are particularly common, and more than half of patients will have distant spread if diagnosed with recurrent disease. To a lesser extent, leiomyosarcomas metastasize via lymphatic channels

The opposite is true for carcinosarcomas in which one-third of patients with clinically stage I tumors will have nodal metastases. Thus, comprehensive pelvic and para-aortic lymphadenectomy is particularly important in staging this disease.

○ **Based on the last FIGO staging recommendations for uterine sarcomas in 2009, how should carcinosarcomas be staged?**

As carcinomas of the endometrium.

○ **What criteria are used to define stage 1 (limited to uterus) leiomyosarcomas versus ESS and adenosarcomas?**

For leiomyosarcomas → the definition is based on the tumor size. Stage 1 A is <5 cm and stage 1B is >5 cm.

For ESS and adenosarcomas → myometrial invasion. Therefore, stage 1 A implies no myometrial invasion, 1B <half of myometrial invasion, and 1C >half myometrial invasion.

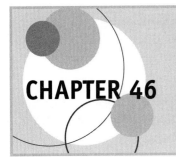

CHAPTER 46

Epithelial and Nonepithelial Ovarian Tumors

Mitchell I. Edelson, MD

○ **Epithelial tumors include what histologic types?**

(1) Serous (46%).

(2) Mucinous (36%).

(3) Endometrioid (8%).

(4) Clear cell.

(5) Brenner.

(6) Undifferentiated carcinomas.

○ **The lifetime risk and mean age for developing epithelial ovarian cancers is?**

1.86% (1/70); 63 years.

○ **Characteristics of ovarian low malignant potential tumors include?**

Tendency to remain confined to the ovary for long periods of time, occurrence predominantly in premenopausal women, associated with an excellent prognosis. There is no need for adjuvant treatment even in those individuals with advanced disease.

○ **Criteria for diagnosis of ovarian low malignant potential tumors include?**

(1) Epithelial proliferation with papillary formation and pseudostratification.

(2) Nuclear atypia and increased mitotic activity.

(3) Absence of true stromal invasion.

○ **What percentage of invasive epithelial tumors spread beyond the ovary?**

75% to 85%.

○ **Psammoma bodies are frequently associated with which type of ovarian tumors?**

Serous.

○ **Serous low malignant potential tumors account for what percentage of all serous tumors?**
Approximately 15%.

○ **Well-differentiated serous adenocarcinoma is histologically defined by?**
A predominance of papillary and glandular cells, round to oval nuclei, and 0 to 2 mitoses per high-power field.

○ **Poorly differentiated serous adenocarcinoma is histologically defined by?**
Solid sheets of cells, nuclear atypia, and 2 to 3 mitoses per high-power field.

○ **What percentage of mucinous tumors of the ovary are malignant?**
<10%.

○ **Mucinous tumors histologically resemble what other cell type?**
Mucinous tumors may resemble either endocervix or gastrointestinal tract.

○ **Which type of ovarian tumors are often associated with similar lesions in the endometrium?**
Endometrioid.

○ **Which ovarian tumors are associated with endometriosis and histologically are composed of cells that project their nuclei to the apical cytoplasm, known as hobnail cells?**
Clear cell tumors.

○ **Clear cell tumors are often associated with which clinical/laboratory findings?**
Hypercalcemia and hyperpyrexia.

○ **A similar constellation of clinical symptoms seen in patients with ovarian cancer is also associated with?**
(1) Mesothelioma.
(2) Primary peritoneal carcinoma.
(3) Tuberculous peritonitis.

○ **This solid tumor type is associated with epithelioid cells that show a coffee bean pattern caused by longitudinal grooving of the nuclei:**
Brenner tumors.

○ **What is the lifetime risk of developing ovarian cancer in BRCA1 and BRCA2 carriers?**
Women with BRCA1 mutations have a 40% to 50% risk of developing ovarian cancer, while women with BRCA2 mutations have a 10% to 25% risk.

○ **What hereditary syndromes of cancer have been associated with an increased risk of ovarian cancer?**
(1) Site-specific familial ovarian cancer.
(2) Breast/ovarian familial cancer syndromes.
(3) Hereditary nonpolyposis colorectal cancer (HNPCC) (formerly known as Lynch II syndrome).

○ **Surgical staging for ovarian cancer should involve what surgical steps?**

Submitting any free fluid for cytology (or peritoneal washings), a systematic exploration of all intra-abdominal surfaces and viscera, biopsy of multiple intraperitoneal sites, biopsy of the diaphragm, infracolic omentectomy, and pelvic and para-aortic lymph node dissection.

○ **What percentage of patients with an ovarian epithelial cancer that appears to be confined to the ovary has occult metastasis?**

Approximately one-third of patients with early stage ovarian epithelial cancer will be upstaged following comprehensive staging with 75% being restaged as having stage III disease.

○ **What are the theories to support the use of cytoreductive surgery for women with an advanced epithelial ovarian?**

Physiologic benefits include alleviation of nausea and early satiety, restoration of adequate intestinal function, and improvement in nutritional status. Improved tumor perfusion and increased growth fraction are additional theoretic benefits.

○ **What is the principal treatment of low malignant potential ovarian tumors?**

Surgical resection alone.

○ **What is the chemotherapeutic treatment regimen of choice for patients with advanced epithelial ovarian cancer?**

A combination of platinum and taxane.

○ **Which chemotherapy regimen recently showed a significant survival benefit among women with optimally debulked epithelial ovarian cancer with a 65.6-month median survival?**

A regimen consisting of intraperitoneal cisplatin and paclitaxel and intravenous paclitaxel demonstrated the longest survival data from a randomized trial in advanced ovarian cancer.

○ **Nonepithelial tumors of the ovary account for what percentage of all ovarian cancers?**

10%.

○ **In the first two decades of life, what percentage of ovarian tumors are germ cell?**

70%

○ **Germ cell tumors commonly secrete what two hormones?**

Alpha-fetoprotein (AFP) and human chorionic gonadotropin (hCG).

○ **What are the different histologic types of germ cell tumors?**

(1) Dysgerminoma.

(2) Teratoma.

(3) Endodermal sinus tumor.

(4) Embryonal carcinoma.

(5) Polyembryoma.

(6) Choriocarcinoma.

(7) Mixed forms.

O   **What is the most common malignant germ cell tumor?**

Dysgerminoma.

O   **What is the second most common malignant germ cell tumor?**

Immature teratoma.

O   **Describe the histologic characteristics of dysgerminomas.**

Large round ovoid or polygonal cells with abundant clear, pale staining cytoplasm, large and irregular nuclei with prominent nucleoli.

O   **What are the most common chemotherapeutic regimens for germ cell tumors?**

(1) BEP (bleomycin, etoposide, and cisplatin).

(2) VBP (vinblastine, bleomycin, and cisplatin).

(3) VAC (vincristine, actinomycin, and cyclophosphamide).

O   **What tumor markers may be elevated in a woman with a dysgerminoma?**

(1) Lactic dehydrogenase.

(2) Beta-hCG.

O   **Endodermal sinus tumors are derived from what structure?**

The primitive yolk sac.

O   **The majority of malignant ovarian germ cell tumors are unilateral except for which type?**

Dysgerminoma tumors can have bilateral involvement in 10% to 15% of cases.

O   **Which stage of ovarian germ cell tumors does not require any further treatment following surgical resection and staging?**

The treatment of choice for a woman with a stage IA dysgerminoma and a stage IA grade 1 immature teratoma is observation.

O   **What is the characteristic microscopic finding of endodermal sinus tumors?**

Schiller-Duval body.

O   **What enzymes are secreted by endodermal sinus tumors?**

AFP and rarely, alpha-1-antitrypsin.

O   **What is the most common malignancy to develop in an initially benign teratoma?**

Squamous cell carcinoma.

O   **How do you distinguish an embryonal carcinoma of the ovary from choriocarcinoma of the ovary?**

There is an absence of syncytiotrophoblastic and cytotrophoblastic cells in an embryonal carcinoma.

○ **What neoplasm closely resembles a similar carcinoma of the adult testes?**

Embryonal carcinoma.

○ **What do the tumors of embryonal carcinomas contain?**

hCG, syncytiotrophoblast-like cells, and AFP in large primitive cells.

○ **Name a rare germ cell neoplasm composed of numerous embryoid bodies resembling morphologically normal embryos.**

Polyembryonal tumors.

○ **Name the three ways choriocarcinomas can arise.**

(1) As a primary gestational choriocarcinoma associated with ovarian pregnancy.

(2) As a metastatic choriocarcinoma from a primary gestational choriocarcinoma arising in other parts of the genital tract.

(3) As a germ cell tumor differentiating in a direction of trophoblastic structures and arising with other neoplastic germ cell elements.

○ **What do choriocarcinomas secrete?**

hCG.

○ **What percentage of choriocarcinomas arise in prepubescent children?**

50%.

○ **What is the most common component of a mixed germ cell tumor?**

Dysgerminoma.

○ **What is the most frequent complication of mature cystic teratomas and when does it most often occur?**

Torsion, most frequently occurring in pregnancy and the puerperium.

○ **In an immature teratoma, which elements correlate with survival and are the basis for the grading of these tumors?**

Neuroepithelium.

○ **What is the most common tumor that secretes estrogen?**

Adult granulosa cell tumors

○ **Describe the histologic appearance of granulosa cell tumors.**

Fibrothecomatous components with scant cytoplasm and coffee bean grooved cells. Mature follicles and Call-Exner bodies are also common.

○ **What other malignancy is commonly associated with granulosa cell tumors of the ovary?**

Endometrioid adenocarcinoma of the uterus.

○   **Individuals with Peutz-Jeghers syndrome have an increase of?**

   (1) Sex cord stromal tumors of the ovary.

   (2) Adenoma malignum (minimal deviation) of the cervix.

○   **Which factors are protective against ovarian carcinomas?**

   (1) Pregnancy.

   (2) Bilateral tubal ligation.

   (3) Hysterectomy.

   (4) Use of oral contraceptives.

CHAPTER 47

Fallopian Tube Neoplasms

Mitchell I. Edelson, MD

○ **What embryologic layer gives rise to the majority of benign tumors of the fallopian tube?**

Mesoderm.

○ **What is a Walthard nest?**

A benign inclusion cyst created in the fallopian tube by invagination of the tubal serosa. It is filled with polygonal epithelial-like cells with distinctive, irregularly ovoid nuclei with longitudinal nuclear grooves that give them a coffee-bean appearance. They are common incidental findings of no clinical importance.

○ **What is the most common benign tubal tumor?**

Adenomatoid tumors (benign mesotheliomas). They appear as small (1–2 cm) nodular masses with multiple, spherical, or slit-like channels lined by an attenuated layer of cells. There is no evidence of cytologic atypia.

○ **What is salpingitis isthmica nodosa and how is it differentiated from primary carcinoma of the fallopian tube?**

Salpingitis isthmica nodosa is a localized diverticulosis of the isthmic portion of the fallopian tube. Grossly, it appears as a firm, nodular dilatation of the isthmus with a diameter of <2 cm. Microscopically, the glandular endosalpinx is seen extending from the lumen deep into the muscularis. It is differentiated from primary carcinoma of the fallopian tube by its lack of cytologic atypia.

○ **What is the most common carcinoma that involves the fallopian tube?**

Metastatic carcinomas from another site in the female genital tract. Almost 50% of women with ovarian cancer and up to 12% of uterine cancers will have spread to the fallopian tube.

○ **What percentage of primary malignancies of the female genital tract arise from the fallopian tubes?**

0.2% to 0.5%.

○ **What is the most common primary malignant neoplasm of the fallopian tube?**

Papillary serous adenocarcinoma, accounting for 90% of all fallopian tube malignancies.

○ **Describe the classic triad of symptoms associated with fallopian tube malignancies.**

Profuse clear or serosanguineous vaginal discharge (hydrops tubae profluens), pelvic pain, and a pelvic mass.

○ **What percentage of patients with fallopian tube malignancies present with the classic triad of symptoms?**

Less than 15%; however, >50% present with vaginal discharge or bleeding and about 60% have a pelvic mass.

○ **How often is bilateral involvement found in adenocarcinoma of the fallopian tube?**

Dependent on the stage of the tumor at the time of diagnosis. For stage I, II, and in situ lesions, the incidence is approximately 7%. In stage III and IV disease, however, bilateral involvement is seen in as many as 30%.

○ **Describe the staging system for fallopian tube tumors.**

Although there are several staging systems for tubal cancers, the most widely used is that of the International Federation of Gynecologists and Obstetricians (FIGO). It is similar to that used to stage ovarian malignancies.

Stage 0	Carcinoma in situ (limited to the tubal mucosa)
Stage I	Growth limited to the fallopian tubes
Stage IA	Growth limited to one tube with extension into submucosa and/or muscularis, but not penetrating the serosal surface. No ascites
Stage IB	Growth limited to both tubes with extension into submucosa and/or muscularis, but not penetrating the serosal surface. No ascites
Stage IC	Tumor either IA or IB but with extension through or onto tubal serosa or ascites containing malignant cells or with positive peritoneal washings
Stage II	Growth involving one or both fallopian tubes with pelvic extension
Stage IIA	Extension and/or metastasis to uterus and/or ovaries
Stage IIB	Extension to other pelvic tissues
Stage IIC	Tumor either IIA or IIB but with ascites containing malignant cells or with positive peritoneal washings.
Stage III	Tumor involving one or both fallopian tubes with peritoneal implants outside pelvis and/or positive retroperitoneal or inguinal adenopathy. Superficial liver metastasis included
Stage IIIA	Tumor grossly limited to true pelvis with negative nodes but with histologically confirmed microscopic seeding of abdominal peritoneal surfaces
Stage IIIB	Tumor involving one or both tubes with negative nodes but histologically confirmed implants of 2 cm or less on abdominal peritoneal surfaces
Stage IIIC	Abdominal implants of >2 cm in diameter and/or positive retroperitoneal or inguinal nodes
Stage IV	Growth involving one or both fallopian tubes with distant metastases. Includes parenchymal liver metastasis and cytologically confirmed malignant pleural effusions

○ **Based on the surgical findings at the time of laparotomy, how common are the four stages?**

Stage I disease accounts for about 29% of all fallopian tube malignancies, stage II for about 23%, stage III 39%, and stage IV for 7%.

○ **What is the 5-year survival for patients with adenocarcinoma of the fallopian tube?**

Overall 5-year survival is approximately 56%, but is dependent on the stage at the time of diagnosis. The associated 5-year survival by stage is as follows: Stage I 81%, stage II 67%, stage III 41%, and stage IV 41%.

○ **What tumor marker is useful in the follow-up of tubal serous carcinomas?**

CA-125.

○ **What is the standard treatment of tubal carcinoma?**

The standard method of treatment is similar to that used for ovarian cancer. Treatment of tubal carcinoma consists of total abdominal hysterectomy, bilateral salpingo-oophorectomy, with comprehensive surgical staging if there is no evidence of metastatic disease. Aggressive cytoreductive surgery, followed by chemotherapy, is performed for advanced disease.

○ **What is the role of cytoreductive surgery?**

Cytoreductive surgery has been demonstrated to have a beneficial effect in the treatment of fallopian tube carcinomas in a similar fashion to that of ovarian malignancies. Patients with a residual tumor mass of <1 cm have a significantly higher survival rate than do patients with larger residual tumors following primary surgery.

○ **What are the most effective chemotherapeutic agents against tubal carcinoma?**

A combination of Taxol and a platinum-based chemotherapeutic agent is currently used.

○ **Name the two most common metastatic tumors that involve the fallopian tube.**

Ovarian and endometrial carcinomas. Peritoneal spread often involves the serosal surface and lymphatic spread from adjacent primary sites may involve the mucosa or muscularis.

○ **What are the histologic criteria often employed in the diagnosis of a primary tubal carcinoma?**

(1) Grossly, the main bulk of tumor is confined to the fallopian tube and arises from the endosalpinx.

(2) Microscopically, the epithelium of the tubal mucosa is involved and shows a papillary pattern.

(3) A transition between benign and malignant tubal epithelium is identifiable.

(4) The ovaries and endometrium are either normal or contain less tumor than the tubes.

○ **A tubal lesion consisting primarily of trophoblastic proliferation in addition to hydropic villi represents what type of fallopian tube tumor?**

Ectopic molar pregnancy. Responsible for approximately 1 in 5000 ectopic pregnancies, they clinically present in a similar fashion to other ectopic gestations, but histologically demonstrate the appearance of either a complete or partial mole.

○ **Describe the methods of spread of tubal carcinomas.**

Tubal carcinomas spread in much the same manner as epithelial ovarian malignancies with transcoelomic exfoliation of cells that implant throughout the peritoneal cavity. Lymphovascular spread to the pelvic and para-aortic nodes is also common.

○ **Although transcoelomic exfoliation was initially suggested as the primary mechanism of spread of tubal carcinomas, why is this theory suspect?**

Typically, the gross appearance of a fallopian tube carcinoma is that of a hydrosalpinx, with a sealed distal end and a dilated tube.

○   **How does depth of invasion relate to survival in fallopian tube carcinomas?**

In a retrospective review, depth of invasion was inversely related to survival. Intramucosal lesions were associated with a crude 5-year survival of 91%, lesions with muscular wall involvement were associated with a 53% survival, and lesions penetrating the serosa were associated with a 25% or less 5-year survival.

○   **Describe the lymphatic drainage of the fallopian tube and its importance in predicting survival.**

The primary lymphatic drainage of the fallopian tube is via the para-aortic lymph nodes. Pelvic or para-aortic lymph node involvement has been found in 10% to 35% of patients at the time of their initial operation, in about 33% of patients at the time of surgery for recurrent disease, and in 75% of patients at autopsy. Survival of patients with positive retroperitoneal or inguinal lymph node involvement (stage IIIC) is lower than that of patients with earlier stages. Finally, the presence of lymphovascular space involvement in early tubal carcinomas is associated with a 5-year survival of only 29% compared with 83% for tumors without identifiable lymphatic or vascular invasion.

○   **What is the prognosis for primary malignant mixed mesodermal tumors of the fallopian tube?**

The overall 5-year survival is 15%, with a mean survival of 17 months.

○   **What percentage of tubal carcinomas involve the ovary at the time of diagnosis?**

Approximately 13% of tubal carcinomas involve the ovary at the time of diagnosis, usually as a result of direct extension.

○   **What percentage of fallopian tube cancers will cause an abnormal cervical cytology specimen?**

Although some series report positive cervical cytology to be as common as 40% to 60%, most series show that only about 10% of patients with tubal carcinomas will have abnormal Papanicolaou smears.

○   **What is the lifetime risk of fallopian tube cancer in women with a BRCA mutation?**

0.6% to 3%.

○   **What percentage of women with a fallopian tube cancer have a mutation in the BRCA1 or BRCA2 gene?**

30%.

○   **Which sites do fallopian tube cancers tend to recur?**

Retroperitoneal lymph nodes and extraperitoneal sites.

○   **What is hydrops tubae profluens?**

A sudden emptying of accumulated fluid in the distended fallopian tube that causes a profuse watery serosanguinous discharge associated with a decrease in the size of a pelvic mass.

○   **Why has the fallopian tube been implicated as the possible origin for pelvic serous carcinomas?**

The presence of a serous tubal intraepithelial carcinoma (TIC) in the fimbria was initially identified in BRCA mutation carriers following risk-reducing salpingo-oophorectomy. Subsequent studies have also identified a coexistent TIC in all forms of pelvic serous carcinomas suggesting its role in the development of ovarian, fallopian tube, and primary peritoneal cancers.

CHAPTER 48

Vulvar and Vaginal Carcinoma

Lauren Abern, MD and
Mitchell I. Edelson, MD

○ **What percentage of gynecologic malignancies originate on the vulva?**

3% to 5%.

○ **What is the average delay in diagnosis of vulvar cancer?**

12 months (6 months patient delay, 6 month physician delay).

○ **What are the borders of the superficial inguinal nodes?**

Inguinal ligament superior.
Border of sartorius muscle laterally.
Border of adductor longus medially.

○ **What is the name of the fascia that is located above the deep inguinal nodes?**

The cribriform fascia that makes up the covering of the femoral sheath.

○ **Observational association of what risk factors have been linked with vulvar cancer?**

(1) Advancing postmenopausal age.
(2) Hypertension.
(3) Diabetes.
(4) Obesity.
(5) Smoking.

○ **What link does the human papilloma virus (HPV) have, if any, with vulvar cancer?**

HPV DNA can be identified in about 70% to 80% of intraepithelial lesions, but is seen in only 10% to 50% of invasive lesions. HPV type 16 seems to be most common, but types 6 and 33 have also been identified.

○ **True or False: Lichen sclerosis has been proven to be a precursor of and leads to invasive vulvar cancer.**

False.

○ **What is the definition of a stage IA vulvar cancer using the latest International Federation of Gynecologists and Obstetricians (FIGO) staging (2009)?**

Tumor confined to vulva or perineum; 2 cm or less in greatest dimension; no nodal metastasis with stromal invasion ≤1.0 mm.

○ **Name the three mechanisms of the spread of vulvar cancer.**

(1) Local growth and extension.

(2) Embolization to regional lymph nodes in the groin.

(3) Hematogenous dissemination to distant sites.

○ **Name the three characteristics that describe the growth pattern of vulvar cancer as these growth patterns influence the rate of lymph node metastasis and survival.**

(1) Confluent.

(2) Compact.

(3) Fingerlike (or spray).

○ **What is the name and location of the last node of the deep femoral nodal group?**

The Cloquet node, or node of Rosenmüller, is located just beneath the Poupart ligament.

○ **Name, in order, the five most common histologic subtypes of vulvar neoplasms.**

(1) Epidermoid (squamous cell).

(2) Melanoma.

(3) Sarcoma.

(4) Basal cell.

(5) Bartholin gland.

○ **True or False: The deep pelvic nodes are essentially never involved with metastatic disease when the more superficial inguinal nodes are uninvolved, even with a clitoral lesion.**

True.

○ **Which vulvar lesion has the classic "cake-icing effect" appearance secondary to hyperemic areas associated with a superficial white coating?**

Paget disease of the vulva.

○ **What underlying malignancy must be ruled out when Paget disease of the vulva is diagnosed?**

Adenocarcinoma of the vulva.

○ **What is the treatment of Paget disease without an underlying adenocarcinoma?**

This is a true intraepithelial neoplasia and can be treated as such with wide local excision.

○ **What is the most frequent histologic subtype seen in Bartholin gland cancer?**

Adenocarcinoma and squamous cell carcinoma occur with equal frequency and comprise 80% of all primary malignant tumors at this site.

○ **How does the lymph node spread pattern of Bartholin gland cancer differ from typical squamous cell vulvar carcinoma?**

The lesion can have a tendency to spread into the ischiorectal fossa and can spread posteriorly directly to the deep pelvic nodes in addition to the typical inguinal lymph node spread pattern.

○ **What is the reported lymph node metastasis rate of stage I squamous carcinoma of the vulva with a thickness of 5 mm or more?**

At least 15%.

○ **Have squamous cell vulvar tumors with a depth of ≤1 mm shown any significant risk of lymph node metastasis?**

No. Tumors of this depth or less carry little or no risk of lymph node metastasis.

○ **What is the name of the vulvar tumor that is a neuroendocrine tumor of the skin, morphologically resembles small-cell carcinomas of neuroendocrine type in other body sites and is associated with frequent lymph node metastasis and a poor prognosis?**

Merkel cell tumor.

○ **What HPV subtype has been associated with verrucous carcinomas of the vulva?**

HPV type 6.

○ **Where is the most common site on the vulva to find an adenoid cystic carcinoma?**

The Bartholin gland. It comprises 15% of all Bartholin gland carcinomas.

○ **Name the most frequent primary vulvar sarcoma identified and its usual location.**

Leiomyosarcoma. It commonly arises in the labium majus or the Bartholin gland area.

○ **What is the single most important prognostic factor in women with vulvar cancer?**

Lymph node metastasis. The presence of inguinal node metastasis routinely results in a 50% reduction in long-term survival.

○ **What is the incidence of positive lymph node involvement in T1 and T2 lesions?**

The incidence of positive inguinal and pelvic lymph nodes varies considerably; however, in the largest study to date it was found that 20% of T1 lesions and 45% of T2 lesions had positive lymph node involvement (higher if adjuvant radiation therapy is administered).

○ **What are the two most common complications associated with radical vulvectomy?**

Wound breakdown occurs in approximately 50% of patients in most series and lymphedema following surgery has been reported in up to 70% of patients.

○ **What is the 5-year survival rate by stage in vulvar cancer?**

Stage I—91%.
Stage II—81%.
Stage III—48%.
Stage IV—15%.

○ **What is the effect of lymph node involvement on survival?**

If lymph node involvement is negative overall, survival is 90% regardless of stage; however, survival rate drops precipitously even if only one lymph node is positive for metastasis (57%).

○ **What is the survival rate with positive deep pelvic nodes in vulvar cancer regardless of stage?**

20%.

○ **How does the International Society for the Study of Vulvar Disease (ISSVD) define microinvasive carcinoma of the vulva?**

A squamous carcinoma having diameter of 2 cm or less, with depth of invasion ≤1 mm. The presence of vascular space involvement would exclude the lesion from this category.

○ **What parameters should be addressed in the pathology report in early superficial vulvar cancer?**

(1) Tumor thickness.

(2) Vascular invasion.

(3) Depth of invasion.

(4) Confluence of invasive neoplastic tongues.

(5) Grade of cell differentiation.

(6) Host response.

○ **What has the term "giant condyloma of Buschke-Lowenstein" been used to describe?**

Verrucous carcinoma of the cervix.

○ **What have postoperative spindle cell nodules on the vulva been confused with?**

Leiomyosarcomas.

○ **What are the most common metastatic tumors to the vulva?**

Squamous cell cancer of the cervix and adenocarcinomas of the endometrium. Other primary sites include the vagina, ovary, urethra, kidney, breast, melanoma, choriocarcinoma, rectum, and lung.

○ **Prior to the treatment of Paget disease of the vulva, what screening should be performed?**

Because of the high incidence of associated carcinomas of the breast and genitalia, a thorough search for such tumors should be performed prior to any consideration of therapy. This should involve breast examination, mammography, cytologic and colposcopic evaluation of cervix, vagina and vulva, and sigmoidoscopy/colonoscopy.

○ **What is the stage of a 3 cm vulvar cancer confined to the vulva with unilateral regional lymph node metastasis of 3 mm?**

Stage IIIA—$T_2 N_{1A} M_0$.

○ **What is the stage of vulvar cancer that is 1 cm in size with adjacent spread to the lower urethra, nodes negative?**

Stage II—$T_2 N_0 M_0$.

○ **What alternatives to radical surgery are available for women with a locally advanced vulvar carcinoma?**

Preoperative chemoradiation has been utilized to reduce the size of many tumors that may be initially invading structures such as the bladder and anus. This treatment plan may allow for limited surgical resection.

○ **Which vulvar cancer has a predilection for hematogenous spread?**

Vulvar sarcomas. In one series 50% had pulmonary metastases.

○ **What is the name of the vaginal tumor that presents as a mass of grapelike nodules most commonly in the first 2 years of life?**

Embryonal rhabdomyosarcoma (sarcoma botryoides).

○ **What is the current acceptable conservative surgical treatment of a vulvar cancer confined to one labia with no central involvement?**

Wide local excision or vulvectomy with ipsilateral groin node dissection that should include all nodes. No attempt should be made to distinguish between superficial and deep inguinal lymph nodes. Groin node dissection cannot be totally dispensed of unless invasion is less than 1 mm.

○ **What is the overall rate of recurrence in treated vulvar cancer, and where does it recur?**

Approximately 25% of patients will recur, and 80% of these recurrences are in the first 2 years. Most recurrences are on the vulva, with a few in the groin.

○ **What is the treatment of node-positive vulvar cancer?**

Two factors appear to be important in the management of regional disease. Radiation therapy can have a significant impact on controlling or eradicating small volume nodal disease, and surgical resection of bulky nodal disease also improves regional control and probably enhances the curative potential of radiation. Patients with positive nodes, particularly more than one positive node, are likely to benefit from postoperative irradiation to the groin and pelvis.

○ **Is surgical debulking of positive pelvic nodes in vulvar cancer superior to radiation for treatment?**

No. Radiation therapy has been found to be superior in the management of patients with positive pelvic nodes.

○ **True or False: Primary cancer of the vagina is one of the rarest of the malignant processes in the human body.**

True.

○ **What is the most common type of vaginal cancer?**

Squamous cell carcinoma.

○ **If a malignant neoplasm involves both the cervix and the vagina and is histologically compatible with origin in either organ, is it classified vaginal or cervical?**

Cervical cancer.

○ **What is the spread pattern of vaginal cancer?**

If it occurs in the upper half of vagina, extension is similar to cervical cancer; if it occurs in the lower part of the vagina, extension is similar to carcinoma of the vulva.

○ **What is the cause of most vaginal tumors/cancer seen?**

Secondary carcinoma from extension of a cervical cancer; primary probably account for the greatest number of so-called vaginal cancers.

○ **What is the histologic distribution of primary vaginal cancers?**

1.	Squamous	85%
2.	Adenocarcinoma	6%
3.	Melanoma	3%
4.	Sarcoma	3%
5.	Misc.	3%

○ **Where is the most frequent location of a primary vaginal carcinoma lesion?**

The predominance of lesions is in the upper third and posterior wall of the vagina.

○ **Have causes of chronic irritation of the vaginal wall, that is, use of a vaginal pessary, prolapse of the vaginal wall, syphilis, leukoplakia, been proven to be a cause of vaginal cancer?**

No. The cause of squamous cell carcinoma of the vagina is unknown.

○ **What is the most frequent presenting symptom of vaginal cancer?**

Vaginal discharge, often bloody, is the most frequent symptom in most series. The signs and symptoms of invasive vaginal cancer are similar to that of cervical cancer.

○ **Are the course and destination of lymphatic channels from different areas in the vagina predictable and consistent?**

No. All lymph nodes in the pelvis may at one time or another serve as a primary site or regional drainage for vaginal lymph and its contents.

○ **How is vaginal cancer staged?**

Clinically similar to cervical cancer. All patients should have a physical examination, chest film, IVP, cystoscopy, and proctoscopy. Optional studies include lymph angiogram and barium enema.

○ **When should a barium enema be definitely included in patients with vaginal cancer?**

In patients with a history of recurrent diverticulitis since it may be important in planning radiation therapy.

○ **What is the primary mode of therapy for vaginal cancer?**

Radiation therapy.

○ **What is the typical radiation treatment plan for larger stage I vaginal cancers and above?**

4000 to 5000 cGy whole pelvis external radiation with an interstitial implant delivery approximately 3000cGy locally.

○ **What is the stage of a vaginal cancer that has extended onto the pelvic sidewall?**

Stage III.

○ **What is typical treatment of a bulky stage I or II vaginal cancer?**

External radiation 4000 to 5000 cGy followed by (in some centers) vaginal ovoids and an intrauterine tandem (Fletcher-Suite). These are used to deliver a surface dose of up to 6000 cGy in 72 hours or 8000 cGy in two applications of 48 hours each separated by 2 weeks, depending on initial thickness and regression of the lesion. Many centers now administer high-dose radiation (HDR) brachytherapy on an outpatient schedule.

○ **In addition to standard radiation therapy, which additional treatments should be considered for a vaginal tumor occurring in the distal third of the vagina?**

Since these tumors frequently metastasize to the inguinal nodes, these nodes are best treated by radical inguinal dissection before radiation therapy.

○ **In clear cell adenocarcinoma of the vagina, what is the precursor lesion found?**

Adenosis.

○ **What has clear cell carcinoma of the vagina and cervix been thought to be associated with?**

Diethylstilbestrol (DES) exposure in utero. Sixty-five percent of clear cell carcinomas of the vagina and cervix have evidence of in utero exposure to DES; however, data does not substantiate that DES intrauterine exposure is a carcinogenic event. It has been shown to be teratogenic with increased adenosis and other uterine anomalies.

○ **What is the treatment of clear cell adenocarcinoma confined to the upper vagina and/or cervix?**

Radical hysterectomy with upper vaginectomy and pelvic lymphadenectomy with retention of the ovaries.

○ **What is the overall survival rate of clear cell adenocarcinoma of the vagina/cervix?**

80%. This is better than 65% crude survival rate for squamous cell cancer of the cervix and much higher than 35% to 40% survival rate reported for squamous cell cancer of the vagina.

○ **Can primary adenocarcinoma of the vagina occur without intrauterine exposure to DES?**

Yes. In both pre- and postmenopausal women.

○ **What is the treatment of malignant melanoma of the vagina?**

Surgical excision (radical excision with nodal dissection). Radiation and chemotherapy have not been found to be effective in the upper two-third of the vagina. An exenterative procedure must be used.

○ **What is the overall survival rate of patients with vaginal melanomas?**

15%.

○ **What is the peak age at presentation of a DES exposure-related clear cell adenocarcinoma of the vagina or cervix?**

19 years old.

○ **What is the histologic finding associated with clear cell adenocarcinomas?**

Hobnails.

○ **Where are clear cell adenocarcinomas of the genital tract in the female most commonly located?**

These tumors appear to arise equally in the ectocervix and upper anterior wall of the vagina.

○ **What is the treatment of sarcoma botryoides in a young child?**

Surgery and adjuvant chemotherapy consisting of a combination of vincristine, actinomycin, and cyclophosphamide that can be used up front permitting more conservative surgery.

○ **What association has been described between the risk of developing vaginal cancer and the time of first exposure in utero to DES?**

The risk was greatest for those exposed in the first 16 weeks in utero and declined for those whose exposure began in the 17th week or later.

○ **What is the incidence of clear cell adenocarcinoma in women prenatally exposed to DES?**

0.14 to 1.4 per 1000.

○ **What is the frequency of recurrence in vaginal cancer by stage?**

Stage I—10% to 20% pelvic recurrence.
Stage II—35% pelvic recurrence/22% distant metastasis.
Stage III—35% pelvic recurrence/23% distant metastasis.
Stage IV—58% pelvic recurrence/30% distant metastasis.

○ **What is the classical gross appearance of adenosis of the vagina?**

Red, velvety grapelike clusters in the vagina.

○ **Name the different types of vaginal cancers.**

Epithelial	Squamous cell
Verrucous	Small cell
Malignant melanoma	Malignant lymphoma
Smooth muscle tumors	Rhabdomyosarcoma
Clear cell adenocarcinoma	

○ **Has chemotherapy been proven to be a useful adjuvant therapy in vaginal cancer?**

No. It has been used only as a salvage agent with poor results.

○ **What is the survival rate with locally recurrent vulvar cancer?**

Recurrence-free survival can be obtained in up to 75% of cases when the recurrence is local and limited to the vulva and can be resected with a gross clinical margin.

○ **Does recurrence of vulvar cancer in the groin have a good prognosis?**

No. Unanticipated recurrence in the groin is almost universally fatal.

○ **What are the major prognostic factors in vulvar cancer?**

Tumor size, depth of tumor invasion, nodal spread, and distant metastasis.

○ **When compared in a randomized prospective study, was radiation to the groin and deep pelvic nodes found to be superior compared with surgical debulking of the deep pelvic nodes in patients with clinically positive inguinal nodes in vulvar cancer?**

Yes. The 2-year survival rates were 59% compared with 31%.

○ **With a malignant melanoma, when can lymphadenectomy be avoided and is not necessary to complete?**

Superficial melanomas (Clark level I–II) as risk of metastatic disease are minimal. A poor prognosis is associated with Clark level IV–V, thickness >2 mm, or mitotic count >10/mm^2.

Radiation Therapy, Chemotherapy, Immunotherapy, and Tumor Markers

CHAPTER 49

Mitchell I. Edelson, MD

○ **What is the dose-limiting toxicity associated with cisplatin?**

Peripheral neuropathy. This is also the most common side effect usually involving the hands and feet.

○ **True or False: Anticancer drugs can kill a fixed number of tumor cells per dose.**

False. Anticancer drugs kill a fixed percentage of tumor cells per dose.

○ **What is the mechanism of action of methotrexate?**

Methotrexate binds dihydrofolate reductase, preventing reduction in folate to tetrahydrofolate, which is necessary for production of thymidine and purines.

○ **What side effects are seen with the use of serotonin antagonists (ondansetron/Zofran, granisetron/Kytril, dolasetron/Anzemet) as antiemetics?**

Headache and constipation.

○ **What is the maximum total cumulative dose of Adriamycin suggested to minimize the risk of cardiomyopathy?**

<500 mg/m^2.

○ **What immediate steps should be taken to minimize tissue damage following extravasation of Adriamycin?**

Stop the infusion, aspirate the drug from the site if possible, apply ice to the affected area, and apply Dimethyl sulfoxide (DMSO) topically and allow to air dry.

○ **While cold packs are recommended for the treatment of most extravasation injuries, with which class of chemotherapy agent should warm soaks be utilized?**

Vinca alkaloids such as vincristine and etoposide.

○ **What is the mechanism of action of paclitaxel?**

Paclitaxel binds and stabilizes intracellular microtubules, leading to abnormal spindle formations that lead to its cytotoxic effect.

○ **Serum albumin levels may be predictive of what toxicity associated with ifosfamide?**

Central nervous system toxicity may occur with serum albumin levels <3.0 mg/dL due to production of chloroacetaldehyde metabolite.

○ **What is the most common secondary malignancy associated with the use of chemotherapy?**

Acute nonlymphocytic leukemia.

○ **What antibiotics should be used initially in a febrile neutropenic patient?**

For low-risk patients with febrile neutropenia, empiric treatment with oral ciprofloxacin and amoxicillin-clavulanate is safe and effective. High-risk patients require monotherapy with an antipseudomonal beta-lactam agent such as Cefepime, meropenem, imipenem-cilastatin, or piperacillin-tazobactam.

○ **How should chemotherapy-induced mucositis be treated?**

Topical solutions containing viscous xylocaine, antacids, and antifungals may be used along with adequate pain relief.

○ **What is the dose-limiting toxicity of paclitaxel?**

Peripheral neuropathy.

○ **Describe steroid premedication for administration of paclitaxel versus docetaxel.**

Dexamethasone 20 mg is given orally the night before and the morning of paclitaxel administration to prevent hypersensitivity reaction.

Dexamethasone 8 mg is given orally bid for 3 to 5 days starting 24 hours prior to docetaxel administration to prevent fluid retention.

○ **What is the best way to avoid cisplatin-induced renal toxicity?**

Aggressive pretreatment hydration.

○ **What is the growth fraction of a tumor?**

The number of cells actively involved in cell division.

○ **Methotrexate is specific for what phase of the cell cycle?**

S phase.

○ **The chemotherapeutic combination with the most documented activity against recurrent squamous cell carcinoma of the cervix is?**

Cisplatin and paclitaxel

○ **The use of chemotherapy concurrently with radiation for primary therapy of cervical cancer is termed?**

Radiosensitization.

○ **What are the most commonly used drugs for primary treatment of advanced ovarian cancer?**

Paclitaxel and carboplatin

○ **What is the dose-limiting toxicity of topotecan?**

Myelosuppression.

○ **What is the most commonly used drug as a single agent for gestational trophoblastic neoplasia?**

Methotrexate.

○ **Pretreatment for prevention of hypersensitivity reactions associated with paclitaxel include the use of?**

Corticosteroids and H1 and H2 blockers.

○ **The etiology of the hypersensitivity reaction to paclitaxel is related to which component?**

Cremophor EL serves as a solvent to allow paclitaxel to be soluble and induces a histamine release, leading to the hypersensitivity reactions observed.

○ **What is the dose-limiting toxicity associated with Vincristine?**

Neurotoxicity.

○ **What is the mechanism of action of 5-fluorouracil?**

Competitive inhibition of thymidylate synthetase.

○ **Cisplatin is associated with depletion of what electrolytes?**

Potassium, magnesium, and calcium.

○ **True or False: Fever is a frequent side effect of bleomycin.**

True. Bleomycin-induced fever occurs within 24 hours of administration.

○ **The purpose of the use of the agent Mesna in conjunction with ifosfamide is?**

Prevention of hemorrhagic cystitis.

○ **Which chemotherapeutic drugs have the most activity against uterine sarcomas?**

Ifosfamide, Taxol, and cisplatin for carcinosarcomas (MMMT) and Adriamycin for leiomyosarcoma.

○ **What is the mechanism of action of vinca alkaloid type drugs?**

Vinca alkaloids bind to tubulin to inhibit normal microtubular polymerization and lead to mitotic arrest.

○ **Ototoxicity associated with cisplatin typically involves what part of the audible range?**

High frequencies.

○ **What is the mechanism of action of topotecan?**

It is a topoisomerase I inhibitor.

○   **True or False: Cyclophosphamide is specific for the M phase.**

False. Cyclophosphamide is an alkylating agent, and is non-cell-cycle specific, although it probably works best in the S phase. M phase-specific agents include the vinca alkaloids

○   **The diagnosis of syndrome of inappropriate antidiuretic hormone (SIADH) associated with cyclophosphamide is made by what lab findings?**

Hyponatremia with less than maximally dilute urine.

○   **True or False: Adriamycin is primarily excreted by the kidney.**

False. Adriamycin is primarily excreted by the liver.

○   **What is the mechanism of action of Etoposide?**

It is an inhibitor of topoisomerase II.

○   **True or False: Methotrexate is primarily excreted by the kidney.**

True.

○   **What is leucovorin?**

Folinic acid. It is used to prevent toxicity by rescuing normal cells from high-dose methotrexate.

○   **True or False: Alopecia is a frequent side effect of vinblastine.**

True.

○   **What is the dose-limiting toxicity of 5-fluorouracil?**

Stomatitis, often with nausea, vomiting, and diarrhea.

○   **Actinomycin D is frequently used as a single agent for therapy of what gynecologic malignancy?**

Gestational trophoblastic neoplasms.

○   **The most significant side effect associated with bleomycin is?**

Pulmonary fibrosis.

○   **What is the mechanism of action of bleomycin?**

It induces single-stranded breaks in DNA by interacting with oxygen and a metal ion cofactor.

○   **Interstitial pneumonitis resulting from bleomycin can be measured by what parameter of pulmonary function testing?**

Decreased diffusing capacity of the lung for carbon monoxide (DLCO).

○   **What is the longest phase of the active cell cycle?**

G1 may last from 4 to 24 hours.

○ **True or False: Dermatitis and nail loss are frequent toxicities of bleomycin.**

True.

○ **What is the mechanism of action of actinomycin D?**

It blocks RNA synthesis by intercalating DNA nucleotide pairs.

○ **What is "radiation recall"?**

Skin erythema and irritation in a previously irradiated field following administration of chemotherapy. Adriamycin and actinomycin D are commonly reported.

○ **For what phase of the cell cycle is cisplatin specific?**

None, but it may be more effective in the S phase. The mechanism of action of cisplatin is poorly understood.

○ **Ifosfamide-induced hemorrhagic cystitis may be treated initially by?**

Hydration and diuresis.

○ **If hemorrhagic cystitis persists despite hydration/diuresis, what is the most effective immediate topical treatment?**

Continuous bladder irrigation.

○ **The toxic metabolite of ifosfamide responsible for hemorrhagic cystitis is?**

Acrolein. Mesna that is given before and after ifosfamide binds this product to prevent cystitis.

○ **What is the dose-limiting toxicity of carboplatin?**

Myelosuppression. (Thrombocytopenia)

○ **For what phase of the cell cycle is paclitaxel specific?**

M phase, since it is an antimitotic.

○ **Retreatment of ovarian cancer with a platinum drug may be appropriate for which patients?**

Patients may be retreated with platinum if they have developed a recurrence at ≥6 months after cessation of their last treatment (platinum sensitive).

○ **The use of a chemotherapeutic agent following definitive treatment of a tumor when a patient is clinically disease free is known as?**

Adjuvant therapy.

○ **Theoretical advantages of intraperitoneal administration of chemotherapy over intravenous administration for ovarian cancer include?**

High concentrations of the drug can be placed in immediate contact with the tumor for longer periods of time, and toxicities may be lessened by liver metabolism as the drug is absorbed into the portal system.

○ **Describe phase I, II, and III studies.**

Phase I studies determine the toxicities and maximally tolerated dose of a therapeutic agent in humans.

Phase II studies are used to obtain efficacy of an agent in order to determine whether further study is advised.

Phase III studies are a randomized controlled trial with the purpose of comparing the efficacy of an investigational agent to a standard therapy.

○ **When used as a radiosensitizer, 5-fluorouracil frequently exacerbates what side effect of radiation therapy?**

Diarrhea, which is a common side effect of both therapies.

○ **Why is intravenous etoposide administered slowly?**

To prevent hypotension.

○ **What agent can be used with ifosfamide to minimize the risk of hemorrhagic cystitis?**

Mesna (2-mercaptoethanesulfonate).

○ **What parameters are used to calculate body surface area?**

Height and weight (BSA = SQRT [ht.wt/3600]).

○ **Why does tumor heterogeneity often result in drug resistance?**

Spontaneous mutations give rise to small numbers of resistant cells that may rapidly reproduce when sensitive cells are killed.

○ **What is the multidrug resistance (MDR) gene?**

The MDR gene is normally present in some human tissues and may be activated in tumors by exposure to certain chemotherapeutic agents, resulting in resistance to many drugs.

○ **Adriamycin-associated cardiotoxicity may be anticipated by the use of what imaging study?**

MUGA scan to estimate ejection fraction at baseline and after every 2 to 3 cycles of treatment.

○ **Tamoxifen is used to antagonize the effect of estrogen on breast cancer, yet may induce endometrial bleeding and cancer. Why?**

Tamoxifen is a mixed estrogen agonist/antagonist, depending on the target tissue.

○ **How long should high-dose progestins be used in patients with recurrent endometrial cancer to obtain maximum clinical response?**

At least 3 months.

○ **What is the most important factor for predicting the efficacy of progestin therapy in endometrial cancer?**

Progesterone receptor status of the tumor.

○ **Marinol (tetrahydrocannabinol) should be used as an antiemetic with caution in what age group?**

Elderly patients may experience dysphoria with the use of Marinol.

○ **What is the dose-limiting side effect associated with liposomal doxorubicin?**

Palmar-plantar eryhrodysesthesia (hand-foot syndrome) is characterized by painful erythema and edema.

○ **Which antimetabolite is a nucleoside analog that can cause myelosuppression and fever as its side effects?**

Gemcitabine.

○ **What agent has the most documented activity in metastatic sex cord tumors of the ovary?**

Cisplatin. It is frequently used in combination with other agents.

○ **The combination of bleomycin, etoposide, and cisplatin (BEP) has been used successfully in what group of female genital tumors?**

Germ cell tumors of the ovary.

○ **Patients undergoing surgery after bleomycin treatment should avoid high-inhaled oxygen concentrations. Why?**

Acute pulmonary decompensation can occur.

○ **In the palliation of primary tumors, what percentage of a curative dose is typically used?**

Relatively high doses, usually 75% to 80% of the curative dose.

○ **What determines the optimal dose of radiation that is used?**

It is determined by the anatomic location, histologic type, stage and other characteristics of the tumor, and relationship of the cancer to other proximal organs.

○ **What are the six major classes of antiemetics used for prevention and treatment of chemotherapy-induced nausea and vomiting?**

(1) Phenothiazines (Compazine).

(2) Gastrointestinal promotility agents (metoclopramide).

(3) Benzodiazepines (lorazepam).

(4) Steroids (dexamethasone).

(5) Serotonin inhibitors (ondansetron, granisetron).

(6) NK-1 receptor blocker (aprepitant/Emend).

○ **From the standpoint of cell burden, what represents a clinical tumor?**

A clinical tumor can be considered to encompass several compartments.

(1) Macroscopic, visible, or palpable.

(2) Microextensions into adjacent tissues.

(3) Subclinical disease, presumed to be present but not detectable even with the microscope.

○ **What constitutes "gross tumor volume (GTV)"?**

GTV is all known gross disease including enlarged regional lymph nodes.

○ **What constitutes the "clinical target volume (CTV)"?**

CTV encompasses the gross tumor volume and the regions proximal to the gross tumor that are considered to harbor potential microscopic disease.

○ **What constitutes the "planning target volume (PTV)"?**

The region around the CTV that allows for variation in treatment setup and breathing motion. It does not, however, include beam characteristics (penumbra).

○ **What are the most commonly used radiation in clinical radiation?**

X-rays and γ (Gamma)-rays. Electrons are also used and heavier particles have been employed in more experimental treatments.

○ **Where do X-rays and γ-rays arise from?**

Their names reflect their different origins. Gamma (γ)-rays arise from within the nucleus (in practice, they are emitted from radioactive isotopes). X-rays arise from outside the nucleus, produced by bombardment of a target with high-speed electrons.

○ **What is the Compton effect?**

The Compton effect is the interaction of a photon with a loosely bound orbital electron in which part of the incident (incoming) photon's energy is transferred as kinetic energy to the electron and the remaining energy is transmitted to another photon. The energy of the incoming photon determines the probability of its interaction with a target atom's outer electrons; as the energy increases, the probability of interaction decreases.

○ **How does ionizing radiation affect damage at the intracellular level?**

Directly and indirectly. In the direct mechanism, the incoming photon displaces on electrons that directly ionize a DNA strand causing a break in the indirect action, and the displaced electron interacts with a water molecule to produce a hydroxyl radical (.OH), a highly reactive free radical that damages the DNA strand.

○ **What occurs following damage to the DNA following ionizing radiation?**

The initial DNA damage brings about a cascade of biologic events that either interfere with mitosis or initiate programmed cell death (apoptosis).

○ **What is the principal target of ionizing radiation?**

DNA is the principal target within the nucleus of the cell.

○ **What type of DNA aberration caused by ionizing radiation is lethal to the cell?**

Most biologic effects of radiation are a result of incorrect joining of breaks in two chromosomes during the repair process. Specifically, two broken chromosomes may recombine to form dicentric (a chromosome with two centromeres) or a centric fragment (a chromosome with no centromeres). These are lethal lesions.

○ **What is the most likely mechanism for radiation-induced carcinogenesis?**

Radiation-induced carcinogenesis likely results from a translocation that moves one oncogene from a quiescent chromosome site to an active one.

○ **What is a cell survival curve?**

It is the relationship between the fraction of cells surviving and the dose of radiation delivered.

○ **In the treatment of malignancy, how is radiation therapy delivered?**

Radiation therapy is usually delivered in three ways:

(1) Teletherapy (external beam).

(2) Brachytherapy in which the source is placed within or close to the organ being treated. (interstitial or intracavitary treatment).

(3) Intracavitary radioisotopes (radioactive chromic phosphate 32P).

○ **Define the term "Growth Delay."**

Growth delay refers to the amount of time following irradiation during which the tumor regrows to the size it was before it was exposed to radiation.

○ **At which point in the cell cycle are cells most sensitive to radiation?**

Cells are more sensitive to radiation during late G_1 and late G_2 phases and more resistant during early G_1 and late S.

○ **What defines "radiosensitivity"?**

The response both in terms of degree and speed of regression of the tumor to irradiation.

○ **What four variables influence the differences in the radiosensitivity of tumors?**

(1) The ability of cells to repair radiation damage (repair), the degree of hypoxia a cell can tolerate (reoxygenation), the proportion of clonogenic cells (repopulation), and cellular (redistribution).

(2) The quality of radiation.

(3) The temperature of tissues.

(4) The presence of various drugs.

○ **Do higher doses of irradiation produce better tumor control?**

Yes. Higher doses of irradiation do produce better tumor control as demonstrated by numerous published dose-response curves. For every increment of radiation delivered, a certain fraction of cells will be killed. However, higher doses do result in greater toxicity to normal tissues.

○ **What radiation dose is typically used for subclinical disease in squamous cell carcinoma or adenocarcinoma of the cervix or endometrium?**

Doses of 4500 to 5000 cGy will result in control of local disease in over 90% of patients.

○ **What doses of radiation are required for <u>microscopic</u> disease of the cervix and endometrium?**

Doses in the range of 6000 to 6500 cGy for epithelial tumors.

○ **What is meant by "subclinical disease?"**

Subclinical disease refers to deposits of tumor cells that are not microscopically detectable but which can, if untreated, progress to clinical disease.

○ **What are the acute effects of whole-body radiation?**

Three types of syndromes can develop depending on the dose:

(1) Cerebrovascular occurring at high doses (10,000 cGy) with death occurring within 1 to 2 hours.

(2) Gastrointestinal injury at moderate doses (500–1200 cGy) resulting in destruction of the gastrointestinal tract and death within several days.

(3) Hematopoetic injury with doses of 250–500 cGy with death occurring within several weeks.

○ **What is the approximate mean lethal whole-body dose for humans?**

Approximately 400 cGy.

○ **Does radiation exposure lead to new mutations or does it just increase the incidence of those mutations that occur spontaneously in a population?**

It increases the incidence of the range of mutations that occur spontaneously.

○ **What is the approximate "doubling dose" of radiation that is required to double the spontaneous mutation rate in humans?**

The best estimate based on mouse data is 100 cGy. The incidence of mutations is essentially a linear function of dose.

○ **What is meant by the "oxygen enhancement effect"?**

Well-oxygenated cells are more sensitive to irradiation because the oxygen molecules react with free radicals that affect biologic damage. That is, a small amount of oxygen will potentiate the effect of irradiation. Inadequately oxygenated cells have a significant impact on the radiosensitivity of a tumor, often necessitating higher doses of radiation.

○ **What is the latency period between exposure to radiation and the development of radiation-induced cancer and leukemia in humans?**

The latency period is usually long with leukemias typically occurring 5 to 7 years following exposure and solid lesions developing after 30 to 40 years.

○ **What concepts have been explored to potentiate radiation therapy and enhance tumor kill?**

(1) Reoxygenation of hypoxic tumor cells between doses of radiation.

(2) The use of radiation sensitizers that selectively increases the effect of ionizing radiation on a tumor.

(3) Hypoxic cell sensitizing compounds that, when administered, sensitize hypoxic cells to radiation.

(4) Bioreductive drugs that specifically kill cells deficient in oxygen.

○ **What do actinomycin D, doxorubicin, mitomycin C, 5-fluorourasil, cyclophosphamide, methotrexate, bleomycin, and cisplatin have in common?**

They are all cytotoxic chemotherapeutic agents that have been shown to interact with radiation to maximize tumor cell killing.

○ **What role does hyperthermia play in radiation therapy?**

Heat selectively kills cells that are hypoxic, nutritionally deficient, and acidosis all being hallmarks of tumor cells. Temperatures above 42.5°C have been demonstrated to enhance the effects of cytotoxic agents.

○ **Which phase in the cell cycle has been shown to be resistant to irradiation?**

The S phase.

○ **What constitutes a rad. and a Gray (Gy)?**

The rad. is a unit that is defined as the absorption of 0.01 joule per kilogram of the medium (1 rad. = 0.01 J/kg). One Gray (Gy) equals 100 rad.

○ **Define "maximum dose."**

The point of maximum dose for high-energy X-rays and γ-rays is several millimeters below the skin. The dose to the point for any given field is referred to as the maximum dose.

○ **The minimal tumor dose is the lowest delivered to the tumor/target volume. The maximum tumor dose should be what percentage above the minimal tumor dose?**

The maximum tumor dose should be no more than 10% to 15% over the minimum dose.

○ **What is the integral dose?**

It is the total dose delivered over the entire volume or to the body of the patient. It is defined in terms of rad-gram or megarad-gram.

○ **What is an isodose curve?**

An isodose curve represents points of equal distance and is used to provide a visual representation of the dose distribution within a single plane. A series of curves are drawn at 10% increments normalized to the dose at the reference depth. The shape of the isodose curve will be influenced by the type of radiation, the size of its source, its field, the filters employed, and integral dose.

○ **What is a dose profile?**

It is the representation of the dose in an irradiated volume as a function of spatial positions along a single line.

○ **What are three distinct types of radiation?**

(1) An alpha (α) or helium nucleus that has a positive charge.

(2) A beta (β) particle or electron that has a negative charge.

(3) Gamma (γ) rays that originate within the nucleus of the atom and have no charge.

○ **How does "intracavitary" differ from "surface-dose" and "interstitial" brachytherapy?**

"Intracavitary" brachytherapy consists of placing applicators with radioactive compounds within a body cavity so as to gain proximity to the target tissue. In contrast, "interstitial" brachytherapy consists of surgically implanting radioactive sources directly into the target tissue. "Surface-dose" brachytherapy consists of an applicator or mold containing radioactive sources designed to deliver a constant dose to a skin or mucosal surface.

○ **The vaginal cylinder, tandem, and colpostat applicators are used in what type of brachytherapy?**

They are used for intracavitary brachytherapy.

○ **How can radiation exposure to nursing and health-care providers be reduced or eliminated?**

Radiation exposure can be greatly reduced by remote afterloading technology.

○ **How do high-dose rate and low-dose rate delivery systems differ from one another?**

Dose rates of 40 to 200 cGy/hour are considered low-dose rates that, in order to deliver clinically useful doses of 1000 to 7000 cGy, must be administered to inpatients over 24 to 144 hours. In contrast, dose rates in excess of 1200 cGy/hour are considered high-dose rates and may be given over several minutes as an outpatient procedure. In general, 2 to 8 high-dose rate fractions must be administered to approximate the therapeutic ratio of a single low-dose rate implant.

○ **What is the inverse square law?**

The absorbed dose at a given point is inversely proportional to the square of the distance from the source of radiation. This forms the basis for intracavitary treatment whereby a high dose can be delivered to local tissues (cervix) with the rapid falloff of dose sparing surrounding tissues (bladder and rectum).

○ **Intracavitary brachytherapy for carcinoma of the uterine cervix traditionally employs the use of an intrauterine tandem and vaginal colpostats. How are they typically positioned?**

The tandem should be in the midline equal distance from the lateral pelvic sidewalls and the vaginal colpostats symmetrically positioned against the cervix. The tandem should be equal distance from the pubis and sacral promontory.

○ **What determines the total milligram hours that are indicated for intracavitary brachytherapy for carcinoma of the uterine cervix?**

Several factors determine the total number of milligram hours to be delivered:

(1) The tumor stage and volume that in turn determine the total dose in cGy to be delivered at point A.

(2) The strength of sources employed in the tandem and vaginal colpostats.

(3) The number of insertions.

(4) Whether whole pelvic radiation will be employed.

○ **Which two radionuclides are commonly used in brachytherapy for the treatment of cervical carcinoma?**

192 Iridium (T1/2 = 74 days) and 137 cesium (T1/2 = 30 years).

○ **What additional radiotherapy has been advocated to increase the parametrial dose after conventional external and intracavitary irradiation?**

Interstitial implantation transvaginally or transperineally into the parametrium or cervix with metallic needles containing ^{226}Ra, ^{60}Co, or ^{137}Cs or with Teflon catheters for insertion of ^{192}Ir wires or seeds.

○ **In treating carcinoma of the endometrium, what three devices are commonly employed for the delivery of intracavitary brachytherapy?**

Heyman-Simon capsules, afterloading tandem, and vaginal colpostats.

○ **What are typical doses of intracavitary brachytherapy for the treatment of carcinoma of the endometrium?**

For preoperative therapy, intracavitary doses of 3500 to 4000 mgh with 2000 mgh to the mucosal vaginal surface. In patients treated with radiation therapy alone, higher doses in the range of 8000 mgh combined with external radiation are given. In postoperative irradiation, doses of 1800 to 2000 mgh to the vaginal mucosa are given.

○ **What three main biologic processes are involved in the "dose-rate effect"?**

(1) Repair of sublethal damage that occurs when radiation is delivered slowly. As the dose rate diminishes, repair of sublethal damage occurs.

(2) Cellular proliferation occurs during protracted radiation exposure if the dose rate is low enough.

(3) Redistribution and accumulation of cells throughout the proliferative cycle. A low-dose rate limits cellular proliferation allowing cells to accumulate in the radiosensitive G2 phase, ultimately leading to greater cell killing.

○ **What are some advantages of low-dose rate remote afterloading brachytherapy for interstitial and intracavitary applications?**

The advantages include reduced radiation exposure to hospital health-care providers, improved control of isodose distributions, and no need for shielded rooms.

○ **What are some advantages of high-dose rate afterloading brachytherapy, what number of fractional doses are used on average and what is the approximate dose per fraction?**

On average, high-dose remote afterloading brachytherapy employs five fractional doses with the dose per fraction ranging between 500 and 800 cGy to point A.

○ **What are some advantages of high-dose rate remove afterloading brachytherapy for interstitial and intracavitary applications?**

(1) The radiation exposure to hospital health-care providers is essentially eliminated.

(2) There are no complications from prolonged bed rest since patient mobilization time is significantly shortened.

(3) Treatment is done on an outpatient basis, eliminating the need for general anesthesia.

(4) Treatment planning and dosimetry are more exact.

○ **What factors predispose a patient to radiation injury?**

The patient's nutritional status, prior collagen-vascular disease, superimposed infection, and physical or chemical trauma.

○ **What doses of radiation will cause skin erythema?**

In general, single doses between 600 and 750 cGy will produce erythema. Dry desquamation appears with doses >5000 cGy and skin ulceration with ulcers over 6500 cGy.

○ **What are some common gastrointestinal complaints following abdominal or pelvic irradiation?**

Adverse side effects include watery diarrhea, abdominal cramping, increased peristalsis, decreased absorption, and transit time. If the rectum is included in the radiation field, rectal discomfort and tenesmus, and bleeding may be experienced.

○ **At what doses of radiation are bowel mucosal ulcerations, fibrosis, stenosis, and fistula formation encountered?**

These adverse changes are seen when the small and large bowel are exposed to doses of 6000 cGy or more.

○ **At what doses of radiation, does radiation cystitis occur?**

Radiation cystitis occurs with moderate doses of irradiation (above 3000 cGy). With doses above 6000 cGy, chronic cystitis, fibrosis, and vesicovaginal fistula may occur.

○ **What doses of radiation will result in ovarian sterilization?**

The dose of radiation that will result in ovarian castration is age dependent, with younger woman requiring larger doses. In general, a single dose of 650 to 800 cGy or fractional doses of 1500 to 2000 cGy will bring about permanent sterilization.

○ **What is the rationale for preoperative radiation therapy?**

The rationale is based on its potential ability to eradicate subclinical disease beyond the anticipated margins of surgical resection, to reduce tumor volume, to sterilize lymph node metastases, and to decrease the possibility for dissemination of clonogenic tumor cells.

○ **What is the rationale for postoperative irradiation?**

The rationale for postoperative irradiation is based on the assumption that subclinical foci of cancer cells will be destroyed along with any residual disease.

○ **How are the effects of combined radiation therapy and chemotherapy helpful?**

The effects of combined radiation therapy and chemotherapy can be independent, additive, and/or interactive. Chemotherapy prior to irradiation results in a diminished tumor load for radiation treatment. Concurrent use of chemotherapy with radiation therapy can bring about additive or supra-additive action, attenuating tumor kill. Chemotherapy after radiation has been used as an adjuvant to control subclinical disease.

○ **What radiation modality provides for the most optimal treatment of carcinoma of the cervix?**

The most optimal treatment combines external beam irradiation (teletherapy) with intracavity or interstitial brachytherapy.

○ **What is the survival rate for stage IA and IB (smaller than 1 cm) cervical carcinoma with radiation therapy?**

Intracavitary irradiation alone results in a 96% survival. External irradiation alone is much less successful, with survival rates two-third of those for combined intracavitary and external beam radiation.

○ **What is the prescribed dose for external beam radiation in the treatment of cervical carcinoma?**

The prescribed dose is dependent on tumor volume and the extent of combined brachytherapy. In general, the relative proportion of external beam radiation increases with tumor volume and stage; it usually precedes intracavitary brachytherapy with paracentral doses ranging between 70 and 85 cGy and pelvic sidewall doses between 45 and 50 Gy.

○ **What are points A and B?**

These are reference points in the pelvis that are used to describe the doses delivered. Point A is 2 cm lateral and 2 cm superior to the external cervical os and anatomically represents the area where the uterine artery crosses over the ureter. Point B is 3 cm lateral to point A and corresponds to the pelvic sidewall.

○ **What is the target "paracentral" or "point A" dose for the treatment of nonbulky stage IB, IIA, or IIB cervical carcinoma?**

The recommended "point A" dose is 75 to 80 Gy of combined external and low-dose rate brachytherapy. One approach would be to administer an initial 20 Gy of "whole pelvic" external beam irradiation in 2 Gy daily fractions followed by 55 to 60 Gy to be delivered by intracavitary means. For more advanced disease, "whole pelvic" external dose of 40 to 45 Gy and intracavitary contribution of 35 to 40 Gy is more appropriate.

○ **For which patients might extended field radiation therapy be indicated in the treatment of cervical cancer?**

The tendency of cervical carcinoma to spread via a stepwise lymphatic route selects for a subset of patients whose disease is contained within the pelvic and aortic lymph nodes outside the conventional pelvic radiation fields. Eradication of tumor in these sites by extended field radiation therapy produces cure rates of 10% to 50%.

○ **Brachytherapy is essential to the successful treatment of cervical cancer. What doses are typically employed to achieve this success?**

The control of bulky pelvic tumor requires minimal doses of 75 to 85 Gy. These doses are not possible with external beam radiation that would easily exceed the rectal and bladder tolerance of 60 to 70 Gy. The inverse square law allows brachytherapy to achieve the required dose gradient over a very short distance.

○ **What isotopes are used in brachytherapy?**

Radium-226 has been replaced by safer isotopes such as cesium-137 for low-dose rate intracavitary administration, iridium-192 for interstitial, and high-dose rate administration, and cobalt-60 for some high-dose rate afterloading applications.

○ **What are 3 indications for interstitial therapy in the treatment of carcinoma of the cervix?**

The three indications for interstitial radiation therapy in cervical carcinoma are:

(1) Centropelvic recurrence after radical surgery.

(2) Distorted anatomy that makes intracavitary insertion difficult.

(3) Bulky parametrial or sidewall disease.

○ **What are the common isotopes used for interstitial implantation?**

The commonly used isotopes are iridium-192 and iodine-125.

○ **Traditional low-dose rate intracavitary brachytherapy is delivered at a dose rate of 0.4 to 0.8 Gy per hour. At what high-dose rate brachytherapy is administered?**

High-dose rate irradiation is, by definition, >0.2 Gy per minute. However, the dose rate is usually much higher in the 2 to 3 Gy per minute range.

○ **What is the role for palliative radiation therapy?**

Using external irradiation single doses of 10 Gy given two to three times per week can help palliate pelvic symptoms such as pelvic pain, vaginal bleeding and discharge, and edema.

○ **What percentage of severe complications occur following radiation therapy for carcinoma of the cervix?**

In general, severe complications occur in 5% to 10% of patients being treated with radiation therapy for cancer of the cervix. Specifically, 2% to 5% of stage IB and IIA, 5% to 10% of stage IIB, and 10% to 15% of stage III.

○ **How is radiation tolerance of an organ or tissue defined?**

It is defined as the dose required to produce a given risk of a life-threatening complication. Accepted nomenclature is expressed as the total dose that produces a 5% incidence of a specified complication within 5 years of treatment or TD 5/5. Published values of TD 5/5 are based on external beam irradiation in fractions of 2 Gy given 5 days a week.

○ **Which two intracavitary brachytherapy techniques are used in the treatment of endometrial carcinoma?**

The two intracavitary brachytherapy techniques that are employed either alone or combined with external pelvic irradiation are the Heyman packing technique (here, the uterine cavity is packed with small capsules loaded usually with cesium-137) and the intrauterine tandem technique.

○ **Which part of the gastrointestinal tract is the most sensitive to radiation injury?**

The small bowel (TD 5/5 = 45 Gy) is the most susceptible, followed by increasing levels of tolerance in the transverse colon, sigmoid colon, and rectum, respectively. The most common site of chronic injury is the anterior rectum.

○ **What are the indications for postoperative irradiation in the endometrial carcinoma patient?**

(1) Deep myometrial invasion.

(2) Invasion of the cervix or vaginal vault.

(3) Metastases to the ovary, tubes, or other pelvic viscera.

(4) High pathologic grade.

(5) Lymph node metastases.

(6) Positive peritoneal washings.

(7) Unresectable tumor.

At present, the role of adjuvant radiation therapy appears to be in reduction of pelvic recurrences in high-risk patients.

○ **What is the basis for preoperative irradiation for adenocarcinoma of the endometrium?**

Radiation therapy can cure 25% of patients with nonresectable tumors confined to the pelvis and 50% of patients with resectable tumors who are medically inoperable.

○ **What is the standard dose for postoperative irradiation in the patient with endometrial carcinoma with either deep myometrial invasion, metastases to the adnexa, or lymph nodes or high pathologic grade?**

Whole pelvis irradiation in a dose of at least 50 Gy given in fractionated doses over 6 to 7 weeks.

○ **What chemotherapy is utilized for neoadjuvant chemoradiation of unresectable vulvar cancer?**

Cisplatin, 5-FU, and mitomycin.

Gestational Trophoblastic Disease

CHAPTER 50

Mitchell I. Edelson, MD

○ **What are the histologically distinct disease entities encompassed by the general terminology of gestational trophoblastic neoplasia (GTN)?**

(1) Hydatidiform moles (complete and partial).

(2) Invasive mole.

(3) Gestational choriocarcinoma.

(4) Placental site trophoblastic tumors (PSTTs).

○ **Describe the characteristics of trophoblastic cells (both normal and abnormal) that allow them to metastasize.**

Trophoblastic cells do not express transplantation antigens (HLA and ABO), allowing them to escape from maternal immunologic rejection. They are thus able to invade into maternal decidua, vessels, and myometrium. Embolization of trophoblastic cells from the endometrial sinuses into the maternal venous system occurs continuously. The maternal pulmonary circulation is responsible for filtering out these cells and thus preventing them access to the system circulation.

○ **What is GTD?**

This is the term used to describe the various diseases with the potential to invade normal tissue and metastasize. This would encompass choriocarcinoma, invasive mole, postmolar GTD, and PSTTs.

○ **What is the incidence of the various forms of GTD in the United States?**

Approximately 1 in 600 therapeutic abortions and 1 in 1500 pregnancies.

○ **What is the incidence of hydatidiform moles in the general population?**

The incidence of complete hydatidiform moles is estimated to be between 0.26 and 13 per 1000 pregnancies. Asian and Latin American women share a twofold increase in risk compared with other populations.

○ **What are the features of complete hydatidiform moles?**

(1) Complete hydatidiform moles lack identifiable embryonic or fetal tissues.

(2) Most commonly results from an ovum that has been fertilized by haploid sperm that then duplicates its own chromosomes.

(3) The most common karyotype is 46XX followed by 46XY (5%)

(4) Diffuse villous edema

(5) Postmolar malignant sequelae 6% to 32%.

○ **What are the features of a partial mole?**

(1) Identifiable embryonic or fetal tissues.

(2) Partial moles usually have a triploid karyotype (69XXX or 69XXY) with the extra haploid set of chromosomes derived from the father.

(3) Focal villous edema.

(4) Postmolar malignant sequelae <5%.

○ **How does age influence the incidence of hydatidiform moles?**

Compared with women 20 to 29 years of age, women over the age of 50 have a marked increase in risk, as well as women under the age of 15. Similarly, increased paternal age (above 45 years of age) also confers an increased risk of a complete molar pregnancy, although the increase is only 4.9 times (2.9 when adjusted for maternal age).

○ **What are the signs and symptoms of an incomplete molar pregnancy?**

In general, these patients present with signs and symptoms of incomplete or missed abortion (amenorrhea, vaginal bleeding, absent fetal heart tones), and the diagnosis may only be possible after histologic review of curettings.

○ **What is the most common presenting symptom in a complete mole?**

Vaginal bleeding

Other symptoms of complete mole include:

(1) Excessive uterine size (50%).

(2) Theca lutein cysts [due to increased serum levels of beta-human chorionic gonadotropin (beta-hCG) and prolactin].

(3) Hyperemesis gravidarum (25%) (due to markedly elevated beta-hCG).

(4) Hyperthyroidism (7%).

(5) Trophoblastic embolization.

(6) The presence of gestational hypertension during the first half of pregnancy should alert the possibility of molar gestation.

○ **What is the term used to describe the sonographic findings of molar pregnancy?**

Snowstorm pattern.

○ **How are patients with hydatidiform moles managed?**

The diagnosis of complete or partial moles is usually made after performing suction D and C for a suspected incomplete abortion. In these cases, patients should be monitored with serial determinations of quantitative hCG values. A baseline postevacuation chest X-ray should be considered.

○ **What is the phantom hCG?**

It is a false-positive test result caused by heterophilic antibodies cross-reacting with the hCG test.

○ **When should Phantom hCG be suspected?**

When the hCG values plateau at relatively low levels and do not respond to therapeutic maneuvers. Heterophilic antibodies are not excreted in the urine; therefore urinary hCG values will not be detectable. Also a false-positive hCG assay will not be affected by serial dilutions of the patient's sera.

○ **Which form of GTD is less sensitive to chemotherapy?**

PSTTs.

○ **How are patients monitored after evacuation of hydatidiform moles?**

Ideally, serum hCG should be obtained within 48 hours after evacuation then every week while elevated until normal for 3 weeks and then monthly until normal for 6 months.

○ **True or False:**

• **Patients with prior partial or complete moles have a 10-fold increase risk of a second hydatidiform mole in a subsequent pregnancy.**

True.

• **Pulmonary complications, such as the syndrome of trophoblastic embolization, are frequently observed around the time of molar evacuation among patients with uterine enlargement of >14 to 16 weeks' gestational size.**

True.

• **IUD is the encouraged contraceptive during the entire interval of hCG follow-up.**

False. In fact they have the potential risk of perforation.

• **Patients with hCG level >100,000, excessive uterine enlargement, and theca lutein cysts larger than 6 cm in diameter are at high risk of postmolar persistent tumor.**

True.

• **The diagnosis of vaginal metastasis should be made with biopsy.**

False. Vaginal metastasis is present in 30% of patients with metastatic disease. These lesions are highly vascular and can bleed vigorously if sampled for biopsy.

○ **The diagnosis of postmolar GTD is made when one of the following occurs?**

(1) Four values or more of plateauing hCG (+/− 10%) over at least 3 weeks.

(2) Rise of hCG >10% for 3 values or more over at least 2 weeks.

(3) Choriocarcinoma confirmed by histology

(4) Persistence of hCG after 6 months following evacuation of a molar pregnancy.

○ **What pretreatment evaluation is required prior to beginning therapy for GTD?**

(1) History and physical examination.

(2) Laboratory evaluation including CBC, serum creatinine, and liver function tests.

(3) Radiographic studies including pelvic ultrasound, CT scan of abdomen and pelvis, chest X-ray or CT of chest, brain MRI, or CT scan.

○ **What percentage of patients have metastatic disease when GTD is diagnosed?**

45%.

○ **What percentage of patients treated for nonmetastatic GTD with negative chest X-ray have pulmonary metastasis noted on chest CT?**

29% to 41%.

○ **What is the most common site of metastasis for GTD?**

Lungs.

○ **What is the preferred single-agent chemotherapy of choice?**

Methotrexate.

○ **Why is methotrexate the preferred method?**

Less toxicity and greater ease of administration make methotrexate a more attractive agent. Dactinomycin is generally reserved for secondline therapy, although both single-agent therapies yield similar response rates.

○ **What is an adequate response to chemotherapy?**

A fall in the hCG level by 1 log after a course of chemotherapy.

○ **Describe the characteristics of gestational choriocarcinoma.**

Gestational choriocarcinoma contains both cytotrophoblast and syncytiotrophoblast elements. Chorionic villi are absent, and if present represent an invasive molar pregnancy. Gestational choriocarcinoma readily invades the maternal venous system, producing metastasis by hematogenous dissemination. Metastases tend to outgrow their blood supply, resulting in central necrosis and often massive hemorrhage.

○ **Describe the characteristics of PSTTs.**

PSTTs are composed of a predominance of intermediate cytotrophoblast cells arising at the site of placental implantation. Because there is only a small proportion of syncytiotrophoblast cells, little beta-hCG is produced. In some patients, human placental lactogen (hPL) is a more reliable marker. These tumors are locally invasive, although a small percentage of patients will develop extrauterine metastasis.

○ **What is the treatment of PSTT?**

These are not sensitive to chemotherapy; therefore, surgery (hysterectomy) becomes the main treatment.

○ **What is the highest risk factor for having a choriocarcinoma?**

A hydatidiform mole in the previous pregnancy confers the greatest risk of the development of a subsequent gestational choriocarcinoma.

○ **Why is induction of labor with oxytocin or prostaglandins not recommended for the evacuation of molar pregnancies?**

Uterine contractions against an undilated cervix theoretically carry an increased risk of the dissemination of trophoblast throughout the systemic circulation.

○ **What type of ovarian cyst can be clinically evident (≥5 cm) in 25% to 35% of women with hydatidiform mole?**

Theca lutein cysts similar to those induced by gonadotropin/hCG ovarian hyperstimulation. These are generally detected pre-evacuation but can arise within the first week after evacuation and can take up to 8 weeks to disappear.

○ **List four possible etiologies for postevacuation associated respiratory distress.**

(1) Trophoblastic deportation.

(2) High-output congestive heart failure secondary to anemia or hyperthyroidism.

(3) Pre-eclampsia.

(4) Iatrogenic fluid overload.

○ **Describe four important steps in the management of respiratory distress associated with molar evacuation.**

(1) Ventilatory support with either supplemental oxygen or mechanical ventilation.

(2) Central monitoring including Swan-Ganz catheter.

(3) Diuresis as indicated by etiology.

(4) Correction of anemia or hyperthyroid etiologies of high output CHF as indicated.

○ **What precaution should be taken prior to evacuation in patients diagnosed with hyperthyroidism as a result of a diagnosis of complete mole?**

Administration of a beta-adrenergic blocker such as propranolol helps to prevent thyroid storm at the time of evacuation or in the postevacuation period.

○ **List three other entities confused with twin gestation complicated by hydatidiform mole.**

Retroplacental hematoma, partial hydatidiform mole, and nonviable twin can have similar presentations.

○ **Of those patients diagnosed with postmolar GTD, what percentage represents patients with persistent or invasive moles versus those patients with choriocarinomas?**

About 70% to 90% of these patients will have persistent or invasive moles, while 10% to 30% will have choriocarcinomas.

○ **Describe the revised International Federation of Gynecologists and Obstetricians (FIGO) 2000 prognostic index score for GTD**

Prognostic Factor	0	1	2	4
Age (year)	≤39	>39		
Antecedent pregnancy	Hydatidiform mole	Abortion		Term pregnancy
Interval[a]	<4 months	4–6 months	6–12 months	>12 months
Pretreatment hCG (mIU/mL)	<1000	1000–10,000	10,000–100,000	>100,000
Largest tumor, including uterine (cm)		3–4 cm	5 cm or greater	
Site of metastases	Lung	Spleen and kidney	GI tract	Brain and liver
Number of metastases	0	1–3	4–8	>8
Prior chemotherapy			Single drug	Two or more drugs

Total score 0–6 = low risk; 7 or higher = high risk.
[a]Interval: time in months from end of antecedent pregnancy to chemotherapy.

○ **Describe the management options by stage.**

(1) Stage I disease (confined only to uterine corpus):

  (a) Patient no longer wishes to preserve fertility—hysterectomy with adjuvant single-agent chemotherapy.

  (b) Patient with PSTT—hysterectomy, as these tumors are resistant to chemotherapy.

  (c) Patient wishes to preserve fertility—single-agent chemotherapy.

  (d) Patient wishes to preserve fertility but tumor resistant to single-agent chemotherapy—combination chemotherapy.

(2) Stage II (metastasis to pelvis and vagina) and III (metastasis to lungs):

  (e) Low-risk patient—single-agent chemotherapy.

  (f) High-risk patient—combination chemotherapy.

(3) Stage IV (distant metastasis).

All these patients should be treated with combination chemotherapy and the selective use of radiation therapy and surgery.

○ **Although most forms of metastatic cancers yield poor survival rates, malignant GTD is considered a curable form of cancer. Describe the life table survival rates for patients with nonmetastatic, metastatic good-prognosis, and metastatic poor-prognosis as defined by the clinical classification system.**

Approximately 100% of patients in the first two categories are cured of disease. However, this rate drops of to approximately 80% in the metastatic poor-prognosis group.

○ **What is considered to be the highest risk factor in the metastatic poor-prognosis group in the clinical classification system?**

Failed prior chemotherapy is the most significant factor. Salvage rates of 14% and 70% have been reported for patients with poor-prognosis metastatic disease treated initially with single-agent and multiagent chemotherapy, respectively.

○ **High-risk/poor-prognosis metastatic GTD is generally treated with a multiagent chemotherapy regimen called EMA-CO. What are the five drugs involved in this regimen?**

Etoposide, methotrexate, dactinomycin, cyclophosphamide, and vincristine are the five chemotherapeutic agents that make up the EMA-CO regimen.

○ **What percentage of remission rate is generally obtainable with the EMA-CO regimen in high-risk/poor-prognosis metastatic patients with GTD?**

Approximately 80% of patients will have their disease put into remission by this treatment regimen.

○ **How long should a woman with nonmetastatic GTD or low-risk metastatic GTD undergo chemotherapy?**

Treatment should continue 1 to 2 cycles after obtaining the first normal hCG value.

○ **How long should treatment continue for a patient with high-risk metastatic GTD?**

Chemotherapy should be continued for at least 3 additional courses after the hCG levels have normalized.

○ **Are women with a complete molar pregnancy at increased risk of a molar pregnancy in future pregnancies?**

Yes. But only 1 in 100 women have at least two molar pregnancies. Even women with two molar pregnancies may still achieve a normal full term pregnancy.

○ **What are the recommendations for women with a prior molar pregnancy when a subsequent pregnancy occurs?**

Obtain a pelvic ultrasound during the first trimester to confirm a normal gestation. Obtain a hCG measurement 6 weeks postpartum to exclude occult trophoblastic neoplasia.

CHAPTER 51 Gynecologic Pathology

Mitchell I. Edelson, MD

○ **What is the sex-determining region Y (SRY) gene?**

The SRY gene is found in the 1A1 region at the distal end of chromosome Yp. Its presence dictates development of testicles, while its absence results in ovarian differentiation.

○ **What two substances are responsible for development of the Wolffian duct system and regression of the Müllerian ducts?**

Testosterone and Müllerian-inhibiting substance (MIS) that are produced by the testes.

○ **What is a hermaphrodite?**

The presence of both ovarian and testicular tissue in a single individual.

○ **What is the most common karyotype in Turner syndrome?**

45X.

○ **What is the most common cause of male pseudohermaphroditism?**

Androgen insensitivity syndrome (testicular feminization).

○ **What is the most common cause of ambiguous genitalia?**

Congenital adrenal hyperplasia.

○ **What are the causative agents of granuloma inguinale and lymphogranuloma venereum?**

Calymmatobacterium granulomatis and *Chlamydia*, respectively.

○ **What is the name of the cytology preparation whereby one scrapes the base of a fresh vesicle, spreads the material on a slide, and stains it in an attempt to diagnose herpes?**

Tzanck prep.

○ **What is the most common cause of a Bartholin cyst abscess?**

Gonorrhea.

○ **What happens to a large number of cases of lichen sclerosus et atrophicus of the vulva in children when they reach puberty?**

A large percentage of these cases involute or regress spontaneously.

○ **What is the most common age of development of lichen sclerosus et atrophicus?**

Postmenopausal women, but it can occur at any age and sex.

○ **What are some ectopic tissues that can occur in the labia?**

Breast (along the milk line), salivary gland tissue, and mesothelial cysts. In addition, various rests of embryonic tissues can occur.

○ **What benign lesion can occur in the vulva and is thought to arise from sweat glands?**

Papillary hidradenoma (hidradenoma papilliferum).

○ **Describe the typical patient who develops papillary hidradenoma.**

This tumor is rare overall; however, it tends to occur in Caucasian females after puberty. This correlates with the development of the apocrine sweat glands that are the origin of this tumor.

○ **What types of human papillomavirus (HPV) are typically recovered from condylomatous lesions of the vulva?**

As in other locations with HPV lesions, the benign appearing condyloma acuminata tend to have HPV types 6 and 11, while squamous cell carcinoma in situ and invasive squamous cell carcinoma of the vulva tend to be associated with types 16, 18, and 31.

○ **What tumor that most commonly occurs in the soft tissue of the vulva of young to middle-aged women, is characteristically well circumscribed, shows positive immunoreactivity for vimentin and desmin, and has been reported to occur in males?**

Angiomyofibroblastoma.

○ **What tumor typically occurs in women <40 and involves the genitalia, is poorly circumscribed, and has distinct myxoid and vascular areas histologically?**

Aggressive angiomyxoma.

○ **What is the most common type of HPV found in vulvar intraepithelial neoplasia (VIN) and invasive squamous cell carcinoma of the vulva?**

HPV type 16.

○ **What is the most common malignant tumor of the vulva?**

Squamous cell carcinoma.

○ **Name three features in the staging of vulvar carcinoma, which are important in determining prognosis.**

(1) Diameter of the tumor.

(2) Depth of invasion.

(3) Status of regional lymph nodes.

○ **What is the classic presentation of bowenoid papulosis of the vulva?**

A pigmented papule in a young pregnant female.

○ **How common is the presence of an underlying, invasive adenocarcinoma in a patient with vulvar Paget disease?**

10% to 20% of the cases.

○ **What are the clinical features of Paget disease of the vulva?**

The lesions may have eczematoid appearance but can develop a raised and velvety appearance with more extensive lesions.

○ **Regarding depth of invasion of squamous cell carcinoma of the vulva, how much invasion is allowed before there is a significant risk of lymph node metastases?**

The so-called microinvasive carcinoma that invades 1 mm or less has almost no risk of lymph node metastases. Those that invade as little as 3 mm show metastatic lymph node involvement in >10% of the cases.

○ **What are some risk factors involved in development of squamous cell carcinoma of the vulva?**

Cigarette smoking, diabetes mellitus, presence of HPV (particularly younger patients), and immunosuppression.

○ **What is the protein produced by HPV infected cells that causes degradation of p53?**

Protein E6.

○ **How common is lymph node metastases in verrucous carcinoma of the vulva?**

While this tumor has a tendency to recur locally, it does not metastasize in the absence of altered, aggressive behavior secondary to radiation therapy. The treatment is local excision.

○ **What tumor, more characteristically found in the salivary glands, can occur in the vulva and is characterized by late hematogenous spread and perineural invasion?**

Adenoid cystic carcinoma.

○ **What percentage of vulvar malignancies are melanomas?**

<5%.

○ **What is Sampson's theory regarding endometriosis?**

This hypothesis states that endometriosis (endometrial glands and stroma) occurs outside of the uterine mucosa via "reflux menstruation" through the fallopian tubes and into the abdominal cavity.

○ **What is Novak's theory regarding endometriosis?**

This theory, favored by many, states that tissue derived from the Müllerian system may undergo metaplasia to become endometrial tissue.

○ **What are the two most common causes of vaginitis?**

Candida albicans and *Trichomonas vaginalis.*

○ **What is the most common cause of bacterial vaginosis?**

Gardnerella vaginalis.

○ **What organism is occasionally seen in Pap smears classically in association with use of an intrauterine device (IUD)?**

Actinomyces israelii.

○ **What is the organism that, in association with the use of tampons, is associated with toxic shock syndrome?**

Staphylococcus aureus. Specifically, the enterotoxin F and exotoxin C produced by the organism and absorbed by the patient are the cause of this syndrome.

○ **What is the name of the rare simple vaginal cyst that is typically found in the lateral or anterolateral wall of the vagina and is lined by a single layer of cuboidal-type cells?**

Gartner duct cyst (mesonephric cyst).

○ **What is the most common benign tumor of mesenchyme in the vagina?**

Leiomyoma.

○ **What is vaginal adenosis and what is it associated with?**

This is a collection of benign mucinous endocervical glands in the vagina and is associated with exposure to diethylstilbestrol (DES) in utero by the patient's mother. Specifically, the critical time of exposure is prior to the 18th week of gestation.

○ **What is the more serious complication associated with in utero exposure to DES?**

Development of clear cell adenocarcinoma of the vagina and cervix.

○ **What is the most common site in the vagina of adenosis and clear cell adenocarcinoma?**

The upper one-third of the vagina on the anterior wall.

○ **What benign polypoid lesion occurs in the vagina and tends to protrude from the introitus and can be confused with sarcoma botryoides?**

Fibroepithelial polyp.

○ **What is the most common malignant vaginal tumor found in children?**

Embryonal rhabdomyosarcoma, also known as sarcoma botryoides.

○ **What is the most common age of presentation of sarcoma botryoides?**

A diagnosis is made at age 5 or less in almost every case. The mean age is about 3 years old. Tumors arising in the cervix occur at a somewhat older age. This tumor has a 90% or greater survival rate.

○ **What is the natural history of VIN?**

The vast majority of lesions will regress following biopsy only. Slightly >10% will persist and <10% will progress to an invasive squamous cell carcinoma.

○ **What percentage of all vaginal malignancies are classified as primary tumors?**

10% to 20% are primary tumors.

○ **What is the most common type of vaginal cancer?**

Secondary cancer from cancer of the cervix.

○ **What is the most common malignant mesenchymal tumor of the vagina?**

Leiomyosarcoma.

○ **What are some of the melanocytic lesions that occur in the vagina?**

Lentigo, blue nevus, cellular blue nevus, and melanoma.

○ **What type of herpes simplex virus (HSV) is typically associated with genital infection?**

Type 2 (HSV-2).

○ **What are some of the potential complications of PID?**

Infertility, bacteremia, abdominal adhesions with resultant bowel obstruction, peritonitis, and chronic pain.

○ **What is the term given to describe the junction of the ectocervix and endocervix?**

The squamocolumnar junction is the point where the columnar epithelium of the endocervical canal meets with the squamous epithelium of the ectocervix. This squamocolumnar junction is constantly changing in relation to puberty, pregnancy, menopause, and hormonal stimulation. The transformation zone is the area between the original squamocolumnar junction and the new squamocolumnar junction that changes depending on the patient's age and hormonal status.

○ **What is the name of the process whereby columnar epithelium of the cervix is replaced by squamous epithelium?**

Squamous metaplasia.

○ **How can you tell where the original squamocolumnar junction was located?**

Identifying nabothian cysts or cervical cleft openings will indicate the presence of columnar epithelium.

○ **What benign glandular proliferative lesion of the cervix is associated with the use of oral contraceptives in young females?**

Microglandular hyperplasia.

○ **What is the most common type of HPV associated with flat condylomas of the cervix?**

Types 6 and 11.

○ **What is the most common type of HPV found in high-grade squamous intraepithelial lesions and invasive carcinomas of the cervix?**

Type 16.

○ **What is the classic colposcopic appearance of a high-grade squamous intraepithelial lesion of the cervix?**

A mosaic pattern.

○ **What is the classic colposcopic appearance of an invasive carcinoma of the cervix?**

Irregular, tortuous blood vessels extending across the cervix.

○ **Is HPV found in association with adenocarcinoma in situ of the cervix?**

Yes. HPV types 16 and 18 have been found in adenocarcinoma in situ of the cervix indicating a possible causal factor in development of adenocarcinoma of the cervix.

○ **What is the most common cause of death in patients with cervical carcinoma?**

Cervical carcinoma tends to spread locally and via lymphatics, not hematogenously. Thus, the ureters are frequently obstructed resulting in hydronephrosis, pyelonephritis, and renal failure that are the most common causes of death.

○ **What types of HPV have been isolated in verrucous carcinoma of the vagina/vulva?**

Types 6 and 16.

○ **Describe the behavior of adenoid cystic carcinoma of the cervix.**

This is a rare cervical tumor that is very aggressive and exhibits local recurrence with distant metastases. The prognosis is similar or worse than the more conventional squamous cell carcinoma of the cervix.

○ **Does the prognosis for adenoid cystic carcinoma of the cervix differ from adenoid basal carcinoma of the cervix?**

Yes. Markedly, therefore it is critical to make the histologic distinction between the two tumors. Adenoid basal carcinomas exhibit a benign behavior with no metastases.

○ **What is the pattern of spread and prognosis in papillary villoglandular adenocarcinoma of the cervix?**

This unusual tumor is found in younger women and, although it can be deeply invasive, it does not appear to metastasize.

○ **What is the name of the benign lesion of the cervix that is composed of a nodular, circumscribed aggregate of dilated endocervical glands that are superficially located beneath the epithelial surface?**

Tunnel clusters.

○ **How common is an associated squamous dysplastic lesion of the cervix found in association with adenocarcinoma in situ of the cervix?**

Very common, ranging from 50% to nearly 100% in a variety of studies.

○ **In an endometrial biopsy, you see pronounced stromal edema, moderate glandular secretions, an absence of stromal/glandular mitoses, markedly tortuous glands, and no significant decidual change. Approximately what day of the 28-day cycle is the biopsy obtained from?**

Approximately day 22. Day 22 is when stromal edema is maximal and glandular secretions are just beyond their peak (day 20 or 21) and predecidual change has not become evident yet.

○ **What is the most common site of endometriosis?**

The ovary.

○ **What is the name of the phenomenon that tends to occur in pregnancy and is characterized by a focus of tightly clustered endometrial glands that appear hypertrophic and demonstrate nuclear pleomorphism and cytoplasmic vacuolization?**

Arias-Stella reaction (which can be confused with clear cell and adenocarcinoma in situ of the cervix.

○ **What substances are produced by the corpus luteum and are important in regulating the secretory phase of the endometrium?**

Estradiol and progesterone.

○ **What is the basic mechanism by which clomiphene citrate is useful as a fertility drug?**

Clomiphene citrate decreases endogenous estrogen thus resulting in secretion of gonadotropin-releasing hormone and then follicle-stimulating hormone (FSH) and luteinizing hormone (LH). This, hopefully, results in ovulation.

○ **What is the most common cause of dysfunctional uterine bleeding in reproductive age women?**

Anovulatory cycles.

○ **What is the most common cause of postmenopausal endometrial bleeding?**

Endometrial atrophy (60%). Remember, endometrial carcinoma must be considered but is the cause in only 10% of the time.

○ **What is the most common etiology of chronic endometritis?**

It is most commonly an ascending infection by way of the cervix following such things as abortion or instrumentation.

○ **What are the most common etiologic agents of chronic endometritis?**

Chlamydia trachomatis and *Neisseria gonorrhoeae.*

○ **What is the name of the endometrial polypoid lesion that has abundant smooth muscle, tends to occur in the lower uterine segment, and occurs in women of reproductive age?**

Atypical polypoid adenomyoma.

○ **What is the relative risk of development of malignancy within the various types of endometrial hyperplasia?**

Simple hyperplasia without atypia—1%.

Simple hyperplasia with atypia—8%.

Complex hyperplasia without atypia—3%.

Complex hyperplasia with atypia—29%.

○ **What are the criteria to make the diagnosis of endometrial intraepithelial neoplasia?**

(1) Lesion must be >1 mm

(2) The area of the glands exceeds the area of the stroma

(3) The cytology is changed relative to the background

(4) Excluded other causes that may mimic condition

○ **What is the mechanism of development of endometrial hyperplasia in obese women?**

Androstenedione is converted to estrone in the adipose tissue that serves as the stimulation for development of hyperplasia.

○ **What is the rate of concurrent endometrial cancer discovered following hysterectomy with prior tissue diagnosis of atypical complex endometrial hyperplasia?**

43% based on a prospective Gynecologic Oncology Group study.

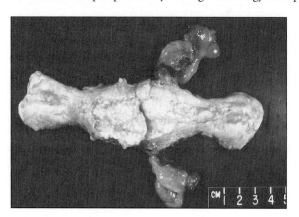

○ **What is the nature of the endometrial carcinomas that develop in obese women secondary to peripheral conversion to estrogens?**

The tumors tend to be well-differentiated, superficially invasive, and have a very good prognosis.

○ **What are some associations with development of adenocarcinoma of the endometrium?**

(1) Obesity.

(2) Diabetes mellitus.

(3) Infertility.

(4) Late menopause.

(5) Any source of continuous unopposed estrogen.

(6) Tamoxifen use.

(7) Hypertension.

○ **What is the prognosis of clear cell carcinoma of the endometrium compared with typical endometrioid carcinoma?**

Clear cell carcinoma tends to occur in older women and carries a poor prognosis.

○ **What is the embryologic origin of the tumor cells in clear cell carcinoma?**

They are of Müllerian origin. Histologically, they are characterized by clear cells, frequently showing a "hobnail" pattern and focal papillary configuration.

○ **Which is more important in the prognosis of endometrial carcinoma, the progesterone receptor status or estrogen receptor status?**

The progesterone receptor status.

○ **Is there a history of estrogen replacement in most patients with clear cell carcinoma of the endometrium?**

No. Most patients are older and do not have that history.

○ **What tumor of the endometrium is characterized by a population of cells that are histologically similar to the stromal cells of a normal proliferative endometrium but exhibit an infiltrative pattern and extensive intravascular involvement by tumor?**

Low-grade endometrial stromal sarcoma.

○ **What is the prognosis in low-grade endometrial stromal sarcoma?**

It is excellent, although it can recur quite late (decades later). The most important factor is stage at presentation.

○ **What is an alternative term for mixed Müllerian tumors?**

Carcinosarcoma that depicts the true nature of the neoplasm—a mixture of carcinoma and sarcoma.

○ **What is the classic clinical presentation for patients with mixed Müllerian tumor?**

They most commonly present with bleeding and on examination have a protuberant polypoid mass protruding through the cervical os.

○ **What do the designations homologous and heterologous elements mean in mixed Müllerian tumors?**

Homologous refers to the state of an undifferentiated sarcoma, while heterologous refers to the presence of differentiated sarcomatous elements that are not derived from the normal uterus such as chondrosarcoma, osteosarcoma, or skeletal muscle differentiation (rhabdomyosarcoma).

○ **What is the prognosis of patients with mixed Müllerian tumor?**

It is very poor, and these tend to occur in older patients. It does not appear that the presence of homologous or heterologous elements markedly affects survival.

○ **What are some of the complications of acute salpingitis?**

- Infertility.
- Small bowel obstruction (secondary to adhesions).
- Pyosalpinx.
- Tubo-ovarian abscess.

○ **What is <u>Gardnerella</u> and what is its importance in the female genital tract?**

It is a small gram-negative rod that can cause vaginitis and is associated with "clue cells" that are epithelial cells covered by bacteria.

○ **What is the best preparation by which one can demonstrate <u>Trichomonas vaginalis</u> at the time of pelvic examination?**

The use of a wet mount is ideal because one can see the flagellated and motile organism swimming in the saline after direct application to the slide from a sampling of the cervix.

○ **What is uterus didelphys?**

This is a congenital abnormality whereby the patient has a double uterus accompanied by a septate or double vagina as a result of lack of complete fusion of the Müllerian ducts.

○ **In a setting of chronic cervicitis, you note a prominent plasma cell infiltrate and distinct germinal center formation. What organism should you suspect most strongly as the etiologic agent?**

Chlamydia trachomatis.

○ **What organism should you suspect in a case of chronic cervicitis where there is significant epithelial spongiosis (intraepithelial edema)?**

Trichomonas vaginalis.

○ **In the pathogenesis of cervical cancer in relation to HPV, what does the E7 viral oncogene do?**

The E7 protein binds to the retinoblastoma gene and displaces some normal transcription factors. This affects normal cell cycle regulation and likely plays a role in the development of carcinoma.

○ **Is there a uniform progression in cervical squamous cell carcinoma from cervical intraepithelial neoplasia (CIN) I to CIN III and subsequent invasive squamous cell carcinoma?**

No. Some lesions clearly do not arise from CIN I. As stated before, the majority of lesions never progress at all.

○ **How commonly do patients with CIN III who have been treated progress to invasive squamous cell carcinoma?**

About 1 in 500.

○ **At what age are you most likely to find a patient with anovulatory cycles?**

They occur most commonly at menarche and in perimenopausal women.

○ **What are the most common sites of endometriosis?**

(1) Ovaries.

(2) Uterine ligaments.

(3) Rectovaginal septum.

(4) Pelvis.

(5) Previous laparotomy scars.

(6) Umbilicus, vagina, vulva, and appendix.

○ **What are some of the typical clinical signs and symptoms of endometriosis?**

Dysmenorrhea, dyspareunia, pelvic pain, gastrointestinal abnormalities, and infertility. The disorder is most common in women in their 20s and 30s.

○ **What is the most common tumor in women?**

Leiomyoma (fibroids).

○ **What is the most reliable indicator of a leiomyosarcoma as opposed to a cellular leiomyoma?**

The mitotic rate is used to differentiate them. Leiomyosarcomas will typically have a mitotic rate exceeding 10 mitotic figures per 10 high-power fields.

○ **Do most leiomyosarcomas arise from a preexisting leiomyoma?**

No. Most believe that leiomyosarcomas arise de novo and that if they do arise within a preexisting leiomyomas, that it is extremely rare (0.1%).

○ **How common is recurrence of leiomyosarcoma following resection?**

Quite common, >50% of cases will metastasize hematogenously most commonly to the lungs.

○ **What is the typical histologic appearance of a benign endometrial polyp?**

These are polypoid portions of endometrial mucosa containing both glands and stroma with thick-walled vessels.

○ **What is the most common bacteria associated with acute salpingitis?**

Chlamydia trachomatis followed by *Neisseria gonorrhoeae*.

○ **How frequently are the fallopian tubes involved when there is tuberculosis involving the female genital tract?**

Essentially always.

○ **What are the histologic features of salpingitis isthmica nodosa?**

This represents bilateral nodules typically in the tubal isthmus, which are composed of tubal epithelial lined channels with admixed, prominent, and smooth muscle bundles.

○ **What are some risk factors for a tubal ectopic pregnancy?**

A history of salpingitis isthmica nodosa, chronic salpingitis, and previous tubal pregnancy.

○ **What is the term given to describe small, simple cysts filled with clear serous fluid that occur commonly next to the fallopian tubes?**

Paratubal cysts, or when larger and near the fimbria, they are called hydatids of Morgagni.

○ **What benign mesothelial-derived tumor can occur in the fallopian tubes?**

Adenomatoid tumor. This is the most common tumor of the epididymis.

○   **How often is primary adenocarcinoma of the tube bilateral?**

One in five cases.

○   **What is the prognosis in tubal adenocarcinoma?**

It is quite poor with about 30% survival at 5 years.

○   **A patient has an ulcerative lesion on the vulva and you are told that microscopically there are Donovan bodies. What are those and what is the disease and organism?**

The disease is granuloma inguinale that is caused by *Calymmatobacterium granulomatis*. The Donovan bodies are vacuolated macrophages that are filled with the organism and are seen with the aid of a Giemsa stain.

○   **By dark-field examination, you are able to detect spirochete organisms taken from a painless ulcer from the genitalia of a female. What is your diagnosis?**

Syphilis (*Treponema pallidum*).

○   **Where in the process of cell division are the oocytes of the ovary at the time of birth?**

They are in a resting stage of the first meiotic division. They will not complete that process until ovulation and fertilization occur.

○   **In a primary follicle of an infant, what are the cells that lie around the oocyte?**

Granulosa cells.

○   **What is a Call-Exner body?**

This is a small, round collection of eosinophilic material that is surrounded by a ring of granulosa cells. These are normal but can be seen in granulosa cell tumors of the ovary.

○   **What is the primary source of estrogen in the preovulatory stage of menses?**

The theca cells.

○   **What is the primary source of progesterone in the ovary that is responsible for regulation of the secretory phase of menses?**

The corpus luteum.

○   **If fertilization occurs, when does primary production of progesterone no longer occur in the corpus luteum?**

After about 8 weeks, the placenta begins taking over primary production of progesterone from the corpus luteum.

○   **What is the name of the benign, non-neoplastic cystic lesion of the ovary that occurs as a result of invagination of the cortex and surface epithelium?**

Epithelial inclusion cyst.

○   **At what age do solitary follicle cysts and corpus luteum cysts occur?**

The solitary follicle cysts occur in perimenopausal women and after menarche, while corpus luteum cysts occur in women of childbearing age.

○ **What is the most common etiologic agent of vaginitis?**

Candida albicans.

○ **Why do leiomyomas often increase in size during pregnancy and decrease in size in postmenopausal women?**

They are estrogen sensitive, thus during the times of high estrogen (pregnancy) they get larger and in times of low estrogen they decrease in size.

○ **What is the name of the condition whereby the patient has numerous follicle cysts in association with oligomenorrhea?**

Polycystic ovarian syndrome (Stein-Leventhal syndrome).

○ **In patients with polycystic ovarian disease, how common is true virilism?**

It is rare. They typically have persistent anovulation, hirsutism, and almost half are obese.

○ **What is the HAIR-AN syndrome?**

Hyperandrogenism (HA), insulin-resistant (IR), and acanthosis nigricans (AN).

○ **At what age does stromal hyperthecosis normally occur?**

Postmenopausal women; however, it can be a part of polycystic ovarian disease in younger women.

○ **What is the microscopic appearance of stromal hyperthecosis?**

It is characterized by nests and groups of luteinized stromal cells with vacuolated cytoplasm.

○ **In polycystic ovarian syndrome, what are the levels of FSH?**

The level of FSH is normal as is 17-ketosteroid production. Androgens, on the other hand, are elevated in the cyst fluid and urine.

○ **Describe the typical clinical presentation in massive ovarian edema.**

The condition is usually unilateral and the patients are young with an average age of 20 years. They present with abdominal or pelvic pain and an associated palpable abdominal mass.

○ **How can you differentiate between fibromatosis and an ovarian fibroma?**

Fibromatosis occurs in younger patients (mean of 25 years) who sometimes have menstrual abnormalities and contains entrapped follicles and their derivatives. In contrast, fibromas are found in older patients, do not contain entrapped normal structures, and are not associated with menstrual abnormalities.

○ **What lesion of the ovary is related to human chorionic gonadotropin (hCG) stimulation, and typically occurs in black multiparous females who are in their 20s or 30s?**

The pregnancy luteoma.

○ **How common is extraovarian spread by ovarian malignancies at the time of initial presentation?**

It is very common (70% of patients), thus the high mortality rate.

○ **What are some of the risk factors for development of ovarian carcinoma?**

Nulliparity, family history, early menarche and late menopause, white race, increasing age, and residence in North America and Northern Europe.

○ **What do recent studies suggest to be the site of origin of high-grade serous epithelial ovarian cancers?**

Fallopian tube mucosa.

○ **What are three syndromes that have been described related to ovarian cancer?**

HNPCC (Lynch II syndrome) cancer of the ovary, endometrium, and colon, breast-ovary syndrome, and ovary-specific syndrome.

○ **Where are the genes located that are responsible for the breast-ovary syndrome?**

The genes are BRCA-1 that is found on chromosome 17q21 and BRCA-2 that is found on 13q12

○ **What serum marker is useful in determining the efficacy of therapy and recurrence of ovarian carcinoma?**

CA-125.

○ **What is the most common cell of origin resulting in ovarian neoplasms (eg, germ cells, stromal cells, and surface epithelium)?**

By far, the surface epithelium gives rise to the most ovarian neoplasms (>60% overall and >90% of malignant tumors).

○ **What is the most common malignant tumor of the ovary?**

Serous cystadenocarcinoma, and it is frequently bilateral (more than half the time).

○ **What are the three general categories, which surface epithelial tumors of the ovary are divided into?**

Benign, low malignant potential, and malignant.

○ **What are some of the histologic features that determine classification into the low malignant potential category?**

These are tumors that are composed of the same cell type but generally lack "high grade" nuclear features, complex architecture, and destructive stromal invasion.

○ **Do ovarian low malignant potential tumors spread beyond the ovary?**

Yes. The majority (60–70%) present confined to the ovary, while up to 40% will spread beyond the ovary, particularly as peritoneal implants. Overall, the prognosis is markedly better than the malignant counterpart with 100% 5-year survival when confined to the ovary and 90% when spread to the peritoneum.

○ **What are the two histologic types of mucinous tumors of the ovary based on histologic appearance?**

In addition to being divided into benign, borderline, and malignant varieties, the mucinous tumors may resemble endocervical mucosa or intestinal epithelium. Thus, the tumors are divided into endocervical type and intestinal type.

○ **What is pseudomyxoma peritonei?**

This is so-called mucinous or gelatinous ascites as a result of implantation of cells in the peritoneal cavity, which produce abundant mucous. This can be a result of a mucinous low malignant potential tumor of the ovary or a mucinous tumor of the appendix. Although benign, death can occur as a result of extensive spreading and compression of abdominal viscera.

○ **Which has a better prognosis, mucinous ovarian low malignant potential tumors of the endocervical, or intestinal type?**

Endocervical type.

○ **What tumor is fairly commonly found concomitantly with an endometrioid carcinoma of the ovary?**

Approximately one-third of patients with an endometrioid carcinoma of the ovary have a coexistent adenocarcinoma of the endometrium. These are thought to be separate primaries.

○ **What ovarian epithelial tumor is characterized by large epithelial cells with abundant intracytoplasmic glycogen and form a so-called "hobnail" appearance as they protrude into the lumen of small tubules/cysts?**

Clear cell carcinoma.

○ **How are most Brenner tumors discovered?**

Incidentally, as about half are microscopic in nature. The vast majority are <2 cm.

○ **How common is bilaterality in endometrioid carcinoma of the ovary?**

It is quite common; up to 50% of patients have bilateral tumors at the time of surgery.

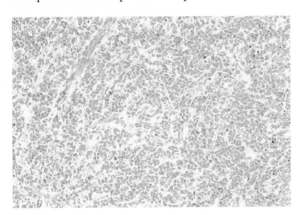

○ **The tumor shown above occurred in the ovary of a 20-year-old female with hypercalcemia that resolved following resection of her ovary. What is the diagnosis?**

Small cell carcinoma.

○ **What is the most common benign tumor of the ovary?**

Dermoid cyst or mature cystic teratoma.

○ **What is the term given to a benign ovarian teratoma where almost all of the tissues are composed of benign thyroid elements?**

Struma ovarii.

○ **Do mature teratoma undergo malignant change?**

The vast majority (99%) do not; however, it can occur and has been well described and is most commonly a squamous cell carcinoma.

○ **What is Meigs syndrome?**

This is the presence of a large ovarian fibroma with associated ascites and pleural effusion both of which resolve upon resection of the fibroma.

○ **What is produced by the majority of granulosa cell tumors that result in "feminizing" signs and symptoms?**

Estrogenic hormones.

○ **What is the characteristic shape of the nuclei of granulosa cells?**

They are round to oval, haphazardly arranged, and frequently contain a longitudinal groove imparting a "coffee bean" appearance.

○ **What ovarian tumor is associated with the basal cell nevus syndrome?**

Fibromas. These tumors are almost universally bilateral, multinodular, and at least focally calcified in these patients.

○ **What is the typical age of presentation in patients with a thecoma?**

They are almost always postmenopausal with a mean age of about 60.

○ **Although this can be true in several ovarian tumors, which sex cord-stromal tumor is associated with the classic yellow gross tumor appearance?**

Thecoma.

○ **In contrast to thecomas, what is the typical age of patients with Sertoli-Leydig cell tumors?**

They occur during reproductive years with a mean of 25 years old.

○ **What syndrome is found in about a third of patients with the sex cord tumor called "sex cord tumor with annular tubules"?**

Peutz-Jeghers syndrome.

○ **What is a so-called Krukenberg tumor?**

This is a gastric carcinoma that is metastatic to the ovary, although it can be of any site of gastrointestinal origin.

○ **What is the ovarian counterpart of the testicular seminoma?**

Dysgerminoma.

○ **In general, what is the prognosis for dysgerminoma?**

It is excellent as the tumor is quite radiosensitive and responsive to chemotherapy. Thus, for a stage I tumor, the 5-year survival is almost 95%. Overall, the 5-year survival is between 70% and 90% for all tumors.

○ **A 17-year-old female has an ovarian tumor that has resulted in an elevated serum alpha-fetoprotein. What is your diagnosis?**

Endodermal sinus tumor.

○ **In an ovarian endodermal sinus tumor, what are some of the characteristic histologic features you would expect to see?**

Schiller-Duval bodies and eosinophilic globules that are PAS-positive and diastase resistant.

○ **What is the typical genotype and phenotype in patients with gonadoblastoma?**

They are usually phenotypic females and genotypic males (have a Y chromosome).

○ **What are some conditions that increase the incidence of hydatidiform mole?**

Poverty, poor nutrition, and extreme ends of reproductive life and consanguinity.

○ **What is the most common karyotype in complete hydatidiform mole (CHM) compared with partial hydatidiform mole (PHM)?**

In CHM, they are almost always 46XX and both "X"s are paternally derived (diandrogenic dispermy), while in PHM, the majority are 69XXY with 69XXX representing up to 40% of cases.

○ **Which is at a greater risk for development of choriocarcinoma—CHM or PHM?**

CHM results in choriocarcinoma in approximately 5% of cases.

○ **Which type of mole is associated with a higher level of beta-hCG?**

The beta-hCG in CHM is usually twice than that of PHM.

○ **What is the most common germ cell tumor to occur bilaterally (approximately 10–20%)?**

Dysgerminomas.

CHAPTER 52 Hypothalamic-Pituitary-Ovarian-Uterine Axis

Chelsea Ward, MD

HYPOTHALAMUS

○ **What structure in the hypothalamus produces the most gonadotropin-releasing hormone (GnRH)?**
Arcuate nucleus in the medial basal hypothalamus.

○ **What is the name of the bundle of nerve cells that carry GnRH to the anterior pituitary?**
Tuberoinfundibular tract.

○ **What is the half-life of GnRH?**
2 to 4 minutes.

○ **How does the pulsatility of GnRH vary in the menstrual cycle?**
Frequency is more rapid in follicular phase, 1 pulse per hour; slower in luteal phase, 1 pulse in 2 to 3 hours.

○ **What can altered frequency and/or amplitude lead to?**
Anovulation (hypothalamic amenorrhea).

○ **Amplitude and frequency of GnRH secretion is regulated by which hormones?**
Ovarian hormones: Estradiol and progesterone
Neurotransmitters: Dopamine, norepinephrine, and serotonin
Neuromodulators: Prostaglandins and opioids
Brain peptides: Neuropeptide Y, melatonin, and leptin

○ **What is the effect of norepinephrine on GnRH release?**
Stimulatory effect.

○ **What are the effects of dopamine and serotonin on GnRH release?**
They inhibit GnRH release.

○ **What role does GnRH have on the anterior pituitary?**

Stimulate release of gonadotrophs: luteinizing hormone (LH) and follicle-stimulating hormone (FSH).

○ **Constant infusion on GnRH has what effect on circulating gonadotrophs?**

Initial increase in both LH and FSH (flare), followed by an inhibition of release for 1 to 3 weeks, called desensitization or downregulation.

○ **What is an important side effect of GnRH agonists?**

Decrease in bone mineral density.

○ **Where do axons from the supraoptic and paraventricular nuclei of the hypothalamus terminate?**

The posterior pituitary or neural lobe.

○ **What hormones are synthesized from the supraoptic and paraventricular nuclei?**

Antidiuretic hormone (ADH) and oxytocin precursors.

○ **What syndrome results from absence of the axonal and GnRH neuronal migration from the olfactory placode?**

Kallmann syndrome (hypogonadotropic hypogonadism).

○ **What are the modes of transmission of Kallmann syndrome?**

X-linked, autosomal dominant, and autosomal recessive.

○ **What are the characteristics of Kallmann syndrome?**

Absence of secondary sexual development, amenorrhea, lack of GnRH, and anosmia.

○ **What is the treatment of Kallaman syndrome?**

Exogenous GnRH.

○ **What are the nonendocrine functions of the hypothalamus?**

Temperature regulation, the activity of the autonomic nervous system, and control of appetite.

PITUITARY

○ **Where is the hypophysis (pituitary gland) located?**

Within the sella turcica.

○ **What is the blood supply to the posterior lobe of the pituitary gland?**

The inferior hypophyseal artery, a branch from the carotid artery.

○ **Who has the larger pituitary gland, men or women?**

The average adult female gland is approximately 20% larger than the average adult male.

○ **Why does the female pituitary gland increase in size by about 10% during pregnancy?**

Because of the hypertrophy of prolactin (PRL) secreting cells.

○ **What percentage of cells in the pituitary gland are gonadotropes?**

Approximately 10%

○ **What six hormones are secreted by the anterior pituitary?**

Growth hormone (GH).
Adrenocorticotropic hormone (ACTH).
Thyroid-stimulating hormone (TSH).
Prolactin (PRL).
Luteinizing hormone (LH).
Follicle-stimulating hormone (FSH).

○ **Which hormones share a similar alpha unit?**

LH, FSH, TSH, (and hCG).

○ **What hormones are secreted by the posterior pituitary?**

Oxytocin and ADH (vasopressin).

○ **What is the action of oxytocin?**

It stimulates uterine contraction during labor and elicits milk ejection by myoepithelial cells of the mammary ducts.

○ **What fold increase in oxytocin receptors occurs throughout pregnancy and labor?**

Number of oxytocin receptors increases 80-fold throughout the pregnancy and doubles during the labor.

○ **What is the time of the peak in oxytocin levels?**

During the LH surge.

○ **What is the action of ADH?**

It causes increased rates of Na+ and Cl− reabsorption and enhances permeability within the collecting ducts of the renal medulla.

○ **What is the function of LH in the adult female?**

Stimulate maturation of the Graafian follicle and its production of estradiol.

○ **What is the half-life of FSH?**

3 to 4 hours.

○ **What is the function of FSH in the adult female?**

Causes follicular rupture, ovulation, and establishment of the corpus luteum.

○   **What is the half-life of LH?**

20 minutes.

○   **What is necessary for midcycle LH surge?**

Increase in estradiol levels above critical concentration and duration (200 pg/mL for 48 hours). The concentration of FSH is greater than LH.

○   **What cells within the pituitary secrete prolactin?**

Lactotrophs.

○   **What is the function of prolactin?**

It initiates and sustains lactation by the breast glands and it may influence synthesis and release of progesterone by the ovary and testosterone by the testis.

○   **What inhibits the release of prolactin?**

Dopamine.

○   **What is the main physiological stimulus for prolactin release?**

Suckling of the breast.

○   **How do drugs such as metoclopramide, haloperidol, chlorpromazine, and reserpine enhance prolactin secretion?**

By interfering with release of dopamine into the pituitary portal circulation.

○   **What are the signs and symptoms of a pituitary neoplasm related to enlargement of the gland?**

Visual field defects (bitemporal hemianopsia), abnormal extraocular muscle movements, and occasionally spontaneous CSF rhinorrhea.

○   **What tests are used to determine gonadotropin deficiency?**

Simultaneous measurement of FSH, LH, and gonadal steroids.

○   **What does low circulating gonadal steroid levels associated with an inappropriately low gonadotropin level suggest?**

A hypothalmic or pituitary disturbance.

○   **What is Sheehan syndrome?**

Postpartum infarction and necrosis of the pituitary.

○   **What are the main clinical features of Sheehan syndrome?**

(1) Postpartum failure to lactate.

(2) Postpartum amenorrhea.

(3) Progressive signs and symptoms of adrenal insufficiency and hypothyroidism.

○ **What are the two most common types of pituitary adenomas?**
Prolactin-secreting and null cell adenomas.

○ **What is the most common functional pituitary tumor?**
Prolactinoma.

○ **Do prolactinomas occur more frequently in men or women?**
Women.

○ **What is the most common presenting symptom of a prolactinoma in a woman?**
Secondary amenorrhea.

○ **In patients with a prolactinoma and secondary amenorrhea, what percentage have an associated galactorrhea?**
50%.

○ **How is the diagnosis of a prolactin-secreting tumor confirmed?**
Radiographic evidence of a pituitary lesion with an elevation of serum prolactin.

○ **What pharmaceutical agent has been shown effective in reducing serum prolactin, reducing tumor, and inhibiting tumor growth?**
Bromocriptine (a dopaminergic agonist).

○ **What is hypersecretion of ACTH by the pituitary referred to as?**
Cushing disease.

○ **Is Cushing disease more common in men or women?**
It is eight times more common in women.

○ **How is the diagnosis of Cushing disease confirmed?**
Increased basal plasma cortisol levels with loss of diurnal variation.
Failure of serum cortisol suppression with the low-dose dexamethasone suppression test.
Increased 24-hour urinary-free cortisol excretion (>100 μg/24 h).

○ **What is the most likely diagnosis in a patient with Cushing syndrome with low plasma ACTH levels?**
An adrenal tumor.

○ **What is the most likely diagnosis in a patient with Cushing syndrome with elevated plasma ACTH levels (>200 pg/mL)?**
An ectopic ACTH-secreting tumor.

○ **What is the most common tumor causing ectopic ACTH secretion?**
Small cell carcinoma of the lung.

○   **What is the most common cause of Cushing syndrome?**

Pituitary microadenoma.

○   **What is the main effect and source of inhibin?**

Inhibits FSH but not LH, secreted by granulosa cells.

○   **What are inhibin A and inhibin B markers of?**

Inhibin A—Corpus luteum function, under control of LH.

Inhibin B—Granulosa cell function, under control of FSH. Elevated in granulosa cell tumors.

○   **What are the effects of activin?**

Upregulates FSH receptor expression, and increases pituitary FSH synthesis and secretion. Also, a physiologic antagonist to inhibin.

○   **What is the main effect and source of follistatin?**

Inhibits FSH and FSH response to GnRH. Product of granulosa cells.

○   **What are the effects of high levels of progesterone?**

Inhibits GnRH pulses at hypothalamus level and subsequently inhibits secretion of gonadotropins.

○   **What is the source of a majority of the circulating testosterone in a nonpregnant woman?**

Peripheral conversion of androstenedione by 17β-hydroxysteroid dehydrogenase. Only 30% to 40% is directly secreted.

○   **What limits peripheral conversion of testosterone to dihydrotestosterone in females?**

Higher levels of sex hormone-binding globulin.

Peripheral conversion of testosterone to estrogen by aromatase.

○   **Accumulation of what substance leads to upregulation of LH receptors?**

FSH-induced cAMP.

○   **Activation of LH receptors in theca cells leads to production of what substance?**

Androstenedione (weak androgen).

○   **In a premenopausal woman, what percentage of estradiol is directly secreted from the ovary?**

95%.

○   **What enzymatic deficiency is associated with most cases of the adrenogenital syndrome (congenital adrenal hyperplasia)?**

21-hydroxylase.

○   **What is the most common enzymatic defect seen in congenital adrenal hyperplasia?**

A deficiency in C-21 hydroxylation.

○ **What is the effect of a C-21 deficiency in females and males?**

It causes pseudohermaphrodites in females and macrogenitosomia praecox (enlarged external genitalia) in males.

○ **What is the most classic symptom of androgen excess?**

Hirsutism.

○ **What test would rule out congenital adrenal hyperplasia?**

Failure of the dexamethasone suppression test.

○ **What is the treatment of congenital adrenal hyperplasia?**

Glucocorticoid administration to suppress ACTH.

○ **What condition results from a G protein mutation that autonomously activates the LH receptor?**

Precocious puberty in males.

○ **What condition results from a G protein mutation that autonomously inactivates the LH receptor?**

Male pseudohermaphroditism.

○ **G protein mutation with resultant inactivation of FSH receptor results in?**

Premature ovarian failure.

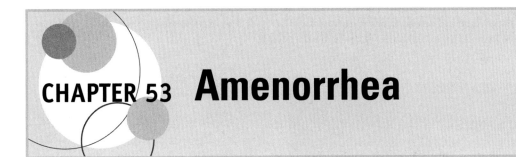

CHAPTER 53 Amenorrhea

Erica L. Borman, DO

○ **Define primary amenorrhea.**

No menses by age 14 in the absence of growth or development of secondary sexual characteristics.

OR

No menses by age 16 with the appearance of secondary sexual characteristics.

○ **Define secondary amenorrhea.**

In a menstruating women, the absence of menstruation for three previous cycle intervals or 6 months.

○ **What is the maximum number of oogonia reached in a female's life cycle?**

6 to 7 million at 16 to 20 weeks' gestation.

○ **What general compartments are evaluated for diagnosis in cases of amenorrhea?**

Compartment I: Disorders of the outflow tract or uterus.
Compartment II: Disorders of the ovary.
Compartment III: Disorders of the anterior pituitary.
Compartment IV: Disorders of the hypothalamus (CNS factors).

○ **What is the number one cause of secondary amenorrhea after pregnancy?**

Anovulation (28%).

○ **A 32-year-old patient develops amenorrhea status post a D & E for a septic abortion. Her transvaginal ultrasound revealed the findings as below. What is the diagnosis?**

Asherman syndrome (thick intrauterine adhesions and calcifications)

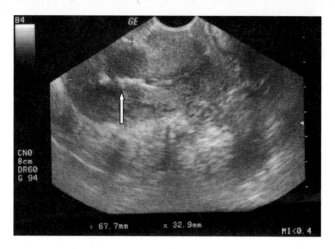

○ **The absence of secondary sexual characteristics indicates that a woman has never been exposed to what?**

Estrogen stimulation.

○ **What laboratory tests should you consider in a patient with primary amenorrhea who does not have a uterus?**

Karyotype and serum testosterone (Müllerian abnormality with 46XX karyotype with normal testosterone versus androgen insensitivity syndrome (AIS) with 46XY karyotype and male serum testosterone levels).

○ **What laboratory tests should you consider in a patient with primary amenorrhea who DOES have a uterus?**

Human chorionic gonadotropin (hCG), thyroid-stimulating hormone (TSH), prolactin (PRL), progestin challenge, follicle-stimulating hormone (FSH), and luteinizing hormone (LH).

○ **When should an MRI be ordered in cases of primary amenorrhea?**

For symptoms of visual changes, headache, or hypogonadotropic hypogonadism.

○ **What is the differential diagnosis of vaginal agenesis?**

Congenital absence of the vagina (with or without uterine structures)
Androgen insensitivity
Transverse septum
Imperforate hymen
17α-hydroxylase deficiency (46XY with complete male pseudohermaphroditism).

○ **In primary amenorrhea, if FSH is elevated and no breast development is present, what is the diagnosis?**

Gonadal dysgenesis (50% of primary amenorrhea cases). Check karyotype next.

○ **What is the first test that should be ordered in a patient with 2° amenorrhea?**

Pregnancy test.

○ **When should you order a karyotype in patients with 2° amenorrhea?**

In all patients age <30 or shorter than 60 inches with ovarian failure.

○ **What is the most common chromosomal abnormality causing gonadal failure and primary amenorrhea?**

45, X (Turner syndrome—50%).

○ **True or False: In Turner syndrome, the specific phenotype relates to the parental origin of the X chromosome and most patients retain the maternal X.**

True.

○ **Partial deletions of the X chromosome can also cause amenorrhea. What is the characteristic of patients who have the deletion in part of the long arm of the X-chromosome (Xq-)?**

Sexual infantilism, normal stature, no somatic abnormalities, and streak gonads.

○ **What is the characteristic of patients with Xp- (deletion of the short arm of the X-chromosome)?**

Phenotypically similar to Turner syndrome.

○ **Primary amenorrhea is associated with various mosaic states 25% of the time, the most common of which is?**

45X/46XX (mixed gonadal dysgenesis).

○ **How does "pure gonadal dysgenesis" differ from "gonadal dysgenesis"?**

Gonadal dysgenesis is absent ovarian function associated with abnormalities in the sex chromosomes. In pure gonadal dysgenesis, individuals have primary amenorrhea, with normal stature and no chromosomal abnormalities. Hence, the gonads are usually streaks.

○ **What is Perrault syndrome?**

46XX gonadal dysgenesis + neurosensory deafness.

○ **What enzyme deficiency may be associated with either 46,XX or 46,XY and cause primary amenorrhea?**

17α–hydroxylase deficiency. Patients with this deficiency have primordial follicles, but gonadotropin levels are elevated because the enzyme deficiency prevents synthesis of sex steroids.

○ **What distinguishes a patient with 46XX 17α-hydroxylase deficiency from one with the same deficiency but an XY karyotype?**

Patients with 46,XY karyotypes lack a uterus. Both of these patients have primary amenorrhea, no secondary sexual characteristics, female phenotypes, hypertension, and hypokalemia.

○ **Name two other enzyme deficiencies that result in a female phenotype with an XY karyotype.**

5α-reductase deficiency and 17–20 desmolase deficiency.

○ **What is the diagnosis of a patient with normal FSH and LH but with a negative progestational challenge test (assuming normal outflow tract)?**

Pituitary-CNS failure (patient needs sella turcica imaging).

○ **What is the most common manifestation of hypogonadotropic hypogonadism?**

Constitutional delay of puberty.

○ **What is the treatment of this?**

Reassurance.

○ **What is Kallmann syndrome?**

Hypogonadotropic hypogonadism due to a lack of gonadotropin-releasing hormone (GnRH) due to failure of migration of the GnRH neuron from the olfactory bulb. These patients are anosmic and have primary amenorrhea.

○ **What is the most common CNS tumor that can lead to primary amenorrhea?**

Craniopharyngioma. It is an extracellular mass that interferes with the production and secretion of GnRH or the stimulation of pituitary gonadotropins. Usually, these patients have disorders of other pituitary hormones as well.

○ **What one test can distinguish hypergonadotropic and hypogonadotropic forms of hypogonadism?**

FSH.

○ **If FSH is elevated, the next appropriate test would be?**

A karyotype.

○ **Is an elevated FSH an absolute indicator of infertility?**

No.

○ **Why does FSH rise prior to menopause?**

Because of decreased inhibin.

○ **In amenorrhea, what are the causes of high gonadotropins?**

- Tumors producing gonadotropins (often lung cancer, but rare).
- Single gonadotropin deficiencies, homozygous mutations in gonadotropin genes.
- Gonadotropin-secreting pituitary adenoma (not associated with amenorrhea).
- Perimenopause, menopause, and premature ovarian failure.
- Resistant or insensitive ovary syndrome and mutations in gonadotropin receptor genes.
- Galactosemia, direct toxic effect of galactose metabolites on germ cell migration.
- 17α-hydroxylase deficiency.

○ **What three tests are helpful in diagnosing 17α-hydroxylase deficiency?**

Serum progesterone—elevated (>3 ng/mL).

17α-hydroxyprogesterone—low (<0.2 ng/mL).

Serum deoxycorticosterone (DOC)—low.

○ **What is the confirmatory test and what is the response in a patient with 17α-hydroxylase deficiency?**

ACTH stimulation test. These patients will have an increase in serum progesterone and no change in 17α-hydroxyprogesterone.

○ **At what age is premature ovarian failure diagnosed?**

<40 years old.

○ **What percentage of women are diagnosed with premature ovarian failure?**

1%.

○ **What other testing should be considered in a patient with premature ovarian failure?**

This is often associated with autoimmune diseases. Check thyroid and adrenal antibodies, TSH, T4, calcium, phosphorus, and fasting glucose. Also, consider fragile X testing and genetic counseling.

○ **What is the next test that should be performed in a patient with premature ovarian failure whose brother has a severe learning disability and suffered from recurrent otitis media as a child?**

FMR1 gene testing. There is an association between fragile X premutation carriers (characterized by 55 to 200 CGG repeats) and premature ovarian failure. Up to a third of premutation carriers have an early menopause.

○ **What other rare conditions are associated with premature ovarian failure?**

Hypoparathyroidism.
Moniliasis.
Myasthenia gravis.
Idiopathic thrombocytopenic purpura.
Rheumatoid arthritis.
Vitiligo.
Autoimmune hemolytic anemia.

○ **What is the treatment of hypergonadotropic hypogonadism?**

Cyclic estrogen and progestin therapy.

○ **In addition to estrogen and progesterone, individuals with 17α-hydroxylase deficiency need what?**

Corticosteroid replacement.

○ **What is the cause of premature ovarian failure?**

The cause is probably accelerated follicular atresia. However, the etiology of this accelerated atresia is unknown. In addition, it can be due to an autoimmune process, infections, or a physical insult such as radiation or chemotherapy.

○ **What infection is a cause of premature ovarian failure?**

Mumps oophoritis

○ **Lymphocytic infiltrate surrounding secondary and antral follicles but not primordial follicles is the hallmark for diagnosis of what cause of premature ovarian failure?**

Autoimmune oophoritis.

○ **A positive test for what antibodies is sufficient to establish a diagnosis of autoimmune ovarian failure?**

Anti-adrenal antibodies and 21-hydroxylase antibodies.

○ **What bad habit is associated with ovarian failure?**

Cigarette smoking.

○ **Why might someone living in Alma, Colorado, undergo menopause earlier than someone in Philadelphia, Pennsylvania?**

Living at high altitude has been shown to be associated with premature ovarian failure—Alma, Colorado, is the highest town with permanent residents in the United States.

○ **What radiation dose will permanently sterilize 100% of women?**

Over 800 rads.

150 rads will give some risk to women over 40. Using 200 to 500 rads, 60% of women aged 15 to 40 will be sterilized. With 500 to 800 rads, 70% of women aged 15 to 40 will be sterilized.

(younger age = increased resistance to radiation)

○ **Which chemotherapeutic agents are most toxic to the ovaries?**

Alkylating agents because they can affect both resting and dividing cells.

○ **What drug, though controversial, may offer protection against chemotherapy-induced ovarian follicular depletion?**

GnRH agonists.

○ **How does hysterectomy contribute to an increased incidence of early menopause?**

The approximate two times increased incidence is thought to occur from disrupting the ovarian blood flow during surgery.

○ **Genetic disorders (ie, mosaicism and deletions) account for a number of patients with premature ovarian failure. What region of the X-chromosome is critical to prevent ovarian failure prematurely?**

Xq26-28.

○ **Name the causes of obstructive amenorrhea.**

Imperforate hymen, transverse vaginal septum, hypoplasia or absence of the uterus, and cervix and/or vagina.

○ **What test can help delineate the female anatomy the best?**

MRI.

○ **How does one differentiate a transverse vaginal septum from an imperforate hymen?**

A transverse vaginal septum lacks distention at the introitus with Valsalva maneuver.

○ **What is the treatment of a vaginal septum?**

Surgical removal followed by Frank dilators to distend the vagina and prevent vaginal stenosis.

○ **The majority of vaginal septums occur in what two areas of the vagina?**

The upper one third (46%) and the middle one third (40%).

○ **What is the karyotype of a patient with Müllerian agenesis?**

46,XX.

○ **In a patient with known Müllerian agenesis, what other system needs to be evaluated and why?**

The renal tract because approximately one-third of patients will have urinary tract abnormalities, and the skeletal system since 12% have skeletal abnormalities including spinal deformities, absent digits, and syndactyly.

○ **Aside from surgical construction of a neovagina, what other method is available?**

Vaginal dilators. Eighty percent of women are able to achieve satisfactory intercourse.

○ **What is the diagnosis of a patient with primary amenorrhea, an absent uterus, and little to absent body hair?**

Complete AIS. It is the third most common cause of 1° amenorrhea.

○ **What is the karyotype of a patient with complete androgen insensitivity?**

46,XY.

○ **Why are there no uterus, tubes, and upper vagina in AIS?**

Anti-Müllerian hormone is present.

○ **How is AIS inherited?**

It is an X-linked recessive gene responsible for the intracellular androgen receptor.

○ **Given that patients with AIS have testes and the high incidence of neoplasia if left in situ, when should the testes be removed?**

After puberty (exception to the rule), at approximately 16 to 18 years of age. This is because the development of secondary sexual characteristics achieved with hormone therapy does not match that with endogenous hormones. In addition, the incidence of gonadal tumors in these patients is rare before puberty.

○ **Do patients with AIS have normal female levels of testosterone?**

No. The levels of testosterone in these phenotypic females are in the normal to slightly elevated male range. Thus, they produce testosterone but are not able to respond to those androgens.

○ **How can one differentiate a patient with androgen insensitivity from one with 5α-reductase deficiency?**

The patient with 5α-reductase deficiency does not develop breasts at puberty. This is due to the levels of testosterone that are present in sufficient amounts to suppress breast development.

○ **What rare enzyme deficiency causes the same clinical picture as AIS?**

17β-hydroxysteroid dehydrogenase that catalyzes the conversion of androstenedione to testosterone in testicular Leydig cells.

○ **A very rare cause of amenorrhea in which both male and female gonadal tissue is present is known as what?**

True hermaphrodite.

○ **What is the diagnosis of a female patient with XY karyotype and palpable Müllerian structures but lack of sexual development?**

Swyer syndrome (remove gonads immediately at diagnosis as they have a high incidence of malignancy).

○ **What is the cause of Swyer syndrome in at least 10% to 15% of affected individuals?**

Mutation in the SRY gene.

○ **What is the most common cause of secondary amenorrhea?**

Pregnancy.

○ **Describe the initial laboratory evaluation for secondary amenorrhea.**

hCG, TSH, PRL, progestin withdrawal, and FSH. Consider testosterone, DHEAS, and pelvic ultrasound for investigating polycystic ovarian disease.

○ **How is a patient's estrogen status and competence of the outflow tract assessed?**

Administer medroxyprogesterone acetate (MPA) 5 or 10 mg for 5 to 10 days, to determine whether the patient bleeds after withdrawal of the medication. Alternatively, can use 200 mg IM progesterone in oil or micronized progesterone 300 mg QD.

○ **How much bleeding is needed for a positive withdrawal response in a progestational challenge?**

Any amount of bleeding no matter how scant.

○ **What percentage of women with amenorrhea and low estrogen levels (from exercise, weight loss, ovarian failure, etc) will actually have a withdrawal bleed from a progestin challenge test, i.e. false-positive results?**

40% to 50%.

○ **If no withdrawal bleed occurs, what is the next step?**

To add estrogen prior to the progestin withdrawal.

(1.25 mg conjugated estrogen or 2 mg of estradiol daily for 21 days with 10 mg of Provera added for the last 5 days).

○ **What is the treatment of Asherman syndrome?**

Hysteroscopy with lysis of adhesions, +/− method to keep the uterine cavity open and high-dose estrogen for 2 months (add MPA 10 mg daily after the third week) and broad-spectrum antibiotics pre-op and 10 days afterward.

○ **Name the methods often used to keep the uterine cavity open.**

IUD or pediatric Foley filled with 3 mL of fluid left in for 7 days.

○ **What percentage of patients with Asherman syndrome have achieved a successful pregnancy after surgical lysis of the intrauterine adhesions?**

70% to 80%.

○ **What complications may these patients then experience with their pregnancy?**

Preterm labor, placenta accreta, previa, and postpartum hemorrhage.

○ **How does hyperthyroidism cause amenorrhea?**

It inhibits gonadotropin release.

○ **How does hypothyroidism cause amenorrhea?**

TRH stimulates prolactin secretion. It works by acting directly on prolactin secreting cells. In addition, the deficiency of thyroid hormones (in hypothyroidism) affects dopamine's inhibitory control of prolactin resulting in hyperprolactinemia.

○ **If elevated TSH and prolactin levels are found in an amenorrhea workup, what do you treat?**

Only the hypothyroidism. The prolactin will normalize with the treatment of the hypothyroidism based on its mechanism of causing amenorrhea.

○ **Hyperprolactinemia causes amenorrhea by what mechanisms?**

Prolactin suppresses the GnRH pulsatile release necessary for ovulation and menstruation and increases opioid activity. It may also act to reduce the granulosa cell number and FSH binding.

○ **What proportion of women with both galactorrhea and amenorrhea will have hyperprolactinemia?**

Two-thirds.

○ **How is galactorrhea confirmed on examination of cloudy or white nipple secretions?**

Microscopic examination of secretions demonstrates lipid droplets.

○ **What test is necessary in women with amenorrhea and hyperprolactinemia once drug induced and physiologic causes of the elevated prolactin have been ruled out?**

MRI of the sella turcica.

○ **In patients with galactorrhea and 2° amenorrhea, how many will have an abnormal sella turcica?**

50%.

○ **What two diseases can cause endometritis and uterine scaring as a result?**

Tuberculosis endometritis and schistosomiasis.

○ **A patient with amenorrhea due to absent FSH receptors or postreceptor defects has what syndrome?**

The resistant ovary syndrome or *Savage syndrome.*

These patients have unstimulated ovarian follicles in their ovaries. In addition, there is no evidence of autoimmune disease (ie, lymphocytic invasion), yet the ovaries are nonfunctional.

○ **Postpartum amenorrhea can be due to what?**

Sheehan syndrome. It is postpartum necrosis of the pituitary from a hypotensive episode also causing failure to lactate and loss of pubic and axillary hair.

○ **What is the classical presenting symptom of Sheehan syndrome?**

Failed lactation.

○ **Which hormone deficiencies are most common in Sheehan syndrome?**

Growth hormone

Gonadotropins

Prolactin

○ **What percentage of body fat is necessary for the initiation of menses and then for the maintenance of menses?**

About 17% and 22%, respectively.

It is thought that decreasing weight can effect GnRH pulsatile secretion.

○ **What three items comprise the female athlete triad?**

Amenorrhea.

Disordered eating.

Osteoporosis/Osteopenia.

○ **Name three causes of amenorrhea that are thought to be caused by abnormalities in neuromodulation in hypothalamic GnRH secretion.**

Anorexia, stress, and exercise.

○ **What is hypothalamic amenorrhea?**

Defect in GnRH pulsatility frequently associated with stressful situations, probably secondary to elevated CRH/cortisol which inhibits gonadal secretion.

○ **How does one diagnose hypothalamic amenorrhea?**

All studies are normal—diagnosis of exclusion (note: gonadotropin may be low or normal) and failure to demonstrate withdrawal bleeding.

○ **What is meant by the term *post-pill amenorrhea*?**

This is the delay in return of menses after a woman stops taking oral contraceptives. Typically the hypothalamic-pituitary suppression should not last >6 months after discontinuation of the pill. At that time the incidence of amenorrhea is about the same as the incidence of secondary amenorrhea in the general population and therefore thought to be unrelated to the use of oral contraceptives.

○ **What are three other causes of secondary amenorrhea due to affected pituitary function?**

Lymphocytic hypophysitis—often occurring during pregnancy or 6 months postpartum.

Carotid artery aneurysm.

Obstruction of aqueduct of Sylvius.

○ **Are leptin levels in anorectic and bulimic patients increased or decreased?**

Decreased.

○ **If a patient has Turner's syndrome clinically, what other things must you evaluate or consider?**

Autoimmune disorders are common and include thyroiditis, type 1 diabetes, autoimmune hepatitis, thrombocytopenia and celiac disease.

Cardiovascular abnormalities- present in ~1/3 and include bicuspid aortic valve, coarctation of the aorta, MVP, and aortic aneurysm.

Renal abnormalities include horseshoe kidney, unilateral renal agenesis or pelvic kidney, rotational abnormalities, and partial or complete duplication of the colleting system.

Karyotype—since 40% are mosaic and may have XY aberrations.

○ **When should evaluation of a patient begin if a patient is amenorrheic after discontinuing oral contraceptive pills (OCPs) and after discontinuing Depo-Provera?**

- 6 months after OCP's discontinued.
- 12 months after the last injection of Depo-Provera.

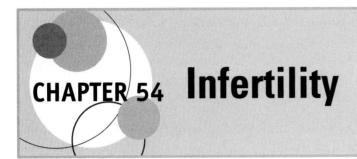

CHAPTER 54 Infertility

Neely N. Nelson, MD

BASIC FACTS AND DEFINITIONS

○ **What is fecundability?**

The probability of achieving a pregnancy within one menstrual cycle.

○ **What is fecundity?**

The probability of achieving a *live birth* within one menstrual cycle.

○ **What is the average fecundability in normal couples?**

20%.

○ **What are the causes of infertility for couples?**

30% to 40% ovarian dysfunction.

30% to 40% tubal/peritoneal pathology.

30% to 40% male factor.

○ **When should a workup for infertility be initiated?**

All couples after 1 year of regular intercourse without conception.

Couples not pregnant after 6 months of regular intercourse and the female partner is >35 years of age, has endometriosis, or has irregular menses, or the male partner has known or suspected poor semen quality.

○ **How long do the egg and sperm have to fertilize in the female reproductive tract?**

Oocytes have a 12- to 24-hour life span, and normal sperm have a 3- to 5-day life span.

○ **Does radiation therapy cause gonadal failure more commonly in males or females?**

Males. Almost all males at any age will have testicular failure.

Females in early reproductive years treated with <700 rads usually do not have ovarian dysfunction. Greater than 2000 rads cause ovarian failure in most women. 15 rads is sufficient to suppress spermatogenesis.

○   **How does chemotherapy affect gonadal function of the in males and females?**

In postpubertal males, approximately 90% will have azoospermia, while women with the same treatment have 50% to 75% chance of ovarian failure. In prepubertal boys, 83% had azoospermia, while 13% of prepubertal girls had ovarian failure.

FEMALE INFERTILITY

○   **What are the primary diagnoses in the infertile woman and what percentage of infertile women have each diagnosis?**

Ovulatory dysfunction (40%).

Tubal and pelvic pathology (40%).

Unexplained (10%).

Unusual problems, that is, anatomic abnormalities, thyroid disease (10%).

○   **How many oocytes are present in each stage of reproductive development?**

16 to 20 weeks' gestation: 6 to 7 million oogonia.

Birth: 1 to 2 million oocytes.

Onset of puberty: 300,000 to 500,000 oocytes.

Age 37 to 38: 25,000 oocytes.

Menopause: 1000 oocytes.

○   **What is the average age of menopause in the United States?**

51 years old.

○   **How many years prior to menopause does follicular loss occur?**

10 to 15 years.

Ovulation

○   **What are the causes of adult-onset anovulation?**

Hypothalamic dysfunction (38%).

Pituitary disease (17%).

Ovarian dysfunction (45%).

○   **Hypothalamic dysfunction may result in anovulation. Name three causes.**

Stress, weight and body composition, and strenuous exercise.

○   **The most common pituitary disorder that causes anovulation is?**

Prolactinoma (empty sella, Sheehan, and Cushing syndromes).

○   **Name the two most common causes of hyperprolactinemia.**

Prolactin-secreting pituitary gland tumors and psychiatric medications.

○ **What is the treatment of infertile women with hyperprolactinemia and anovulation?**

Bromocriptine 2.5 to 7.5 mg daily or cabergoline 0.25 to 1 mg twice a week.

○ **When should prolactin levels be retested after beginning dopamine agonist therapy?**

4 weeks after initiating therapy or changing the dosage.

○ **What imaging study is used for the diagnosis of a prolactinoma?**

MRI of the sella turcica.

○ **What percentage of women will ovulate after establishment of euprolactinemia?**

80%.

○ **What BMI is associated with an increased risk of ovulatory infertility?**

>27.

○ **What is the mechanism by which anorexia nervosa causes anovulation?**

Hypothalamic amenorrhea, decreased follicle stimulating hormone (FSH) and luteinizing hormone (LH) with apulsatile or low-amplitude, low-frequency pulsatile hormone secretion.

○ **The most common ovarian causes of anovulation are?**

Ovarian failure and polycystic ovary syndrome (PCOS).

○ **How can you test for ovulation in women with regular menses?**

(1) Progesterone level 1 week before expected onset of menses.

(2) Basal body temperature (BBT) increase occurs 24 hours after ovulation, useful for establishing a pattern.

(3) LH predictor kits predict ovulation within 24 to 48 hours from the time of the surge, best if use kit with first morning void when urine is most concentrated, testing is then repeated late afternoon/early evening, good timing for intercourse or intrauterine insemination (IUI), and false-positive tests occur in 7% of cycles.

(4) Serial transvaginal ultrasound (TVUS) provides the most reliable estimate for detecting when ovulation occurs.

(5) Endometrial biopsy (EMB)-anovulatory women are always in the proliferative phase, secretory endometrium implies ovulation in the absence of exogenous progesterone/synthetic progestin, also important in patients with irregular menses to rule out hyperplasia and to diagnose endometritis.

○ **What is a luteinized follicle?**

An unruptured follicle, ovulatory women trying to conceive should be advised to limit nonsteroidal anti-inflammatory drug (NSAID) use to the menstrual phase of the cycle due to suspected interference with normal ovulation; NSAIDs predispose patients to a luteinized or unruptured follicle.

○ **What is clomiphene citrate (CC)?**

A nonsteroidal estrogen agonist/antagonist.

○   **What is the initial dose of CC?**

50 mg for 5 days starting on day 3, 4, or 5 of the cycle.
50% of women will ovulate at the 50-mg dose.

○   **How is ovulation induction with gonadotropins performed?**

Start FSH or LH/FSH at 75 IU or 150 IU daily starting day 2 or 3 of a cycle. Measure estradiol at day 6 or 7 and if adequate (500–1500 pg/mL) perform TVUS until diameter of largest follicle is 16 to 18 mm. Then administer 5000 to 10,000 IU of human chorionic gonadotropin (hCG) and around the time of intercourse or insemination.

○   **Who should be evaluated for diminished ovarian reserve (DOR)?**

Infertile women over 35 years of age, women who have a family history of early menopause, women with a history of ovarian surgery or chemotherapy/radiation treatment, or women who are smoker or have a long history of smoking.

○   **What causes an elevation in FSH?**

Decreasing feedback inhibition from a shrinking follicular pool.

○   **What does an elevated FSH result in?**

As FSH levels rise, the follicular phase shortens because FSH stimulates a more rapid follicular development and estradiol levels rise earlier in the cycle.

○   **What is the menopausal transition?**

Marked by onset of irregular cycles, average age is 46 but ranges between 34 and 54; when this occurs, menopause can be expected in 5 to 6 years.

○   **What is DOR?**

Currently, there is no accepted definition of DOR; however, ovarian reserve tests screen for those at risk of lower than expected fertility potential.

○   **Are screening tests diagnostic for DOR?**

No. They are used to identify women more likely to have a poor response to gonadotropin stimulation. Testing should be limited to women at risk of DOR to maximize positive predictive value (PPV) and maximize specificity to avoid false-positive test results that would categorize a woman with normal ovarian reserve as having DOR.

○   **What is the most effective treatment of DOR?**

In vitro fertilization (IVF) with donor egg.

○ **What are the screening tests for DOR?**

(1) Anti-Müllerian hormone (AMH)—a promising screening test, low levels are associated with poor response to ovarian stimulation; however, threshold values have not yet been determined to be used confidently in clinical practice.

(2) Antral follicle count (AFC)—2 to 10-mm follicles are counted in both ovaries on TVUS, this is an indirect measure of ovarian reserve because as the number of small antral follicles decreases, the supply of primordial follicles decreases.

(a) AFC correlates well with oocyte yield in IVF cycles, a threshold of 3 to 4 has high specificity for poor response to ovarian stimulation.

(3) Inhibin B concentrations and ovarian volume have limited clinical utility as ovarian reserve tests.

(4) Basal FSH concentration on days 2 to 4 of the cycle is the simplest and most widely used test of ovarian reserve, levels >10 IU/L had high specificity for poor response to IVF, levels >18 are 100% specific for failure.

(b) Sometimes increased estradiol levels suppress FSH in patients with DOR, if the estradiol is >60 to 80 pg/mL, the FSH may be normal, and if both estradiol and FSH are elevated, there is poor prognosis for success with IVF.

(c) Measuring a stimulated FSH level on day 10 of the cycle using CC 100 mg po qd from day 5 through day 9 of the cycle has increased sensitivity but decreased specificity for DOR compared with a basal FSH concentration.

○ **Can testing be combined for higher detection rates for DOR?**

No. Use the tests individually because combining various tests does not result in higher detection rates for poor performance.

Cervical Factors

○ **How does estrogen affect cervical mucus?**

As estrogen increases, cervical mucus becomes more copious and watery allowing sperm to penetrate.

○ **How does progesterone affect cervical mucus?**

Progesterone inhibits production causing mucus to become more viscous.

○ **Is there a role for postcoital testing to look for cervical factor infertility?**

No longer recommended!

○ **Which uterine abnormalities affect fertility and also affect pregnancy outcomes?**

(1) Submucosal leiomyoma—Can distort anatomy interfering with sperm and egg transport, can affect implantation causing glandular atrophy overlying myoma from mechanical pressure, causes threefold increased risk of miscarriage and may decrease IVF success by up to 70%.

(2) Intramural leiomyoma—Decreases IVF success by 30%, myomectomy should be considered in women who fail IVF treatment.

(3) Subserosal fibroids have *no* effect on fertility.

(4) Asherman syndrome—Any insult that causes destruction or removal of the endometrium can result in adhesions, endometrium most fragile between 2 and 4 weeks postpartum, 90% of adhesions due to curettage, in developing countries, genital tuberculosis (TB) causes adhesions.

(5) Polypectomy may improve reproductive performance in infertile women.

○ **How is the uterine cavity evaluated?**

(1) Hysterosalpingogram (HSG)—Also identifies tubal pathology

(2) TVUS or saline sonohysterography—Also recommended in cases of menorrhagia or intermenstrual spotting

(3) Hysteroscopy—Reserved for treatment

○ **How do abnormalities appear on HSG?**

Developmental uterine anomalies have characteristic filling patterns, myomas or large polyps produce curvilinear filling defects, and intrauterine adhesions produce grossly irregular contours and filling defects.

○ **TVUS may be helpful to diagnose?**

- Narrowed discontinuous stripe may represent intrauterine adhesions.
- Overall or focal increase in endometrial stripe may represent polyp or myoma.
  - (Use sonohysterography to further delineate)
- Differentiate between septate and bicornuate uteri by evaluation of fundus.
- Endometrial stripe trilaminar pattern poor predictor of receptivity.
  - Proliferative phase, described as hypoechoic.
  - Secretory phase, has increased echodensity.

○ **What is the treatment of intrauterine adhesions?**

Hysteroscopic lysis of the adhesions.

○ **The overall pregnancy rate following treatment of intrauterine adhesions is?**

60% to 75%.

○ **After lysis of adhesions, what medical therapy is initiated to inhibit further development of adhesions?**

Placement of IUD, pediatric Foley, and/or post procedure hormone therapy which assists the endometrium in re-epithelializing.

○ **What patient history is concerning for tubal pathology?**

(1) Pelvic inflammatory disease (PID): risk of tubal infertility after first episode 10%, second episode 25% to 35%, and third episode 50% to 75%.

(2) Septic abortion.

(3) Ruptured appendix.

(4) Tubal surgery.

(5) Ectopic pregnancy.

(6) Endometriosis.

(7) Inflammatory bowel disease (IBD)

○ **When should HSG be completed?**

Immediately after end of menses, recommend prophylactic antibiotic: doxycycline 100 mg bid starting 2 days before procedure.

○ **Is chromotubation done with indigo carmine or methylene blue?**

Indigo carmine is the recommended prophylactic treatment as methylene blue can cause methemoglobinemia in patients with G6PD deficiency. Also, the patient should be treated with doxycycline 100 mg orally twice daily for 5 days.

○ **When is a chlamydial antibody test used?**

In patients with a normal HSG, a positive chlamydial antibody test may be useful in unexplained infertility to detect tubal dysfunction.

○ **How is distal tubal occlusive disease diagnosed?**

Laparoscopy is the gold standard for diagnosis.

○ **What is the percentage of patients that regret having a tubal ligation?**

7% and 1% request reversal.

○ **What is the percentage of patients who request reversal but have irreparable tubes?**

<5%.

○ **Which type of tubal ligation has the greatest and the least success with reversal?**

Reversal has greatest success with pins or clips in patients with no other infertility factors.
Low success with cauterized tubes.

○ **What is the risk of ectopic pregnancy after tubal reversal?**

1% to 7%. Ectopic rates are higher with isthmic-ampullary anastomoses compared with isthmic-isthmic anastomoses.

○ **What is the process of separating adherent fimbriae?**

Fimbriolysis.

○ **What is the process of correcting the phimotic or partially obstructed fimbriated end of tube?**

Fimbrioplasty.

○ **What is neosalpingostomy?**

Surgically reopening an obstructed tube with the understanding that patency may be restored but function may not and if pregnancy does not occur in 1 year, patient will need IVF.

○ **Does performing a salpingectomy in the presence of large hydrosalpinges increase the success rate of IVF?**

Yes, there is a twofold increase in success with IVF.

○ **How is proximal tubal occlusive disease diagnosed?**

HSG, one-third of all obstructions found on HSG located at the proximal tube but 20% to 40% of the time it is a false-negative result, and repeat HSG often reveals patency.

○ **What are the common histologic diagnoses in tubal occlusive disease?**

(1) Obliterative luminal fibrosis.

(2) Salpingitis isthmica nodosa that is diverticulosis of the fallopian tube.

(3) Chronic inflammation.

(4) Intratubal endometriosis.

○ **Does assisted reproductive technology (ART) have the same outcomes compared with tubal reconstruction?**

Yes. Advances in ART equal or exceed outcomes with tubal reconstruction.

○ **What are the poor prognostic factors for successful pregnancy in regard to tubal disease?**

Tubal diameter >20 mm.

Absence of visible fimbriae.

Dense pelvic adhesions.

Ovarian adhesions.

Advanced age of male partner.

Duration of infertility problem.

○ **What is the treatment of endometriosis in the infertile patient?**

Surgical removal/ablation of endometriomas/endometrial implants.

○ **Fecundability is highest up to how many months after the first surgery?**

6 to 12 months.

○ **When there is documented ovulatory function, normal uterine cavity and patent tubes, as well as a normal semen analysis, what are the most likely causes of occult infertility?**

Abnormal gametes.

Abnormal implantation.

○ **What is the first-line treatment of unexplained infertility?**

Ovulation induction and IUI; IUI alone demonstrates no significant improvement and Clomid alone demonstrates no significant improvement. In cases refractory to Clomid and IUI, use gonadotropins and IUI.

○ **What is the most effective treatment of unexplained infertility?**

IVF.

○ **What percentage of couples with unexplained infertility for <3 years duration will become pregnant with 3 years of expectant management?**

60%.

○ **Is artificial/donor insemination first-line treatment of male factor infertility?**

No! Artificial/donor insemination is now the treatment of last resort.

○   **What is the process of sperm development and maturation?**

Each day about 3 million spermatogonia begin to develop into primary spermatocytes.
Spermatocytes complete first meiotic division to become secondary spermatocytes.
Secondary spermatocytes complete second meiotic division to become spermatids.
Spermatids undergo maturation process to spermatozoa (mature sperm).
Final maturation step takes place in female genital tract, process called capacitation.
Entire process takes 70 days, and every day 50% of the potential sperm are lost.

○   **How long does it take for spermatozoa to travel from the testes to the ejaculatory ducts?**

2 to 3 weeks, semen analysis reflects conditions that occurred weeks earlier. For example, febrile illness results in transient but dramatic drop in sperm concentration.

○   **What testicular cells are analogous to the theca cells of the ovary?**

Leydig cells that produce testosterone and are located in the testicular interstitium.

○   **What testicular cells are analogous to the granulosa cells of the ovary?**

Sertoli cells are located in the seminiferous tubules and form the blood-testes barrier as well as provide metabolic support to the developing sperm by concentrating testosterone in the tubules

○   **What is the function of FSH in the testicle?**

Increases LH receptors on the Leydig cells, inhibin from the Sertoli cells, and inhibits FSH secretion through a negative feedback mechanism.

○   **What is the function of LH in the testicle?**

Increases testosterone production by the Leydig cells. Testosterone and estradiol produce a negative feedback mechanism to the hypothalamus and pituitary resulting in decreased LH production.

○   **When should a male infertility evaluation be initiated?**

After 1 year of regular intercourse without success but may be initiated earlier if the female partner is >35 years of age or the man has a concerning history of mumps, cryptorchidism, trauma, diabetes, inguinal hernia repair, or is taking medication that could cause ejaculatory dysfunction such as alpha-blockers, phentolamine, methyldopa, guanethidine, and reserpine.

○   **How should a semen specimen be collected and analyzed?**

Collect after 3 days of abstinence and examine specimen within 1 hour of collection, best to give specimen at the lab.

○   **What are the major parameters of semen analysis?**

Concentration.
Motility.
Morphology.

○   **What are normal semen parameters?**

Traditional World Health Organization (WHO) reference values for normal semen analysis:

- Volume 1.5 to 5 mL.
- pH >7.2.
- Viscosity <3 on scale 0 to 4.
- Sperm concentration >20 million/mL (probability of conception rises then plateaus at concentrations >50 million/mL).
- Total sperm count >40 million/ejaculate (multiply semen volume by sperm concentration to determine count, may be normal in oligospermia if volume is high or may be normal if the volume is low but the concentration of sperm is high).
- Percentage motility >50%.
- Forward progression >2 on scale of 0 to 4 (scale based on percentage of sperm moving forward, be it slow-grade 2, or rapid, grades 3-4, probability of conception increases up to 60% then plateaus).
- Normal morphology ("Kruger strict criteria") >14%, sperm morphology remains *the best* predictor of sperm function.
- Round cells <5 million/mL, epithelial cells, prostate cells, immature sperm, and leukocytes are all considered "round cells."
- Sperm agglutination <2 on scale of 0 to 3.

○   **What was changed by the 2010 WHO revised reference value for lower limits of normal?**

Lowered lower limit of normal sperm concentration to >15 million/mL.

Lowered percentage motility to >40%.

Lowered percentage normal morphology to >3 to 4%.

○   **What is the etiology of low volume acidic semen?**

- Fact: Semen is made up of secretions from the seminal vesicles that are alkaline and contain fructose.
- Prostate secretions are acidic.
- Low volume could be due to incomplete collection or short abstinence interval.
- Congenital bilateral absence of the vas deferens (CBAVD) results in hypoplastic or absent seminal vesicles, resulting in low-volume acidic ejaculate.
- This is also found with ejaculatory duct obstruction; complete obstruction results in ejaculate with no fructose or sperm.
- When androgen levels are low, secretions from the seminal vesicles and the prostate are decreased.
- Postejaculatory urinalysis should be completed whenever the semen volume is <1cc to look for retrograde ejaculation.

○   **What is azoospermia?**

- Absence of sperm, affects 1% of all men and 10% to 15% of men with infertility.
- Obstructive versus nonobstructive azoospermia, 40% of the time obstructive.
- Must be confirmed on repeat semen analysis.

○   **What is oligospermia?**

- Sperm concentration <20 million/mL, considered severe if <5 million/mL.
- Associated with varicocele, hypogonadism, and microdeletions in the Y chromosome.
- An endocrine and genetic evaluation is recommended in men with oligospermia.

○ **What is asthenospermia?**

- Poor sperm motility.
- Associated with sperm autoantibodies, genital tract infection, varicocele, partial obstruction, and prolonged abstinence.
- Kartagener syndrome—primary ciliary dyskinesia resulting in poor sperm motility, also affects cilia of the respiratory tract.
- Nonmoving sperm can be viable—tests for viability include a dye test and the hypoosmotic sperm swelling test.

○ **What is teratospermia?**

- High percentage of morphologically abnormal sperm.
- Considered severe if there is only 4% morphologically normal sperm by traditional WHO standards.
- Associated with varicocele and primary or secondary testicular failure.
- Most labs do not complete a "strict" morphology evaluation, this is done at specialized andrology labs using specific criteria; most labs do a basic morphology assessment.

○ **Semen morphology may be graded using what "strict" criteria?**

Kruger strict morphology. This assessment results in a more rigorous systematic evaluation of sperm morphology.

○ **What test is available to assess sperm function—attachment, penetration, and fertilization of ova?**

There is no reliable test of sperm function!

○ **What should happen when abnormal semen parameters are found?**

(1) Physical examination by urologist.

(2) Endocrine evaluation—particularly low sperm concentration or sexual dysfunction.

(3) Genetic evaluation—particularly for azoospermia or severe oligospermia.

○ **What are the four categories of male infertility?**

- Hypothalamic-pituitary problems (1–2%).
- Primary gonadal disorder (30–40%).
- Disorder of sperm transport (10–20%).
- Idiopathic.

○ **What is cryptorchidism and what is it a possible sign of?**

Cryptorchidism—failure of testicular descent.

Testicular descent is an androgen-dependent process; therefore, it is more common in men with abnormal testosterone production such as Klinefelter syndrome

○ **What are varicoceles?**

A varicocele is a dilated pampiniform plexus, more common on the left than on the right.

○ **What is the treatment of clinically evident varicoceles?**

Surgical repair may improve semen parameters and fertility rates in up to 40% of cases.

○ **How does aging affect male fertility?**

- As a man ages, there is a decrease in semen volume, sperm motility, and proportion of morphologically normal sperm.
- Pregnancy rates decrease and time to conception increases as men age.
- IVF data, however, is inconclusive in couples using donor eggs where male partner age is the dependent variable: some studies show no impact of male age where others demonstrate an age impact.
- Male germ cells, (spermatogonia), undergo more mitotic replications than female germ cells; however, it is not clear whether there is any increased risk of miscarriage with age;
- Sperm overproduction thought to buffer affects of aging as there is no measurable decrease in male fertility before age 45 to 50.

○ **A male with low testosterone and serum gonadotropin values <5 IU/L or lower would have what diagnosis?**

Hypogonadotropic hypogonadism.

○ **What should be done when hypogonadotropic hypogonadism is diagnosed?**

Check a prolactin level and obtain an MRI of the brain to look for an adenoma.

○ **How is congenital versus adult onset hypogonadotropic hypogonadism treated differently?**

If spermatogenesis was never initiated as in prepubertal/congenital hypogonadotropic hypogonadism, the patient must be treated with LH (hCG) and FSH.

If azoospermia occurs after puberty, spermatogenesis can be resumed and maintained with hCG alone.

○ **What is the treatment of adult hypogonadotropic hypogonadism?**

hCG 2000 IU IM three times per week for 6 months followed by 37.5 IU of FSH IM three times per week, or pulsatile administrations of gonadotropin-releasing hormone (GnRH) 4 µg q 3 hours by an infusion pump.

○ **What is the most common cause of retrograde ejaculation and how is it diagnosed?**

The most common cause is prostatectomy. The second most common cause is testicular carcinoma. Diagnosis is made by finding ejaculate of low volume with azoospermia or severe oligospermia and multiple sperm in urine specimen postejaculation.

○ **How do you treat retrograde ejaculation?**

Phenylpropanamide 75 mg bid or ephedrine sulfate 25 mg qid or urine can be collected and sperm can be harvested from the urine for insemination.

○ **Exposure to which drug toxins is hypothesized to produce disorders of sperm production?**

Chemotherapeutic agents.

Sulfasalazine.

Alcohol.

Cimetidine.

Lead, cadmium, mercury.

Carbon disulfide industrial solvent.

Nematocide (DBCP).

Beta-blockers.

○ **What is the likely cause of azoospermia with a negative fructose test?**

Obstruction. Causes include infection, surgery, and CBAVD as is seen in up to 80% of males with cystic fibrosis. Fructose is produced in the seminal vesicle and would be present in the semen if at least one tract is patent.

○ **What is the pregnancy rate after vasovasostomy (vasectomy reversal)?**

Within 3 years of vasectomy: 70–97%.
Within >3 or <15 years of vasectomy: 30%.

○ **What is the treatment of gonadal failure associated with Klinefelter syndrome (47,XXY)?**

Typically donor sperm. However, there are now reports of healthy deliveries now using IVF, testicular sperm aspiration, and preimplantation genetic diagnosis to identify euploid embryos.

CHAPTER 55 Assisted Reproductive Technology

Erin M. Murphy, MD

○ **What are assisted reproductive technologies (ART)?**

A large number of techniques that bring the sperm and oocytes closer together in order to increase the chance of pregnancy.

○ **What are the types of ART?**

IVF or in vitro fertilization—The eggs are aspirated from the ovary, mixed with the sperm in a dish, and the fertilized eggs (embryos) are transferred to the uterus 3 to 5 days later.

ICSI (intracytoplasmic sperm injection)—Single sperm is directly injected into oocyte.

Gestational carrier surrogacy—Fertilized egg placed into the uterus of a surrogate.

Egg donation—Use of a woman's oocytes in order to achieve pregnancy in an infertile woman or a woman at risk of maternally transmitted genetic disease.

GIFT or gamete intrafallopian transfer—The eggs are aspirated from the ovary and deposited with the sperm in the fallopian tube via laparoscopy.

ZIFT or zygote intrafallopian transfer—Eggs are aspirated from the ovary, mixed with the sperm in a dish, and the fertilized eggs (embryos) are transferred to the fallopian tube.

GIFT and ZIFT are much less commonly performed recently due to relative invasiveness of this procedure as compared with IVF.

○ **What are the indications for IVF?**

Tubal factor infertility, endometriosis, mild-to-moderate male factor infertility, diminished ovarian reserve, ovulatory dysfunction, and unknown/idiopathic infertility.

○ **What are normal semen parameters?**

Volume >2 mL
Sperm concentration ≥20 million/mL
Motility >50%
Morphology >4% WHO

○ **What are oligospermia, asthenospermia, and teratospermia?**

Oligozoospermia—Low concentration of sperm.

Asthenozoospermia—Decreased motility.

Teratozoospermia—Abnormal sperm morphology.

○ **What is the most severe case of male infertility?**

Azoospermia—No sperm in ejaculate (prevalence 1%).

○ **What are the two types of azoospermia?**

Obstructive azoospermia—Due to obstruction of outflow; occurs with absence of vas deferens or surgical ligation of vas deferens as well as severe infection.

Nonobstructive azoospermia—No obstruction identified; testicular failure.

○ **What are the four types of procedures used to obtain sperm from patients with obstructive azoospermia?**

TESA: Testicular sperm aspiration

PESA: Percutaneous epididymal sperm aspiration

MESA: Microepididymal sperm aspiration

TESE: Testicular biopsy

○ **What is a varicocele? How does it affect fertility?**

Dilation of the pampiniform plexus of the spermatic vein is known as a varicocele (ie, a varicosity of the spermatic vein). Approximately 40% of men have a varicocele commonly occurring on the left side because the right spermatic vein drains into the inferior vena cava (a shorter distance); however, a severe varicocele can cause a decrease in sperm production by increasing the temperature of the left testes, which then heats up the right testes.

○ **What is ovarian reserve? How is it assessed?**

Ovarian reserve is essentially the quantity and quality of the remaining egg supply that a woman has. Women are born with approximately 2 million oocytes and do not generate any new eggs. Men constantly produce new sperm. By the age of 37, approximately 200,000 or 10% of the original egg supply remains.

The three most commonly used tests of ovarian reserve are the "Day 3 FSH level," the "Clomiphene Challenge Test," and the "Basal Antral Follicle Count." Essentially, if the pituitary is secreting comparatively high levels of FSH in order to achieve normal follicular development, this indicates a poor egg supply. The Basal Antral Follicle Count is an estimate of the number of small follicles seen without any stimulation.

○ **How is an IVF cycle performed?**

(1) Supraphysiologic doses of gonadotropins (follicle-stimulating hormone, FSH and luteinizing hormone, LH) are given to stimulate the ovaries to produce multiple eggs.

(2) Ultrasounds are performed to monitor the growth of the follicles containing the oocytes as well as the rising serum estradiol levels resulting from multifollicular development.

(3) Human chorionic gonadotropin (hCG) is given to simulate an "LH surge."

(4) Just prior to the time that ovulation would have occurred, the eggs are aspirated from the ovary under transvaginal ultrasound guidance and sedation anesthesia.

(5) In the IVF laboratory, the oocytes are incubated or injected with sperm.

(6) Embryo development is carefully observed for the next 2 to 5 days. Using criteria such as the rate of cleavage, cell symmetry, fragmentation rate, etc, the embryologist attempts to choose the embryos with the highest probability of implantation.

(7) The selected embryos are transferred into the uterus under ultrasound guidance

(8) The remainder of the embryos may be frozen for the patient's future use.

○ **How do you prevent the patient from having a spontaneous LH surge?**

One of two possible additional medications is typically giving in addition to gonadotropins

(1) A gonadotropin-releasing hormone (GnRH) agonist. The GnRH agonist is started in the midluteal phase of the preceding cycle and will cause ovarian suppression by downregulation and desensitization of pituitary gonadotropin receptors. Once the ovaries are suppressed, the gonadotropins are administered concomitantly with the GnRH agonist until the day of hCG injection. The most widely used GnRH agonist is leuprolide acetate. The GnRH agonist "turns off" the pituitary.

(2) A GnRH antagonist. The antagonist competes with native GnRH molecules for pituitary binding sites, thus causing an immediate suppressive action and requires a shorter administration period. The GnRH antagonist "blocks" the pituitary from seeing GnRH.

○ **How is multifollicular recruitment monitored?**

Recruitment is monitored with daily estradiol measurements and ultrasound.

○ **Why is hCG administered instead of LH to simulate the "LH surge"?**

hCG is given at a dosage of 5,000 to 10,000 IU to aid in final maturation of the oocytes. hCG binds to the LH receptors, having the same effect but with a longer half-life.

○ **What is ICSI? What is "conventional insemination"?**

A single sperm is injected into a mature oocyte. Typically, this is done if the partner has a very low sperm count, low motility, or poor morphology. With conventional insemination, a microdroplet of media is placed in a Petri dish containing both the oocytes and a sample of washed sperm diluted to about 1 to 1.5 million/cc.

○ **How can you tell if the eggs fertilized?**

Oocytes are examined approximately 17 hours after ICSI or insemination. A normal fertilized oocyte will contain two polar bodies and two pronuclei, which will be visible under the light microscope. The presence of one polar body indicates nonfertilization (no male pronucleus), while three polar bodies suggests polyspermy (two male pronuclei).

○ **How many embryos are transferred back to the uterus?**

In general, the younger the patient and the better the prognosis, the fewer the embryos that are transferred. This is because the older the patient, lower the likelihood that the embryo will implant and develop into a normal pregnancy.

The American Society of Reproductive Medicine guidelines recommend in general, for cleavage-stage embryos:

Under age 35—one to two.
Age 35 to 37—two to three.
Age 38 to 40—three to four.
Over age 40—five.

○ **Approximately how many live births result in singletons, twins, and triplets?**

Singletons: 60%.

Twins: 29%.

Triplets or more: 5%.

Unreported/miscarriage: 6%.

○ **What is the age of IVF patients?**

More than two-third of IVF patients are 30 to 39 and 20% are over 40.

○ **How does frozen embryo live birth rates compare with fresh embryo live birth rates?**

Frozen embryo rates are approximately 10% lower than fresh embryo live birth rates.

○ **What is ovarian hyperstimulation syndrome (OHSS)?**

Ovarian enlargement in response to exogenous gonadotropin therapy.

○ **What are symptoms of OHSS?**

Abdominal distention/pain, ascites, gastrointestinal problems, respiratory distress, oliguria, hemoconcentration, electrolyte imbalance, and thromboembolism.

○ **What is the pathophysiology of OHSS?**

Increased vascular permeability with the loss of fluid, protein, and electrolytes into the peritoneal cavity; thought to be the result of vasoactive substances produced by the corpus luteum (VEGF).

○ **What is preimplantation genetic diagnosis (PGD)?**

It is a procedure available to couples whose offspring may be at risk of genetic abnormality. This technique allows couples to have their embryos screened prior to uterine transfer.

○ **How is PGD performed?**

PGD begins by using the technique of embryo biopsy. A single cell is removed from a day 3 embryo containing six to eight cells.

○ **What type of disorder can be detected by PGD?**

X-linked disorder.

Single gene defects.

Age related chromosomal aneuploidies.

○ **What are two detection techniques currently used in PGD?**

Fluorescence in situ hybridization (FISH) and polymerase chain reaction (PCR).

○ **What is the definition of aneuploidy?**

Any deviation from an exact multiple of the haploid number of chromosomes, whether more or less.

○ **What are the most common aneuploidies in newborns?**

Trisomy 21.

Sex chromosome aneuploidies.

Trisomy 18.

Trisomy 13.

○ **Can ART or PGD be used for sex selection?**

Yes. For example, if a woman is a carrier of a sex-linked disease such as Duchenne muscular dystrophy, PGD may be performed using FISH to identify the sex of the embryos with the goal of transferring only female embryos.

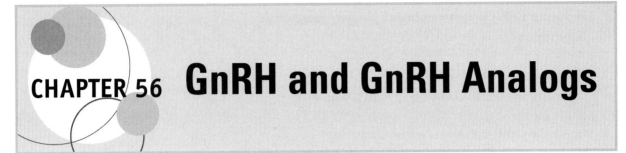

CHAPTER 56 GnRH and GnRH Analogs

Stephanie J. Estes, MD, FACOG

○ **What is the olfactory placode?**

The olfactory placode is a plate of ectoderm from which the olfactory organ and gonadotropin-releasing hormone (GnRH) neurons originate.

○ **How many cells migrated from olfactory area will produce GnRH?**

1000 to 3000.

○ **What syndrome develops as a result of olfactory axons and GnRH neurons failure to migrate from the olfactory placode?**

Kallmann syndrome.

○ **What is the primary unique symptom of Kallmann syndrome?**

Anosmia (or hyposmia).

○ **What is the most common mode of transmission of Kallmann syndrome?**

X-linked. Transmission can also be autosomal dominant or autosomal recessive.

○ **What is GnRH and where is it produced?**

GnRH is gonadotropin-releasing hormone that is produced by the arcuate nucleus of the hypothalamus.

○ **What is the half-life of GnRH?**

2 to 4 minutes.

○ **What is the cause of the short half-life of GnRH?**

The short half-life of GnRH is due to rapid cleavage of the bonds between amino acids 5 to 6, 6 to 7, and 9 to 10.

○ **What are the modes of administration of GnRH agonists?**

IV, SQ, nasal spray, sustained-release implants, and IM injections of biodegradable microspheres. The GnRH analogues cannot escape destruction if administered orally.

○ **How many GnRH receptors are in each pituitary gonadotrope?**

10,000 receptors.

○ **What is the structure of GnRH?**

GhRh is 10 amino acid decapeptide arranged in a "hair pin" loop.

○ **How is the GnRH delivered to portal circulation?**

Via an axonal pathway.

○ **What reproductive hormone measurement is used as an indication of GnRH pulsatility?**

Luteinizing hormone (LH).

○ **How is GnRH pulsatility described in the follicular phase?**

Pulsatile secretion is more frequent but lower in amplitude during the follicular phase compared with the luteal phase.

○ **How is GnRH pulsatility described in the luteal phase?**

Higher amplitude compared with follicular phase. Slower pulsatile secretion, especially toward the end of the luteal phase, which favors FSH synthesis that is required for the next cycle.

○ **What is the regulatory mechanism responsible for GnRH pulsatility?**

Pulsatile, rhythmic activity is an intrinsic property of GnRH neurons, although various hormones and neurotransmitters modulate that action.

○ **What is the effect of norepinephrine on GnRH pulsatile release?**

Stimulatory.

○ **What is the effect of dopamine and serotonin on GnRH pulsatile release?**

Inhibitory.

○ **What is the effect of neuropeptide Y on GnRH pulsatile release?**

Stimulatory.

○ **What is the effect of melatonin on GnRH pulsatile release?**

Inhibitory.

○ **What is the effect of endogenous opiates on GnRH pulsatile release?**

Inhibitory.

○ **True or False: Each pulse of LH measured in the peripheral blood corresponds to a hypothalamic pulse of GnRH into the portal system in a one-to-one relationship.**

True. Of note, although FSH is released with LH, FSH pulses are much more difficult to detect because the half-life of FSH is longer than the interval between GnRH pulses.

○ **What is the effect of high progesterone levels on the release of GnRH?**

Progesterone inhibits GnRH pulses at the level of the hypothalamus, and also antagonizes pituitary response to GnRH by interfering with estrogen action.

○ **What is the effect of low progesterone on GnRH pulsatile release?**

Low progesterone enhances the LH response to GnRH at the pituitary level, and allows the FSH midcycle surge.

○ **What are the two phases of GnRH therapy?**

Agonist phase.
Antagonist phase.

○ **What are the three primary positive actions of GnRH on gonadotropins?**

Synthesis and storage.
Self-priming so that gonadotropins are ready for direct secretion.
Immediate release.

○ **What are the FDA-approved indications of GnRH agonist therapy?**

Endometriosis.
Anemia (preoperatively with iron therapy for uterine leiomyomas).
Central precocious puberty.

○ **What are the non-FDA-labeled indications of GnRH agonist therapy?**

Hirsutism.
Induction of amenorrhea in special clinical situations (eg, in thrombocytopenic patients and prior to bone marrow transplant).
Breast cancer.
Ovarian cancer.
IVF.
Premenstrual dysphoric disorder.
Leiomyoma.

○ **What is the FDA-approved medication given with GnRH agonists as "add-back" therapy?**

Norethindrone 5 mg daily.

○ **What other medications have been given clinically as "add-back"?**

Low-dose estrogen with low-dose progestin.

○ **What benefit does low-dose estrogen treatment have compared with higher dose estrogen when treating endometriosis in pelvic pain patients with add-back therapy?**

Less pelvic pain and higher continuation rate of treatment.

○ **When can add-back therapy begin in relationship to GnRH analogues?**

At the same time.

○   **Does add-back therapy decrease the effectiveness of the GnRH agonist?**

No.

○   **Is GnRH agonist therapy effective for the treatment of pelvic pain due to endometriosis in patients who failed treatment with NSAIDs or oral contraceptives (OCPs)?**

Yes.

○   **Which GnRH agonists are FDA-approved in the United States for the treatment of endometriosis?**

Leuprolide, nafarelin, and goserelin.

○   **What is the total time (in months) approved by the FDA to utilize GnRH agonists?**

12 months. The dose may be initiated for 6 months and then repeated or continued for an additional 6 months.

○   **According to ACOG guidelines, should empiric GnRH agonist treatment be used in adolescents <18 years old for presumed endometriosis?**

No.

○   **True or False: GnRH agonists can be used in the treatment of leiomyomatosis peritonealis disseminata and adenomyosis.**

True.

○   **What are the contraindications to GnRH agonist therapy?**

Pregnancy, undiagnosed abnormal uterine bleeding, breastfeeding, undiagnosed pelvic mass, and reproductive tract neoplasia.

○   **What change in the circulating levels of FSH and LH is seen shortly after initiation of the GnRH agonist treatment?**

An increase in FSH and LH (flare effect).

○   **What is the duration of initial agonist phase of GnRH?**

1 to 3 weeks.

○   **What are the mechanisms that cause a hypogonadotropic, hypogonadal state after prolonged administration of GnRH antagonist?**

Desensitization, downregulation of the receptors, and secretion of biologically inactive gonadotropins.

○   **Desensitization is?**

The uncoupling of GnRH peptide/receptor complex from any intracellular actions.

○   **Downregulation refers primarily to?**

The decrease in the number of cell surface GnRH receptors.

○ **When do desensitization and downregulation occur?**

1 to 3 weeks after initiation of treatment.

○ **When is GnRH agonist therapy initiated to avoid a flare effect?**

Midluteal phase.

○ **Will a patient who has started a GnRH agonist in the midluteal phase (approximately day 21) get her menses?**

Yes. Ovulation has occurred and therefore withdrawal from progesterone will result in menses. Thereafter, ovulation (and menses) will likely be suppressed.

○ **How can GnRH therapy be monitored?**

The patient may be seen monthly. Check baseline E2, FSH, and progesterone. Recheck serum E2 after 2 months of therapy. Repeat bone density if treatment ≥6 months. Appropriate testing for specific sex steroid-dependent diseases after 3 months of therapy.

○ **When does the GnRH therapy become effective in downregulating estradiol levels?**

4 to 6 weeks. Patient should be amenorrheic by that time.

○ **What are the adverse effects of GnRH?**

Hot flashes: >75%.
Irregular (light) vaginal bleeding: 30%.
Headache, mood changes, vaginal dryness, and arthralgias/myalgias: 5% to 15%.
Allergic reaction: <10%.
Bone loss: long term.

○ **At what estradiol level is suppression with GnRH therapy adequate?**

<30 pg/mL.

○ **True or False: GnRH agonist treatment can delay the diagnosis of leiomyosarcoma.**

True. However, its incidence is extremely low, especially in premenopausal women.

○ **What percentage of women going for myomectomy will end up having hysterectomy?**

10% to 30%.

○ **What is the usefulness of GnRH therapy in fibroids?**

Reduction in size of the fibroids and improvement in bleeding symptoms by 6 to 8 weeks of therapy. It also increases the hemoglobin and hematocrit concentration.

○ **Which hormones are the endometrium and fibroid dependent for growth?**

Estrogen (and perhaps progesterone for fibroids).

○ **What is the change in mean uterine volume seen with GnRH agonist treatment?**

30% to 64% decrease in mean uterine size after 3 to 6 months of treatment.

○ **When is maximal response usually noted?**

By 3 months.

○ **How long does it typically take for menses to return after cessation of GnRH agonist treatment?**

4 to 10 weeks.

○ **How long does it typically take for myoma and uterine size to return to pretreatment levels after cessation of GnRH agonist treatment?**

3 to 4 months.

○ **Why might a GnRH agonist be useful in the treatment of hyperandrogenism?**

The assumption is that the hyperandrogenism is at least in part gonadotropin-dependent, and that long-term treatment with GnRH agonists will inhibit LH and to a lesser extent FSH leading to a decline in ovarian function and consequently ovarian androgen production.

○ **Why is GnRH agonist therapy not the recommended first-line treatment of ovarian hyperandrogenism?**

GnRH agonist therapy should be considered only after failure of OCP therapy with or without spironolactone, because GnRH agonist treatment causes severe hypoestrogenism, and add-back therapy is necessary if treatment is continued for more than a few months. Also, agonist is expensive compared with OCPs, and must be given parenterally.

○ **Does the GnRH agonist therapy decrease adrenal androgen secretion?**

No.

○ **What are the pros and cons of evoking a midcycle LH surge using GnRH agonists?**

Decreased probability of ovarian hyperstimulation is a possible benefit. It is still not certain whether corpus luteum function following ovulation induction by GnRH agonists is adequate to sustain nidation and continuation of pregnancy or if pharmacological luteal support is mandatory.

○ **What percentage of bone loss occurs in women on GnRH therapy for 6 months?**

5% to 10%.

○ **How are the GnRH antagonists synthesized?**

With multiple amino acid substitutions that allow binding of the antagonist to GnRH receptor and competitive inhibition.

○ **How long does it take to produce suppression by GnRH antagonists?**

It is an immediate action resulting in therapeutic effects within 24 to 72 hours.

○ **Why is response to antagonist treatment faster than to agonist?**

Because there is no initial flare response.

○ **What are the treatment indications of use of GnRH antagonists?**

Endometriosis, prostate cancer, precocious puberty, and female infertility.

○ **What are the disadvantages of using GnRH antagonists?**

Cost, lack of potency, and undesirable effects due to histamine release.

○ **GnRH analogs currently in the use have half- lives ranging (in hours).**

1.5 to 6 hours.

○ **After binding GnRH, the GnRH receptor peptide complexes do what?**

They migrate toward each other, then internalize, then are degraded and recycled to the cell surface.

○ **GnRH acts on its cell surface receptor on the gonadotrope to increase the release of LH and FSH by which mechanisms?**

Mobilization of calcium from internal sources.
Calcium influx to intracellular sites from the extracellular space.
Calmodulin binding within the cell.

○ **GnRH acts on its cell surface receptor on the gonadotrope to increase the synthesis of LH and FSH by which mechanism?**

Activation of protein kinases to achieve cytosolic protein phosphorylation.

○ **Can hirsutism be treated with GnRH on a long-term basis?**

Yes. If add-back therapy is used.

○ **Are there differences in the isoforms of LH produced by the pituitary during GnRH treatment?**

Yes. There is a large decrease in biologically active LH compared with total immunoreactive LH and thus the ratio of bioactive to total LH is greatly reduced.

○ **What is one of the rare risks of GnRH therapy for submucous myoma?**

There is a small risk (2%) that heavy vaginal bleeding will occur usually 5 to 10 weeks later, due to hemorrhage from degenerating submucous myomata.

○ **What effect does treatment with GnRH have on menstrual bleeding?**

At least 70% of women will achieve amenorrhea; however, some women will have light intermittent bleeding or frequent spotting.

○ **What is the major disadvantage of starting GnRH treatment in the follicular phase of the cycle?**

There is a greater tendency for a "flare effect" and a longer delay prior to downregulation.

○ **What is the major disadvantage of starting GnRH treatment in the late luteal phase of the cycle?**

The patient may have an early pregnancy and GnRH is contraindicated in pregnancy.

○ **Can GnRH analogues be utilized for fertility preservation in women undergoing chemotherapy?**

Yes. However, this is one of the most debated topics in fertility preservation discussions. Protective effect was seen in early animal studies and mostly nonrandomized evidence. Many others studies, including the German Hodgkin Study Group randomized trial, do not show an effect or others indicate mixed results. A summary in peer-reviewed papers of patients receiving GnRH analogues versus controls revealed a rate of premature ovarian failure of 11.1% in the GnRH group and 55.5% in the control group; however, only one of these was a randomized trial.

○ **Has triptorelin been shown to decrease the incidence of chemotherapy-induced early menopause in women with breast cancer?**

Yes. The absolute reduction was 17% in one recent open-label, randomized superiority study.

○ **What is the theoretical biologic problem with giving GnRH analogues as fertility preservation in women being treated for breast, ovarian, or endometrial cancer?**

Some suggest that since breast, ovary, and endometrium express GnRH receptors that it cannot be determined at this point that GnRH analogues do not reduce the efficacy of chemotherapy either by effect on GnRH receptors or by inducing glutathione S-transferases.

○ **Can GnRH analogues be utilized for fertility preservation in women undergoing radiation therapy?**

No.

CHAPTER 57

Laparoscopy and Infertility Surgery

Jacqueline Kohl, MD, MPH

○ **When might diagnostic laparoscopy be indicated during an infertility workup?**

In young women with a history of pelvic inflammatory disease, ectopic pregnancy, pelvic surgery, or chronic pelvic pain.

○ **Which patients do not benefit from laparoscopic surgery for infertility?**

Older women and those with multiple infertility factors: these patients are likely to do better with in vitro fertilization (IVF).

○ **What types of pathology can be treated via laparoscopy?**

Pelvic adhesions, endometriosis, endometrioma, mild hydrosalpinx, distal tubal occlusion, and leiomyoma.

○ **What are the relative contraindications to laparoscopic surgery?**

Extremes of body weight, inflammatory bowel disease, presence of large abdominal mass, and advanced intrauterine pregnancy.

○ **What is the size range of laparoscopes?**

2 to 12 mm.

○ **What are the differences between unipolar and bipolar electrocoagulation systems?**

In a unipolar system, the current passes from the generator through the instrument to a ground plate and then back to the generator.

The bipolar system uses the two insulated jaws of the instrument to carry the current to and from the generator. The tissue between the jaws completes the circuit.

○ **What is capacitive coupling?**

The ability of two conductors to transmit or receive electrical flow while separated by an insulator. It is done in unipolar coagulation.

○ **What is the disadvantage of capacitive coupling?**

The energy may be transferred to intraperitoneal tissues such as bowel and cause an inadvertent burn.

○ **How far out can lateral tissue damage occur?**

2 to 3 cm for unipolar and 1 to 2 cm for bipolar.

○ **What are the differences between cutting and coagulation currents?**

Cutting current provides a constant high-energy waveform.

The coagulation waveform creates an initial high-voltage peak that quickly dissipates and results in desiccation of the outer layer of the tissue and increased tissue resistance.

○ **Define tissue fulguration, coagulation, and desiccation.**

Fulguration means heating the tissue without contacting it. This is beneficial for superficial hemostasis with minimal tissue penetration.

Coagulation means heating the tissue to the extent that the protein loses its innate configuration and becomes solid.

Desiccation means that the liquid component of the tissue evaporates and the tissue becomes dry.

○ **What are the major types of lasers used in surgery, and how are they used?**

CO_2, argon, 532-nm potassium-titanyl-phosphate (KTP/532), and neodymium:yttrium-aluminum-garnet (Nd:YAG).

CO_2 is used mostly for tissue vaporization, whereas KTP and YAG mostly for coagulation.

○ **What preferentially absorbs the energy each laser?**

Water preferentially absorbs CO_2, while hemoglobin and hemosiderin preferentially absorb KTP and YAG.

○ **What is the approximate depth of penetration of CO_2 laser?**

Approximately 0.1 to 0.2 mm is achieved.

○ **What are the advantages of using CO_2 laser in laparoscopy?**

It cuts quickly, produces very little thermal damage, and can be used for vaporization, coagulation, and excision.

○ **What are the disadvantages of using CO_2 laser in laparoscopy?**

Poor hemostasis, cumbersome equipment, too much laser plume produced, difficulty aligning the beam, and identifying the helium-neon beam.

○ **What is the depth of penetration of argon and KTP lasers?**

0.4 to 0.8 mm.

○ **What are the advantages of using fiber-optic lasers in laparoscopy?**

Less cumbersome equipment, very accurate targeting, less plume, better hemostasis, smaller channel needed for fibers, and better visualization against abdominal organs.

○ **What are the disadvantages of using fiber-optic lasers in laparoscopy?**

They do not cut as well as CO_2 lasers and are less safe because of penetration of both tissue and water.

○ **What is the depth of penetration of YAG laser?**

0.6 to 4.2 mm.

○ **Why is CO_2 used preferentially over nitrous oxide for achieving pneumoperitoneum?**

CO_2 is rapidly absorbed by blood and therefore less likely to lead to gas embolism.

○ **How do you confirm adequate hemostasis during operative laparoscopy?**

Examine the surgical site under water or without the pneumoperitoneum.

○ **What are some of the benefits of laparoscopic surgery compared with laparotomy?**

Decreased hospital utilization, recovery time, patient discomfort, and overall cost.

○ **What are the alternatives to the standard umbilical insertion sites for Verres or trocar placement?**

Open laparoscopy, LUQ (beneath the costal margin of the ninth intercostal space at the edge of the lateral rectus or anterior axillary line), posterior cul-de-sac, or transfundal.

○ **Which patients may be good candidates for port placement in the LUQ?**

Patients who have undergone multiple abdominal surgeries or are known to have extensive adhesions or in whom insufflation is not attainable in the conventional spaces.

○ **What are desired intraperitoneal pressures during laparoscopy?**

Upon entry, ≤10 mmHg → after insufflation, ≤20 to 25 mmHg.

○ **Describe the "hanging drop test."**

Rapid intake of the drop of fluid as well as the inability to reaspirate the media. It suggests intraperitoneal location of the Veress needle.

○ **Which vessels can usually be identified by transillumination?**

Superficial epigastric vessels.

○ **The inferior epigastric artery is a branch of what artery?**

External iliac.

○ **When viewed from the laparoscope, the landmarks used to locate the inferior epigastric vessels are?**

The inferior epigastric vessels lie medial to the round ligament and lateral to the obliterated umbilical artery (lateral umbilical ligament).

○ **What are some common complications associated with gynecologic laparoscopy?**

Vascular and bowel injury, urinary tract injury, thermal injury, peripheral neuropathy due to poor positioning, hematoma and post-op bowel herniation.

○ **When is a patient most likely to sustain injury during laparoscopy?**

Entry access injuries account for over 50% of complications, especially small bowel and retroperitoneal vessels.

○ **What is the classic cardiac murmur associated with a gas embolism?**

Millwheel; it is described as a churning cardiac murmur.

○ **What is the primary concern in a patient that reports increasing abdominal pain after laparoscopy?**

Injury to the bowel or GU tract (ureter, bladder). Bowel injury in particular is often missed at the time of surgery.

○ **True or False: Hemostatic injuries to the bowel serosa do not need to be repaired.**

True.

○ **If after the initial trocal placement visualization reveals small bowel mucosa, what is your next step?**

With the trocar in place, a laparotomy is performed and the enterostomy is closed in a purse string fashion. This may also be done laparoscopically.

○ **What bladder injuries can be managed expectantly?**

Lacerations smaller than 5 mm may heal spontaneously if a Foley catheter is maintained for 4 to 5 days postoperatively.

○ **Which test can confirm ureteral injury?**

Intravenous indigo carmine is injected and cystoscopy should reveal dye from the ureteral orifices within 5 minutes.

○ **What test would you order on a patient who presents with a fever and right-sided abdominal and flank pain 2 days after undergoing a laparoscopic procedure?**

Intravenous pyelogram is the procedure of choice to rule out ureteral injury.

○ **How can one prevent a post-laparoscopy incisional hernia from occurring?**

By fascial closure in ports larger than 7 mm and/or the Z-track method (trocar insertion through skin then moving trocar slightly to create a separate entry through the fascia (ie, not "straight-in" insertion).

○ **What is the size range of diagnostic and operative hysteroscopes?**

Diagnostic: 4 to 5 mm.
Operative: 7 to 10 mm.

○ **What is the high-viscosity distension medium used in hysteroscopy?**

Hyskon (32% dextran 70 in dextrose).

○ **What are the low-viscosity distension media used in hysteroscopy?**

Normal saline, glycine (1.5% and 2.2%), 3% sorbitol, and 5% mannitol.

○ **What is the osmolarity of these solutions?**

1.5% glycine and 3% sorbitol: Hypo-osmolar.

5% mannitol and 2.2% glycine: Iso-osmolar.

○ **What is the safest hysteroscopic medium?**

Normal saline (0.9% sodium chloride).

○ **What is a dangerous fluid deficit with the use of glycine?**

A fluid deficit of ≥500 mL is associated with increased risk of hyponatremia and hypo-osmolality.

○ **What is the advantage of Hyskon over other media?**

It is immiscible with blood. This allows for excellent visualization, even during active bleeding.

○ **What are potential complications of Hyskon use?**

Idiosyncratic anaphylactoid reaction, hypervolemia, hyponatremia, pulmonary edema, and bleeding diathesis.

○ **What is the maximum volume of Hyskon that can be used during a single case?**

500 mL. Above that, the incidence of pulmonary edema has been described as high as 1.4%.

○ **Name four conditions that can be treated hysteroscopically.**

Submucosal fibroid, endometrial polyp, uterine adhesions, and uterine septum.

○ **What is the recurrence rate of endometriomas after surgical treatment?**

The recurrence rate is approximately 10% to 20%.

○ **Name two laparoscopic procedures for management of chronic pelvic pain.**

LUNA (laparoscopic uterosacral nerve ablation) and presacral neurectomy.

○ **What is the term pregnancy rate following laparoscopic salpingoneostomy?**

Rates vary widely but average around 15%.

○ **What is the ectopic pregnancy rate following laparoscopic salpingoneostomy?**

Up to 40% of all pregnancies.

○ **What is the incidence of finding pelvic pathology during a laparoscopy for an infertility evaluation?**

It is reported between 25% and 75%.

○ **Does laparoscopic treatment of endometriosis increase pregnancy rates?**

This is a controversial area. In early-stage disease, there is some evidence that pregnancy rates improve postoperatively.

○   **What percentage of patients experience improvement in pelvic pain after laparoscopic ablation of early-stage endometrial implants?**

Approximately 70%. However, in a significant proportion, pain will recur.

○   **What is depicted below and what surgical technique is used to correct it?**

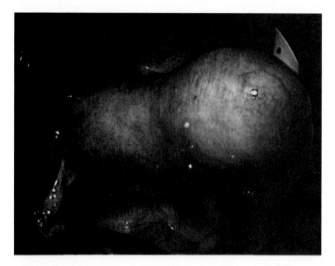

This is a bicornuate uterus with divergent horns. Strassman metroplasty is the classic technique used to unify the horns through wedge resection and apposition of the myometrium.

○   **What surgical techniques are available to correct the uterine anomaly seen below (and what anomaly is pictured)?**

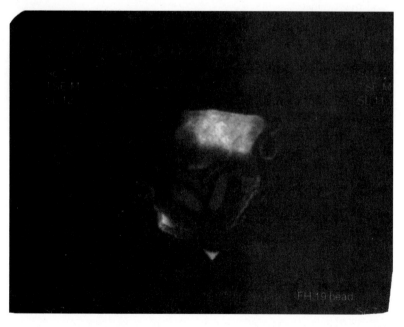

A uterine septum is pictured. Hysteroscopic resection is the procedure of choice. A Jones metroplasty (wedge resection) is the classic abdominal procedure.

○   **What is the condition seen below?**

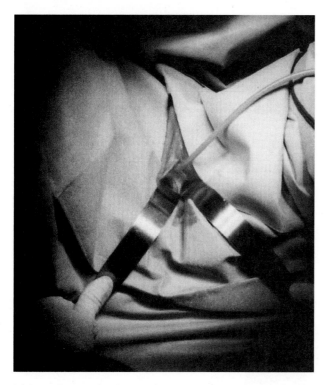

This is a longitudinal vaginal septum. Surgical removal is indicated with complaints of dyspareunia. This is also associated with duplication of the cervix and uterus.

○   **How is proximal tubal occlusion corrected?**

With either fluoroscopic or hysteroscopic fallopian tube catheterization.

○   **Describe the technique that is used to treat the condition seen below.**

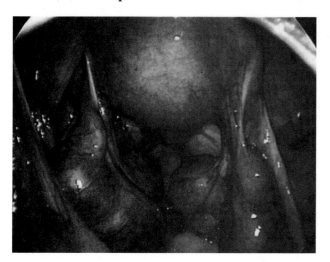

Hydrosalpinx is pictured. Radial incisions are made in the distal tube. The flaps are then folded back onto the tubal serosa either by heat (Bruhat technique) or sutures. Otherwise consider salpingectomy and proceed with IVF.

O   **True or False: Hydrosalpinges should not be surgically removed in patients undergoing IVF.**

False. Rates of implantation and pregnancy are improved with salpingectomy.

O   **What is the overall live birth rate following tubal reanastomosis?**

40% to 80%.

O   **What is the ectopic pregnancy rate following tubal reanastomosis?**

Approximately 5%.

O   **Under what circumstances can tubal anastomosis be attempted?**

In patients <37 with 4 cm of residual tube and with prior ring or clip sterilization.

O   **What are the advantages of the da Vinci telerobotic system?**

It may help to convert a laparotomy to a laparoscopic procedure. It has an EndoWrist with 7 degrees freedom of motion whereas laparoscopically 4 degrees of motion. There is also three-dimensional view.

O   **What portion of the tube is being anastomosed using the da Vinci telerobotic system?**

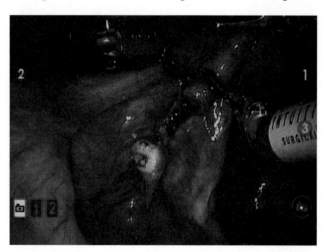

This is an isthmic-isthmic anastomosis procedure showing the grasper holding the proximal cut portion of the left fallopian tube.

CHAPTER 58 Hyperandrogenism

Erica L. Borman, DO and
Stephen G. Somkuti, MD, PhD

○ **What are the three sources of androgen production?**

Ovary (25%), adrenal (25%), and periphery (50%).

○ **What is the first step in adrenal steroid synthesis?**

The first step in adrenal steroid synthesis is the combination of acetyl CoA and squalene to form cholesterol, which is then converted into pregnenolone.

○ **In what disease process or syndrome is androstenedione secreted primarily by the ovary compared to normal premenopausal women who have equal production from the ovaries and the adrenals?**

Polycystic ovary syndrome (PCOS).

○ **What is the most potent circulating androgen?**

Testosterone.

○ **What are the effects of excess androgen in prepubertal boys?**

- Penile enlargement, growth of hair in androgen-dependent areas, deepening of the voice, and development of other secondary sexual characteristics.
- Increases height velocity, somatic development, and skeletal maturation.
- Premature epiphyseal fusion leading to short adult height.

○ **What are the effects of excess androgen in prepubertal girls?**

- Hirsutism, acne, and clitoromegaly (eg, heterosexual precocious puberty).
- Increases height velocity, somatic development, and skeletal maturation.
- Premature epiphyseal fusion leading to short adult height.

○ **What are the effects of excess androgen in pubertal boys?**

Increases the rate of progression of puberty and skeletal maturation, and decreases adult height.

○ **What are the effects of excess androgen in pubertal girls?**

Virilization, primary or secondary amenorrhea, and increased skeletal maturation.

○ **What are the effects of excess androgen in adult males?**

Inhibits gonadotropin secretion that may lead to decreased testes size, testicular testosterone secretion, and spermatogenesis.

○ **What are the effects of excess androgen in adult females?**

Hirsutism, acne, male pattern baldness, menstrual irregularities, oligomenorrhea or amenorrhea, and infertility.

○ **Define clitoromegaly.**

Clitoral length >10 mm or a clitoral index (length times width) >35 mm.

○ **Which of the following increase SHBG (the others decrease it)? (1) Estrogens, (2) danazol, (3) OCPs, (4) androgens, (5) liver disease, (6) pregnancy, and (7) hyperthyroidism.**

1, 3, 6, 7.

○ **Low levels of sex hormone binding globulin (SHBG) during pregnancy have been associated with the risk of developing what pregnancy complication?**

Gestational diabetes.

○ **How does danazol treatment (in endometriosis) result in hyperandrogenism?**

Danazol (an isoxazol derivative of 17α-ethinyltestosterone) decreases SHBG production and therefore elevates free testosterone levels. It also cross reacts with the androgen receptor.

○ **What happens to SHBG concentration in hyperandrogenic women with PCOS and how does it affect total and free testosterone?**

Low SHBG levels result in normal to slightly increased total testosterone and increased free testosterone.

○ **What percentage of testosterone is unbound or free in the circulation in normal females, hirsute females, and males?**

1%, 2%, and 3%.

○ **What percentage of circulating testosterone is bound to SHBG in normal females, hirsute females, and males?**

80%, 79%, and 78%.

○ **What percentage of circulating testosterone is bound loosely to albumin?**

19%.

○ **What is the immediate precursor to testosterone and what is the enzyme, present in most tissues, that aids its conversion to testosterone?**

Androstenedione, which is converted by 17β-hydroxysteroid dehydrogenase (17-ketosteroid reductase) to testosterone.

○ **What are the metabolic excretory products of testosterone?**

17-ketosteroids.

○ **In ovulatory women, which ovarian cell types are involved in androstenedione (1) secretion and (2) conversion to estrone and estradiol, and which (3) hormone is directly involved in stimulating this cascade?**

(1) Theca cells, (2) granulosa cells, and (3) luteinizing hormone (LH).

○ **What happens to LH pulse frequency and amplitude in patients with PCOS?**

They are increased.

○ **Which enzyme is involved in the conversion of androstenedione to estrogens, and what is the activity level of this enzyme in PCOS and the resulting effects?**

Aromatase, which is deceased, and as a result excessive amounts of androstenedione are secreted into the circulation, which can be converted peripherally to testosterone by most tissues.

○ **Which hormone stimulates the granulosa cells to produce aromatase that converts androgen to estrone and estradiol?**

Follicle-stimulating hormone (FSH).

○ **True or False: The low or normal FSH levels found in patients with PCOS are due to increased inhibin levels.**

False. Inhibin levels are not increased in patients with PCOS.

○ **Anovulation and follicular atresia seen in patients with PCOS results from?**

High androgen levels inhibiting aromatase activity, and an androgen dominant microenvironment ensues in the follicle inhibiting further maturation.

○ **Dehydroepiandrosterone sulfate (DHEA-S) is exclusively secreted from which gland?**

Adrenal.

○ **What is the normal circulating range of DHEA-S in women?**

Ranges are dependent on age and each individual laboratory but typically range from 100 to 350 μg/dL.

○ **What is the active form of testosterone and what enzyme converts testosterone to its active form?**

Dihydrotestosterone and 5α-reductase.

○ **What is the effect of insulin-like growth factor 1 (IGF-1) on the enzyme 5α-reductase?**

5α-Reductase activity is increased. In anovulatory patients with insulin resistance and hyperinsulinemia, this can intensify hirsutism.

○ **What is the metabolite of dihydrotestosterone that reflects 5α-reductase activity?**

3α-Androstanediol glucuronide (3α-AG).

O   **Drugs associated with hirsutism include?**

Cyclosporine, glucocorticoids, minoxidil, diazoxide, and phenytoin.

O   **True or False: Anabolic steroids used by female athletes may be a cause of hirsutism.**

True.

O   **Typical endocrine profiles of athletes engaged in sports such as swimming or rowing differ from those typical of dancers in what way?**

Sports that emphasize strength over leanness such as swimming or rowing have athletes with mildly elevated LH levels, elevated LH/FSH ratios and mild hyperandrogenism rather than hypoestrogenism from disruption of GnRH pulsatility, and decrease in LH, causing decrease in ovarian stimulation.

O   **What is the effect of estradiol on hair growth?**

Estradiol retards the rate and initiation of growth leading to finer, less pigmented and slower growing hair.

O   **In women with PCOS, most estrogen is derived from?**

Extraglandular aromatization of androstenedione to estrone.

O   **Long-standing amenorrhea associated with PCOS may predispose to?**

Endometrial hyperplasia and more rarely atypia and carcinoma.

O   **What are some theories driving the PCOS picture with increased ovarian androgen production?**

Increased volume of theca cells, increased LH stimulation of theca cells, potentiation of the action of LH by hyperinsulinemia, different biological activity of the beta-subunits of LH, increased LH receptor expression on thecal cells of patients with PCOS, decreased FSH secretion resulting in decreased aromatase activity leading to decreased potential estrogen production and increased androgen production as a result, and genetic predisposition.

O   **What is the relationship between hyperinsulinemia and hyperandrogenism?**

Insulin amplifies androgen production and both insulin and IGF-1 can enhance the ovarian androgen response to gonadotropin stimulation. Insulin also inhibits hepatic synthesis of SHBG and inhibits hepatic production of IGF-binding protein 1 (IGF-BP-1).

O   **What are the three phases of hair growth?**

Telogen (resting phase), anagen (active), and catagen (period of regression).

O   **What are the ovarian sources of hyperandrogenism?**

PCOS, stromal hyperthecosis, and tumors.

O   **Virilizing tumors of the ovary include?**

Sertoli-Leydig, lipoid cell, sex cord tumor with annular tubules (SCTAT), thecoma, and Gynandroblastoma (rare tumor producing both ovarian and testicular cells or tissues).

○ **What is the typical age Sertoli-Leydig tumors are seen?**

Age 25 with the vast majority being benign.

○ **Virilization occurring in pregnancy should raise suspicion for?**

The presence of a luteoma that is an exaggerated reaction of the ovarian stroma to human chorionic gonadotropin (hCG). Hyperreactio luteinalis (functional androgen-producing theca-lutein cysts), also a nonneoplastic condition resulting in bilateral ovarian enlargement, is more commonly seen in conditions of high hCG such as multiple gestations, fetal hydrops, hydatidiform mole, and gestational trophoblastic disease.

○ **What are the typical findings seen in stromal hyperthecosis?**

It is similar to PCOS but typically more severe and long standing. Serum testosterone is typically >200 ng/dL, both ovaries are enlarged, and the ovary rarely responds to stimulation or suppression.

○ **What is the histologic appearance of hyperthecosis?**

Patches of luteinized theca-like cells scattered throughout ovarian stroma. This results in more intense androgenization and a greater degree of insulin resistance.

○ **An ovarian or adrenal androgen-secreting tumor should be suspected when?**

Suspect clinically by history and physical examination, sudden as opposed to gradual onset of symptoms; virilization, ovarian tumors tend to be unilateral with testosterone levels >150 ng/dL, adrenal tumors typically have DHEA-S levels >700 μg/dL.

○ **What percentage of DHEA is produced by the testes or ovaries?**

About 20%.

○ **In men compared with women, what is the percentage of testosterone derived from the adrenals or adrenal precursors?**

Less than 5% in men compared to 40% to 65% in women depending on the menstrual phase of the cycle.

○ **What are some of the causes of adrenal hyperandrogenism?**

Primary ADRENAL: Premature adrenarche; adrenal tumors, androgen-secreting carcinomas

Adrenocorticotropic hormone (ACTH)-dependent causes: Congenital adrenal hyperplasia (CAH) (21-hydroxylase deficiency and 11β-hydroxylase deficiency), ACTH-dependent Cushing syndrome, glucocorticoid resistance.

Other causes: Hyperprolactinemia and placental enzyme deficiencies (deficient in placental aromatase or sulfatase).

○ **Name characteristics of an adrenal mass that are typical for an adenoma and for a carcinoma.**

Adenomas are small, usually <4 cm in diameter, have smooth borders and low unenhanced CT attenuation values. Carcinomas are larger, and have irregular margins, necrosis, hemorrhage, or calcifications.

○ **How can hyperprolactinemia cause hyperandrogenism?**

Prolactin receptors have been identified in the human adrenal and prolactin can increase adrenal DHEA production.

○   **What is the daily dose of exogenous androgen intake (DHEA) that can cause signs of hyperandrogenism in female?**

DHEA in daily dose of 50 to 100 mg taken chronically.

○   **What is premature adrenarche?**

The appearance of pubic or axillary hair before age 8 years old in girls and 9 years old in boys, without other signs of puberty or virilization and without an advance in bone age.

○   **What is the treatment of choice for adrenal tumors?**

Surgery.

○   **What is the treatment of choice for adrenal carcinomas?**

Surgical exploration followed by chemotherapy.

○   **True or False: Treatment of adrenal hyperandrogenism depends on the diagnosis.**

True. Specifically adrenal tumors need surgery and adrenal carcinomas are highly malignant, with cure uncommon; glucocorticoid resistance should be treated with dexamethasone (a glucocorticoid with no intrinsic mineralocorticoid activity) and likely an androgen-blocking agent (spironolactone or flutamide); congenital adrenal hyperplasia (CAH) is treated with a glucocorticoid and usually a mineralocorticoid.

○   **Adrenal sources of hyperandrogenism are best treated with?**

Low-dose steroids including dexamethasone (0.25–0.5 mg/day) or prednisone (2.5–5 mg/day). However, used alone, they are not very effective.

○   **Frequency of Cushing syndrome causes?**

Diagnosis	Percentage of Patients
Cushing disease	68
Ectopic ACTH	12
Ectopic CRH	<1
Adrenal adenoma	10
Adrenal carcinoma	8
Micronodular/macronodular hyperplasia	1
Major depression/alcoholism	1

○   **What are signs of Cushing syndrome?**

Menstrual irregularities, progressive central obesity, skin atrophy, easy bruising, purple striae, hyperpigmentation (due to increased ACTH-usually ectopic production), fungal infections of the skin and nail (tinea versicolor), psychological changes (emotional lability, agitated depression, mild paranoia, insomnia), hypertension, decreased glucose tolerance, ophthalmologic findings, and osteoporosis.

○ **Why is osteoporosis common in Cushing syndrome?**

Because there is decreased bone formation and increased bone resorption due to decreased intestinal calcium absorption and decreased renal calcium absorption, approximately 20% have vertebral compression fractures.

○ **What are the ophthalmologic findings and why are they concerning?**

Increased intraocular pressure in approximately 25% of patients, which is reversible; however, it can worsen preexisting glaucoma. Therefore, patients with glaucoma should not receive high-dose glucocorticoid treatment as they can have sudden irreversible deterioration of vision. In addition, posterior subcapsular cataracts can be caused by chronic hypercortisolism.

○ **What are three screening tests for Cushing syndrome?**

(1) Overnight dexamethasone suppression test (1 mg between 11pm-midnight followed by 8 AM cortisol- <1.8 µg/dL is nml).

(2) Urinary-free cortisol >250 µg/24 hours or three times above the upper limit of normal.

(3) Late-night salivary cortisol level.

If the tests are equivocal, then a midnight serum cortisol and/or dexamethasone-CRH test may clarify the diagnosis.

In addition, plasma ACTH concentration will help determine if the diagnosis is ACTH dependent or not.

○ **What things can falsely elevate salivary cortisol levels?**

Licorice, chewing tobacco, and smoking.

○ **What common medication can cause false-positive dexamethasone suppression test?**

Oral contraceptives (OCPs). Estrogen can increase cortisol-binding globulin concentration and since serum assays measure total cortisol, OCPs can cause false-positive results.

○ **What is the treatment for Cushing disease?**

Surgery or pituitary irradiation.

○ **What are the three distinct zones of the adrenal cortex and the corresponding steroids they produce?**

The outer zona glomerulosa (mineralocorticoids), the middle zona fasciculata (glucocorticoids), and the inner zona reticularis (sex steroids).

○ **Who should be screened for adult onset CAH?**

Those having early onset of hirsutism, high androgen levels, strong family history of hirsutism, those of high risk ethnic groups (Hispanic, Mediterranean, Slavic, or Ashkenazi Jewish heritage), and those with hypertension.

○ **What enzyme converts 17-hydroxyprogesterone to 11-deoxycortisol and when deficient accounts for >90% of cases of CAH?**

21-hydroxylase (CYP21A2).

○ **What does 21-hydroxylase deficiency pathophysiologically cause?**

Decreased cortisol synthesis resulting in increased ACTH (corticotropin), causing adrenal stimulation leading to increased androgen production.

○ **What are the different clinical presentations/syndromes of 21-hydroxylase deficiency?**

(1) Classical form: Simple virilizing form (genital ambiguity—female infants have pseudohermaphroditism; males have normal sexual development)/salt-wasting form (two-third of infants), may cause sexual precocity in children—if not virilized at birth and disorder is overlooked.

(2) Nonclassical form/late-onset form: During childhood or early adolescence, they may present with precocious puberty. Symptoms at time of puberty or soon thereafter include acne, hirsutism, menstrual irregularity, and infertility issues.

○ **What percentage of hirsute patients may have 21-hydroxylase enzyme deficiency?**

5%.

○ **The genetic inheritance pattern of CAH due to 21-hydroxylase deficiency is?**

Autosomal recessive. It is the most common autosomal-recessive disorder (more common than sickle cell and cystic fibrosis).

○ **What percentage of Caucasian hyperandrogenic women have late-onset CAH?**

1% to 2%.

○ **The complete form of 21-hydroxylase enzyme deficiency results in a lack of what two important glucocorticoid and mineralocorticoid steroids?**

Cortisol and aldosterone.

○ **How do you screen for 21-hydroxylase deficiency for late-onset form?**

Obtain 8 AM follicular phase 17-hydroxyprogesterone level. It should be <200 ng/dL. If >800, nonclassical CAH is diagnosed. If it is 200 to 800 ng/dL, then an ACTH stimulation test should be performed—synthetic ACTH (cosyntropin) is given and in most affected patients 17OHP levels rise to above 1500 ng/dL (43 nmol/L); if borderline results, genotyping should be done.

○ **What is the treatment of CAH?**

A glucocorticoid and usually a mineralocorticoid.

○ **Other rare enzyme deficiencies that result in hirsutism include?**

3β-hydroxysteroid dehydrogenase (3β-HSD) and 11β-hydroxylase deficiency.

○ **How can a 3β-HSD enzyme defect be diagnosed?**

By performing an ACTH stimulation test and finding an elevated 17-hydroxypregnenolone to 17 hydroxyprogesterone ratio (usually >6.0). You will also see an increase in DHEA-S levels. There is now gene sequence testing available as well.

○ **How do you diagnose an 11β-hydroxylase enzyme deficiency?**

Presence of hypertension and an elevated serum 11-deoxycorticosterone.

○ **Between what gestational weeks does exposure to androgen excess result in female sexual ambiguity?**

Between gestation weeks 7 and 12.

○ **Which chromosome is the gene for the androgen receptor located on?**

The X chromosome. Defects may result in incomplete masculinization of males.

○ **According to the Rotterdam criteria, the diagnosis of PCOS requires the presence of?**

Any 2 of the following three criteria: (1) Oligomenorrhea and/or anovulation, (2) clinical or biochemical signs of hyperandrogenism (free testosterone is most sensitive), (3) polycystic ovaries by U/S [2 or more follicles in each ovary, 2–9 mm in diameter; and/ or >10 mL ovarian volume per ovary (0.5 × length × width × thickness)]; note: other etiologies must be excluded (CAH, androgen-secreting tumor, Cushing syndrome, etc).

○ **Measurement of what hormone could be used to replace ultrasound or other imaging that show polycystic ovaries while still satisfying the third Rotterdam criteria?**

Anti-Müllerian hormone (AMH) correlates with the number of antral follicles and has been shown to be elevated in both adolescents and adults with PCOS as well as adolescents with oligomenorrhea without evidence of hyperandrogenism.

○ **Which criteria are not needed in the NIH definition of PCOS?**

Polycystic ovaries by US. Must have the first two criteria of the Rotterdam definition.

○ **What percentage of normal women meet ultrasonographic criteria for polycystic ovaries?**

8% to 25%.

○ **What are the definitions of amenorrhea and oligomenorrhea?**

Amenorrhea is no menstrual periods for 3 consecutive months or more.
Oligomenorrhea is <9 menstrual periods per year.

○ **Define hirsutism.**

Excess terminal, thick pigmented, body hair in a male distribution; commonly on upper lip, chin, periareolar area, and midsternum, along the linea alba of the lower abdomen.

○ **What is idiopathic hirsutism?**

Hirsute women with regular menstrual cycles and normal serum androgen levels. The most logical explanation is an increased sensitivity to androgens mediated by increased peripheral 5α-reductase activity.

○ **What percentage of women with PCOS have hirsutism?**

Roughly 70% but its prevalence depends on race/ethnicity.

○ **Do Asian women with PCOS typically have hirsutism? Why or why not?**

No. The concentration of hair follicles differs between races and ethnic groups. Asian and Native American women generally have little body hair. This probably also reflects racial and ethnic differences in local levels of 5α-reductase activity.

○ **What lipid abnormalities are typically found in patients with PCOS?**

Decreased high-density lipoprotein (HDL) cholesterol and increased triglycerides.

○ **What test should be ordered in suspected diagnosis of PCOS and why?**

Fasting blood sugar or oral glucose tolerance test to rule out type II diabetes (FBS >125/OGTT >199) or impaired glucose tolerance (FBS 101–125/OGTT 140–199); free testosterone, if not clinically hyperandrogenic to help with diagnosis; total testosterone, if with hirsutism, to help rule out adrenal or ovarian androgen-secreting tumor (>200 concern for ovarian tumor—pelvic U/S; >500–800 concern for adrenal tumor—CT scan or MRI); DHEA-S if with hirsutism, to rule out adrenal source with CAH or tumor; 17-OH progesterone if with hirsutism, to rule out CAH (5% of PCOS with hirsutism); prolactin if with hirsutism (hyperprolactinemia can cause hirsutism); and TSH to rule out thyroid disease.

○ **What is the normal range of total serum testosterone in women?**

Between 20 and 80 ng/dL.

○ **What range of total serum testosterone is typically seen in patients with PCOS?**

Just above normal, typically <100 ng/dL.

○ **What are the abnormal feedback signals that may result in anovulation in the patient with PCOS?**

Estradiol levels may not fall low enough to allow sufficient FSH response for the initial growth stimulus of oocytes. This may result from excess estrogen production due to peripheral conversion in adipose cells of androgens (principally androstenedione) to estrogens. The levels of estradiol may also be inadequate to induce the ovulatory surge of LH.

○ **What happens to the surface area of the ovary in PCOS?**

It typically doubles and the volume may increase up to 2.5-fold.

○ **Histologically, the PCOS ovary is characterized by?**

Multiple atretic and cystic follicles, a thickened tunica (outermost layer), and a fivefold increase in stroma.

○ **How does weight loss in the obese patient with PCOS improve hyperandrogenism and anovulation?**

Weight loss increases SHBG concentrations, thereby decreasing androgen levels; it also decreases the amount of androgen converted to estrogen in adipose tissue. These effects combine to give a more normal pattern of gonadotropin secretion leading to regulation of ovulation.

○ **What percentage of patients with PCOS placed on clomiphene citrate will ovulate?**

80%, with pregnancy rates being approximately 40% to 60%.

○ **The spontaneous abortion rate in patients with PCOS is increased and may be as high as?**

50%.

○ **What effects may the insulin-sensitizing agent metformin have in obese women with PCOS?**

It has been reported to lower serum insulin, decrease serum free testosterone, increase serum SHBG levels, and decrease ovarian 17α-hydroxylase and 17,20-lyase activity. However, further studies remain to be done to confirm the clinical utility of metformin in this population of women. The weight loss experienced in these women may also account for the observed effects.

○ **What are metformin's mechanisms of action?**

(1) To suppress hepatic glucose output; (2) to decrease intestinal absorption of glucose; (3) to increase insulin-mediated glucose utilization in peripheral tissues; and (4) has an antipolytic effect that decreases fatty acid concentrations, as a result decreasing gluconeogenesis.

○ **What are the therapeutic effects of combined OCPs?**

(1) A decrease in LH secretion and as a result a decrease in ovarian androgen production; (2) increased hepatic production of SHBG with decreased free testosterone as a result; (3) decrease in adrenal androgen secretion; (4) regular menses, resulting in preventing endometrial hyperplasia; and (5) progestins inhibit 5α-reductase activity in skin that decreases DHT.

○ **Why should a birth control method always be used with spironolactone?**

It has anti-androgen effects and may inhibit normal development of the external genitalia in a male fetus.

○ **For women who desire pregnancy and have PCOS with infertility, what would be some management options?**

(1) Weight loss and dietary modification, (2) Clomid, and (3) metformin and combined Clomid/metformin.

○ **What is the effect of metformin treatment during IVF in women with PCOS?**

Metformin has been shown to improve pregnancy and live birth rates as well as reduce the risk of ovarian hyperstimulation syndrome.

○ **How should metformin be dosed and what are some contraindications?**

Because of GI side effects, the dose should be increased slowly to a maximum of 2000 mg qd with 1 to 2 weeks elapsing between increases in doses. Contraindications: avoid in renal insufficiency, CHF, sepsis; it should be stopped prior to IV contrast; should not be given with cimetidine as it competes for renal clearance; and creatinine should be checked prior to starting metformin (and should be <1.4) and make sure normal fluid intake.

○ **What surgical treatments are available for the treatment of PCOS/hirsutism?**

Historically, wedge resection was used, now in disfavor due to postoperative adhesions. Laparoscopic YAG laser drilling of the ovary has been used with some success in otherwise medically refractory patients to induce ovulation. Laparoscopic ovarian diathermy (electrocautery) was compared with gonadotropin therapy in two randomized controlled trials, resulting in similar success rates (approximately 55% pregnancy rates), with lower multiple gestation rates.

○ **When should surgical treatments be used?**

When the only cause of infertility is PCOS and additional tubal factors, endometriosis and oligospermic male partners have been excluded. Then the pregnancy rates are 80% to 87% compared with 14% to 29%. In addition, Clomid and metformin should first be attempted, BMI should be <30, and women should have an increased LH concentration of >10 IU/L.

○ **What are the possible treatments of hirsutism?**

Hair removal and weight loss.

Vaniqa (eflornithine hydrochloride cream 13.9%).

OCP.

Spironolactone.

Flutamide.

Finasteride.

Cyproterone acetate.

Gonadotropin-releasing hormone agonist.

Glucocorticoid therapy.

Combined therapy with an estrogen-progestin contraceptive, metformin plus flutamide.

○ **What complementary/alternative therapy has been shown in randomized controlled trials to decrease androgen levels?**

Acupuncture.

○ **What is the mechanism of action of spironolactone?**

It blocks the effects of androgens in the periphery at the receptor (by competing with DHT for binding to the receptor) and has a suppressive effect on enzymes important in the biosynthesis of androgens.

○ **What is the recommended dose of spironolactone for the treatment of hirsutism?**

50 to 100 mg bid.

○ **What is the difference between finasteride and dutasteride?**

Dutasteride (Avodart) inhibits both isoforms of 5α-reductase, type I and type II, whereas finasteride (Propecia or Proscar) inhibits only type II.

○ **What is the minimum period of treatment necessary to see a clinical improvement in hirsutism?**

3 to 6 months.

○ **What is leptin?**

A protein hormone produced by adipocytes that increases general metabolism. Abnormalities may contribute to the metabolic disturbances in patients with PCOS.

○ **What percentage of women with PCOS meet the criteria for type II diabetes and for impaired glucose tolerance?**

7% to 10% and 35%.

○ **Define android obesity.**

A waist:hip ratio >0.85. Visceral fat is more metabolically active than subcutaneous fat and results in higher free fatty acid concentrations leading to hyperglycemia.

○ **Define the metabolic syndrome.**

Diagnosis requires three of the following five criteria: (1) increased waist circumference: >88 cm, (2) increased BP: ≥130/85, (3) increased triglycerides: ≥150, (4) decreased HDL: <50, and (5) increased fasting glucose ≥100 or previously established diabetes mellitus.

○ **What is "HAIR-AN" syndrome?**

Hyperandrogenism, insulin resistance, and acanthosis nigricans.

○ **What is acanthosis nigricans?**

Gray-brown, velvety, occasionally verrucous discoloration of the skin (neck, groin, axillae) associated with hyperinsulinemia. It is characterized histologically by papillomatosis and hyperkeratosis.

○ **What are the two types of hair and which are most affected by androgens?**

Vellus (fine, soft, short, and unpigmented) and terminal (long, coarse, and pigmented). The vellus hair that covers the body of infants is called lanugo.
Terminal hair is most affected by androgens.

○ **True or False: One's total endowment of hair follicles is determined prior to birth.**

True. Hair follicles develop at approximately 8 to 10 weeks of gestation and are completed by 22 weeks of gestation

○ **What is hypertrichosis?**

Excess terminal or vellus hair in areas not androgen dependent

○ **What drugs may cause hypertrichosis as an adverse effect?**

Phenytoin, penicillamine, diazoxide, minoxidil, or cyclosporine.

○ **What medical conditions may be associated with hypertrichosis?**

Hypothyroidism, anorexia nervosa, malnutrition, porphyria, and dermatomyositis.

○ **Is there a place for gonadotropin-releasing hormone agonist therapy in the treatment of hirsutism?**

Yes. Typically only in the HAIR-AN or hyperthecosis patient who has been resistant to conventional first-line therapies. Regimen consists of low-dose add-back using HRT or OCPs to avoid hypoestrogenism.

○ **Hair loss after pregnancy is explained by?**

The anagen phase of hair growth is prolonged by estrogens thus increasing the absolute number of hair follicles in this phase. Once the high estrogen levels end, many hair follicles enter telogen simultaneously, and are shed as new hairs begin to grow.

○ **What is the Ferriman-Gallway score?**

A grading system (1–4) scoring amount of hair growth and the location. This then can be used to follow objectively and quantitate hair growth. Scores <8, 8–15, >15 generally indicate mild, moderate, and severe hirsutism, respectively. However, because most women have scores <8, scores of 3 or higher fall outside the norm.

CHAPTER 59

Disorders of Prolactin Secretion

Stephanie J. Estes, MD, FACOG

○ **What are the pituitary causes of hyperprolactinemia?**

Pituitary disease (most common 50%).

- Prolactinomas
- Lymphocytic hypophysitis
- Empty sella syndrome
- Cushing disease
- Growth hormone-secreting tumors
- Plurihormonal adenoma

○ **What are other causes of hyperprolactinemia?**

Hypothalamic disease (rare)

- Craniopharyngiomas, meningiomas, metastasis of other tumors
- Vascular
- Pituitary stalk section
- Suprasellar surgery or mass extension
- Irradiation

Granulomas, infiltrations

Neurologic

- Chest wall lesions (chest trauma, herpes zoster; with neural mechanism similar to suckling)
- Spinal cord lesions
- Breast stimulation
- Epileptic seizures

Medications

- Phenothiazines
- Tricyclic antidepressants, SSRI's
- Narcotics
- Centrally acting antihypertensive agents (methyldopa, reserpine)
- Verapamil (unknown mechanism; does not occur with other Ca channel blockers)
- Oral contraceptive pills
- Antiemetics (metoclopramide)

Idiopathic hyperprolactinemia

Decreased clearance of prolactin

- End-stage renal disease
- Big prolactin=macroprolactinemia (prolactin circulates in large aggregates)

Other

- Pregnancy
- Hypothyroidism
- Cirrhosis
- Adrenal insufficiency
- Polycystic ovary syndrome (PCOS)

○ **What is the most common cause of mildly elevated prolactin levels?**

Stress.

○ **What other causes of a mildly elevated prolactin level must be considered?**

Recent meal, breast stimulation, coitus, exercise, or if the patient has just awakened.

○ **What is the predominant physiologic prolactin inhibitory factor?**

Dopamine.

○ **What are other prolactin inhibitory factors?**

Gonadotropin-releasing hormone (GnRH)-associated protein

GABA

○ **Name five prolactin releasing "factors."**

Serotonin

Thyrotropin-releasing hormone (TRH)

Vasoactive intestinal peptide (VIP)

Opioid peptides

Prolactin-releasing peptide (PRLrP)

Estrogens and the hormonal milieu of pregnancy

Growth hormone-releasing hormone (GHRH)

GnRH

○ **What is the most common pituitary tumor?**

Prolactin-secreting adenoma.

○ **How does elevated prolactin cause amenorrhea?**

Prolactin inhibits the pulsatile secretion of GnRH.

○   **What conclusions can be made based on prolactin serum levels?**

- Normal values are generally <25 ng/mL (µg/L).
- Slightly increased values (21–40 ng/mL) may be rechecked as they may reflect response to physiologic stimuli rather than true hyperprolactinemia.
- 20 to 200 ng/mL can be found in any patient with hyperprolactinemia.
- >250 ng/mL usually indicates the presence of a prolactinoma.
- >500 ng/mL is diagnostic of a macroprolactinoma (>1 cm in diameter).
- >1000 ng/mL is suggestive of macroadenomas >2 cm in diameter.

○   **According to the 2011 Endocrine Society Clinical Guidelines, how many prolactin levels should be obtained to diagnose hyperprolactinemia?**

One. A single measurement of prolactin at a level above the upper limit of normal confirms the diagnosis as long as the serum sample was obtained without excessive venipuncture stress.

○   **True or False: Are dynamic tests of prolactin secretion using TRH, L-dopa, nomifensine, or domperidone superior to a single prolactin measurement?**

False.

○   **What specific medications can cause prolactin levels to be >200 ng/mL?**

Risperidone and metoclopramide.

○   **True or False: Do symptoms of hyperprolactinemia correlate with its severity?**

True.

- Severe hyperprolactinemia (>100 ng/mL): Typically associated with overt hypogonadism, subnormal estradiol levels and its consequences: Amenorrhea, hot flashes, and vaginal dryness.
- Moderate hyperprolactinemia (50–100 ng/mL) usually causes amenorrhea or oligomenorrhea.
- Mild hyperprolactinemia (20–50 ng/mL) may cause only insufficient progesterone secretion and thus short luteal phase. Even without menstrual abnormalities these levels of prolactin are associated with infertility.

○   **What is the association between hyperprolactinemia and galactorrhea?**

Premenopausal women: Most patients with hyperprolactinemia do not have galactorrhea; most patients who have galactorrhea have normal prolactin levels.

Postmenopausal women: As they are markedly hypoestrogenemia the galactorrhea is rare. In this group of patients, hyperprolactinemia is recognized only when adenoma becomes so large that causes headache or visual disturbances.

○   **What percentage of women with high prolactin levels have galactorrhea?**

33%.

○   **What percentage of circulating prolactin is monomeric?**

85%. There are "big prolactin" (dimer) and "big big prolactin" (polymeric).

○   **What occurs to the prolactin concentration in pregnant women?**

It increases from the normal range 10–25 ng/mL to 200–400 ng/mL, as estrogen suppresses the hypothalamic dopamine.

○ **What are the physiologic prolactin concentrations after delivery and in response to suckling?**

Basal rate is high comparing with nonpregnant state and may further increase in response to suckling (up to few hundreds ng/mL). Over 4 to 12 weeks, the prolactin level decreases to normal and there is no longer a rapid release of prolactin with each suckling episode.

○ **Does breast examination or nipple stimulation increase prolactin secretion in nonlactating women?**

No. The magnitude of the increase in prolactin level is directly proportional to the degree of preexisting lactotroph hyperplasia due to estrogen.

○ **Can prolactin adenomas secrete other hormones?**

Yes. Approximately 10% secrete growth hormone as well.

○ **Can other pituitary hormone levels be affected by a mass lesion in the area of sella turcica?**

Yes. Thus, levels of all pituitary hormones should be checked in such situation.

○ **Are lactotroph adenomas more frequent with multiple endocrine neoplasia type 1?**

Yes. Prolactinomas occur in 20%.

○ **Are lactotroph tumors benign in nature?**

In most cases yes, but rare tumors can be malignant and metastasize.

○ **What is the natural history of microadenomas?**

Studies with 4 to 6 years of follow-up show that 95% of microadenomas do not enlarge.

○ **True or False: Progression from microadenoma to macroadenoma is rare?**

True.

○ **What is the treatment of hyperprolactinemia?**

First-line treatment is dopamine agonists as they decrease hyperprolactinemia due to any cause and decrease the size and secretion of most lactotroph adenomas.

○ **What is the rationale for treatment of hyperprolactinemia?**

Existing or impending neurologic symptoms due to the size of lactotroph adenoma.

Endocrine effects of hypogonadism: In women infertility, oligomenorrhea or amenorrhea, hypoestrogenemia (which may lead to osteoporosis); in men decreased libido and energy, impotence, loss of sexual hair, osteoporosis, possibly loss of muscle mass.

Galactorrhea may not be sufficiently bothersome to require treatment.

○ **What improvements in symptoms are expected in the majority of patients treated with dopamine agonists?**

Resolution of visual field defects.

Resolution of amenorrhea.

Resolution of infertility.

Improvement in sexual function.

○ **Which dopamine agonists are available for treatment of hyperprolactinemia?**

Cabergoline—used once or twice weekly, probably more effective and less nauseating than bromocriptine, effective in patients resistant to bromocriptine as well.

Bromocriptine—often used twice a day. It has been on the market for more then 20 years, which makes it a safe choice for pregnant patients

Pergolide—no longer recommended as it has been shown to cause valvular heart disease

Quinoglide, bromocriptine depo—are still being studied

○ **True or False: Does cabergoline have a higher frequency of pituitary tumor shrinkage compared with other dopamine agonists?**

True. It is hypothesized that cabergoline has a higher affinity for the dopamine receptor binding sites.

○ **When can one expect prolactin level to fall after initiation of dopamine agonist therapy?**

Usually it happens within 2 to 3 weeks.

○ **Dopamine agonists restore ovulation in what percentage of cases?**

90%.

○ **What percentage has cessation of galactorrhea after bromocriptine therapy?**

50% to 60% have cessation; 75% have reduction in galactorrhea. Thus, cessation of galactorrhea is slower and may not occur as frequently as resumption of ovulation/menses.

○ **When can one expect decrease in size of adenoma after initiation of dopamine agonist therapy?**

It is always preceded by fall in prolactin levels. One may see tumor shrinking after 6 weeks, though usually it is observed within 6 months.

○ **When can one expect improvement in visual symptoms after initiation of dopamine agonist therapy?**

Patient should be reassessed within 1 month, although improvement may occur within a 24 to 72 hours.

○ **What are the side effects of therapy with dopamine agonists?**

Most common is nausea. Others include postural hypotension, headache, dizziness, constipation, and fatigue. Less common are vomiting, nasal congestion, depression, and Raynaud phenomenon. Rare cardiovascular events.

○ **How can side effects of dopamine agonists be minimized?**

Start with half dose, take it with food, give medication at bedtime, and then add second dose in the morning after the patient is tolerating the night dose. In women, nausea can be avoided by vaginal administration.

○ **What is the regimen for bromocriptine therapy?**

Start at 1.25 mg after dinner or at bedtime for 1 week, then increase to 1.25 mg twice a day. After 1 month, evaluate for side effects and prolactin levels. May increase the dose up to 5 mg bid. The dose that results in normal serum prolactin level should be continued.

○   **What is the regimen for cabergoline therapy?**

Start 0.25 mg orally twice weekly, increase by 0.25 mg twice weekly at 4-week intervals; maximum 1 mg twice weekly.

○   **What is the definition of a microadenoma and a macroadenoma?**

Microadenoma is <10 mm in diameter.

Macroadenoma is 10 mm in diameter or greater.

○   **In asymptomatic patients with hyperprolactinemia, what laboratory test should be assessed to see if the elevated prolactin level consists of less bioactive forms?**

Macroprolactin

○   **What percentage of hyperprolactinemic women achieve pregnancy with dopamine agonist therapy?**

80%.

○   **What group of patients with prolactin adenomas should undergo surgery?**

Patients with symptoms of hyperprolactinemia that did not respond to medical therapy, and patients with adenomas that do not shrink during therapy or patients with giant lactotroph adenomas (>3 cm) wishing to become pregnant.

○   **True or False. Women are more common than men to be dopamine agonist resistant.**

False.

○   **What percentage of patients are resistant to bromocriptine and to cabergoline?**

25% and 10%.

○   **What clinical risk is present in patients with long-term use of high-dose cabergoline?**

Cardiac valvular regurgitation. But, most studies have shown no evidence of clinically significant heart valvular disease in patients receiving the usual doses of cabergoline.

○   **What is the best single predictor of persistent cure of prolactin adenoma with surgery?**

Serum prolactin concentration of 5 ng/mL or less on the first postoperative day.

○   **What is the role of radiation therapy in patients with lactotroph adenomas?**

It decreases the size and secretion of adenoma, but it occurs slowly and prolactin may be elevated many years after treatment. Radiation is limited to patients after the debulking surgery of very large macroadenomas. With this treatment, there is 50% chance of loss of anterior pituitary hormone secretion during subsequent 10 years.

○   **Should patients with asymptomatic medication-induced hyperprolactinemia be treated?**

No.

○ **Is there a place for estrogen therapy in patients with hyperprolactinemia?**

There is a narrow group of patients that may benefit from estrogen therapy: patients with lactotroph microadenomas causing hyperprolactinemia and hypogonadism, not responding or not tolerating dopamine agonist treatment; patients with hyperprolactinemia and amenorrhea due to antipsychotic agents. In such patients, prolactin levels should be monitored regularly as there is a small risk of increasing the size of adenoma.

○ **What are the risks of complications of microadenomas versus macroadenomas during pregnancy?**

The risk is small for microadenomas at about 5% to 6% level, whereas for macroadenomas it might be as high as 36%. Complications are increase in adenoma size, headache, visual impairment, and diabetes insipidus.

○ **What is the treatment of lactotroph microadenomas before and during pregnancy?**

Treatment is with dopamine agonists; bromocriptine is the preferred medications as there is longer history of its safe usage during pregnancy. The goal is to decrease prolactin level to normal before conception (patient should attempt pregnancy after a few months of normal menses and prolactin levels) and stop the medication once pregnancy is confirmed. Medication may be restarted (and is effective) if complications arise.

○ **Should serum prolactin measurements be performed in pregnant women with prolactinomas?**

No.

○ **For asymptomatic pregnant patients with prolactinomas, what clinical testing is indicated?**

None. If severe headaches or visual field changes occur, then MRI and visual field testing are recommended.

○ **Is the management of patients with macroadenomas any different from those with lactotroph microadenomas before and during pregnancy?**

Patients with a macroadenoma and those with evidence of compression of optic chiasm should be treated with transsphenoidal surgery with possible post-op radiation before pregnancy. If complications arise during pregnancy, the treatment of choice is bromocriptine. If the adenoma does not respond to medical therapy and vision is severely impaired, patients undergo surgery in the second trimester or after delivery if it is diagnosed in the third trimester. Pregnancy should be discouraged in patients not responsive to medical therapy. Follow-up depends on size of adenoma and complications.

○ **What therapeutic options should be considered in patients desiring pregnancy but not responding to dopamine agonists?**

Transsphenoidal surgery or ovulation induction.

○ **May patients with prolactin adenomas breastfeed? Does this depend on the size of tumor?**

It is safe to breastfeed with a microadenoma or if there is an asymptomatic macroadenoma. Symptomatic patients with macroadenomas should be treated. If patients are receiving dopamine agonists, nursing should be stopped.

○ **Do patients with microadenomas or macroadenomas have increased incidence of spontaneous miscarriage or other complications of pregnancy?**

No.

○   **What are two treatment options for patients with amenorrhea caused by a microadenoma who do not desire pregnancy?**

Dopamine agonist

Oral contraceptive pill

○   **When may treatment with dopamine agonists for hyperprolactinemia be stopped?**

If the prolactin levels have been normal for 2 years and there is no evidence of adenoma on MRI, then cessation of therapy can be considered. Prolactin level should be checked periodically as there is a significant rate of recurrence (26% to 69% recurrence rate depending on the cause and study during 4–5 years of follow-up).

○   **Within what time period would one expect a recurrence in hyperprolactinemia for patients who have stopped their dopamine agonists after having normal levels for 2 years?**

Most common to have recurrence within 1 year.

○   **What is the recommended follow-up for patients for whom dopamine agonists have been tapered or discontinued?**

Prolactin level every 3 months for 1 year and then yearly prolactin level.

○   **What is the treatment of hyperprolactinemia secondary to hypothyroidism?**

Thyroid hormones, only.

○   **Does the decidual endometrium have any endocrine function?**

Yes. The secretion of prolactin.

○   **During pregnancy, what areas contribute to prolactin secretion?**

The uterus, maternal and fetal pituitaries.

○   **Is the decidual secretion of prolactin affected by dopamine agonist treatment?**

No.

○   **What area is typically being invaded in patients with prolactin levels >2000?**

Cavernous sinuses.

○   **When treating macroadenomas, is it necessary to check frequent (every 3 months) MRIs?**

No. Serum prolactin can be followed alone. MRI should be obtained 6 months after treatment.

○   **What is the classic visual field impairment seen in patients with macroadenomas?**

Bitemporal hemianopsia.

○   **What is a malignant prolactinoma?**

A prolactinoma that has metastases outside of the CNS (very rare).

○ **What medication is recommended to treat malignant prolactinomas?**

Temozolomide therapy.

○ **What is the empty sella syndrome?**

A syndrome associated with the incomplete development of the sellar diaphragm that allows the subarachnoid space into the fossa of the pituitary.

○ **Does the empty sella syndrome progress eventually resulting in pituitary failure?**

No.

○ **What is Sheehan syndrome?**

Panhypopituitarism following infarction and necrosis of the pituitary secondary to postpartum hemorrhage.

○ **How does the hypothalamus maintain suppression of the pituitary prolactin secretion?**

The hypothalamus delivers a prolactin-inhibiting factor through the portal circulation.

○ **How does suckling affect prolactin secretion?**

Suckling inhibits the production of prolactin inhibiting factor.

○ **How does dopamine suppress prolactin?**

Dopamine binds lactotroph cells and blocks prolactin secretion.

○ **If medication is the cause of galactorrhea, will discontinuation of the medication resolve the galactorrhea?**

Yes. Usually within 3 to 6 months.

○ **How is hypothyroidism associated with galactorrhea?**

Excess TRH is released and acts as prolactin releasing factor, stimulating prolactin release from the pituitary.

○ **Can excessive estrogen lead to galactorrhea?**

Yes. Estrogen can suppress the hypothalamus reducing the production of prolactin inhibiting factor.

○ **Can prolonged suckling stimulate release of prolactin and subsequent galactorrhea from a nonpregnant patient?**

Yes.

○ **Can mild hirsutism occur with ovulatory dysfunction caused by hyperprolactinemia?**

Yes.

○ **Can breast implants lead to galactorrhea in women with normal levels of prolactin?**

Yes, due to the stimulation of the sensory afferent nerves.

○ **Do normal ovulatory menstrual periods occur in women with hyperprolactinemia if they are given exogenous GnRH?**

Yes.

○ **What are the most common tumors associated with delay in pubertal development?**

Prolactinomas and craniopharyngiomas.

○ **What is the most common symptom patients report with intrasellar expansion?**

Headache.

○ **Can primary hypothyroidism appear similar to a pituitary tumor in imaging studies?**

Yes, due to the hypertrophy of the thyrotrophs.

○ **Is galactorrhea more suspicious for malignancy if produced from a single alveolar duct?**

Yes.

○ **What is the "hook effect" (when interpreting prolactin levels)?**

In the presence of a macroadenoma, markedly elevated prolactin levels (5,000 ng/mL) can appear as mildly elevated levels (20–200 ng/mL) that is from the hook effect. This occurs because both the capture and signal antibodies in the sandwich immunoassays are saturated giving an artificially low result.

○ **How would one evaluate for a hook effect when prolactin levels are not as high as expected?**

(1) Repeat the test with a 1:1000 serum sample dilution.

  OR

(2) Washout can be performed to eliminate excess unbound prolactin after binding to the first antibody.

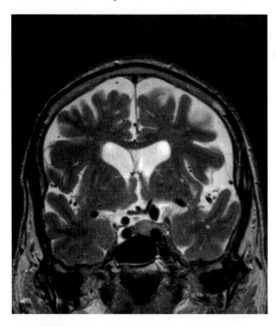

Microadenoma: Coronal T2W

(Reproduced, with permission, from Dan TD Nguyen, MD. Department of Radiology, Penn State Milton S. Hershey Medical Center. Hershey, PA.)

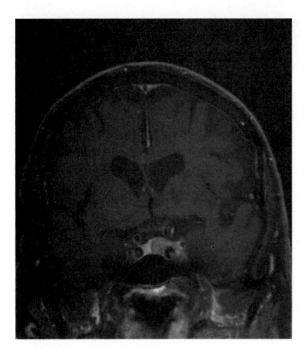

Microadenoma: Postcontrast T1W

(Reproduced, with permission, from Dan TD Nguyen, MD. Department of Radiology, Penn State Milton S. Hershey Medical Center. Hershey, PA.)

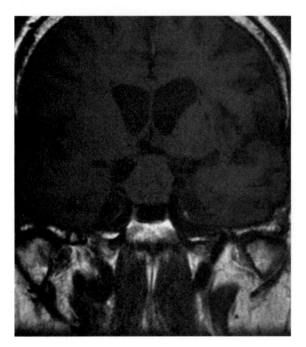

Macroadenoma: Noncontrast coronal T1W

(Reproduced, with permission, from Dan TD Nguyen, MD. Department of Radiology, Penn State Milton S. Hershey Medical Center. Hershey, PA.)

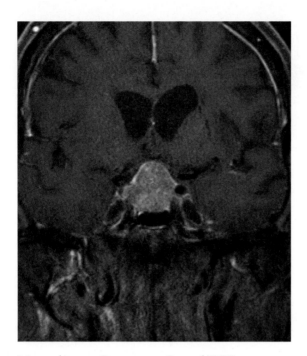

Macroadenoma: Postcontrast Coronal T1W

(Reproduced, with permission, from Dan TD Nguyen, MD. Department of Radiology, Penn State Milton S. Hershey Medical Center. Hershey, PA.)

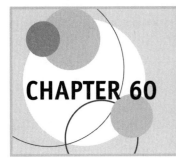

Miscarriage, Recurrent Miscarriage, and Pregnancy Termination

CHAPTER 60

Victoria Myers, MD

○ **What is the definition of miscarriage? Pregnancy loss before 20 weeks gestational age.**

Involuntary termination of pregnancy before the pregnancy reaches viability. This is typically considered <22 weeks of gestation (dated from LMP) or below a fetal weight of 500 g.

○ **What is "habitual aborter" or recurrent pregnancy loss?**

Three or more consecutive spontaneous abortion (SAB).

○ **What percentage of pregnancies end in SAB?**

12% to 20% of clinically recognized pregnancies end in SAB, whereas 13% to 26% of unrecognized pregnancies end in SAB.

○ **What is the incidence of two or more consecutive SABs?**

0.4% to 2%.

○ **What is the risk of subsequent SAB in a patient with three consecutive miscarriages?**

30% to 45%.

○ **What is the risk of subsequent SAB in a patient with three consecutive miscarriages and with at least one liveborn?**

30%.

○ **Name three independent risk factors for SAB.**

Increasing parity, maternal age, and paternal age.

○ **What are causes of recurrent SAB?**

Genetic, anatomic, immunologic, inherited thrombophilias, infectious, endocrine, and environmental.

○ **What is the prevalence of major chromosomal abnormalities being present in either partner of a couple with two or more pregnancy losses?**

Four to eight percent of couples with recurrent pregnancy loss one or the other partner may have a chromosomal abnormality, usually a balanced translocation.

○ **What is the most common single type of karyotypic abnormality present in SAB?**

Aneuploidy especially trisomies.

○ **What percentage of first-trimester SABs have karyotypic abnormalities?**

50%.

○ **What percentage of second trimester?**

30%.

○ **What percentage of stillbirths?**

3%.

○ **What are the most common types of abnormal karyotypes found?**

Trisomy (50%), monosomy 45,X (20%), triploidy (10%), and structural abnormalities (5%).

○ **What is the most common single chromosomal abnormality?**

45,X.

○ **What is the occurrence of uterine anomalies in those with repeated abortion?**

10% to 15%.

○ **What is the most common uterine anomaly?**

Septate uterus.

○ **What is the etiology of uterine anomalies?**

Müllerian ducts fusion defects that occur between 6 and 10 weeks in fetal development

○ **Is the prevalence of urinary tract anomalies increased in patients with all uterine malformations?**

Only for those with unicornuate/bicornuate uterus or uterus didelphys, NOT in those with septate uterus.

○ **What is the approximate incidence of SAB associated with the unicornuate uterus?**

34%.

○ **What is the SAB rate for those with a bicornuate uterus?**

Only slightly higher than the normal population

○ **What is the SAB rate for those with a septate uterus?**

21% to 44%.

○ **What is the SAB rate following surgical correction of septate uteri?**

It decreases to 15%.

○ **What effect does DES exposure have on patients who are able to conceive?**

It may have an increased SAB rate, preterm labor and delivery, as well as an increase in the ectopic pregnancy rate.

○ **What percentage of recurrent aborters have abnormal placentation?**

6%. Most are of the circumvallate type.

○ **What percentage of habitual aborters conceive post-myomectomy?**

Approximately 50%.

○ **Name three endocrinologic abnormalities associated with SAB?**

Thyroid diseases (both hyper and hypo), uncontrolled diabetes mellitus, and hyperprolactinemia.

○ **Name FIVE organisms associated with SAB.**

Chlamydia, *Toxoplasma gondii*, herpes, *Listeria*, and cytomegalovirus.

○ **Name tests for evaluation of fetal loss caused by antiphospholipid syndrome**

Lupus anticoagulant and anticardiolipin antibody.

○ **What is the effect of smoking on the abortion rate?**

Those who smoke >10 cigarettes daily have a greater chance of SAB. Relative risk 1.2 to 3.4.

○ **What is the risk of abortion in those women who have more than two drinks/day of alcohol?**

A twofold greater abortion risk.

○ **Does caffeine influence fertility or SAB rates?**

There is little evidence to support a clear detrimental effect of moderate to high amounts of caffeine intake on fertility or spontaneous miscarriage rates.

○ **What effect will 5 rads have on the abortion rate?**

Irradiation of <5 rads will have no effect.

○ **What percentage of intrauterine adhesions are caused by spontaneous and induced abortions?**

More than two thirds.

○ **Does high hyperglycemia affect miscarriage rates?**

Yes. Studies suggest that achieving euglycemia may lower the miscarriage rate.

○ **What androgens have been associated with miscarriage rates?**

Androstenedione and testosterone.

○ **Patients experiencing spontaneous, recurrent abortion would benefit from what established testing?**

Category	Recommended Tests	Other Tests
Genetic	Karyotype, both parents	
Anatomic	HSG or sonohysterogram or hysteroscopy	MRI as indicated
Immunologic	Lupus anticoagulant Anticardiolipin antibody	
Thrombophilias	Factor V Leiden Prothrombin gene mutation Activated protein C resistance Homocysteine MTHFR[a] Protein C Protein S Antithrombin III	
Endocrine	TSH, fasting blood glucose, HbA1c Prolactin	
Infectious	Gonorrhea and *Chlamydia* cultures	*Listeria* and TORCH titers if indicated
Environmental	History	

[a]Methylenetetrahydrofolate reductase.

○ **When is the appropriate time to do such a workup?**

After three SABs or in women above 35 after two SABs.

○ **What is the risk of ectopic pregnancy in those experiencing repetitive SAB?**

A fourfold increased risk.

○ **What is the miscarriage rate if embryonic cardiac activity is seen sonograpically at 6 weeks' gestation and at 8 weeks' gestation?**

6% to 8% and 2% to 3%.

○ **What is the occurrence of threatened miscarriage and what percentage results in abortion?**

Threatened miscarriage occurs in 30% to 40% of human gestations leading to abortion in half of these.

○ **How many weeks after fetal death with retained products of conception may consumptive coagulopathy with hypofibrinogenemia occur?**

5 weeks.

○ **What percentage of SABs become infected?**

1% to 2%.

○ **What is the risk of death from abortion?**

0.6/100,000 for elective abortions.

○ **Nonsurgical methods can be used to terminate pregnancies at which gestational ages?**

<7 to 9 weeks.

○ **Surgical methods are used to terminate pregnancies at which gestational ages?**

<7 to 23 weeks typically; however, the upper gestational limit varies according to each state.

○ **Are prophylactic antibiotics recommended for pregnancy termination?**

ACOG recommends use of 100 mg doxycycline prior to procedure followed by 200 mg post-op.

○ **What are the most common complications of surgical abortions?**

Less than 1% of cases will develop hemorrhage, fever, infection, and retained products of conception.

○ **What is the optimal management for postabortal pain, bleeding, and fever?**

Oral antibiotics and ergot medications followed by repeat uterine evacuation performed under local anesthesia in an ambulatory center, if retained products are suspected.

○ **How effective is RU 486 when used with misoprostol in first-trimester medical pregnancy termination?**

Ninety-seven percent had successful pregnancy termination if given by 49 days from the last menstrual cycle.

○ **How effective is methotrexate when used with misoprostol in first-trimester medical pregnancy termination?**

Ninety-six percent had successful pregnancy termination if given by 63 days from the last menstrual cycle.

○ **What agent is commonly used for multifetal, selective reduction to prevent cases of extreme prematurity?**

Intracardiac KCl (0.05 to 3 mL).

○ **What percentage of abortions are performed within the first 12 weeks of pregnancy?**

90%.

○ **Why is local anesthesia preferable to general anesthesia with pregnancy termination?**

General anesthesia is associated with greater risk of perforation, visceral injury, hemorrhage, and death.

○ **What morbid events can occur with the use of local anesthetics?**

Convulsions, syncope, and fever have been associated with the use of local anesthetics.

○ **What is the risk of surgical perforation in the first-trimester patient?**

9.4/100,000 induced abortions.

○ **Which country has the highest abortion rate among all Western nations?**
The United States of America.

○ **Suction curettage accounts for what percentage of all abortion procedures?**
90%.

○ **What is the predominate method of abortion beyond the first trimester?**
Dilatation and evacuation.

○ **Name another method used to induce contractions to perform abortion in the second trimester.**
Prostaglandin induction.

○ **What are two important determinants of abortion complication?**
Gestational age and method of abortion chosen.

○ **What are the associated causes of hemorrhage after pregnancy termination?**
Uterine atony, a low-lying implantation site, a pregnancy of more advanced gestational age, or perforation.

○ **What percentage of pregnancy terminations are done in the first trimester?**
In 1990, approximately 88% were done in the first trimester, 11% between 13 and 20 weeks, and 1% were done at 21 weeks or greater.

○ **Which groups of medical agents have been found extremely useful for pregnancy termination?**
Prostaglandin E2 (dinoprostone) and prostaglandin E1 (misoprostol) as well as the antiprogestin RU 486 (mifepristone) and the antimetabolite methotrexate have been very useful for this purpose.

○ **RU 486 is an analogue of which steroid used frequently in oral contraceptive pill formulations?**
Norethindrone.

○ **Under what conditions is hysterotomy indicated?**
Failed abortion when uterine anomaly is suspected.

○ **Which landmark Supreme Court decision concludes that the state may not interfere with the practice of abortion in the first trimester?**
Roe v. Wade.

○ **What percentage of abortions are obtained by married women?**
25%.

○ **What effect does laminaria japonicum have on the morbidity associated with forcible dilation during D&E?**
Fivefold reduction in cervical laceration.

CHAPTER 61

Family Planning and Sterilization

Karen T. Feisullin, MD

○ **What are the failure rates during first year of use in United States?**

Method	Percentage of Women with Pregnancy		Percent of Women Continuing use at 1 Year
	Typical	Lowest Expected	
No method	85	85	
Spermicides	29	18	42
Withdrawal	27	4	43
Fertility awareness-based methods	25		51
Standard Days Method		5	
Two Day Method		4	
Ovulation		3	
Sponge			
Parous women	32	20	46
Nulliparous women	16	9	57
Diaphragm with spermicide	16	6	57
Condom			
Female (reality)	21	5	49
Male	15	2	53

(continued)

Method	Percentage of Women with Pregnancy		Percent of Women Continuing use at 1 Year
	Typical	Lowest Expected	
Combined and progestin only pill	8	0.3	68
Ortho Evra patch	8	0.3	68
NuvaRing	8	0.3	68
DepoProvera	3	0.3	56
Intrauterine device (IUD)			
Copper T	0.8	0.6	78
Levonorgestrel	0.2	0.2	80
Sterilization			
Female	0.5	0.5	100
Male	0.15	0.10	100
Implanon	0.05	0.05	84

○   **What are the methods to measure the contraceptive efficacy?**

Pearl index and life table analysis.

○   **True/False. The failure rates increase with duration of use with most contraceptive methods.**

False. Failure rates actually decline with duration of use. The Pearl index is calculated as the pregnancy rate in a population divided by 100 years of user exposure and therefore fails to accurately compare methods at various durations of exposure. This limitation is overcome by using the method of life table analysis that gives the failure rate for each month of use.

○   **What are the recommendations following vasectomy?**

Barone et al. 2003 reported that azoospermia is more likely after 12 weeks (60%) than after 28 ejaculations (28%). A more reliable way to document azoospermia is semen analysis. Other forms of contraception are recommended until two semen samples show no motile sperm.

○ **What is the pregnancy rate after vasectomy reversal?**

70% to 80%. However, the prospect of pregnancy decreases with time elapsed from vasectomy decreasing to 30% after 10 years.

○ **What are the most common adverse effects of vasectomy?**

Hematomas, pain, and infection.

○ **Does vasectomy increase the risk of prostate cancer?**

Current data does not support an association between prostate cancer and vasectomy. Therefore, screening for prostate cancer should be no different in men who had a vasectomy.

○ **Describe the 10-year cumulative failure rates for female tubal sterilization.**

Unipolar coagulation	0.75
Postpartum partial salpingectomy	0.75
Silastic/Falope ring	1.77
Interval partial salpingectomy	2.01
Bipolar coagulation	2.48
Hulka-Clemens Clip	3.65
Hysteroscopic sterilization—microinsert	0.1
Hysteroscopic sterilization—polymer matrix	1.1

○ **What is the tubal sterilization technique with lowest failure rate?**

Postpartum partial salpingectomy has the lowest failure rate.

○ **What is the mortality rate of tubal sterilization?**

Mortality rates in the United States have been calculated in one to four deaths per 100,000 procedures. Most deaths are attributable to complications from general anesthesia, operative trauma, sepsis, and myocardial infarction. Long-term mortality is due to ectopic pregnancies.

○   **Describe the different methods of postpartum or interval mini-laparotomy tubal sterilization.**

Pomeroy	Double ligation at the base of a loop of isthmic portion of tube followed by excision of the knuckle of tube
Modified Pomeroy	Excision of segment of isthmic portion of tube after separate ligation of cut ends
Irving	Double ligate and sever tubes. Bury proximal stump into uterus and put distal stump into mesosalpinx
Uchida	Leaves of broad ligament and peritubal peritoneum injected with saline. Divide muscular part of tube/excise 3 to 5 cm. Bury proximal tube in leaves of broad ligament and include distal stump in line of closure
Fimbriectomy	Excision of fimbria of tube
Parkland	Midsegment of tube is separated from mesosalpinx at an avascular site; separated tubal segment is ligated proximally and distally and excised

○   **Which method is associated with increased risk of ectopic pregnancy after tubal sterilization?**
Bipolar tubal coagulation (17.1/1000).

○   **How long after tubal sterilization does the risk of ectopic pregnancy increase?**
The annual rate of ectopic pregnancies following tubal ligation is similar in the first 3 years and in the 4th through 10th year after sterilization.

○   **Does the patient's age at the time of sterilization determine the risk of ectopic pregnancy after tubal sterilization?**
Yes. Except for postpartum partial salpingectomy women sterilized before age 30 years are twice as likely to have an ectopic pregnancy than older women.

○   **True/False. Women who undergo tubal sterilization are more likely to have menstrual abnormalities.**
False. Current evidence indicates that tubal sterilization does not cause menstrual abnormalities.

○   **How many sterilized women will eventually undergo tubal anastomosis?**
1.1%, but this does not include women undergoing in vitro fertilization.

○   **What determines the pregnancy rates after tubal anastomosis?**
Pregnancy rates correlate with the length of the remaining tube; a length of 4 cm or more is optimal. Age of patient, time from sterilization, and sterilization technique may also influence success rates.

○   **What is ESSURE?**
ESSURE is a method of transcervical/hysteroscopic permanent sterilization that causes tubal blockage by encouraging local tissue growth with polyethylene terephthalate fibers (PET). An attached outer-coiled spring is released that molds to the shape of interstitial portion of each fallopian tube.

○ **What are advantages of ESSURE?**

ESSURE can be done in the physician's office without the need for conscious/general anesthesia. It is a transcervical approach with no incision required and may be preferred for obese women, women with abdominal adhesions, and women with risk factors for general anesthesia.

○ **What is the follow-up post ESSURE?**

Hysterosalpingogram must be done 3 months post-procedure to ensure complete tubal blockage. The couple must use another form of contraception in the interim.

○ **What is the effectiveness of ESSURE?**

99.8% effective after 3 years (1 pregnancy in 100 women in 3 years after placement).

NATURAL METHODS

○ **Name fertility awareness-based methods of contraception.**

Calendar charting (Standard Days Method, Two Day Method), basal body temperature charting, cervical mucus charting, sympto-thermal charting, and electronic methods (mini microscopes, hand held computers to evaluate cervical mucus).

○ **Does pre-ejaculate contain sperm?**

No. It is fluid produced by local glands. However, a previous ejaculate may leave sperm hidden within the urethral lining.

HORMONAL CONTRACEPTION

○ **Are combined oral contraceptives (COC) contraindicated in patients with a history of benign breast disease or a family history of breast cancer?**

No. Only if the woman has current or recent breast cancer.

○ **What positive test prevents women with lupus from taking COC?**

Positive antiphospholipid antibodies. This is associated with an increased risk of both arterial and venous thrombosis. Unless there are other cardiovascular risk factors, women with lupus are good candidates for hormonal contraceptives.

○ **Can women with migraines take COCs?**

Women under 35 who have migraines without aura, and without other risk factors for stroke can take COCs. Women of all ages who have migraines with aura should not take them.

○ **At what age should women stop using COCs?**

Women without medical problems who are nonsmokers may continue COCs until menopause.

○ **Should COCs be prescribed to women with diabetes and/or hypertension?**

Patients who are compliant with follow-up and management of their hypertension and diabetes may be started on a trial of COC, provided they have no additional cardiovascular risk factors.

○ **Is depression a contraindication for COCs?**

No. Symptoms are not exacerbated by them.

○ **What precautions should women with epilepsy on anticonvulsants take?**

They should take a pill with at least 30 µg ethinyl estradiol because of the decreased effectiveness of the COC in women taking these medications. Use of other contraception should be encouraged.

○ **Should COCs be discontinued prior to major surgery?**

It is suggested that oral contraceptives be discontinued approximately 6 weeks prior to any major surgery with prolonged immobilization. If they are continued, heparin prophylaxis should be provided.

○ **Can women with dyslipidemia use COCs?**

Yes, provided that their disease is well controlled. The parameters for poor disease control include LDL >160 mg/mL, triglycerides >250 mg/day or comorbidities of the disease. The patients who meet criteria should be started on a low-dose estrogen pill.

○ **Should patients on depot medroxyprogesterone acetate (DMPA) be assessed for bone mineral density (DXA scan)?**

No. At this time, the short-term data does not support the need for DXA for patients on DMPA.

○ **Name the conditions where progestin-only methods may be more appropriate than combination contraceptives.**

The conditions include migraine headaches, smokers, obesity, hypertension, hyperlipidemia, history of thromboembolism, thrombogenic mutations, SLE (use with caution in those with positive antiphospholipid antibodies and thrombocytopenia), sickle cell disease, cardiovascular, and cerebrovascular disease.

○ **Which anticonvulsants may decrease the effectiveness of COCs?**

Barbiturates, carbamazepine, felbamate, phenytoin, topiramate, primidone, and vigabatrin.

○ **What are the regimens available for emergency contraception?**

The most commonly used oral emergency contraception regimens are the progestin-only regimen, which consists of two 0.75 mg levonorgestrel pills taken at the same time (Plan B), and the combined estrogen-progestin regimen, which consists of two doses—each containing 100 µg of ethinyl estradiol plus 0.5 mg of levonorgestrel—taken 12 hours apart. If there is low risk of sexually transmitted infections, placement of a copper IUD can be used for emergency contraception with the added benefit of being a highly effective method for up to 10 years after placement.

○ **How long after exposure can emergency oral contraceptives be given?**

Up to 120 hours. It is most effective if initiated in 12 to 24 hours.

○ **What is the most common side effect of oral contraceptives when used for emergency contraception?**

Nausea. It occurs in 50% to 70% of those treated. Up to 22% may vomit.

○ **When should the woman prescribed emergency contraception expect her menses?**

Within a few days of her normal menses. It may be a few days early or late. If >2 weeks pass with no menses, she should take a pregnancy test.

○ **What to do when pills are missed?**

Scenario	What to Do?	Backup Method Needed?
1 pill is missed	Take pill as soon as possible and resume schedule	None needed
2 pills missed in the first 2 weeks	Take 2 pills on each of the next 2 days and finish pack	Need for backup method minimal but recommended for 7 days
2 pills missed in the 3rd week	Start new pack or if Sunday start—take one pill until Sunday and start new pack	Start immediately and for 7 days
More than 2 active pills are missed at any time	Start new pack or if Sunday start—take one pill until Sunday and start new pack	Start immediately and for 7 days

○ **What are noncontraceptive benefits of COCs?**

Treats menstrual cycle disorders, acne, hirsutism; reduces risk of ovarian and endometrial, and colon cancers; improves pain from endometriosis; and prevents development of functional ovarian cysts.

○ **How much is menstrual blood flow decreased by pill use?**

Up to 43%. It is less effective than the levonorgestrel IUD (see section on IUD).

○ **Pill use decreases the incidence of functional cysts by?**

80% to 90%. Oral contraceptives suppress follicle-stimulating hormone (FSH) and luteinizing hormone (LH) ovarian stimulation. They do not make an existing cyst regress more quickly.

○ **For the treatment of PMS, which type of pill is more effective?**

Oral contraceptives containing progestin, drospirenone, and those with a shorter pill-free interval are more effective than placebo.

○ **For women using oral contraceptives, what is their reduction in risk of ovarian cancer?**

The relative risk of developing ovarian cancer in women with any use of oral contraceptives is 0.73. Additionally, the protective effect lasted 30 years after discontinuing the pills.

○ **For women using oral contraceptives for at least 2 years, what is the reduction in risk of endometrial cancer?**

Women who use oral contraceptives for at least 12 months had a relative risk of 0.6. The protective effect lasted for at least 15 years after discontinuing the pills.

○ **In lactating women, how soon after delivery can COC pills be started?**

COCs may be started once milk production is well established, usually 6 weeks postpartum. Progestin only pills, however, are a better choice because they are not associated with decreased milk production, although studies have not shown less weight gain in babies whose mothers take COCs.

○ **In nonlactating postpartum women when should combination pills be started?**

After 4 weeks postpartum. This avoids the immediate postpartum hypercoagulable state.

○ **Among nonlactating postpartum women when does the first ovulation occur?**

On average 45 to 94 days postpartum.

○ **How effective is breastfeeding alone in preventing pregnancy?**

Ninety-eight percent for the first 6 months in women who have not resumed their menses and are exclusively breastfeeding.

○ **Are women more likely to gain or lose weight with oral contraceptive use?**

Both are equally likely. The effect on weight is small.

○ **What is NuvaRing?**

It is a combined hormonal contraceptive. The ring is placed in the vagina for 3 weeks and then removed for a week to allow withdrawal bleeding. A new ring is then placed 7 days later.

○ **How does NuvaRing work?**

NuvaRing releases 15 μg ethinyl estradiol and 120 μg etonogestrel daily.

○ **Is it necessary to remove NuvaRing for sexual intercourse?**

No. The ring should not be removed for sexual intercourse. However, if the ring is displaced outside the vagina during intercourse, it may be rinsed and should be placed back in the vagina within 3 hours.

○ **How does the transdermal contraceptive patch work?**

Ortho Evra patches deliver 20 μg of ethinyl estradiol and 150 μg of norelgestromin daily. The patch is changed once a week for 3 weeks, followed by 1 week of no patch.

○ **What are the most frequent side effects of the patch?**

Breast symptoms, headache, application site reaction, and nausea. Few women considered these side effects a reason to discontinue the patch. Reaction at the application site is the leading cause to stop using the patch.

○ **Is the patch more effective than OCPs?**

No. The efficacy of these methods is similar. However, the efficacy may decrease in women with weight >90 kg.

○ **What should be recommended if the patch becomes detached?**

A partially detached patch for <24 hours duration should be reattached or replaced if it has lost its stickiness. For longer detachment, a new patch should be applied and 7-day backup contraception should be provided.

○ **True/False. The transdermal patch has a better compliance than OCP?**

True.

○ **What is the Seasonale pill?**

A 91-day extended cycle OCP. It consists of 84 active pills followed by 7 inactive pills, resulting in 4 withdrawal bleeds per year.

○ **What is the hormonal component of Seasonale?**

The pill contains 30 μg of ethinyl estradiol and 150 μg of levonorgestrel.

○ **What is Seasonique and how does it differ from Seasonale?**

Seasonique is also a 91-day extended cycle OCP. It consists of the same 84 active pills followed by 7 pills containing 10 μg of ethinyl estradiol, which may result in less breakthrough bleeding.

○ **Is the efficacy of Seasonale pill comparable with conventional OCP?**

Yes. The Seasonale pill has similar effectiveness to 28-day cycle combined OCP.

○ **Is the breakthrough bleeding more frequent with the Seasonale pill?**

Yes. Compared with traditional combined OCP, women who take Seasonale have more unplanned bleeding. However, it decreases after the fourth cycle.

○ **Do the side effects increase with Seasonale?**

No. The side effects and contraindications of Seasonale are similar to other combined OCP.

○ **How does DepoProvera work?**

It inhibits gonadotropin secretion, which inhibits follicle maturation and ovulation. Endometrial proliferation is then inhibited.

○ **What is the effect of progestin on the uterus?**

It results in a shallow atrophic endometrium, making it less receptive to implantation. It also thickens cervical mucus and reduces tubal motility.

○ **What is the "grace" period with DepoProvera?**

2 weeks. A 150-mg injection actually provides >3 months protection.

○ **What is the average weight gain per year of use of DepoProvera?**

2 to 5 pounds.

○ **What is the expected period of time for return of fertility after DepoProvera?**

6 months to 1 year.

○ **What is Implanon?**

Implanon is a progestin (etonogestrel)-containing implant placed in the upper arm. It protects against pregnancy for 3 years.

○ **When should Implanon be inserted to minimize pregnancy risk?**

Within 5 days of the onset of menstruation or 3 to 4 weeks after delivery.

○ **In progestin-only pill users, which women are at greatest risk of pregnancy?**

Those who take their pill >3 hours late. The main mechanism of action is thickening of cervical mucus and thinning the lining of the endometrium, which depends on taking the pill daily at the same time every day. Menstrual cycles prior to pill use were ovulatory and whose cycles are least disturbed.

BARRIER METHODS

○ **Do all condoms protect against all sexually transmitted diseases (STDs)?**

No. Condoms may permit the passage of viruses such as human papilloma virus (HPV) and herpes simplex virus (HSV).

○ **What is the method failure rate of the condom?**

Perfect use has a 2% failure rate versus actual use rates of about 18%.

○ **Are spermicidal condoms as effective as a condom plus intravaginal spermicide?**

No. The dose delivered by a lubricated condom is much less than intravaginal spermicide.

○ **What is the rate of pregnancy after a condom breaks?**

About 1 per 23 breaks. Rates of breakage are about 1 to 2 per 100 condoms used.

○ **What lubricants increase breakage?**

Oil-based lubricants such as Vaseline, baby oil, and lotions. Heat can also break down condoms, so storing them in a wallet or hot car is not recommended.

○ **What are the two components of spermicides?**

Base or carrier (foam, cream, or jelly) and spermicidal chemical, usually nonoxynol-9.

○ **How do spermicides work?**

They are surfactants that destroy the sperm cell membrane.

○ **How much time does it take for spermicidal suppositories to be effective?**

10 to 15 minutes. The act of intercourse should ideally occur <20 minutes after insertion of the spermicide and no >30 minutes after.

○ **How quickly can sperm enter the cervical canal?**

As soon as 15 seconds after ejaculation.

○ **Can oil-based products be used with female condoms?**

Yes. The synthetic material it is made with (nitrile or polyurethane) is stronger than latex and is less susceptible to deterioration.

○ **When should a diaphragm be inserted?**

Ideally, <2 hours before intercourse. If placed 3 to 6 hours before intercourse, an additional dose of spermicide should be inserted. For every act of intercourse after the diaphragm has been inserted, another dose of spermicide should be placed.

○ **After insertion, how long does the diaphragm provide effective contraception?**

A diaphragm should be left in place for 6 hours following intercourse. For longer intervals, additional spermicide is recommended.

○ **What is the failure rate with diaphragm?**

6% with perfect use, 16% with typical use.

○ **How much spermicide should be used with the cervical cap?**

The dome should be one-third full. Additional spermicide is not necessary for up to 48 hours.

○ **Are female condoms, diaphragms, and caps equally effective for nulliparous and parous women?**

For nulliparous women, yes. For parous women, the cap is less effective.

○ **How frequently should women using cervical caps have Pap smears?**

The FDA recommends a pap after 3 months of use. Otherwise women using vaginal barriers need no special follow-up.

INTRAUTERINE DEVICE (IUD)

○ **What percentage of women use an IUD?**

In the United States, about 7% of contraceptive users chose an IUD. Worldwide, up to 50% of contraceptive users use them.

○ **Who are the candidates of an IUD?**

Candidates of IUD:
- Multiparous and nulliparous women at low risk of STDs
- Women who desire long-term reversible contraception
- Women with the following medical conditions:
  - Diabetes
  - HIV-positive women
  - Immediately postabortal or spontaneous abortion
  - Thromboembolism
  - Menorrhagia/dysmenorrhea—levonorgestrel only preferred
  - Breastfeeding
  - Breast cancer—copper only within first 5 years of diagnosis

○ **What are the contraindications to IUD use?**

- Current pregnancy
- Pelvic inflammatory disease (current or within the past 3 months)
- STDs (current)
- Puerperal or postabortion sepsis (current or within the past 3 months)
- Mucopurulent cervicitis
- Unexplained abnormal uterine bleeding
- Malignancy of the genital tract
- Anatomic abnormalities including bicornuate uterus, cervical stenosis, or fibroids severely distorting the uterine cavity
- Wilson disease, or allergy to any component of the IUD
- Current breast cancer is a contraindication to the levonorgestrel IUD

○ **Is routine screening for STDs (eg, gonorrhea and chlamydia) required before insertion of an IUD?**

Current data do not support routine screening in women at low risk of STDs.

○ **Is antibiotic prophylaxis before IUD insertion recommended?**

Routine use of prophylactic antibiotics at the time of IUD insertion is not recommended.

○ **When should an IUD be removed in a menopausal woman?**

At least 1 year after the cessation of menses.

○ **If actinomyces is found on a Pap smear of an IUD user, what should be done?**

First a culture to confirm the diagnosis. If confirmed, the infection should be treated. The IUD does not have to be removed.

○ **What is the mean menstrual blood loss associated with the copper IUD use?**

70 to 80 mL. This compares with 35 mL for a normal menstrual cycle.

○ **With the progesterone releasing IUD, what is the mean menstrual blood loss?**

25 mL per cycle.

○ **What is the risk of ectopic pregnancy in a woman using an IUD compared with a woman using other forms of contraception or no contraception?**

Because the possibility of pregnancy is reduced, the overall risk of ectopic pregnancy with a failed IUD is only 5%. However if pregnancy does occur with an IUD in place the chances of it being an ectopic are higher than in those who use other forms of contraception or none at all.

○ **Which method of reversible contraception has the highest 1-year continuation rate?**

The IUD. This is because discontinuation necessitates a visit to a health-care facility for removal.

○ **When is a woman using an IUD at greatest risk of PID?**

At insertion and in the first 3 months of use.

○ **What is the rate of IUD expulsion?**

2% to 10% in the first year.

○ **When should the IUD be inserted in the postpartum period?**

Within the first 10 minutes after the placenta delivers, or at 6 to 8 weeks. If the IUD is inserted 1 to 2 days after delivery, the risk of expulsion increases. Women who are immediately postabortal or spontaneous abortion may also have an IUD placed.

○ **For postcoital contraception, when should the IUD be inserted?**

The copper IUD may be used within 120 hours of unprotected intercourse.

○ **What is the incidence of uterine perforation with IUD insertion?**

1/1000. The string may still be visible in the os.

○ **What are the noncontraceptive benefits of the IUD?**

The IUD reduces the risk of endometrial and cervical cancer. The levonorgestrel IUD reduces the risk of PID, reduces dysmenorrhea and menstrual bleeding, can treat endometrial hyperplasia and cancer, and may decrease endometriosis pain. The levonorgestrel IUD can also be used to protect the endometrium in women on estrogen replacement.

REFERENCE

Barone MA, Nazerali H, Cortez M, et al. A prospective study of time and number of ejaculations to azoospermia after vasectomy by ligation and exicision. *J Urology* 2003;170(3):892-96.

CHAPTER 62

Lesbian, Gay, Bisexual, and Transgender Health

Lauren Abern, MD

○ **What is gender identity?**

A person's innate identification as male or female, which may or may not correspond to the person's body or designated sex at birth.

○ **What is sexual orientation?**

Refers to the gender(s) of people an individual is attracted to.

○ **Is a person's sexual orientation distinct from their gender identity?**

Yes. One's gender identity does not imply sexual orientation. For example, a transgender woman (male to female) may be attracted to other women and identify as a lesbian.

○ **What is the definition of transgender?**

It is a broad term used for people whose gender identity or expression differs from their assigned sex and includes transsexuals, cross-dressers, androgynous people, genderqueer, and anyone that identifies as neither female nor male and/or as neither a man nor as a woman. It does not refer to sexual orientation.

○ **What is the definition of transsexual?**

This refers to individuals who seek hormonal and possibly surgical treatment to modify their bodies so they may live full time as members of the sex category opposite to their birth-assigned sex.

○ **What is the definition of female to male?**

This refers to someone who identifies and portrays his gender as male but was identified as female at birth. Also, trans man, or transman.

○ **What is the definition of male to female?**

This refers to someone who identifies and portrays her gender as female but was identified as male at birth. Also, trans woman or transwoman.

○ **What is the definition of genderqueer?**

This refers to someone who defies or does not accept stereotypical gender roles and may choose to live outside expected gender norms. Genderqueer people may or may not partake in hormonal or surgical treatments.

○ **What does it mean to transition?**

Making changes to one's life in order to live in an affirmed gender. This may include social and/or medical changes such as changing one's name, revising legal documents to reflect one's gender identity, taking hormones, or having surgery.

○ **Do the majority of transgender people have genital surgery?**

No. Not all transgender people desire surgery, and many who do cannot afford them.

○ **In regards to fertility, what is important to discuss prior to initiation of hormone therapy?**

Hormone use may reduce fertility and can even cause permanent infertility even if hormones are discontinued. There is a need for good reproductive counseling.

○ **What can transgender women do prior to hormone therapy if they desire a biological child?**

They can utilize sperm banking for potential future use.

○ **What can transgender men do prior to hormone therapy to preserve fertility?**

They can freeze their eggs or embryos for future implantation. Those that do not ovulate on their own after stopping hormone therapy can attempt pregnancy with the eggs or embryos that were preserved prior to treatment. It is important to recognize that not all transgender men regain fertility.

○ **Are transgender people at a higher risk of acquiring HIV?**

Yes, four times the risk is highest in transgender women of color.

○ **Are transgender men on hormones at risk for pregnancy if they have unprotected intercourse with nontransgender men?**

Yes. Even though testosterone reduces their fertility, testosterone is not a form of contraception.

○ **What is the percentage of transgender men who do not receive annual pelvic examinations?**
50%.

○ **What are the reasons for transgender men to not receive annual pelvic examinations?**

Discomfort with the physical examination, lack of money or insurance, lack of a medical provider that they feel comfortable with, and the belief that they do not need pelvic examinations.

○ **What are absolute contraindications to androgen therapy?**

Pregnancy, breastfeeding, uncontrolled coronary artery disease, active endometrial cancer, active known androgen sensitive breast cancer

○　**What are some relative contraindications to androgen therapy?**

Migraines, polycythemia, heart failure, renal failure, history of uterine cancer, history of DVT, and severe hypertension.

○　**What is the half-life of testosterone in the blood?**

70 minutes.

○　**What are some irreversible effects that occur with testosterone?**

Clitoromegaly, deepened voice, and facial and body hair growth.

○　**What are some reversible effects that may occur with testosterone?**

Increased libido, muscle mass, appetite, weight gain, and fluid retention, acne, increased cholesterol, and vaginal dryness.

○　**How often do transgender men need pelvic examinations?**

Annually, regardless of whether they have had a hysterectomy and bilateral salpingo-oophorectomy.

○　**What gynecologic syndrome is seen more frequently in transgender men?**

PCOS.

○　**Up to how many months can it take for a transgender man to become amenorrheic?**

5 months.

○　**Can menses return if a transgender man stops taking testosterone?**

Yes. Therefore, it is possible to get pregnant. Contraception should be initiated if pregnancy is not desired.

○　**If a transgender man has vaginal bleeding after 5 months of testosterone use, what evaluation should be taken?**

Endometrial biopsy and luteinizing hormone (LH) level.

○　**What do low levels of LH indicate in a transgender man with vaginal bleeding?**

Adequate testosterone dosing. Therefore, it is not an inadequate dose that is causing the bleeding.

○　**What can happen to the ovaries of transgender men after years of testosterone use?**

The ovaries develop a PCOS morphology.

○　**For a transgender man on testosterone, what is the benefit of having an oophorectomy?**

The amount of testosterone needed to cause masculinization and amenorrhea can be decreased.

○　**What can help alleviate vaginal dryness in transgender men?**

Vaginal estrogen.

○ **Do transgender men need mammograms if they have had a mastectomy?**

If the patient has a family history, residual tissue, or risk factors, they will need yearly mammograms. All transgender men should continue to have annual chest tissue exams.

○ **After a hysterectomy, do transgender men need Pap smears?**

Only if they have a history of cervical cancer or high-grade cervical dysplasia. If they had a supracervical hysterectomy, then pap guidelines should be followed.

○ **What changes will occur in transgender women using estrogen?**

Gynecomastia, redistribution of fat, reduced testicular volume, and reduced hair growth.

○ **What should be screened for annually in transgender women on estrogen?**

Prolactin levels and visual field examinations to check for prolactinomas.

○ **What are some risk factors that would require a transgender woman to need a mammogram after the age of 50?**

BMI >35, estrogen and progesterone use >5 years, and family history.

○ **Are Pap smears needed in a transgender woman with a neovagina?**

No.

○ **What medication can be used in transgender children to delay puberty?**

Gonadotropin-releasing hormone (GnRH) agonists.

○ **At which tanner stage should GnRH agonists be started in children?**

Tanner Stage 2 of puberty.

○ **Is HIV a contraindication for hormone treatment in transgender individuals?**

No.

○ **What percentage of women in the United States identify as lesbian?**

1.1%.

○ **What percentage of women in the United States identify as bisexual?**

3.5%.

○ **What are some risk factors for bacterial vaginosis in women that have intercourse with women?**

Higher number of lifetime female partners, shared use of vaginally inserted sex toys, and a female partner with bacterial vaginosis.

○ **Should a woman who has intercourse with other women be screened for bacterial vaginosis?**

No.

○ **Should the partner of a woman diagnosed with bacterial vaginosis be treated if they do not have symptoms?**

No.

○ **What percentage of lesbians get Pap smears?**

44% to 56%.

○ **Should Pap smear guidelines differ for lesbians?**

No.

○ **Can HPV be transmitted between two women?**

Yes.

○ **What other sexually transmitted infections can be passed between female partners?**

Trichomoniasis, syphilis, HSV, HIV, and hepatitis.

○ **Should lesbians be screened for *Chlamydia*?**

Yes. Chlamydial infections have been reported in women who have intercourse with other women.

○ **What factors place lesbians at a greater risk of developing gynecologic cancers?**

Smoking, obesity, nulliparity, and less frequent gynecologic examinations.

○ **What are some barriers preventing lesbians from accessing health care?**

Lack of patient education materials aimed at lesbians, lack of knowledge of health-care providers, low socioeconomic status, absence of spousal insurance benefits, and prior negative experiences with the health-care system.

○ **Are lesbians and bisexual women at an increased risk of lung cancer?**

Lesbians are more likely to smoke than heterosexuals. As a result, this places them at an increased risk.

○ **Are lesbians at a higher risk of cervical cancer?**

Lesbians are less likely to get Pap smears, which can result in undiagnosed cervical dysplasia and cancer.

○ **Are lesbians at a higher risk of breast cancer?**

Lesbians are less likely to undergo mammography, which lowers their chances of discovering the cancer in early stages.

○ **What are some of the reasons lesbians and bisexual women are less likely to report domestic violence?**

Fewer services available, threats of being outed, fear of discrimination, and concerns of losing their children in custody battles.

○ **True or False: Lesbian and bisexual women are more likely to abuse alcohol and drugs than straight women.**

True.

○ **What are some of the reasons for lesbians and bisexual women to develop anxiety and depression?**

Rejection by friends and family, lack of health insurance, social stigma, unfavorable treatment by the legal system, hate crimes, and violence and abuse.

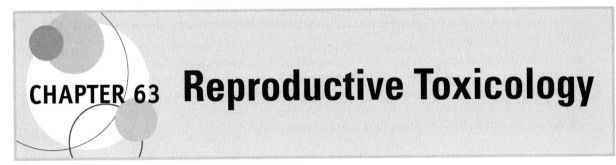

CHAPTER 63 Reproductive Toxicology

Emese Zsiros, MD, PhD

○ **What are the FDA drug labeling categories for use during pregnancy?**

The FDA-assigned five pregnancy categories as used in the Drug Formulary are as follows:

Category A: Adequate and well-controlled studies have failed to demonstrate a risk to the fetus in the first trimester of pregnancy (and there is no evidence of risk in later trimesters).

Category B: Animal reproduction studies have failed to demonstrate a risk to the fetus and there are no adequate and well-controlled studies in pregnant women.

Category C: Animal reproduction studies have shown an adverse effect on the fetus and there are no adequate and well-controlled studies in humans, but potential benefits may warrant use of the drug in pregnant women despite potential risks.

Category D: There is positive evidence of human fetal risk based on adverse reaction data from investigational or marketing experience or studies in humans, but potential benefits may warrant use of the drug in pregnant women despite potential risks.

Category X: Studies in animals or humans have demonstrated fetal abnormalities and/or there is positive evidence of human fetal risk based on adverse reaction data from investigational or marketing experience, and the risks involved in use of the drug in pregnant women clearly outweigh potential benefits.

○ **What is the risk of birth defect in the general US population?**

Every woman in the general population has a 3% risk of having a child with a birth defect. Birth defect is the leading cause of infant mortality in the United States, accounting for 20.1% of all infant deaths.

○ **A 21-year-old female requests counseling because she was taking birth control pills without knowing she was pregnant. What do you tell her?**

Extensive epidemiologic studies have revealed no increased risk of birth defects in women who have used oral contraceptives prior or during pregnancy. It is recommended for any patient who has missed her period that pregnancy should be ruled out before continuing oral contraceptive use. Oral contraceptive use should be discontinued if pregnancy is confirmed.

○ **Patient comes to the office complaining that she got pregnant with her recently placed intrauterine device (IUD). How do you advise her?**

Among IUD users, there are on average about 6 pregnancies per 1000 woman-years. The rare intrauterine pregnancies that occur in women using an IUD generally end in miscarriage. About 25% of these pregnancies end in a live birth if the device is left in place, compared with about 90% if the device is removed. Early IUD removal appeared to improve outcomes but did not entirely eliminate risks. Ectopic pregnancies are rarer in IUD users than in women who do not use contraception. However, about 1 in 20 pregnancies that occur in women using an IUD is ectopic.

○ **Is the spermicide nonoxynol-9 a teratogen?**

No. Literature demonstrates that vaginal spermicide use before or during pregnancy is not associated with increased rates of pregnancy loss or abnormal offspring.

○ **Your patient with a history of infertility conceived with clomiphene citrate (CC) and now she is concerned the potential risk of birth defect associated with the use of medication. How do you counsel her?**

In the United States an estimated 1.6% of pregnancies are conceived with the use of CC, reflecting >67,000 exposed pregnancies per year. Two types of birth defects that have been most commonly reported to be associated with CC exposure are neural tube defects and hypospadias; however, results regarding the association between CC and these birth defects have been inconsistent. Because of the small number of cases, the inconsistency of some findings and the potential unknown reason of subfertility, these associations should be interpreted cautiously.

○ **What is pica?**

Pica is an *appetite* for non-nutritive substances or food ingredients (eg, ice, *coal, soil, chalk,* flour, raw potato, and starch). Symptoms must persist for >1 month. Pica is seen in all ages, particularly common in *pregnant women.* The condition's name comes from the *Latin* word for the *magpie,* a bird that is reputed to eat almost anything.

○ **Does the month of contraception matter in the United States in respect to birth defect?**

Birth defect rates in the Unites States were found to be highest for women conceiving in the spring and summer (maternal LMPs in April–July). This increase was significant for 11 of the 22 categories of birth defects reported in the CDC natality database from 1996 to 2002. This has been attributed to elevated concentrations of agrichemicals (nitrates, atrazine, and other pesticides) in surface water during those months.

○ **What advice do you give pregnant women about fish consumption?**

According to the U.S. Food and Drug Administration and the Environmental Protection Agency, a pregnant woman can safely eat up to 12 ounces (two average meals) a week of a variety of fish and shellfish. Nearly all fish contain trace amounts of methyl mercury, which are not harmful to humans. However, long-lived, larger fish that feed on other fish accumulate the highest levels of methyl mercury and pose the greatest risk to people who eat them regularly. Hence, pregnant and nursing women and also young children should not eat the following fish:

    Shark
    Swordfish
    King mackerel
    Tilefish

○ **What are the major adverse effects of smoking during pregnancy?**

The Surgeon General warns women of the dangers of smoking on every pack they buy. Smoking causes intrauterine growth restriction (IUGR) and increases the incidence of preterm delivery in a dose-dependent manner. The incidence of placenta previa, abruptio placentae, and spontaneous abortion also increased in smokers.

○ **A patient asks you about caffeine intake during pregnancy. What do you tell her?**

Studies about the effects of caffeine on pregnancy report conflicting results. Of the studies that do show that caffeine is harmful to pregnancy, the effects seem to be most significant when caffeine intake is >300 mg/day (about three cups of coffee per day). Caffeine may be associated with IUGR when consumed in these quantities.

○ **Is the hot tub or sauna dangerous to pregnancy?**

The American College of Obstetricians and Gynecologists (ACOG) states that becoming overheated in a hot tub or sauna is not recommended during pregnancy and its use in the first trimester is associated with neural tube defect (RR 2.8). The ACOG also recommends that pregnant women never let their core body temperature rise above 102.2° F. If a pregnant woman wishes to use the hot tub, then its temperature should be lowered, and she should not spend >10 minutes in the warm water.

○ **What are the special concerns of flying during pregnancy?**

The ACOG recommends women not to fly after their 36th week of pregnancy. Airlines have their own flight restrictions for pregnant women, which can vary according to whether she is flying domestically or internationally. Most airlines won't take pregnant women past 36 weeks, even on short-haul flights of 2 hours, and most of the travel insurance won't cover her late in pregnancy, usually from around 32 weeks.

Also a single, long international flight due to thinner portion of the atmosphere increases radiation exposure to a week's worth of natural background radiation, however, is far from a health concern, even for pregnant women. But aviation workers can easily exceed the recommended safe limits, which is 20 millisieverts (mSV) a year. (For scale, a person at ground level gets about 2.4 mSv of natural background radiation a year.) Other risks from flying result from cramped seating, dehydration, which increases the risk of deep vein thrombosis.

○ **Your dermatologist colleague asks you if he can prescribe tetracycline to a pregnant patient for her severe acne. What do you advise him?**

Tetracycline and its derivatives should not be used after 16 weeks' gestation and in childhood up to the age of 8 due to its effects on calcium-containing tissue, particularly teeth. Tetracycline might cause permanent discoloration of the teeth (yellow or brown) and enamel hypoplasia (a small pit or dent in the tooth or can be widespread that the entire tooth is small and/or mis-shaped). There are no adequate and well-controlled studies in pregnant women regarding the topical use of tetracycline solutions; however, animal studies have shown no harm to the fetus with topical applications.

○ **Your pregnant patient is complaining of severe acne and asks your advice on safe treatment options. What do you recommend?**

Many women have trouble with acne during pregnancy because of overproduction of sebum due to hormonal changes. Acne treatment in pregnancy starts with self-care, such as cleaning the face twice a day with lukewarm water and avoiding resting hand on the face or picking/scratching acne sores. Patient should be advised to use oil-free cosmetics that are noncomedogenic.

Second-line treatment involves topical erythromycin (Erygel), which is the drug of choice for pregnancy acne. Azelaic acid (Azelex, Finacea) may be another topical option. Opinions about using benzoyl peroxide to treat pregnancy acne are mixed and its potential teratogenic risk is undetermined, but there are no case reports about benzoyl peroxide and birth defects in the literature.

○ **What should you tell the patient who is thinking about starting an isotretinoin (Accutane) treatment of her acne?**

Patients who are taking oral isotretinoin treatment, even for short periods of time, have an extremely high risk of severe birth defects. Before prescribing Accutane the patient must had a negative pregnancy test and sign the she understands that she must not get pregnant 1 month before, during the entire time of her treatment as well as for 1 month after the end of her treatment. She must avoid sexual intercourse completely or she must use two separate effective forms of *birth control* at the same time.

○ **Describe the pattern of congenital malformations caused by isotretinoin (Accutane).**

Affected offspring develop severe ear defects, cardiovascular anomalies (conotruncal malformations), CNS defects, and disturbances in development of the thymus. Another retinoid, vitamin A when ingested in quantities >10,000 IU/day has also been shown to increase the incidence of cranioneurofacial anomalies in exposed fetuses. Beta-carotene (a vitamin A precursor) is safe in pregnancy.

○ **Is topical retinoid treatment also teratogenic?**

There are no adequate and well-controlled studies in pregnant women regarding the teratogenic effect of topical retinoid treatment; however, applied at higher doses resulted malformations in rats and rabbits (Category C). Thus, this only should be used during pregnancy if the potential benefit justifies the potential risk to the fetus.

○ **What is the current recommendation treating epilepsy during pregnancy?**

According to studies, 90% of the pregnant women on antiepileptic medication deliver normal infants. Antiepileptic drugs (AEDs) should not be discontinued in patient in whom the drug is administered to prevent major seizures, because of the strong possibility of precipitating status epilepticus. All commonly used AEDs have been associated with congenital malformations, although some of the newer anticonvulsants have not been used in large enough numbers to have meaningful data. In general, using multiple agents at higher doses is associated with the increased incidence of birth defects. A single anticonvulsant at the lowest possible dose for efficacy is recommended whenever possible.

○ **Is the antiepileptic phenytoin (Dilantin) safe in pregnancy?**

Children of women receiving phenytoin can develop fetal hydantoin syndrome. This consists of prenatal growth deficiency, microcephaly, mental retardation nail and digit hypoplasia, and midfacial abnormalities. Some of the AEDs' side effect is related to folate deficiency. Phenytoin, carbamazepine, barbiturates, and valproate are linked to folate malabsorption or they interfere with folate metabolism. Thus, increased dose of folic acid supplementation (4 mg daily) prior to conception and during pregnancy is recommended to patients who are using seizure medicines such as phenytoin (Dilantin, Phenytek), carbamazepine (Tegretol, Tegretol XR, Carbatrol), and phenobarbital. The same applies to women who take at least 1000 mg per day of Depakote (valproate).

○ **What is folate deficiency associated with pregnancy? What is the recommended folate intake during pregnancy?**

Folate deficiency is associated with neural tube defects (ie, spina bifida and anencephaly). Women of reproductive age should ingest 400 μg of folate per day. If they have had a child with neural tube defect in the past, they should take 4 mg of folate daily periconceptionally. Ideally women should start folate supplementation prior to trying to conceive.

○ **Is lithium use for manic depression indicted in pregnancy?**

Lithium is a category D drug and its use in the first trimester can result in Ebstein anomaly (tricuspid value is abnormal and has only two leaflets). Although there is a strong association between the drug and the cardiac lesion, it is very rare and does not warrant routine pregnancy termination.

○ **How does thalidomide affect the developing fetus?**

Thalidomide is a *sedative, hypnotic,* and *anti-inflammatory medication,* which was prescribed during the late 1950s and early 1960s to *pregnant* women as an *antiemetic* to combat *morning sickness* as well as a sleep aid. It was sold in almost 50 countries under at least 40 names, including Distaval, Talimol, Nibrol, Sedimide, Quietoplex, Contergan, Neurosedyn, and Softenon. From 1956 to 1962, approximately 10,000 children were born with severe malformations, about 5000 survived beyond childhood. Malformations were amelia (absence of limbs), phocomelia (short limbs), hypoplasticity of the bones, absence of bones, external ear abnormalities, facial palsy, eye abnormalities, and congenital heart defects, because their mothers had taken thalidomide during pregnancy. The medication never received approval for sale in the United States, but 2.5 million tablets had been given to >1200 American doctors during Richardson-Merrell "investigation," and nearly 20,000 patients received thalidomide tablets, including several hundred pregnant women. In the end, 17 American children were born with thalidomide-related deformities.

○ **What is the mechanism behind thalidomide-induced teratogenesis?**

The mechanism of action of thalidomide is not fully understood. Thalidomide possesses immunomodulatory, anti-inflammatory, and anti-angiogenic properties. Available data from in vitro studies and clinical trials suggest that the immunologic effects of this compound can vary substantially under different conditions, but may be related to suppression of excessive tumor necrosis factor-alpha (TNF-α) production and down-modulation of selected cell surface adhesion molecules involved in leukocyte migration. Thalidomide is racemic—it contains both left- and right-handed *isomers* in equal amounts. One *enantiomer* is effective against morning sickness. The other is *teratogenic* and causes birth defects.

○ **Is thalidomide still on the market in some countries?**

Yes. Thalidomide is currently used in three countries: Mexico, Brazil, and in the United States. The current indication of thalidomide use is erythema nodosum leprosum (ENL), a severe and debilitating complication of leprosy (Hansen's disease) and multiple myeloma. Effective contraception must be used for at least 4 weeks before beginning thalidomide therapy, during thalidomide therapy, and for 4 weeks following discontinuation of thalidomide therapy.

○ **What are the risks of amphetamine use during pregnancy?**

Infants born to mothers dependent on amphetamines have an increased risk of premature delivery and low birth weight. Also, these infants may experience symptoms of withdrawal as demonstrated by *dysphoria,* agitation, and significant *lassitude.* However, there is no known association with structural abnormalities.

○ **Are all social and illicit drugs associated with increased rates of placental abruption?**

No. Only cocaine and smoking are known to cause increased rates of placental abruption. Alcohol, coffee, heroin, marijuana, and amphetamines have no such association.

○ **Does amphetamine use in pregnancy cause congenital abnormalities?**

Amphetamine use in pregnancy has not been associated with congenital abnormalities; however, its use correlates to a reduction in birth weight, prematurity, postpartum hemorrhage, and retained placenta. Because of anorectic impact of the drug, amphetamines may severely affect maternal nutrition.

○ **How does cocaine affect pregnancy?**

The most common complication caused by cocaine during pregnancy is abruptio placentae due to vasoconstriction and extreme high blood pressures. In addition, brain anomalies, intestinal atresia, congenital heart defects, and limb reductions have been described. Cocaine may cause these effects by vasoconstrictions and subsequent infarction.

○ **What is the neonatal abstinence syndrome, and what agents cause it?**

It is caused by maternal heroin addiction or maternal methadone treatment during pregnancy. It results from neonatal withdrawal and consists of tremulousness, hyper-reflexia, high pitch cry, sneezing, sleepiness, tachypnea, yawning, sweating, fever, and seizures. The onset of symptoms is at birth.

○ **What is fetal alcohol syndrome?**

Infants suffer from IUGR, mental retardation, and develop characteristic facies, which consists of short palpebral fissures, a flat midface, a thin upper lip, and hypoplastic philtrum.

○ **At what time during gestation is the fetus most susceptible to alcohol toxicity?**

Probably in the second and third trimesters. In a study of 60 women, those who were heavy drinkers but stopped after the first trimester had children with normal mentation and behavioral patterns.

○ **Your 28-year-old pregnant patient expresses concerns about the ultrasound examination you have prescribed. How do you counsel her?**

Ultrasound has no documented harmful effect on developing fetuses with the use of current ultrasound techniques. High-level ultrasound energy could potentially cause harm to the fetus by two mechanisms—thermal damage and cavitation. However, these effects are not seen at the low levels of ultrasound energy used during diagnostic studies.

○ **What recommendations would you make to a woman who requires a magnetic resonance imaging (MRI) study during pregnancy?**

MRI has not been shown to be harmful in pregnancy. However, based on a lack of evidence that supports the safety of MRI during pregnancy, the National Radiological Protection Board has recommended that women in the first 3 months of pregnancy be excluded from MRI examinations. There is no evidence to recommend termination of pregnancy after an inadvertent first trimester exposure.

○ **What is the time of gestation during which a fetus is most susceptible to the effects of ionizing radiation?**

The fetus is most susceptible to radiation between 8 and 15 weeks of gestation. Before 8 weeks if the exposure does not result in a spontaneous abortion, the fetus will be unaffected. Between 16 and 25 weeks postfertilization, the fetus is less vulnerable to radiation effects. After the 26th week of pregnancy, the radiation sensitivity of the unborn baby is similar to that of a newborn.

○ **How would a significant radiation exposure affect a fetus?**

Doses of >100 rads (cGy) have been associated with microcephaly, which may or may not be associated with mental retardation. Growth retardation is also seen in exposed fetuses. From epidemiologic and animal studies, it does not appear that exposures of <10 rads could affect a pregnancy at any gestational age.

○ **Does radiation from diagnostic studies present a risk to pregnant women?**

Aside from the emotional distress induced by this exposure, probably not. The risk of teratogenesis with exposures of <5 rads is minuscule. The following table presents radiation doses presented to the uterus by various radiographic procedures.

Study	View	Dose/Study (mrad)
Chest	AP and lateral	0.05
Abdomen	AP and lateral	125
IVP		1000
Upper GI series		50
Barium enema		2000–4000
CT abdomen		2500

○ **Pregnant patient in her second trimester presents to the emergency room with acute abdominal pain. She is refusing any imaging studies and asks about the risks of radiation. How would you counsel her?**

The potential risks of in utero radiation exposure of a developing fetus include prenatal death, IUGR, small head size, mental retardation, organ malformation, and childhood cancer. The risk of each effect depends on the gestational age at the time of exposure, fetal cellular repair mechanisms, and the absorbed radiation dose level. However, in general from typical radiologic examinations the fetal risks are minimal and, therefore, that radiologic and nuclear medicine examinations that may provide significant diagnostic information should not be withheld from pregnant women.

○ **What immunizations are contraindicated during pregnancy?**

In general, live virus vaccines are contraindicated during pregnancy. These include measles, mumps, rubella, varicella, and yellow fever. However, all toxoids, immunoglobulins, and killed virus vaccines are considered safe in pregnancy and should not be withheld, if indicated.

○ **What is the current recommendation for giving influenza vaccine to pregnant women?**

The influenza vaccine is an inactivated live vaccine and so far no risks from immunization have been described. According to the current ACOG guidelines, all women who are pregnant in the second and third trimester during the flu season (October-March) and women at high risk of pulmonary complications regardless of the trimester should receive the influenza vaccination.

○ **Is breastfeeding a contraindication to immunization?**

Breastfeeding is not a contraindication to immunizations. Live and inactivated vaccines and toxoids can all be given during this time.

○ **What are the hazardous effects of rubella vaccination during embryogenesis?**

Even though the vaccine contains live attenuated virus, there are no known cases of congenital rubella syndrome (malformations of the heart and CNS, deafness, cataracts, mental retardation) as a consequence of inadvertent vaccination during early pregnancy. However, to be safe, all women receiving the vaccine should be advised to postpone pregnancy for 3 months.

○   **Is varicella infection during pregnancy innocuous?**

No. Varicella (chicken pox) is a known teratogen. Maternal infection in the first half of pregnancy results in congenital varicella syndrome in 1% to 5% of cases. This syndrome consists of CNS and skeletal abnormalities and mental retardation. Maternal varicella infection late in pregnancy (within 5 days before and after delivery) may result in chicken pox skin lesions, pneumonia, and other complications. Approximately 30% of infected children develop disseminated disease.

○   **What factors affect the ability of a drug or a chemical to cross the placenta and reach the embryo?**

These include molecular weight, lipid solubility, degree of ionization, and protein binding. Compounds with low molecular weight, high lipid affinity, low degree of ionization, and low protein binding affinity will cross the placenta easily and rapidly. Also placental blood flow, pH gradient between the maternal and fetal serum and tissues, and placental metabolism of the chemical significantly affect drug transport.

○   **How does pregnancy affect an individual's susceptibility to toxins?**

Increased ventilation enhances absorption of toxic gasses.

Progesterone decreases gut motility and may enhance absorption of certain agents.

Hypoalbuminuria results in decreased serum protein binding and thus increased bioavailability of protein-bound toxins.

Increased GFR may increase clearance of some agents.

Increased blood volume and body fat results in increased distribution and sequestration

○   **What criteria are necessary to establish that a drug or chemical exposure causes congenital abnormalities?**

Epidemiologic studies should consistently display an adverse association in exposed individuals.

Secular trends consistently display a relationship between the incidence of a particular malformation and human exposures. An animal model mimics the human malformation at clinically comparable exposures. The teratogenic effects should increase in relation to the dose.

The observed teratogenic effect should be consistent with biologic and scientific principles of occurrence.

○   **In general, during which time during pregnancy is the fetus most susceptible to teratogens?**

During the embryonic period, this lasts from 2 to 12 weeks postconception. This is the time of organogenesis.

○   **What are the fetal toxic effects of the agents listed in the left hand column?**

1.	Benzodiazepines	A.	Orofacial clefting
2.	Lithium	B.	Epstein anomaly
3.	Valproic acid	C.	Neural tube defects
4.	DES	D.	Vaginal adenosis, uterine malformations
5.	ACE inhibitors	E.	Renal dysplasia

○   **What are the categories of fetal development defects?**

There are malformations, disruptions, and deformations.

○ **What are malformations, disruptions, and deformations?**

A *malformation* is a defect that results from a developmental process, which has been abnormal from the beginning of conception at very early in the life of the embryo. Its impact may be seen in a single or in multiple developmental regions.

A *disruption* is a developmental defect that results from an intrinsic or extrinsic factor that interferes with the originally normal development process. In the absence of the effects of this factor, the development would have been normal. It cannot be inherited.

A *deformation* is an abnormal form, shape, or position of a part of the body due to the effect of mechanical force acting on that area during development.

○ **What are the differences between a sequence, syndrome, and association?**

A *sequence* is multiple anomalies resulting from a single known of presumed malformation, deformation, or disruption.

A *syndrome* is multiple anomalies due to a single malformation.

An *association* is the occurrence of multiple anomalies associated with a known or unknown malformation in two or more people.

○ **What steps are required to assess a person's risk of an adverse reproductive outcome?**

The first step is identifying whether the agent can cause a defect, and if so, the type of defect caused. The next step is characterization of the hazard to assess the critical amount of an exposure needed to produce the result being studied. Thirdly, the degree, type, and timing of the exposure are identified. Finally, how likely it is that the defect resulted from the exposure being studied and not from other internal or external causes or from chance.

○ **What does the word *teratogenesis* mean?**

Teratogenesis is a medical term, literally meaning *monster-birth*, which derives from teratology, the study of the frequency, causation, and development of congenital malformations—misleadingly called *birth defects*. Teratogenesis has gained a more specific usage for the development of abnormal cell masses during fetal growth, causing physical defects in the fetus. The study of teratogenesis is called teratology.

○ **What are Wilson general principles of teratology?**

The Six Principles of Teratology provides a framework for understanding how structural or functional teratogens act. These principles were developed by James G. Wilson and are as follows:

(1) Susceptibility to teratogenesis depends on the genotype of the conceptus and the manner in which this interacts with environmental factors.

(2) Susceptibility to teratogenic agents varies with the developmental stage at the time of exposure.

(3) Teratogenic agents act in specific ways (mechanisms) on developing *cells* and tissues to initiate abnormal embryogenesis (pathogenesis);

(4) The final manifestations of abnormal development are death, malformation, growth retardation, and functional disorder.

(5) The access of adverse environmental influences to developing tissue depends on the nature of the influences (agent).

(6) Manifestations of deviant development increase in degree as dosage increases from the no-effect to the totally lethal level.

○ **What are the adverse reproductive outcomes associated with occupational and environmental exposure?**

These include infertility, single gene defects, chromosome abnormalities, spontaneous abortions, congenital malformation, IUGR, perinatal deaths, developmental disabilities, behavioral disorders, and malignancies.

○ **What is "recall bias" in reproductive toxicology?**

Women with an adverse pregnancy outcome such as spontaneous abortion, fetal or neonatal demise, or a congenital malformation are more likely to recall exposure to environmental or occupational or infectious agents. However, those with satisfactory pregnancy outcomes tend to forget such exposures.

○ **What is "selection bias" in reproductive toxicology?**

When studying a particular outcome or teratogenic agent, there are potential problems that can affect the interpretation of reported results. Some examples include (i) inaccurate or incomplete information about single or multiple exposures and confounding exposures, (ii) incomplete, inaccurate or absent survey responses, (iii) not validating the reproductive history, (iv) recall bias, (v) inaccurate methods of data collection, and (vi) investigators' bias toward one of the possible outcomes of a study.

○ **Who is more susceptible to carbon monoxide (CO) poisoning, a mother or her fetus?**

The fetus. CO causes toxicity by asphyxiation. It binds to hemoglobin to form carboxyhemoglobin (COHb). Fetal COHb levels tend to be 10–15% higher than maternal levels. If a woman has a significant enough exposure to cause unconsciousness, >50% of fetuses will die in utero and the many of the remainder suffer from significant impairment.

○ **How do you treat a patient with suspected CO poisoning?**

High-dose O_2 displaces CO from Hb and causes it to diffuse out of tissues. Hyperbaric oxygen therapy will more significantly reduce the half-life of CO in the bloodstream and it is the treatment of choice when available. The half-life of CO in maternal blood is approximately 230 minutes and it is longer in the fetus. The half-life is reduced to 90 minutes with 100% and can be safely reduced to <30 minutes with hyperbaric oxygen therapy.

○ **What maternal blood level of lead is toxic to her fetus?**

Maternal blood lead levels as low as 10 μg/mL have been linked to neurobehavioral disturbances in their offspring. The CDC has defined blood levels above 25 μg/mL as elevated, because this is when toxic effects are seen in adults, but the fetus appears to be more susceptible to lead poisoning.

○ **What effect does lead have on the human body?**

Lead can affect multiple organ systems and may cause death in adults when blood concentrations exceed 300 μg/mL. The central nervous system, GI tract, kidneys, joints, and reproductive systems may all be affected. Studies vary whether lead causes structural malformations in exposed fetuses, but it is clear that lead causes learning disabilities and other behavioral disturbances.

○ **Which women today are most at risk of mercury poisoning?**

Fish-eaters. The only real human exposure to organic mercury is through consumption of fish. Fetuses are more susceptible to toxic effects of mercury than their maternal hosts, so extra care must be taken when working with pregnant patients. Large exposures to methyl mercury have resulted in infants with microcephaly, mental retardation, cerebral palsy, and blindness.

○ **Is working as a medical resident harmful during pregnancy?**

Overall, residency training has not been shown to cause spontaneous abortion, preterm birth, or low birth weight. However, when women worked >100 hours/week, preterm birth rate was slightly increased. Mild preeclampsia that was not associated with adverse pregnancy outcome was also increased in women residents.

○ **Should pregnant anesthetists and nurses be allowed to administer anesthetic agents?**

Yes. Provided there is adequate ventilation and a functioning gas scavenger system in the operating room so that any possible fumes or vapors are quickly dissipated to the outside environment.

○ **What are the major reproductive hazards facing pregnant health-care worker?**

Working with antineoplastic and carcinogenic drugs in improperly ventilated areas has been associated with increased risk of pregnancy loss and congenital anomalies. Anesthetic agents may increase the risk of pregnancy loss, but do not appear to increase malformation rates. Infectious diseases such as hepatitis and HIV pose a risk to workers and their fetuses. Chemical sterilants widely used in operating rooms, pharmacies, and laboratories may have reproductive toxicity. Lastly, the stress on residents imposed by long working hours may increase the risk of preterm delivery and preeclampsia.

○ **To which toxins are a ceramic artist or a painter exposed?**

Ceramics artists and painters may be exposed to lead and other heavy metals. Kilns emit toxic gases including CO. In general, you won't know what her exposures are at work or at home if you don't ask!

○ **In which occupation do workers face the greatest risk of job-related violence?**

In a 1996 report, OSHA stated that more assaults occur against health-care workers and social workers than in any other industry. Pregnancy does not offer any protection against violence.

○ **What is the primary problem facing women who become pregnant while living at high altitude (>1600 m)?**

IUGR. The average birth weight decreases by 100 g per 100 m of elevation for term pregnancies. Smoking appears to exacerbate the effects of high altitude on fetal growth. As far as traveling, it seems probable that a 2-week visit to moderate altitude (<3000 m) is unlikely to affect the final birth weight of a baby.

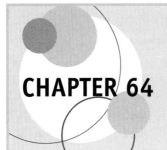

CHAPTER 64

Basic Epidemiology and Clinical Biostatistics

Mary C. Naglak, PhD, RD

The purpose of this chapter is to familiarize the reader with the basic principles of descriptive and analytic epidemiology, as well as basic clinical biostatistics.

○ **Define epidemiology.**

Epidemiology is the study of the distribution and determinants of disease in human populations. There are two types of epidemiology: descriptive and analytic.

○ **How is epidemiology applied to obstetrics and gynecology?**

Epidemiology can be used for descriptive purposes, such as surveillance of the occurrence (incidence) of a particular illness. It can also be used for analytic purposes, such as studying risk factors for disease development. Epidemiologic methods can be used to assess the performance of diagnostic tests, determine the progression or natural history of a disease, study prognostic factors, and evaluate treatments for a disease.

○ **What are risk factors?**

Risk factors are attributes or agents suspected to be related to the occurrence of a particular disease.

○ **Define epidemic.**

An epidemic is a sudden and great increase in the occurrence of a disease within a population.

○ **Define pandemic.**

A pandemic is a rapidly emerging disease outbreak that affects a wide range of a geographically distributed population.

○ **What does the phrase "sentinel cases" refer to?**

The first few affected patients identified in a disease outbreak are referred to as sentinel cases.

○ **What does it take for a disease outbreak to occur?**

A pathogen of sufficient quantity, a susceptible population, and a mode of transmission.

○ **Define attack rate of a disease outbreak.**

It is the number of persons affected by the disease among the persons at risk of the disease.
It is calculated as follows:
Attack rate (AR) = (number of new cases/persons at risk) × 100

○ **What are the two primary modes of transmission of a disease outbreak?**

Disease can be spread *person-to-person* and by *common sources of exposure* (contact with a risk factor originating in a shared environment of people).

○ **When should a disease outbreak be investigated?**

Consideration should be given to the number and severity of affected persons, an unknown, cause and public health concerns.

○ **What is the term used for the time duration from diagnosis to death?**

Survival time; the median survival time is the duration of time from diagnosis to death that is exceeded by 50% of subjects with a particular disease.

○ **How is "survival" defined in epidemiologic terms?**

Survival is the likelihood of remaining alive for a specified period of time after the diagnosis of a particular disease. It can be estimated as follows:

S = A-D/A where S is survival, *A* is the number of newly diagnosed patients under observation, and *D* is the number of deaths observed in a specified period of time. It can be expressed as a decimal or converted to the corresponding percentage.

○ **How do you define premature death?**

Premature death measures the years of potential life lost to a particular disease.

○ **Define descriptive epidemiology.**

Descriptive epidemiology includes activities related to characterizing the distribution of diseases in a population.

○ **What is disease frequency?**

Disease frequency is the amount of disease or morbidity in a population expressed as incidence or prevalence.

○ **What types of measures are used to describe disease frequency?**

Incidence rate, prevalence, and risk are used to describe disease frequency.

Incidence rate measures how rapid newly affected cases of the disease of interest develop. It is useful for tracking changes in the occurrence of disease over time. It can be calculated as follows:

IR = A/PT, where IR is incidence rate, *A* is the number of *new cases* of the disease in a population, and PT is the measure of net time that persons in the population at risk of developing the disease is observed. PT is also known as person time; usually expressed as number of cases per 100,000 per year.

Prevalence is the proportion of a population that is affected by a disease or condition at a given time. It includes *new, existing, and recurring cases* in a population. It can be calculated as follows:

P = C/N; where P is prevalence, *C* is the number of *new, existing, and recurring cases* at a given point in time, and *N* is the total population at risk.

Risk is the likelihood or probability that a person will contract a disease. A simple formula for calculating this is as follows:

R = A/N where R is risk, *A* is the number of *newly* affected persons, and *N* is the number of unaffected persons under observation.

○ **How is the number of newly diagnosed cases per year for a disease determined?**

Numbers of newly diagnosed cases are affected by (1) the frequency with which the disease occurs, (2) how the disease is defined, (3) the size of the population from which cases develop, and (4) completeness of case reporting.

○ **Why is disease screening performed?**

It is done in order to detect a disease at an earlier stage than would occur through routine methods. Screening can detect people who either have a disease that can be treated in the early stages or those individuals at high risk of the disease who would benefit from early intervention to reduce risk of developing the disease.

○ **Why is it important for a screening test to be reliable and valid?**

A reliable test gives the same results when the test is repeated on the same person several times; results are reproducible. A valid test measures what it is designed to measure. A reliable and valid screening test minimizes the number of false-positive and false-negative test results.

○ **How is the validity of a screening test assessed?**

Sensitivity and specificity are used to assess the validity of a screening test. Sensitivity is the proportion of people with a disease or condition with a positive test result. Specificity is the proportion of people without a disease or condition with a negative test result. The goal is to maximize both sensitivity and specificity to minimize false positives and false negatives. Sensitivity and specificity are also used to assess diagnostic tests.

○ **What is the predictive value and how does it relate to a screening test?**

The predictive value of a test is the ability of the test to accurately distinguish people with and without a disease or condition. The positive predictive value is the probability of disease given a positive test result. The negative predictive value is the probability of no disease or condition given a negative test result. Positive and negative predictive values are also used to assess diagnostic tests.

○ **What is a likelihood ratio?**

Unlike predictive values, likelihood ratios are not influenced by the prevalence of the disease in the population being studied. A positive likelihood ratio is how likely it is to obtain a given test result among people with the disease. A negative likelihood ratio is how likely it is to obtain a given test result among people without the disease.

○ **What is a likelihood ratio nomogram?**

A likelihood ratio nomogram is a graphical scale used to determine the posttest probability of disease. It utilizes the likelihood ratio of a diagnostic test and the pretest probability of a disease (disease prevalence in a population) to determine the posttest probability of a patient having the disease.

○ **What is an ROC curve used for?**

A receiver operating characteristic (ROC) curve is used to evaluate the properties of a diagnostic test. It is a plot of the true-positives (sensitivity) on the y-axis and the false-positives (1-specificity) on the x-axis. The area under the ROC curve (AUC) is calculated and compared to 1. Values closest to 1 indicate a good diagnostic test.

○ **What biases are present in the screening process?**

The three types of bias present in the screening process are volunteer (selection) bias, lead-time bias, and length-time bias. Volunteer bias refers to the fact that volunteers tend to be better educated and in better health than the general population. Lead-time bias refers to the increased survival duration introduced by early recognition of the disease (lead-time) through the screening process. Length-time bias refers to the fact that screening preferentially identifies more slowly progressing diseases that tend to have a better prognosis.

○ **How are patterns of disease occurrence characterized in epidemiology studies?**

Patterns of disease are characterized by person, place, and time.

○ **What study designs are used for descriptive epidemiology studies?**

Correlational studies, case-reports or case-series, surveys, and surveillance studies. The results of descriptive epidemiology studies can form hypotheses for analytic research.

○ **What are correlational studies?**

Correlational studies are used to identify associations between risk or causative factors and disease. They cannot determine causation.

○ **What are case-reports or case-series?**

A case-report is a unique experience of one patient. A case-series is a small group of patients with a similar diagnosis.

○ **What are survey studies?**

Survey studies provide an overview of people studied at one point in time for a wide variety of descriptive information. Survey data cannot answer questions about disease etiology.

○ **What is disease surveillance?**

Disease surveillance refers to a systematic method for monitoring patterns of disease occurrence and health outcomes in a population.

○ **What is SEER?**

SEER is an acronym for Surveillance, Epidemiology, and End Results program. It is a population-based registry utilized and managed by the U.S. National Cancer Institute as one way of monitoring the incidence of cancer by geographic area.

○ **Define analytic epidemiology.**

Analytic epidemiology attempts to explain possible causes for the occurrence of a disease.

○ **Analytic epidemiology must first establish if an association exists between a specific factor and the disease in question. What are measures of association?**

Relative risk (RR), odds ratio (OR), attributable risk (AR), and population attributable risk (PAR) are all measures of association.

○ **How is RR calculated?**

RR is the cumulative incidence in the exposed subjects divided by the cumulative incidence in the unexposed subjects.

○ **How is OR calculated?**

The OR is the number of exposed cases times the number of unexposed controls divided by the number of unexposed cases times the number of exposed controls.

○ **How is AR calculated?**

AR is the cumulative incidence in the exposed subjects minus the cumulative incidence in the unexposed subjects.

○ **How is PAR calculated?**

PAR is the cumulative incidence in the population (exposed and unexposed) minus the cumulative incidence in the unexposed.

○ **What study designs are used to study associations?**

Observational study designs are used to study association. Observational study designs include cohort studies, cross-sectional studies, surveillance studies, and case-control studies (see definitions below).

○ **What is causation?**

A possible causal relationship is suggested when studies of disease provide evidence for a significant association between a specific factor and a disease outcome. *Experimental studies* are designed to test whether a causal relationship exists between a specific factor and the disease.

○ **What types of experimental study designs are used to study causation?**

Experimental study designs used to study causation include randomized controlled trials (RCTs), group-randomized trials, and multicenter RCTs (see definitions below).

○ **What issues decrease the strength of analytic epidemiology studies?**

Selection bias, incidence-prevalence bias, measurement bias, confounders, and effect modifiers can all decrease the strength of studies.

○ **What is selection (volunteer) bias?**

Selection (volunteer) bias refers to the differences between characteristics of people selected for a study and those who are not selected. For example, volunteers for a study tend to be healthier and better educated.

○ **What is incidence-prevalence bias?**

Incidence-prevalence bias occurs where there is a loss of cases (by death or recovery) due to significant periods of time between exposure and development of the disease or condition.

○ **What is measurement bias?**

Measurement bias occurs when individual measurements or classifications of disease or exposure are inaccurate.

○   **What are confounders?**

Confounding relationships are relationships where the factor of interest is related to another factor that is also influencing the outcome of interest.

○   **What are effect modifiers (or interactions)?**

An effect modifier (or interaction) is a third variable that alters the association between an exposure and a disease outcome. With an effect modifier, the exposure may not have the same effect in all settings or subgroups.

○   **What is age adjustment?**

Age adjustment takes summary rates for various populations and removes differences in age distributions so that the adjusted rate is independent of age. Age adjustment is used when the age profiles of the populations being compared are quite different.

○   **What is a cohort study?**

A cohort study is an observational study that tracks health information over a period of time. It provides information on disease development and allows study of the natural history of a disease. Cohort studies are good for studying common diseases where exposure and risk factors result in measurable disease outcome in a reasonable amount of time following exposure.

○   **What is meant by the phrase, "natural history" of an illness?**

Natural history of an illness is the progression of a disease through successful stages, often used to describe the course of an illness for which no effective treatment is available.

○   **Define case fatality.**

It is a way of characterizing the natural history of an illness. It is represented as the percentage of patients with a disease who die within a specified observation period. Case fatalities are estimated in the following way:

CF = D/A where CF is case fatality, D is the number of deaths, and A is the number of diagnosed patients. The resulting estimate can be left as a proportion or multiplied by 100 to convert it to a percentage.

○   **What is a cross-sectional study?**

Cross-sectional studies are observational studies that collect descriptive information about subjects; all subjects are measured at the same point in time. It is a relatively simple and inexpensive study design because there is no follow-up involved.

○   **What is a case-control study?**

A case-control study is an observational study in which subjects are sampled based on the presence (case) or absence (controls) of a disease of interest. Information is collected about earlier exposure to risk factors of interest.

○   **What is a RCT?**

A RCT is an experimental study in which subjects are randomly assigned to treatment groups. It is the most robust design for investigating a causal relationship between a treatment and its effect. Randomization overcomes selection bias and ensures confounders are equally distributed among groups.

○ **What are group-randomized trials?**

They are randomized trials where identifiable groups (eg, physician practices) rather than individuals are allocated to treatment or control conditions.

○ **What are multicentered randomized trials?**

They are RCTs conducted at multiple centers rather than a single center.

○ **Define clinical biostatistics.**

Clinical biostatistics is the application of study design and statistical analysis in clinical medicine.

○ **What are the essential characteristics of a research question?**

A research question must be feasible to study, interesting to both the researcher and the clinician, novel or innovative, ethical, and relevant or worth doing.

○ **What are the essential characteristics of a hypothesis?**

A hypothesis must be measurable, it should specify the population being studied, identify the time frame, indicate the type of relationship being examined, include the variables (see below) being studied, and define the statistical level of significance (defined later in chapter).

○ **What are variables?**

Variables are characteristics of interest in a study that have recorded value(s) for each patient in the study. There are two types of variables: quantitative and qualitative.

○ **What are quantitative variables?**

Quantitative variables are also called continuous variables. They are measured on a scale in which a value could be placed between any two numbers (can be measured to the decimal place).

○ **What are the two types of qualitative variables? Define each.**

The two types of qualitative variables are nominal and ordinal.

Nominal variables have no defined order. Numerical values are assigned to represent individual items, for example, marital status: 1 = married, 2 = divorced, 3 = single. The order (number assigned) has no meaning for a nominal variable. Nominal data are reported as proportions (percentages and ratios).

Ordinal variables have an inherent order, for example, pain severity, 1 = no pain, ... 10 = worst pain ever. Ordinal variables allow us to rank order individual items.

○ **What is a binary observation?**

It is a nominal measure that has only two outcomes (eg, amenorrhea: yes or no)

○ **What is the difference between an explanatory/predictor variable and an outcome variable?**

An explanatory/predictor variable is the independent variable and the outcome variable is the dependent variable in a study. Qualitative or quantitative variables can be independent or dependent variables.

○   **What are confounding variables?**

Confounding variables are extraneous factors (variables) related to both the outcome of interest and the exposure of interest, for example, age, sex, tobacco use, and history of tobacco use. Confounding variables can be addressed through the study design or data analysis.

○   **What is an alpha (α) level of significance?**

The alpha (α) level of significance, often set at 0.05, is the chance a researcher is willing to take that there is actually no significant relationship between variables when the statistical test indicates that there is a relationship. In other words, an alpha of 0.05 indicates the researcher is willing to take the chance that a "statistically significant" result is incorrect 5% of the time; 95% of the time the relationship indicated by the statistical test (p-value) would be correct.

○   **What is a p-value?**

A p-value is the probability that the observed difference or relationship between variables occurred by chance ("luck of the draw"). The higher the p-value, the lower the chance that an observed relationship actually exists. The researcher sets the p-value less than or equal to the alpha (α) level chosen (see above). Typically, the p-value is set at ≤ 0.05. If the researcher wants a lower probability of a statistical relationship occurring by chance, they may set a significance (α) level ≤ 0.01 or ≤ 0.001. A p-value ≤ 0.001 indicates there is only a 0.1% chance that a statistically significant relationship occurred by chance.

○   **What is the difference between clinical and statistical significance?**

A clinically important finding is a conclusion that has possible implications for patient care. A statistically significant finding is a conclusion that there is evidence against the null hypothesis.

○   **What is meant by a null hypothesis?**

It represents the hypothesis being tested about a population. Null means "no difference," and refers to a situation in which no difference exists between variables (eg, no difference between the means in a treatment and control group).

○   **What is bias?**

Bias is an error related to the way the targeted and sampled populations differ. Bias threatens the validity of a study.

○   **What is a type I error?**

A type I error results if a true null hypothesis is rejected or if a difference is concluded when no actual difference exists. A type I error is also known as an alpha (α) error.

○   **What is a type II error?**

A type II error results if a false null hypothesis is not rejected or if a difference is not detected when a difference exists. A type II error is also known as a beta (β) error.

○   **What are the two general types of study designs used in medical research?**

The two general types of study designs are observational and experimental.

○   **What is an observational study?**

An observational study is one that does not involve an intervention or manipulation. There are several types of observational studies including cross-sectional, cohort, and case-control studies.

○ **Describe the various types of observational studies.**

An observational study may be forward looking (cohort), backward looking (case-control), or looking at simultaneous events (cross-sectional). Cohort studies generally provide stronger evidence than case-control or cross-sectional study designs. Historical cohort studies are retrospective cohort studies of data collected in the past. Observational studies cannot establish cause and effect.

Cross-sectional study: An observational study that examines a characteristic in a group of subjects at one point in time (provides a "snap-shot" in time). For example, surveys and studies to describe the prevalence of disease and/ or exposure in a specific population at one point in time are cross-sectional studies.

Case-control study: A type of study that examines patients who have the outcome or disease of interest and compares them to control subjects who do not have the outcome or disease.

Cohort study: A longitudinal study composed of two groups of people; one group having a risk factor or exposure, and the other group who do not have the risk factor or exposure. Both groups are followed prospectively through time to learn how many people in each group develop the outcome or consequence of interest.

○ **Describe an experimental (intervention) study.**

An experimental study is a comparative study involving an intervention or manipulation. RCTs are examples of experimental studies. Subjects with the disease or problem of interest are randomly assigned to the treatment or control group. Comparisons between the groups are made for any differences in the outcome of interest as a result of the intervention (treatment). It is the most robust design for investigating a causal relationship between a treatment and its effect.

○ **What is a box plot?**

A box plot is a graph that displays both the frequencies and distributions of observations. It is useful for comparing two distributions. It is also called a "box and whisker" plot.

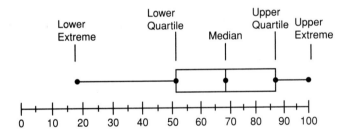

○ **Define frequency distribution.**

In a set of numerical observations, the list of values occurs along with the frequency of their occurrence. It can be displayed as a graph or table. Frequency distributions are used to condense the data into a more manageable form.

Height (cm)	Frequency
170	7
172	2
174	3
176	1
178	4

○ **What is meant by the phrase "measures of central tendency"?**

Measures of central tendency refer to summary numbers that describe the middle of a distribution such as the mean, median, or mode. The mean is the sum of the X values divided by the total number in the sample (n). The median is the middle observation. The mode is the value of a numerical variable that occurs the most frequently.

○ **Define confidence interval.**

The interval calculated from sample data that has a given probability (eg, 95%) that the unknown parameter (eg, a mean or proportion) is contained within the interval. The confidence interval is the estimated range within which it is likely (eg, with 95% probability) that the true point estimate (eg, the true population mean) exists. Confidence intervals are usually expressed as 90%, 95%, or 99%. The width of the confidence interval is inversely related to the sample size, indicating that as the amount of information about the population increases, the precision in the estimate increases.

○ **What is meant by the effect size?**

It is the magnitude of a difference or relationship. It is used in sample size calculations and for combining results across studies as in a meta-analysis.

○ **What is the independent sample t-test?**

The independent sample t-test (also known as the student's t-test) is used to test the null hypothesis that two independent (or unrelated) samples have the same mean. The t-test is used for quantitative data.

○ **What does ANOVA stand for?**

ANOVA stands for analysis of variance; it is similar to but more robust than the t-test. It is a statistical procedure that compares the means of two or more groups of subjects on one or more variables to determine if they are (statistically) significantly different.

○ **What is a paired or dependent-sample t-test?**

The paired (or dependent sample) t-test is used to compare the means of two paired observations on the same individuals. Quantitative data collected in a before and after study design are analyzed using the paired t-test.

○ **What is the chi-square test (χ^2)?**

It is a statistical test for contingency tables used to determine whether factors or characteristics are independent or not associated with each other. It is also used to test the null hypothesis that proportions are equal.

○ **Describe the Fisher's exact test.**

It is a statistical test for contingency tables that are used when the sample size is too small to use the chi-square test. A contingency table is used to display counts, or frequencies for two or more qualitative variables.

○ **What is the Mantel-Haenszel test?**

The Mantel-Haenszel test is a statistical test of two or more 2 × 2 tables. It is used to compare survival distributions or to control for confounding factors.

○ **What is RR?**

RR is the ratio of the incidence of a given disease in an exposed or at-risk population to the incidence of the disease in unexposed persons. It is calculated in cohort or prospective studies.

○ **What is a control event rate (CER)?**

The number of subjects in a control group who develop the outcome being studied.

○ **What is an experimental event rate (EER)?**

The number of subjects in the experimental or treatment group who develop the outcome being studied.

○ **Define relative risk reduction (RRR).**

RRR is the reduction in risk *with a new therapy;* it is the absolute value of the difference between EER and the CER divided by the CER.

○ **Define absolute risk reduction (ARR).**

Reduction in risk *with* a new therapy compared with the risk *without* a new therapy. It is the absolute value of the difference between the EER and the CER.

○ **Define absolute risk increase.**

The increase in risk *with* a new therapy compared with the risk *without* the new therapy.

○ **What is meant by a hazard ratio?**

Ratio of risk of an outcome (such as miscarriage) occurring at any time in one group compared with another group.

○ **What does NNT stand for?**

NNT stands for the number needed to treat. NNT is the number of patients who need to be treated with a proposed therapy in order to prevent, or cure one person. It is the reciprocal of the absolute risk reduction (1/ARR).

○ **What does NNH stand for?**

NNH stands for number needed to harm. NNH is the number of patients who need to be treated with a proposed therapy in order to cause one undesirable outcome (1/ARI).

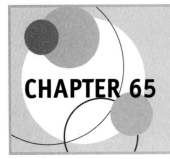

ACOG Screening Guidelines Since 2007

CHAPTER 65

Laura E. Martin, DO

○ **Why is cervical cancer screening important?**

About 60% of cervical cancer cases are found in patients who have had inadequate screening.

○ **What is the incidence of cervical cancer in the United States?**

Approximately 12,000 persons per year.

○ **What is the incidence of death from cervical cancer?**

4220 persons per year.

○ **How many women age 15 to 19 have cervical cancer?**

1 to 2 in 1,000,000 per year.

○ **What percentage of women over 65 years old have cervical cancer?**

19%.

○ **When should screening begin?**

21 year of age.

○ **How does the immune system respond to human papilloma virus (HPV) in a healthy patient?**

85% to 90% of imunocompetent women clear the virus in 8 to 24 months. The remainder of women will develop cervical dysplasia and possibly cervical cancer.

○ **Which screening methods are appropriate?**

Both the liquid prep and the conventional technique (cells prepared on a slide) are appropriate with or without HPV DNA testing.

○ **What is the benefit of the liquid based prep?**

It also tests for gonorrhea and *Chlamydia*.

○   **What are the most common HPV types that lead to cervical carcinoma?**
HPV 16, 18.

○   **How is High Risk HPV testing used in screening tests?**
An adjunct to cytology in women 30 to 65 years old and in ASCUS pap reflex testing to determine the need for colposcopy.

○   **What is co-testing?**
Cytology plus HPV testing.

○   **Which genotypes are tested in reflex HPV testing?**
16, 18.

○   **What is the time from HPV infection to cervical cancer?**
A median of 15 to 25 years.

○   **Why were the screening guidelines changed from screening every 3 to 5 years?**
There was a negligible difference in the risk of cancer with increase in colposcopic procedures.

○   **Why is co-testing for women aged 21 to 29 not recommended?**
In this population, HPV testing usually detects transient infection without carcinogenic potential.

○   **How often should you screen for cervical cancer?**
Screening is age dependent.
21 to 29 years old cytology alone every 3 years.
30 to 65 years old cytology alone every 3 years or co-testing every 5 years.
Over 65 years old, no screening if negative adequate test results. If the patient has a history of CIN 2-3 or adenocarcinoma, then continue screening for 20 years.

○   **What is an adequate negative test result?**
Defined as three negative, consecutive cytology results or two consecutive co-test results in 10 years with the last one being in the past 5 years.

○   **Which is the preferred method of screening in the age of 30 to 65?**
Co-testing is preferred because it is more sensitive in detection of CIN 3 and adenocarcinoma.

○   **How do you manage a positive HPV test and negative cytology in women over 30 years old?**
(1) Repeat HPV testing in 1 year and if repeat test is positive perform colposcopy or
(2) Reflex to HPV genotype and if positive for HP 16, 18 perform colposcopy, if negative repeat co-testing testing in 12 months.

○ **Which populations should be screened more frequently?**

HIV positive
DES exposed
Immunocompromised
History of CIN2-3 and carcinoma

○ **How should women with HIV be screened?**

Women with HIV should be screened at the age of diagnosis, twice in that first year and yearly thereafter.

○ **Why is screening over the age of 65 years old ineffective?**

There is a very low risk of progression to cancer in women with newly inquired infections and there are more false positives 2/2 vaginal atrophy in postmenopausal women

○ **When is it appropriate to discontinue screening in women with a hysterectomy?**

When the woman has never had CIN2 or higher and the cervix is removed.

○ **When should women with a hysterectomy with a cervix or history of CIN2 or higher stop cervical cancer screening?**

Women should be screened for 20 years with cytology every 3 years after the treatment of CIN 2 or greater.

○ **What carcinoma is the leading cause of death in women in the United States?**

Lung cancer.

○ **What carcinoma is the second leading cause of death in women in the United States?**

Breast cancer.

○ **What is the lifetime risk of developing female breast cancer?**

12% or 1 in 8 women.

○ **How many women are diagnosed with breast caner each year?**

Approximately 200,000.

○ **What are the components of breast cancer screening?**

Breast imaging, clinical breast examination, and self-awareness or self-examination.

○ **What is the difference between breast self-examination and self-awareness?**

Breast self-examination describes monthly self-breast examinations and breast awareness describes familiarity with one's own breast without scheduled self-examination.

○ **Which organizations endorse breast imaging, breast self-awareness, and clinical examination as the standard screening modality?**

ACOG, National Comprehensive Cancer Network, and American Cancer Society.

○ **How large does a breast mass generally have to be before it is palpable?**

Approximately 2 cm.

○ **What size tumor can mammography detect?**

1 mm.

○ **What is the description of the time a mass is detected by screening to the time it is palpable?**

Sojourn time.

○ **What factors decrease the sojourn time?**

Patient's advanced age and the aggressiveness of the cancer.

○ **When does ACOG recommend beginning screening?**

Clinical breast examination should start at the age of 20 and breast imaging should start at the age of 40.

○ **How many women aged 39 to 49 must be screened to prevent one cancer death?**

1 in 1904 women.

○ **How many women aged 50 to 59 must be screened to prevent one cancer death?**

1 in 1339 women.

○ **What are the imaging modalities available for screening?**

Mammography, ultrasound, and MRI.

○ **Why is mammography the preferred method of screening?**

Mammography has a high sensitivity 79% and specificity 90% for detecting breast lesions (National Cancer Institute. "Breast Cancer Screening Modalities" www.cancer.gov/cancertopics/pdq/screening/breast/healthprofessional/page4).

○ **What are the potential adverse consequences of mammographic screening?**

False negative mammograms, false positive mammograms, and radiation exposure.

○ **What are the consequences of a false-positive test?**

20% to 30% of patients will have an unnecessary biopsy and undue stress.

○ **When should mammography stop?**

Women aged 75 and older should consult with their physician on an appropriate time to stop screening.

○ **What role does ultrasound play in screening for breast cancer?**

It allows for evaluation of inconclusive mammographic results by identifying cystic versus solid masses, by evaluating dense breast tissue, and by guidance in core-needle biopsy.

○ **Who should receive MRI screening modality?**

Patients with a 20% lifetime risk of breast cancer.

Personal history of breast and ovarian cancer.

Personal history of ovarian cancer and a close relative with ovarian cancer or premenopausal breast cancer.

Personal history of ovarian cancer with an Ashkenazi Jewish ancestry.

Personal history of breast cancer at the age of 50 years or younger with a close relative with ovarian cancer or male breast cancer.

Personal history of breast cancer at the age of 40 years or younger and Ashkenazi Jewish ancestry.

Personal history of BRAC1 and BRAC2 or a close relative with BRAC positive testing.

Personal history of Li-Fraumeni syndrome, Cowden syndrome, or Bannayan-Riley-Ruvalcaba syndrome or one of these syndromes in a first-degree relative.

Personal history of radiation to the chest from 10 years old to 30 years old.

(Close relative is defined as a first- or second-degree relative)

○ **What is the difference between breast self-examination and breast self-awareness?**

Breast self-examination is a monthly breast examination performed by the patient, and breast self-awareness is becoming familiar with ones breast so that changes can be detected.

○ **Why is breast self-awareness preferred by ACOG over breast self-examination?**

The Shanghai Breast Self-Examination Study enrolled 266,000 women aged 29 to 72 and showed no change in breast cancer deaths for patients who performed breast examinations versus those who did not.

○ **How many women are the first to identify breast cancer in themselves?**

Up to 70% of women <50 years old and 50% of women >50 years old.

○ **What is the significance of clinical breast examinations?**

Clinicians detected 5 cases of cancer per 1000 patients examined and also detected 7.4 cases of cancer per 1000 patients screened when mammography was normal.

○ **What is the frequency of clinical breast examination?**

For those aged 20 to 39 examine every 1 to 3 years and those over 40 should be examined yearly.

○ **What is the incidence of breast cancer in women aged 40 to 49?**

1 in 69.

○ **What is the incidence of breast cancer in women aged 50 to 5?**

1 in 38.

○ **How many women <50 years are diagnosed with breast cancer per year?**

Approximately 50,000.

○ **What are the risks of breast cancer?**

Age, early onset menarche, low parity, late menopause, Ashkenazi Jewish heritage, and familial disease: BRAC, Li-Fraumeni syndrome, Cowden syndrome, or Bannayan-Riley-Ruvalcaba syndrome.

○ **What is the Gail model and what is it used for?**

It is a risk assessment tool that incorporates the patient's age, family history of breast cancer, history of breast biopsy, and reproductive factors to assess the 5-year risk of breast cancer. If the risk is 1.7% or greater, this indicates a need for increased screening.

○ **What patients are in need of increased screening?**

Patients who have a lifetime risk of breast cancer of 20% or greater, and history of breast biopsy with atypical hyperplasia and lobular carcinoma in situ.

○ **What is appropriate for increased screening?**

Self-breast examinations, biannual clinical breast examinations, annual mammography, and annual MRI.

○ **What is the triple screen and how sensitive is it in detecting Down syndrome?**

The triple screen is a test performed prior to 20 weeks' gestation that incorporates maternal serum alpha fetal protein (MSAFP), estriol, and human chorionic gonadotropin (hCG) to calculate the risk of aneuploidy. The test is 70% effective in detecting Down syndrome.

○ **What is the quad screen and how sensitive is it in detecting Down syndrome?**

The quad screen incorporates the triple screen in addition to testing inhibin A levels, which increases the sensitivity to 80%.

○ **What changes are seen in analytes of a Down fetus?**

MSAFP decreases by 0.74, estriol decreases by 0.75, hCG increases by 2.06, and inhibin increases by 1.77.

○ **What analytes are used in evaluation of trisomy 18 and how are these markers affected?**

MSAFP, estriol, and hCG are all decreased, while inhibin A is not used in screening for trisomy 18.

○ **What is the integrated screen?**

This study measures the nuchal translucency (NT) (fluid collection on the fetal neck) plus PAPP-A and β-hCG in the first trimester and combines these results with second-trimester measurements of inhibin A, MSAFP, and unconjugated estriol.

○ **What is the sensitivity of the integrated screen and the sequential screen with NT?**

94% to 95%.

○ **What is the disadvantage of the integrated screen?**

Patients have to wait 3 to 4 weeks for results, lose the opportunity for CVS, and possibly become lost to follow-up.

○ **What is the difference between the stepwise sequential screen, the contingent sequential screen, and the integrated screen?**

The stepwise sequential screen reports the results of the first-trimester analyte screen with NT and the combined second-trimester analyte screen.

The contingent sequential screen reports the first part of the sequential and does not test low-risk patients in the second trimester.

The integrated screen incorporates the first- and second-trimester analytes plus or minus the NT in one final report.

○ **Which tests should be offered?**

If a patient presents in the first trimester, integrated testing should be offered and if they present in the second trimester, a quad screen should be offered.

○ **When can an NT be performed?**

Between 10.4 and 13.6 weeks.

○ **How many fetuses with an increased NT will have a chromosomal abnormality?**

One-third.

○ **Why is first-trimester screening preferred?**

If there is a positive screen before 14 weeks, CVS may be offered and early termination may be preformed if desired.

○ **What should be offered to patients with increased risk of aneuploidy?**

Genetic counseling and chorionic villous sampling or amniocentesis.

○ **What should be offered if a patient has an NT >3.5 cm?**

The patient should be offered a targeted fetal ultrasound and fetal echocardiogram because heart defects, abdominal wall defects, and genetic syndrome may be associated with this finding.

○ **What are other markers of aneuploidy in the first trimester?**

Absent nasal bone, crown-rump length, femur and humeral length, head and trunk volumes, and umbilical cord diameters.

○ **What are other markers of aneuploidy in the second trimester?**

Echogenic bowel, cardiac echogenic focus, and dilated renal pelvis.

○ **How is aneuploidy screening affected in multiple gestations?**

It is less accurate in both the first and the second trimester but can still be performed.

○ **What are the WHO criteria for diagnosing osteoporosis using dual-energy X-ray absorptiometry (DXA) bone mineral density (BMD) measurement?**

Category	T-Score
Normal	≥−1.0
Low bone bass (osteopenia)	<−1 or >−2.5
Osteoporosis	≤2.5

- T-Score is the BMD measurement (preferably the femoral neck, total hip, and lumbar spine) of the patient compared with the mean BMD of a young, healthy cohort of females.
- A Z-score is also reported; it compares the patient's BMD with the mean BMD of women her age. This score can be of value when it demonstrates that a woman's BMD is significantly below than that of her peer group. It is NOT used to diagnose osteoporosis.

○ **How do you make a clinical diagnosis of osteoporosis in the absence of DXA imaging?**

- Medical history of low-trauma fracture (especially vertebral or hip) in an at-risk woman.
- History of low-trauma fractures that occur in a situation that would not be expected to cause fractures in most individuals (eg, a vertebral fracture from opening a window).

○ **What is the fracture risk assessment tool (FRAX)?**

- A tool that predicts the risk of osteoporotic fracture for a person in the next 10 years.
- Used as an aid in decision making regarding treatment initiation when a patient's BMD score is in the low bone mass range.
- Clinical risk factors used in the tool include, age, sex, BMI, previous fragility fracture, parental hip fracture, current smoking status, corticosteroid use (≥5 mg prednisolone per day for 3 months), alcohol intake ≥3 units per day, rheumatoid arthritis, and other secondary causes of osteoporosis.
- Results are specific for gender and race for various countries where fracture data were available to incorporate into the tool.
- Limitations: can only be used in postmenopausal, who are not receiving osteoporosis treatment, and have no prior hip or vertebral fracture.

○ **How does FRAX help in clinical decision making?**

- Treatment for osteoporosis should be initiated in women who have a T-score from −1 to −2.5 and a FRAX score ≥3% for risk of hip fracture or a FRAX score ≥20% for risk of a major osteoporotic fracture (defined as forearm, hip, shoulder, or clinical spine fracture) or both in the next 10 years.
- The tool can be used to determine if screening is necessary prior to age 65.
- It can be a useful tool for a concerned patient who does not meet criteria for a DXA scan.
- FRAX should be used on an annual basis to monitor the important effect of age on fracture risk.

○ **When should bone density screening be initiated?**

- Begin at the age of 65.
- Postmenopausal women younger than 65 years with other risk factors for fracture.
- FRAX can be used in women younger than 65 years to determine which women should have a DXA scan; women with a FRAX 10-year risk of major osteoporotic fracture of 9.3% can be referred for DXA because that is the risk of fracture found in a 65-year-old Caucasian woman with no risk factors.

○ **What factors are considered high risk for fracture in postmenopausal women <65?**

- Medical history of a fragility fracture.
- Body weight <127 lb.
- Medical causes of bone loss (medications or diseases).
- Parental medical history of hip fracture.
- Current smoker.
- Alcoholism.
- Rheumatoid arthritis.

○ **Is BMD monitoring necessary for patients taking depot medroxyprogesterone acetate (DMPA)?**

No because partial or full recovery of BMD occurs at the spine and at least partial recovery occurs at the hip after discontinuation of DMPA. The short-term loss of BMD associated with DMPA is recovered and unlikely to place an adolescent or adult woman at risk of fracture during use or in later years.

○ **How often should DXA scan be repeated if a woman older than 65 years does not have osteoporosis?**

If FRAX does not indicate a high risk of fracture:

- Interval screening every 15 years for a woman older than 65 years with a normal BMD or mild bone loss (T-score ≥−1.5).
- Interval screening every 5 years for a T-score from −1.5 to −1.99.
- Interval screening annually for a T-score between −2.0 and −2.49.

○ **When should treatment for osteoporosis be recommended?**

- Women who have a BMD T-score of <−2.5.
- Women in the low bone mass with a high-risk FRAX assessment (a 10-year risk of major osteoporotic fracture ≥20% or a risk of hip fracture ≥3%).
- Women who have had a low-trauma fracture (especially of the vertebra or hip) are candidates for treatment even in the absence of DXA diagnosed osteoporosis.

○ **How is treatment effect monitored?**

- After treatment initiation, one DXA scan 1 year or 2 years later can be used to assess the effect of treatment.
- If BMD is stable or improved, the DXA does not usually need to be repeated in the absence of new risk factors.
- Testing should not be undertaken before 2 years after initiation of treatment because it often takes 18–24 months to document a clinically meaningful change.